Etiology of Parkinson's Disease

NEUROLOGICAL DISEASE AND THERAPY

Series Editor

WILLIAM C. KOLLER

Department of Neurology
University of Kansas Medical Center
Kansas City, Kansas

1. Handbook of Parkinson's Disease, *edited by William C. Koller*
2. Medical Therapy of Acute Stroke, *edited by Mark Fisher*
3. Familial Alzheimer's Disease: Molecular Genetics and Clinical Perspectives, *edited by Gary D. Miner, Ralph W. Richter, John P. Blass, Jimmie L. Valentine, and Linda A. Winters-Miner*
4. Alzheimer's Disease: Treatment and Long-Term Management, *edited by Jeffrey L. Cummings and Bruce L. Miller*
5. Therapy of Parkinson's Disease, *edited by William C. Koller and George Paulson*
6. Handbook of Sleep Disorders, *edited by Michael J. Thorpy*
7. Epilepsy and Sudden Death, *edited by Claire M. Lathers and Paul L. Schraeder*
8. Handbook of Multiple Sclerosis, *edited by Stuart D. Cook*
9. Memory Disorders: Research and Clinical Practice, *edited by Takehiko Yanagihara and Ronald C. Petersen*
10. The Medical Treatment of Epilepsy, *edited by Stanley R. Resor, Jr., and Henn Kutt*
11. Cognitive Disorders: Pathophysiology and Treatment, *edited by Leon J. Thal, Walter H. Moos, and Elkan R. Gamzu*
12. Handbook of Amyotrophic Lateral Sclerosis, *edited by Richard Alan Smith*
13. Handbook of Parkinson's Disease: Second Edition, Revised and Expanded, *edited by William C. Koller*
14. Handbook of Pediatric Epilepsy, *edited by Jerome V. Murphy and Fereydoun Dehkharghani*
15. Handbook of Tourette's Syndrome and Related Tic and Behavioral Disorders, *edited by Roger Kurlan*
16. Handbook of Cerebellar Diseases, *edited by Richard Lechtenberg*
17. Handbook of Cerebrovascular Diseases, *edited by Harold P. Adams, Jr.*
18. Parkinsonian Syndromes, *edited by Matthew B. Stern and William C. Koller*
19. Handbook of Head and Spine Trauma, *edited by Jonathan Greenberg*
20. Brain Tumors: A Comprehensive Text, *edited by Robert A. Morantz and John W. Walsh*

21. Monoamine Oxidase Inhibitors in Neurological Diseases, *edited by Abraham Lieberman, C. Warren Olanow, Moussa B. H. Youdim, and Keith Tipton*
22. Handbook of Dementing Illnesses, *edited by John C. Morris*
23. Handbook of Myasthenia Gravis and Myasthenic Syndromes, *edited by Robert P. Lisak*
24. Handbook of Neurorehabilitation, *edited by David C. Good and James R. Couch, Jr.*
25. Therapy with Botulinum Toxin, *edited by Joseph Jankovic and Mark Hallett*
26. Principles of Neurotoxicology, *edited by Louis W. Chang*
27. Handbook of Neurovirology, *edited by Robert R. McKendall and William G. Stroop*
28. Handbook of Neuro-Urology, *edited by David N. Rushton*
29. Handbook of Neuroepidemiology, *edited by Philip B. Gorelick and Milton Alter*
30. Handbook of Tremor Disorders, *edited by Leslie J. Findley and William C. Koller*
31. Neuro-Ophthalmological Disorders: Diagnostic Work-Up and Management, *edited by Ronald J. Tusa and Steven A. Newman*
32. Handbook of Olfaction and Gustation, *edited by Richard L. Doty*
33. Handbook of Neurological Speech and Language Disorders, *edited by Howard S. Kirshner*
34. Therapy of Parkinson's Disease: Second Edition, Revised and Expanded, *edited by William C. Koller and George Paulson*
35. Evaluation and Management of Gait Disorders, *edited by Barney S. Spivack*
36. Handbook of Neurotoxicology, *edited by Louis W. Chang and Robert S. Dyer*
37. Neurological Complications of Cancer, *edited by Ronald G. Wiley*
38. Handbook of Autonomic Nervous System Dysfunction, *edited by Amos D. Korczyn*
39. Handbook of Dystonia, *edited by Joseph King Ching Tsui and Donald B. Calne*
40. Etiology of Parkinson's Disease, *edited by Jonas H. Ellenberg, William C. Koller, and J. William Langston*

Additional Volumes in Preparation

Etiology of Parkinson's Disease

edited by

Jonas H. Ellenberg
National Institute of Neurological Disorders and Stroke
National Institutes of Health
Bethesda, Maryland

William C. Koller
University of Kansas Medical Center
Kansas City, Kansas

J. William Langston
The Parkinson's Institute
Sunnyvale, California

Marcel Dekker, Inc. New York • Basel • Hong Kong

Library of Congress Cataloging-in-Publication Data

Etiology of parkinson's disease / edited by Jonas H. Ellenberg, William C. Koller, J. William Langston.
p. cm. -- (Neurological diseases and therapy ; v. 40)
Includes bibliographical references and index.
ISBN 0-8247-8823-0 (hardcover : alk. paper)
1. Parkinsonism--Etiology. I. Ellenberg, Jonas H. II. Koller, William C. III. Langston, J.W. (James William)
IV. Series.
[DNLM: 1. Parkinson Disease--etiology. W1 NE33LD v. 40 1995 / WL359 E84 1995]
RC382.E87 1995
616.8'33071--dc20
DNLM/DLC
for Library of Congress 94-49181
CIP

The publisher offers discounts on this book when ordered in bulk quantities. For more information, write to Special Sales/Professional Marketing at the address below.

This book is printed on acid-free paper.

Marcel Dekker, Inc.
270 Madison Avenue, New York, New York 10016

Current printing (last digit):
10 9 8 7 6 5 4 3 2 1

PRINTED IN THE UNITED STATES OF AMERICA

Preface

In the latest version of his book *Parkinson's Disease: A Guide for Patient and Family*, Roger C. Duvoisin writes unequivocally that "the cause of Parkinson's disease is unknown." While there have been many intriguing hypotheses and studies on its etiology over the 150 years since James Parkinson first described the disease, we are still unable to point to a factor or set of factors that cause this neurodegenerative disorder. There is, however, an enormous literature on the topic. This book reviews the literature relevant to etiology with several goals: (1) to critically assess the body of research on putative etiologic hypotheses with a focus on methodological issues and to evaluate the degree to which study conclusions are justified based on the data presented and the biological justification for conclusions or speculations; (2) to assess the potential interaction of the environmental and genetic hypotheses (exploring, for example, the possibility that a genetically determined defect predisposes to a toxic insult); and (3) to set the stage for future research in an era of very exciting new technology that promises to bring new insights into the neurodegenerative process. In this book, critical overviews are presented as guides to areas of most promising research and the most promising methodologies to pursue that research.

The book is divided into five parts, beginning with the clinical and pathological descriptions of Parkinson's disease. The first part focuses on the differentiation between Parkinson's disease and parkinsonism and includes a discussion of other forms of parkinsonism and an overview of the mechanisms of cell death. Part II covers the role of possible hereditary factors in the etiology of Parkinson's disease. Classic genetic concepts are discussed, as are inherited risk factors that might enhance susceptibility to exogenous toxins and endogenous factors that might relate to the etiology of Parkinson's disease. Part III gives an overview of the methodological problems in studies of Parkinson's disease, some inherent and some avoidable, and approaches to assessment of information from epidemiological studies of Parkinson's disease. In Part IV research is covered that relates to the putative environmental or exogenous agents that may be related to the etiology of Parkinson's disease. We conclude in Part V with an exhaustive compilation of the world literature on the etiology of Parkinson's disease and related literature.

The extensive literature on the etiology of Parkinson's disease over the past 150 years has never been critically reviewed as a whole. There have been only sporadic individual reviews of specific etiologic agents or areas. This book brings together, for the first time, a comprehensive overview of what we know and do not know about the etiology of Parkinson's disease in an integrated rather than fragmented approach. Based on this overview, strategies for future research into the cause and prevention of Parkinson's disease are presented. The concepts presented will also apply to other neurodegenerative disorders and diseases of the aging. Combining both basic research and clinical insights, this book should be of interest to the entire neurological community as well as those researchers and practitioners involved in all aspects of central nervous system disorders that involve the basal ganglia.

This work will be a valuable reference source for anyone working in the area of neurodegenerative disease and, more specifically, Parkinson's disease.

Jonas H. Ellenberg
William C. Koller
J. William Langston

Contents

Contributors

Patricia G. Butterfield, R.N., Ph.D. Research Fellow, Center for Research on Occupational and Environmental Toxicology, Oregon Health Sciences University, Portland, Oregon

Jonas H. Ellenberg, Ph.D. Chief, Biometry and Field Studies Branch, National Institute of Neurological Disorders and Stroke, National Institutes of Health, Bethesda, Maryland

Lysia S. Forno, M.D. Neuropathologist, Department of Veterans Affairs Medical Center, and Professor Emerita of Neuropathology, Department of Pathology, Stanford University School of Medicine, Palo Alto, California

Lawrence I. Golbe, M.D. Associate Professor, Department of Neurology, University of Medicine and Dentistry of New Jersey–Robert Wood Johnson Medical School, New Brunswick, New Jersey

Ian Irwin, B.A., B.S. Chief, Neurotoxicology and Neuropharmacology Laboratories, The Parkinson's Institute, Sunnyvale, California

William C. Koller, M.D., Ph.D. Professor and Chairman, Department of Neurology, University of Kansas Medical Center, Kansas City, Kansas

J. William Langston, M.D. President, The Parkinson's Institute, Sunnyvale, California

Rajesh Pahwa, M.D. Assistant Professor, Department of Neurology, University of Kansas Medical Center, Kansas City, Kansas

Gustavo C. Román, M.D., F.A.C.P., F.R.S.M. Former Chief, Neuroepidemiology Branch, National Institute of Neurological Disorders and Stroke, National Institutes of Health, Bethesda, Maryland

Peter S. Spencer, Ph.D., F.R.C. Path. Professor of Neurology and Director and Senior Scientist, Center for Research on Occupational and Environmental Toxicology, Oregon Health Sciences University, Portland, Oregon

Caroline M. Tanner, M.D. Director, Department of Clinical Research, The Parkinson's Institute, Sunnyvale, California

Adrian Williams, M.D. University Department of Clinical Neurology, Queen Elizabeth Hospital, Edgbaston, Birmingham, England

Matthew M. Zack, M.D., M.P.H. Medical Epidemiologist, Division of Chronic Disease Control and Community Intervention, Centers for Disease Control and Prevention, Atlanta, Georgia

Zhen-Xin Zhang, M.D. Neuroepidemiologist, Neuroepidemiology Branch, National Institute of Neurological Disorders and Stroke, National Institutes of Health, Bethesda, Maryland, and Peking Medical College Hospital, Beijing, China

Introduction

Jonas H. Ellenberg

National Institute of Neurological Disorders and Stroke, National Institutes of Health, Bethesda, Maryland

William C. Koller

University of Kansas Medical Center, Kansas City, Kansas

J. William Langston

The Parkinson's Institute, Sunnyvale, California

The cause of Parkinson's disease remains unknown. This simple fact accounts for the length of this volume and its concluding bibliography. Despite the missing pieces of the puzzle that are still needed to discover the cause of the disease, the intensity of research in this arena is at an all-time high. For this reason, we believe that a book on the etiology of Parkinson's disease is both timely and warranted. In this Introduction, a brief history of the origins of this volume is provided, which in turn will help explain its scope and aims. In addition, an overview of the organizational structure is presented with summaries of each section to help direct readers as they make their way through this book.

I. BACKGROUND

In 1986, one of the editors (JWL) received a grant from the Centers for Disease Control to investigate the etiology of Parkinson's disease. Rather than utilizing the grant for a specific research project, he decided to organize an eclectic committee of individuals from a variety of disciplines relevant to current theories on the cause and epidemiology of Parkinson's disease. Backgrounds of committee members ranged from neurochemistry and neurotoxicology to environmental health, neurology, and biostatistics. This group, known as the Parkinson's Epidemiology Research Committee (PERC), held its first meeting in February 1988 at The Parkinson's Institute (known then as the California Parkinson's Foundation). The original goal of PERC was to review all of the epidemiological studies on Parkinson's disease, assess their validity, determine gaps in current knowledge, and make recommendations for future research in this area.

As the Committee delved more into the myriad theories and investigations on the cause(s) of Parkinson's disease, it evolved both in scope and in nature. By 1989, PERC had shifted its emphasis from a "think tank" structure to much more of an action-oriented group, with a long-term goal of stimulating projects on the epidemiology and etiology of Parkinson's disease. Specific goals included (1) generating new hypotheses regarding the cause of Parkinson's disease, (2) reviewing and assessing previously proposed hypotheses and examining the strengths and weaknesses of these hypotheses, (3) developing priorities for current and proposed epidemiological efforts in Parkinson's disease and related disorders, (4) examining methodologies and generating protocols for future epidemiological studies, (5) organizing symposia on issues related to the cause of Parkinson's disease (the first such symposium was held in Miami in 1989, and a second took place in Santa Cruz in 1994), and (6) fostering, facilitating, and initiating specific projects. To achieve this last goal, working committees were set up to plan and obtain funding for specific projects. A number of projects have been successfully implemented, including a study of twins who served in World War II. This study provides an unparalleled opportunity to look at gene-environment interaction in Parkinson's disease.

One of these working committees was assigned the project of reviewing the entire English-speaking literature on the epidemiology of Parkinson's disease; this committee, which is composed of the Editors of this book, began its labors in late 1989. As the literature review progressed, it became increasingly apparent that an enormous body of literature was being identified and critically reviewed. This was due in part to the fact that the scope of the committee had been expanded to include all articles that might be relevant to the cause of Parkinson's disease. As the number of articles obtained and reviewed continued to increase, the Bibliography Subcommittee, as it was called, realized that it would be worthwhile to make the results of this labor available to the general scientific and medical community. Therefore, a decision was made to publish the bibliography.

However, as work continued on the bibliography, it began to take on a life of its own. It became apparent that a "bare bones" bibliography would lack substance and would not be wholly satisfactory. Therefore, a decision was made to expand the scope of the project to an annotated bibliography, with a goal of providing a brief discussion for each category of references cited. However, with time, even this approach seemed too limited, and a decision was made to expand the bibliography into a comprehensive book, with chapters designed to cover each of the major areas relating to the cause of Parkinson's disease.

In the process of inviting PERC members to contribute chapters, authors were encouraged to provide commentary on the current relevance of the material covered to the etiology of Parkinson's disease. A second goal was to provide a critical review of the work published to date, highlighting the strengths and weaknesses of the research methodology, data analysis, and/or conclusions drawn from the evidence presented. Contributors were also asked to summarize future directions for research on the cause of the disease.

Because the original conception of this book came from an epidemiologically oriented group, there may be some bias toward an environmental etiology for Parkinson's disease. To at least some degree, this emphasis reflects current thinking regarding its cause. On the other hand, there has been a concerted effort to leave all doors open when it comes to considering the etiology of the disease, and an entire section of the book is devoted to considering the importance of genetics in Parkinson's disease. Perhaps the most likely possibility, that the disease represents an outcome of the interplay between environmental and inherited factors, is a prominent theme when the book is considered as a whole.

II. ORGANIZATION AND CONTENT

This volume has been carefully orchestrated to achieve a logical order of presentation. It is divided into five parts. Part I contains general information that is relevant to all of the remaining parts and provides what the Editors consider essential background information for anyone interested in the cause of Parkinson's disease. Chapter 1 provides an overview of current concepts regarding Parkinson's disease as a disease entity. Approaches to and accuracy of diagnosis are reviewed, and issues relating to terminology and variability of disease expression are addressed. In addition, other forms of parkinsonism are discussed. This chapter is a critical primer for any investigation into the cause of the disease because of the obvious need to characterize the disorder to be studied. The second chapter, on the other hand, deals with the vexing possibility that what we call Parkinson's disease might comprise multiple diseases or, alternatively, might be a single disease with multiple causes. This brief chapter is provided because these possibilities, if true, are likely to enormously confound research. Until the cause is known, all possibilities must be considered. To completely ignore the possibility of a multifactorial origin could represent a major pitfall for anyone considering research in this area.

The third chapter moves from clinical concepts to the neuropathological aspects of Parkinson's disease and other parkinsonian syndromes. A general knowledge of neuropathology provides an anchor for anyone interested in the study of neurological disease, both in regard to diagnosis (Parkinson's disease is defined here, at least, as an identifiable clinicopathological entity) and as yet another place to look for clues to the cause of the disease, which is a critical focus of the chapter. The final chapter in Part I focuses on mechanisms of cell death. Even though much of the material covered in this chapter is not directly related to Parkinson's disease, cell death remains the essential underlying feature of the disease. For this reason, an in-depth review of the current body of knowledge in this area is provided as another indispensable component of background information.

Part II of this volume deals with the genetics of Parkinson's disease. The possibility that Parkinson's disease is inherited has been intermittently considered for well over a century. Indeed, the tides of opinion have seemed to ebb and flow in 10- to 20-year cycles as to whether the disease is primarily genetic or acquired in origin. This history, along with current views on the genetic aspects of the disease, is described in detail in Chapter 5. As will become apparent on reading this chapter, there has been a resurgence of interest in the possibility that genetics may play an important role in Parkinson's disease.

Chapter 6 delves into the possibility that a genetic predisposition is a key component in Parkinson's disease. This chapter was added in view of recent evidence that one or more endogenous risk factors might exist in patients who contract Parkinson's disease. We are pleased that Dr. Adrian Williams, the only contributor to this volume who is not a member of PERC, accepted our invitation to contribute such a chapter, which deals with abnormalities of xenobiotic metabolism as possible risk factors for Parkinson's disease. Since this is likely to become an area of intensive investigation during the remainder of this decade, it seemed appropriate to include such a chapter.

The final chapter (Chapter 7) in Part II deals with the possibility that one or more endogenous sustances in the brain have in some way gone awry, thereby causing damage to neuronal structures. This area has recently come under increasing scrutiny as more and more endogenous compounds with neurotoxic potential have been identified in the brain. A discussion of these compounds is placed in the section on genetics since, as naturally occurring substances in the brain, they must be under genetic control.

Part III of the book deals with the epidemiology of Parkinson's disease. The chapters in Part III examine the observational associations in regard to the occurrence of Parkinson's disease and their relationships to demographic and other clinical factors. There is an emphasis in Part III on the issues involved in the design, implementation, and analysis of epidemiological studies of the etiology of Parkinson's disease. The first chapter in Part III (Chapter 8) reviews the difficulties in defining, and then ascertaining with some reasonable level of certainty, the presence of both the disorder and the putative risk factors. A comprehensive review of the worldwide data on the incidence and prevalence of Parkinson's disease is utilized to examine geographic and racial variation, age-related morbidity, mortality, and changes of the frequency of the disorder over time in an attempt to pinpoint clues to the etiology of Parkinson's disease.

Chapter 9 examines the literature on the association of other diseases, conditions, disabilities, and injuries that may have preceded the onset of Parkinson's disease and may possibly be considered part of the etiologic process. Since there is currently no indicator for subclinical Parkinson's disease, determining the temporal relationship of a premorbid or coexisting condition is difficult, if not impossible, for most conditions. Nonetheless, understanding of the mechanism of parallel or similar etiologic processes leading to the coexistence of Parkinson's disease with another disorder should not be summarily dismissed, since it may represent an important avenue for developing insights into the etiology of the disease.

Chapter 10 reviews in detail several precepts of conventional wisdom such as racial and gender differentials in frequency of Parkinson's disease. It is concluded that the evidence, although abundant, is not very convincing. The chapter is perhaps more important for its cautionary note and advice regarding the pro forma weight that peer-reviewed reports are often given without careful scrutiny of the methodological approaches used and the appropriateness of the inferences drawn.

The final chapter of Part III (Chapter 11) begins with a cursory examination of methods that may be used by investigators in the evaluation of possible predictors of Parkinson's disease in their own work and in assessment of putative predictors in the reported work of others. Most of the chapter is devoted to describing the problems of selection bias in epidemiological studies of the association of risk factors for Parkinson's disease and the potential for such bias to produce observed results that under- or overestimate the strength of the actual association. In the case of the negative association of smoking with onset of Parkinson's disease, it is demonstrated that while this result has been observed by many authors, a type of selection bias could produce such a result when in reality the association was nonexistent or even positive.

Part IV reviews exogenous agents that might cause Parkinson's disease. This is a particularly rich area since environmental causes of parkinsonism have been recognized since the 1800s. The wide variety of chemicals and metals that have been reported to cause parkinsonism are covered comprehensively in Chapter 12. This chapter also deals with the complex issues involved in identifying and confirming the role of exogenous agents as the putative causes of neurological disorders. Epidemiological studies implicating environmental agents in the cause of Parkinson's disease are also reviewed in this chapter, with a critical eye toward methodological strengths and weaknesses. Chapter 13 is dedicated entirely to MPTP, since it was this compound that ignited interest in exogenous agents as a cause of parkinsonism. To this day, MPTP remains unique in its ability to consistently induce pure parkinsonism after systemic administration. Studies on mechanism of action of this compound have opened a remarkable number of new research avenues into the cause of nigrostriatal degeneration. While an MPTP-like substance that might actually be the cause of Parkinson's disease has yet to be identified in the environment, this remains an avenue of research worthy of intensive pursuit.

The final chapter in Part IV examines yet another potential environmental cause of Parkinson's disease, infection. The possibility that an infectious agent is a cause of the disease dominated thinking for much of the earlier and middle parts of this century. This, of course, was stimulated by a phenomenon known as postencephalitic parkinsonism, which followed von Economo's encephalitis, a condition that appeared to be pandemic in 1918–1920. The phenomenon was so striking that it was eventually proposed that all cases of Parkinson's disease were postencephalitic (the so-called "cohort hypothesis"). While few today would suggest that infection is a leading candidate as an etiologic agent, it remains a possibility that should not be discarded. Hence, a chapter on infection and Parkinson's disease is included.

III. THE BIBLIOGRAPHY

Part V brings us full circle to the origin of this book. Chapter 15 comprises the bibliography and represents our best attempt at compiling all of the articles in the English language (and other languages for which English abstracts were available) that have some bearing on the cause of Parkinson's disease. One can say with near certainty that references have been omitted that should have been included. There are also a small number of references that are not directly relevant to the cause of Parkinson's disease, but that were added because they will be useful for those interested in designing or reviewing studies of the etiology of Parkinson's disease (for example, references on basic free radical chemistry). Despite these problems, we believe that this list is one of the most comprehensive ever assembled on the cause of Parkinson's disease, and as such, it should serve as an in-depth reference source for those interested in the etiology of Parkinson's disease.

Although this bibliography will always be useful when searching for references that antedate its publication date, it is also very clear that the bibliography will become outdated quickly because new and relevant references are appearing almost daily. Indeed, this presented a problem for the Editors, because of the difficult question as to when to "close down" the process of adding new references, which continued to pour in while the chapters were being written and even edited. With the explosion of information sources and the development of the so-called "information superhighway," perhaps it will be possible to find a way to constantly update this section. The editors are investigating the possibility of putting the bibliography "on line" via E-mail or possibly providing a CD-ROM on an annual basis. Regardless of whether or not this can be achieved, this final chapter is intended to provide a timely and useful tool for those who are interested in learning more about the cause of Parkinson's disease. It is the hope of the editors that this volume will provide not only a resource for past research on the cause of Parkinson's disease, but also a road map to the future.

1

Defining Parkinson's Disease and Parkinsonism

Rajesh Pahwa and William C. Koller

University of Kansas Medical Center, Kansas City, Kansas

I. INTRODUCTION

The view that Parkinson's disease is a specific morbid entity was introduced by James Parkinson (1) in 1817, and accepted by the founding fathers of neurology, such as Charcot (2) and Gowers (3). In this chapter, classic concepts of the disease and its pathological substrate are presented. In addition, the large number of disorders that can cause signs and symptoms similar to Parkinson's disease are described. As will become evident, distinguishing these many forms of parkinsonism from Parkinson's disease can be a formidable task. We conclude by considering the current difficulties in making an accurate clinical diagnosis. The overall goal of this chapter is to provide a thorough knowledge of these concepts as a starting point for investigating the cause of Parkinson's disease and related disorders, and as critical background information for the chapters that follow.

II. PARKINSON'S DISEASE

In the following section the classic features of Parkinson's disease as a unitary clinicopathological entity are described. From time to time, this concept has been challenged, an important issue that is dealt with in Chapter 2 of this volume. Synonyms for Parkinson's disease include idiopathic Parkinson's disease and idiopathic Lewy body parkinsonism. However, the latter term requires knowledge of the neuropathology of the disease and, therefore, is not particularly useful for clinical purposes. Although some investigators also refer to Parkinson's disease as idiopathic parkinsonism, this term has the disadvantage of being relative nonspecific, referring to parkinsonism of any unknown cause.

A. Signs and Symptoms

The cardinal features of Parkinson's disease are resting tremor, rigidity, bradykinesia, and postural instability. The characteristic tremor is present at rest, often involving the thumb and forefinger (pill-rolling), with a frequency of 4–6 Hz; the arms, legs, head, and even the jaw may be involved. Postural and action (kinetic) tremor may also occur in Parkinson's disease.

Bradykinesia, defined as the inability to initiate or perform common motor movements with normal speed, is one of the most incapacitating features of the disease. Other features of bradykinesia include a delay in arresting movement, a decrease in amplitude and speed of repetitive movements, difficulty in shifting from one movement to another (often resulting in freezing), and the inability to execute simultaneous or sequential tasks. A peculiar feature of bradykinesia is the transient ability to reach normal levels of activity under certain circumstances, such as when emotionally stressed (''akinesia paradoxica'') (14). Regular eye blinking, facial movements, associated movements of the arms while walking, and assuming a relaxed posture while sitting are impaired and cannot be accomplished without conscious effort.

Rigidity is typically present in both the flexors and extensors of a joint, and it can affect both appendicular and axial musculature. The posture of a Parkinson's disease patient is typically flexed, with the head bowed, trunk bent forward, the shoulders drooped, arms flexed at the elbow, with hands in front of the body and the knees flexed (5). This causes the center of gravity to be displaced forward, leading to a tendency to lose balance with either propulsion or retropulsion. Postural righting reflexes are lost as the disease progresses. This loss, when severe enough, typically leads to falling.

Although tremor is frequently the first symptom to attract diagnostic attention, subtle symptoms, such as slowness of movement, loss of agility, tremulousness, and depression, are often present early in the disease process. Other early manifestations include loss of dexterity of finger movements (e.g., buttoning shirts), infrequent blinking, lack of facial expression, micrographia, flexed posture of the trunk, poverty of associated movement, dragging of a leg, and the sensation of tightness, stiffness, and aching in the limbs (6). These and other symptoms may be of such gradual onset that 1–2 years often pass before a diagnosis of Parkinson's disease is first entertained.

The nonmotor manifestations that also occur in Parkinson's disease are shown in Table 1. Their prevalence and severity varies markedly among patients and, in a few of them, it may be the presenting complaint. However, the diagnosis of

Table 1 Nonmotor Manifestations in Parkinson's Disease

Sensory phenomena
Loss of smell
Dementia
Depression
Autonomic nervous system dysfunction

Parkinson's disease cannot be made until the motor manifestations are clinically present. Furthermore, most clinicians will not make a diagnosis of Parkinson's disease until there is evidence of progression (see Section II.C, this chapter).

Subjective sensory disturbances, such as pain, tingling, numbness, and burning have been reported in approximately 40% of patients with Parkinson's disease (7). An intriguing recent observation is that the sense of smell is decreased in 75–90% of patients (8). The physiological basis of this finding is unknown, but this loss of smell may be present many years before the onset of motor symptoms (8). Assuming this is not an inherited trait [as suggested by twins studies (9)], this observation has several interesting hypothetical implications: (a) because olfactory receptors are directly exposed to the outside environment, they could represent a portal of entry for a putative environmental agent to make its way from the nasal cavity to the brain, or (b) the underlying disease process may decrease the resistance of the olfactory epithelium, such that an environmental agent can more easily damage the olfactory epithelium. On the other hand, it is also possible that the olfactory system is predisposed to destruction from degenerative process associated with Parkinson's disease itself (8,10,11).

Dementia is not unusual in Parkinson's disease (12–15), but its prevalence and cause are both matters of some debate. The prevalence of dementia in Parkinson's disease has been reported to occur in 10–40% of cases (16–21). The prevalence rate probably varies between studies because of several factors, including the use of different criteria for the diagnosis of dementia, as well as the use of different psychometric assessment scales. Another reason is that many of these studies employ a clinic-based population, rather than population-based survey (17).

The relation between dementia and the etiology of Parkinson's disease is unknown. Marder et al. (22) found that first-degree relatives of demented patients with Parkinson's disease had at least six times the risk of dementia compared with nondemented patients with Parkinson's disease. Glatt et al. (23) found a slight male predominance (not statistically significant) and an older age in patients with dementia, than for those without this disorder. These investigators also reported that patients with Parkinson's disease had a high prevalence of dementia and a high prevalence of Parkinson's disease in first-degree relatives, raising the possibility of shared genetic risk factors.

One of the major affective symptoms associated with Parkinson's disease is depression, which has been reported to occur in 37–90% of the patients with this disease (24,25). Depression may occur early in the disease (26), and there is a controversy over whether the depression is endogenous or reactive, although many investigators favor the former (see Chapter 9).

A variety of autonomic nervous system symptoms have been reported in Parkinson's disease. They include orthostatic hypotension, gastrointestinal problems (namely swallowing difficulties, delayed gastric emptying, excessive salivation, and constipation), sexual dysfunction, dermatitis, excessive sweating, and urinary problems (27).

B. Disease Onset

An important issue concerning the natural history of Parkinson's disease (and theories on its cause) is determining when the pathological process begins. It is generally accepted that there is a long presymptomatic phase in Parkinson's disease (28,29). Support for a long latent period for Parkinson's disease comes partly from the nonmotor symptoms of the disease, which may antedate the motor signs by many years (30). For example, depression can occur years before the onset of the motor signs of Parkinson's disease (26). Autonomic symptoms, such as constipation and dermatitis, may predate Parkinson's disease. Primary sensory complaints may be present for months or years before its onset (7,31,32). Patients often complain of loss of olfaction years before the onset of Parkinson's disease, sometimes for periods of up to 10–20 years.

All of these observations point out the difficulties in early diagnosis, but they also indicate a long latency period for this disease. If such a period exists, identifying its onset is likely to greatly facilitate the search for the cause. Unfortunately, there is as yet no way to accomplish presymptomatic diagnosis; therefore, the exact time of disease onset and duration of the presymptomatic phase (assuming one exists) is unknown. Finding ways to diagnosis presymptomatic disease remains one of the major goals of research on the cause of the disease.

C. Disease Progression

Parkinson's disease is a progressive disorder, and most clinicians will not make a firm diagnosis without evidence of such progression. Since there is as yet no way to monitor underling disease progress at the neuropathological level, virtually all studies of disease progression are, by necessity, based on clinical observation. These studies have indicated a marked individual variability. Traditionally, Parkinson's disease has been divided into five clinical stages according to the extent of disability (33), and the rate of change from stage to stage can be used as a rough indicator of progression. These stages, originally described by Hoehn and Yahr (34) are defined as follows: stage I, unilateral involvement, with minimal or no functional impairment; stage II, bilateral or midline involvement, without impairment of balance; stage III, moderate generalized dysfunction and early impairment of equilibrium on standing and walking; stage IV, significant disability, although the patient is still able to walk and stand unassisted; stage V, confinement to bed or wheelchair unless aided.

In their initial study, Hoehn and Yahr (34) reported that 37.1% of their patients whose illness had been present for less than 5 years had reached stage III or beyond. By 5–9 years, this had increased to 63%. Of all their patients who had had their illness 10 years or longer, 33.9% were still in stage I and II; although Hoehn and Yahr referred to these patients as having atypical primary parkinsonism, they may have represented Parkinson's disease with an unusually benign course. Marttila and Rinne (34) studied the rate of progression and found that bilateral symptoms appeared an average of 2.9 years after onset (stage I); subsequent stages were reached at intervals of about 2–2.5 years. They also identified a small subset of patients with rapid progression of the disease (''malignant course''), who were in stages III–V within 3 years of onset, or reached stages IV–V before 5 years. Because about 30% of newly diagnosed patients present in stage II, it cannot be known with certainty whether or not all patients initially have unilateral signs or symptoms.

More recent studies have used the Unified Parkinson's Disease Rating Scale (UPDRS) to gauge the progression of the disease (35,36). In patients not requiring antiparkinsonian medications, Tetrud and Langston (35) reported that the motor scale of the UPDRS examination deteriorated at a rate of 13.4 points per year and the Parkinson Study Group (36) reported a deterioration of 8.6 points per year. Diamond et al. (37) reported the results of long-term experience with levodopa and its effects on the progression of the disease. Their results suggested that the patients treated with levodopa had a steady progression of disease, but at a level of severity much lower than that before treatment. Other studies have reported similar results (38–41).

Birkmayer et al. (42) used rate of progression to divide Parkinson's disease patients into two groups: benign or malignant. They found that the benign cases responded very well to levodopa treatment and showed a long-lasting (7 years) decrease in disability, whereas, in the malignant cases, the drop in disability resulting from introduction of antiparkinsonian therapy lasted for only a year. The malignant type was seen more often in the older group of patients. It is possible that the patients diagnosed with the malignant type of Parkinson's disease might have had one of the neurodegenerative forms of atypical parkinsonism (see Section III on parkinsonism). For this reason, a note of caution should probably be entertained in accepting the results of any study on ''malignant Parkinson's disease'' unless such cases are pathologically verified.

Goetz et al. (43) studied the risk factors for progression of Parkinson's disease among those patients with slowly progressive versus rapidly progressive disease. They found that patients with rapidly progressive disease were older at disease onset than those whose disease progressed more slowly. Marttila and Rinne (33) found that patients who presented predominantly with tremor carried a better prognosis than those with other parkinsonian signs. However, these results were not duplicated by Goetz and his co-workers (43). Zetusky et al. (44) have also found that tremor along with relative preservation of mental status, earlier age of onset, and family history of parkinsonism is associated with a favorable prognosis. There has been no association with the rate of progression and family history of parkinsonism, trauma, stress, lack of smoking, lack of early measles infection, chemical or herbicide exposure, well water as primary drinking source, rural living, or daily vitamin ingestion (34,43).

D. Parkinson's Disease with Onset Younger than Aged 40

Occasionally Parkinson's disease occurs before the age of 40 years. Although historically this has been referred to as the ''juvenile'' from of the disease (45), most investigators now prefer the term *young-onset* when the disease begins between the ages of 20 and 40 years, reserving the term *juvenile* for parkinsonism beginning before the age of 20.

Several groups have attempted to identify subpopulations of patients based on age and on the clinical and pharmacological features of the disease. For example, Narabayashi et al. (45) classified patients with the disease beginning younger than age 40 as follows: group I, with onset in the 30s and a clinical picture and course similar to Parkinson's disease; and group II, with an average onset age of 12 years and the clinical signs of dystonia, rigidity, and tremor. Both groups have a good clinical response to levodopa.

Furukawa et al. (46) compared ventricular cerebrospinal fluid (CSF) biopterin levels in patients with classic Parkinson's disease with those with onset younger than 40 years. They divided their patients younger than 40 into two groups: those with good response to levodopa, followed by marked motor fluctuations and dopa-induced dyskinesias (type I), and those with a milder response to levodopa, with less fluctuations (type II). They found that the mean ventricular CSF biopterin levels were markedly lower in the type I patients than in classic Parkinson's disease or type II patients. They concluded that the type II group represented early-onset classic Parkinson's disease, but that the type I group was a distinct subgroup, having a different physiopathology from classic Parkinson's disease.

Familial incidence of parkinsonism is higher in patients with young-onset Parkinson's disease than in patients with onset after the age of 40 years. Yokochi et al. (47) reported a familial incidence of 40.7% in patients with onset between

21 and 40 years of age and 46.2% in those with onset at aged 20 or below. A joint survey by seven neurological hospitals in Japan, revealed familial incidence of 47.8% in the aged group below 30, 29.7% in the aged group 30–39, 5.2% in the aged group 40–49, 6.7% in the aged group 50–59, 3.2% in the aged group 60–69, and 0% in the aged group older than 70 (45).

Genetic forms of juvenile parkinsonism (JP) have been described, and tyrosine hydroxylase activity has been reported to be decreased in several subcortical nuclei in brains of hereditary juvenile parkinsonism patients (48), which raises the possibility that it might be a candidate gene for PD.

E. Neuropathology

The neuropathology of Parkinson's disease is well defined and will not be discussed in detail, since it is the subject of an entire chapter in this volume (see Chapter 3, this volume). In brief, the disease is characterized by loss of neurons in the substantia nigra and other pigmented nuclei, including the locus ceruleus (49). The loss of cells in the zona compacta of the substantia nigra results in a profound dopamine depletion in the striatum, which is responsible for most, if not all, of the motor symptomatology of the disease. Importantly, other nonpigmented areas of the brain may also be involved in Parkinson's disease, including the nucleus basalis of Mynert. Another cardinal feature of the disease is the Lewy body, a round, concentric, eosinophilic inclusion found within degenerating neurons. Although not unique to Parkinson's disease, these inclusions are highly characteristic of the disease at the pathological level, and many (though not all) neuropathologists will not make a diagnosis of classic Parkinson's disease without their presence (hence, the term "idiopathic Lewy body parkinsonism"). As a clinicopathological entity, a diagnosis is not made unless both the clinical and pathological features are present.

The neuropathological correlates of dementia in Parkinson's disease have not been fully clarified. Ross et al. (50) have suggested that there are three subtypes of dementia in Parkinson's disease: (a) a subcortical dementia caused by a dopamine deficiency; (b) a more marked dementia associated with atrophy of nucleus basalis, which presumably results in a cortical cholinergic deficit (51); and; (c) Alzheimer's disease (AD) pathology with features of both cortical and subcortical dementia.

A complicating issue is the entity referred to as diffuse Lewy body disease (52,53). It has been suggested that Lewy body disease can be divided into three types: Type A diffuse distribution of Lewy bodies, involving brainstem and cortex; type B, a transitional form; type C, Lewy bodies confined to the brainstem (Parkinson's disease). In the diffuse form, dementia may be the sole presenting feature, often accompanied by marked psychiatric disturbances. Some investigators have been so impressed with the range of Lewy body-associated disease that they have suggested there is a clinical and pathological spectrum of the Lewy body that constitutes one disease. Sage and Mark (54) point out that, even within a familial cluster, there is both a clinical spectrum (parkinsonism–dementia) as well as a pathological spectrum of Lewy body disease. In one pathological study of patients with the clinical diagnosis of AD, but without known parkinsonism, in 11% of the cases there was nigral neuronal loss and Lewy bodies sufficiently severe to make the additional pathological diagnosis of Parkinson's disease (55). Given this overall picture, the relation between dementia, Parkinson's disease, Lewy bodies, and Alzheimer's disease now remains somewhat murky, particularly in very elderly individuals. Until more clinicopathological studies are performed, determination of the exact cause of dementia when present in Parkinson's disease is likely to be a difficult task.

F. Neuropathologic Evidence for a Prolonged Presymptomatic Phase

As noted earlier, most investigators believe that Parkinson's disease begins well in advance of the onset of symptoms. Several pathological studies support this proposition. First, there are the intriguing reports of Lewy bodies in the sympathetic ganglia of patients without motor signs of Parkinson's disease, a finding that strongly suggests the presence of preclinical Parkinson's disease (56,57). Second, Scherman et al. (58) performed a study of tritiated α-dihydrotetrabenazine (^{3}HTBZOH) in the caudate nucleus of 57 patients with Parkinson's disease with age at death of 73.0 ± 1 years. Extrapolation of a regression model of their observed data indicated that striatal dopaminergic innervation might be about 55% lower in Parkinson's disease patients than in the control population at 60 years. The authors suggest that these results indicate that the pathological process begins about 20–30 years before the first symptom. However, Agid et al. (59) have pointed out that this assumption is valid only if the death rates of dopamine neurons in both parkinsonian and control subjects are constant during that period. These issues are also discussed in Chapter 3.

G. The Aging Nigrostriatal System: Clues to the Etiology of Parkinson's Disease?

That the same cells (substantia nigra) that are affected in Parkinson's disease, an age-related disorder, are also thought to decline with normal aging, has attracted the attention of investigators for years. The same statement can be made about changes in striatal dopamine, as there have been numerous reports of loss of striatal dopamine with advancing age as well (60–63). Postmortem studies on binding to dopamine receptors have also shown a decrease in the substantia nigra and caudate at a rate of about 50% over 70 years (63). Studies have shown a decline in neuronal counts with advancing age. McGeer et al.

(64) reported a steady loss of nigral neurons, at a rate of 7% per decade, between the ages of 10 and 80 years. Mann and his associate reported a 7% decline between the ages 15 and 65 (1.4% per decade), with a subsequent fall of 21% between the ages of 65 and 84 years (11% per decade) (65,66).

Given these observations, it has been hypothesized that Parkinson's disease occurs secondary to a subclinical, environmentally induced damage to the substantia nigra, followed by the continued age-related attrition of the nigral neurons, a process that should eventually lead to expression of the disease. As shown in Figure 1, Langston (67) has put forward four different theories concerning the

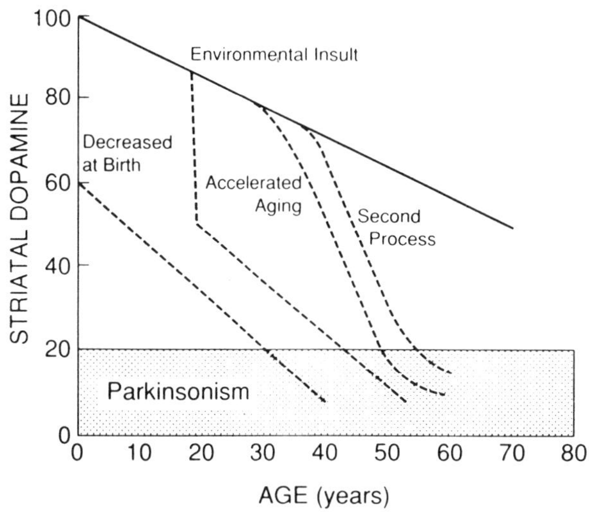

Figure 1 Four different theories concerning the sequence of events that lead to Parkinson's disease. They are based on two assumptions: (a) striatal dopamine declines slowly with normal aging (solid line), and (b) an 80% decrease of striatal dopamine is required for parkinsonism to develop. Decreased at birth: This broken line depicts the consequence of decreased striatal dopamine at birth. As can be seen, an age-related decline is striatal dopamine would lead to the development of parkinsonian symptoms later in life. Environmental insult: A similar sequence of events might occur if an environmental insult produced a partial reduction in nigrostriatal dopaminergic neurons. If we assume the loss of striatal dopamine was less than 80%, symptoms would not develop until the normal age-related decline resulted in an 80% depletion of dopamine (second broken line). Accelerated aging: The third broken line shows the events that might occur if age-related decline began to accelerate abnormally. We do not know why an age-related decline occurs, much less why this process might begin accelerating to produce parkinsonism later in life. Second process: A final possibility is that a second, entirely different process, unrelated to normal aging is responsible for Parkinson's disease, as shown by the fourth broken line. (From Ref. 67.)

sequence of events that lead to Parkinson's disease. This is based on two assumptions: the striatal dopamine declines slowly with normal aging, and an approximately 80% decrease of striatal dopamine is required for parkinsonism to develop. There might be decreased striatal dopamine at birth and, hence, an age-related decline in striatal dopamine would lead to the development of parkinsonian symptoms later in life. Second, an environmental insult might lead to a similar sequence of events by producing a partial reduction in nigrostriatal dopaminergic neurons. Another possible scenario is that the age-related decline might accelerate secondary to an unrelated (and yet to be determined) factor. In this instance, understanding the mechanism of normal aging of the nigrostriatal system would have direct relevance to the cause of Parkinson's disease. Finally, an entirely different process, unrelated to normal aging, might be responsible for Parkinson's disease.

On the other hand, several studies have not supported a relation between normal aging of the dopaminergic nigrostriatal system and Parkinson's disease. Gibb and Lees (68) showed that the nigral loss was greater in 12 young-onset parkinsonians compared with 22 late-onset cases. However, Scherman et al. (58) found that the rate of decrease of dopaminergic innervation in the caudate nucleus was similar whether onset occurred before or after 60 years of age. McGeer et al. (69), using special stains to visualize human leukocyte antigen (HLA)-DR–bearing microglia, found that the number of nigral neurons undergoing phagocytosis in Parkinson's disease patients was six times greater than in age-matched control subjects. This indicated the presence of a pathological process that was much more active than could be explained on the basis of normal aging alone. Recently, Fearnley and Lee (70) studied the microarchitecture of the substantia nigra in controls and patients with Parkinson's disease. The pars compacta was divided into a ventral and a dorsal tier, and each tier was further subdivided into three regions. In 36 controls, they found a linear fallout of pigmented neurons with advancing age in the pars compacta of the caudal substantia nigra, at the rate of 4.7% per decade (21–91 years). The ventral tier was relatively spared compared with the medial ventral and dorsal tiers. However, in Parkinson's disease patients, there was an exponential loss of pigmented neurons with a 45% loss in the first decade after the diagnosis of Parkinson's disease. Regionally, the loss was greatest at the lateral ventral tier (opposite that of normal aging), followed by the medial ventral and dorsal tiers.

This debate is likely to continue until there is a way to monitor nigral cell loss in living humans. However, the hypothesis that a subclinical environmental insult to the substantia nigra could eventually lead to the expression of parkinsonism owing to subsequent normal aging is subject to direct testing. This is because a large cohort of humans who were exposed to 1-methyl-4-phenyl-1,2,3,6-tetrahydropyridine (MPTP) in 1982, remained asymptomatic. Presumably some, if not all, of these individuals sustained damage to their substantia nigra; these individuals are currently enrolled in a long-term follow-up program to see if the aging process will eventually lead to expression of parkinsonism.

III. Parkinsonism

We now turn to those disorders which, because they also affect the nigrostriatal system (either directly or indirectly), can cause signs and symptoms similar to those seen in Parkinson's disease. When present, and not obviously caused by Parkinson's disease, this constellation of clinical features is referred to as parkinsonism (or a parkinsonian syndrome). The usual definition is that *parkinsonism* is a motor syndrome consisting of the following signs: tremor, rigidity, bradykinesia, and postural instability or impairment of postural reflexes (34,72). In the following section, the many forms of parkinsonism that are not due to Parkinson's disease are reviewed. A classification of common parkinsonian syndromes is given in Table 2.

A. Other Neurodegenerative Disorders that Characteristically Manifest as Parkinsonism

The other conditions that can manifest as parkinsonism have been categorized under a variety of terms, including atypical parkinsonism, parkinson-plus syndromes (because they manifest parkinsonism plus other signs and symptoms), and the multiple-system atrophies (see Table 2). The latter term implies knowledge of the underlying pathology and, therefore, may not be the best for clinical use. Parkinson-plus certainly captures some of the syndromes for which nonparkinsonian signs are prominent (e.g., progressive supranuclear palsy), but it is not unusual for these disorders to present as relatively pure parkinsonism, at least in their earlier stages (e.g., striatonigral degeneration). For these reasons, the term atypical parkinsonism may be preferable for these parkinsonian neurodegenerative disorders. For most of these diseases, this issue is a problem only in the earlier disease stages, because with time, a more precise diagnosis can be made as other nonparkinsonian features become manifest.

Before proceeding to a description of these disorders, it should be noted that Quinn (73) has recently suggested a somewhat different way of categorizing the disorders described in the following section. Specifically, he suggests that the term *multiple-system atrophy* be used to refer to "sporadic adult-onset degenerative disease of the central and autonomic nervous system characterized by cell loss and gliosis (without Lewy bodies, unless incidental) in a selection of the following structures: striatum, nigra, olives, pons, cerebellum and intermediolateral cell columns, and Onuf's nucleus in the spinal cord." He specifically excludes hereditary olivopontocerebellar atrophies (OPCA) from the multisystem atrophies, and suggests that the oligodendroglial cytoplasmatic inclusions may

Table 2 Classification of Parkinsonian Syndromes

A. Hereditary diseases of CNS associated with parkinsonism
Wilson's disease
Huntington's disease
Hallervorden–Spatz disease
B. Multiple system atrophies with parkinsonian features
Progressive supranuclear palsy
Olivopontocerebellar atrophy
Striatonigral degeneration
Shy-Drager syndrome
C. Other degenerative diseases of the CNS with parkinsonian features
Primary pallidal atrophy
Idiopathic dystonia–parkinsonism
Corticodentatonigral degeneration
Hemiatrophy–hemiparkinsonism
Parkinsonism–ALS–dementia complex of Guam
Atherosclerotic
Alzheimer's and Pick's diseases
Creutzfeldt–Jakob disease
D. Other CNS disorders
Normal pressure hydrocephalus
Stroke
Tumor
Trauma
Subdural hematoma
Syringomesencephalia
E. Infectious and postinfectious
Encephalitis lethargica
Encephalitides
Syphilis
F. Toxic
Manganese
Carbon monoxide
Carbon disulfide
Cyanide
Methanol
MPTP
G. Pharmacological
Neuroleptics
Reserpine, tetrabenazine
α-Methyldopa
Lithium
Fluphenazine
H. Metabolic causes
Hypoparathyroidism and basal ganglia calcification
Chronic hepatocerebral degeneration

represent a unifying pathological feature. Progressive supranuclear palsy is excluded from the multisystem atrophies, since these inclusions are not present in that disease entity nor in patients with hereditary OPCA. This concept of multisystem atrophies as a specific entity, with multiple expressions (striatonigral degeneration, olivopontocerebellar atrophy, or Shy–Drager syndrome) may or may not stand the test of time, but it is mentioned here, since anyone dealing with these syndromes is going to have to be familiar with all of the different approaches to classification.

1. Progressive Supranuclear Palsy

In 1963, Richardson and associates (74) reported a series of eight cases of parkinsonism in combination with a progressive supranuclear palsy (PSP). A year later they presented a more extensive study of this newly identified disorder (75). Sixty-two percent of the patients initially presented with gait difficulties and 22% with mental changes. Other initial complaints included slowness or stiffness of movement, abrupt falls, poor or blurred vision, dysphagia, or dysarthria (75).

Supranuclear ophthalmoplegia is the hallmark of PSP. In addition to the gaze palsy, which typically affects vertical (downward) conjugate eye movements, there is a marked increase in axial tone, particularly of the neck, which is less prominent in the extremities. The disease responds poorly to traditional antiparkinsonian therapy. The pathology of PSP clearly differs from Parkinson's disease, both in distribution of the lesions and type of pathology (neurofibrillary tangles, rather than Lewy bodies; see Chapter 3).

The etiology of PSP remains unknown. Steele et al. (75), in their original report, postulated that it was either a primary central nervous system degeneration or a postinfectious degenerative neurological disorder following a viral infection. This was based on the pathological features of PSP, which resembled postencephalitic parkinsonism, with numerous neurofibrillary tangles present in affected areas.

Several authors have since raised the possibility of a viral cause (761–80); however, inflammatory changes that would indicate a viral origin have rarely been observed (75–77,79–83). Efforts in transmitting PSP to primates have also been unsuccessful (77,78). Furthermore, the ultrastructure of the neurofibrillary tangles observed in PSP is different from that seen in neurological diseases accepted as being postinfectious (84–86) Finally, none of the PSP patients have a history of encephalitis (77).

Dubinsky and Jankovic (87) studied 58 patients with PSP and found that 32.8% of patients had computed tomography (CT), magnetic resonance imaging (MRI), or autopsy evidence of multi-infarct state. This compares with 12.9% of their Parkinson's disease patients. It is not clear to what extent the imaging findings of infarcts accounted for the clinical findings, and few investigators currently consider PSP to have a vascular cause.

There have also been reports of patients developing PSP following head trauma (88–90). There is no evidence to indicate that genetic factors play a role in the etiology. There has been only a single report of family history of PSP (90). The disorder does not seem to have a proclivity for any racial or ethnic group.

Recently, Davis et al. (91) conducted a case–control study to find the possible risk factors for PSP. They found no significant differences between cases and controls for occupation; well water use; exposure to radiation, lead, aluminum, chemicals, or pesticides. There was no significant difference between smoking, alcohol ingestion, head trauma, menopause, or type of personality. The other factors that were compared and for which no significant differences were found are listed in Table 3.

2. *Olivopontocerebellar Atrophy*

The olivopontocerebellar atrophies (OPCAs) encompass a large group of disorders that cause cerebellar ataxia. The term permits the clinical description of patients who demonstrate a combination of cerebellar and basal ganglia syndromes. A wide variety of neurological features aside from cerebellar signs (gait ataxia, limb dysmetria, or other) can be present, including corticospinal defects, extrapyramidal features (dystonia, chorea, myoclonus), cranial nerve palsies, autonomic nervous system dysfunction, and peripheral nervous system abnormalities (amyotrophy fasciculations). The pathological changes can also be quite varied, including cerebellar, basal ganglia, brainstem, and spinal cord abnormalities. The term olivopontocerebellar atrophy (OPCA) was first used by Dejerine and Thomas (92), in the year 1900, to describe two cases of sporadic late adult-onset cerebellar syndromes. Even though the term does not describe all the pathological changes that may be present in the disorder, it has survived the test of time.

Dominant and recessive hereditary forms, as well as sporadic cases of OPCA, have been described. Berciano (93) reviewed 132 cases of OPCA from the literature and found that 67 of them were familial and 65 were sporadic. Destunis (94) reported 45 cases of OPCA, of which 16 were hereditary. Eleven of these 16 cases had an autosomal dominant mode of transmission, and the remaining 5 cases had autosomal recessive inheritance.

Following a report by Yakura et al. (95) of a possible linkage of hereditary ataxia to the HLA loci on chromosome 6, many linkage analyses have been performed. In the pedigrees initially reported by Currier et al. (96) and Schut and Haymaker (97), there was convincing evidence that familial OPCA locus was linked to the HLA loci. However, subsequent studies on the remaining families failed to confirm those results (93).

There are various classifications for OPCA. Koningsmark and Weiner (98) have divided the inherited OPCAs into five types: OPCA I, Menzel type, is an autosomal dominant disorder, with age of onset between 14 and 58 years, and

Table 3 Factors Not Associated with Progressive Supranuclear Palsy

Education
Living in a rural area
Lived on farm
Living outside United States
Occupations
Exposure to potential toxins
Smoking
Alcohol
Contact sports
Head trauma
Type A personality
Menopause
Hypertension
Stroke
Meningitis or encephalitis
Seizures
Herpes zoster
Thyroid disease
Cold sores
Peptic ulcer
Fractures
Meniere's disease
Psychiatric illness
Surgery
Blood transfusion
Dentures
Dental procedures and surgery
Glaucoma
Exposure to pets, wild animals, livestock
Mother's age older than 40
Born first in family
Family history of Down syndrome, dementia, epilepsy, stroke, essential tremor, Parkinson's disease

Source: Ref. 93.

death occurring between 32 and 60 years. Clinical findings include unsteady gait, dysarthria, clumsiness of hands, tremor of body and extremities, sensory loss, involuntary movements, and pyramidal signs. OPCA II, Fickler-Winkler type, is an autosomal recessive disorder, with age of onset between 20 and 80 years, and death occurring between 33 and 84 years. It is characterized by ataxia, normal sensations, and depressed reflexes. OPCA III, with retinal degeneration, is autosomal dominant, with age of onset between 1 and 34 years, and death occurring between 1.5 and 75 years. Clinically, it consists of ataxia, tremor of arms and head, dysarthria, progressive visual loss, and blindness. OPCA IV, Schut-Haymaker type, is autosomal dominant, with age of onset between 17 and 30 years, and death occurring between 26 and 48 years, characterized by ataxia, dysarthria, laryngeal and facial palsy, dysphagia, and hypoactive to hyperactive reflexes. OPCA V is an autosomal dominant disorder, beginning between the ages 7 and 45 years, and death occurring between 11 and 63 years. It is characterized by dementia, ophthalmoplegia, and extrapyramidal signs.

Olivopontocerebellar atrophy is a group of heterogenous disorders, with a probable diverse etiology. There have been studies that have described an association between OPCA and abnormalities of the enzyme glutamate dehydrogenase (GDH) (99–108). Some studies have shown that there is deficiency of GDH in late-onset forms of OPCA; however, the mode of inheritance is not uniform. In 1980, Plaitakis et al. (99) reported a subject with juvenile-onset spinocerebellar and extrapyramidal syndrome and two siblings with adult-onset spinocerebellar syndrome and found that there was a decrease in GDH in the cultured skin fibroblasts and homogenates of leukocytes in all three cases. Yamaguchi et al. (100) found a decrease in GDH activity in leukocytes and platelets from five OPCA patients with sporadic disease. In 1983, Duvoisin et al. (101) reported a deficiency of GDH in leukocytes of patients with late-onset OPCA manifested by parkinsonian features, ataxia, supranuclear oculomotor dysfunction, and peripheral neuropathy and, in some cases, amyotrophy. Their data suggested autosomal dominant inheritance with low penetrance.

Plaitakis et al. (102) measured GDH activity in leukocytes from 88 patients with various types of neurodegenerative disorders affecting primarily the cerebellum or the basal ganglia. They found 12 of their patients had partial deficiency of the enzyme and abnormal systemic glutamate metabolism (102,103). The majority of these patients had signs consistent with the diagnosis of OPCA, although there were a few with atypical neurological manifestations. Seven cases of GDH deficiency were familial and five were sporadic. The genetic pattern of their data was compatible with autosomal recessive inheritance. Another interesting finding in this study was that the decrease in GDH activity was limited to the "particulate heat-labile" component of the enzyme and not the "particulate heat-stable" component.

Sorbi et al. (104) studied GDH activity in platelets from four patients with nondominant form of adult-onset OPCA and in affected and nonaffected members of two families with a dominant form of OPCA. They reported partial deficiency of GDH activity in three patients with nondominant OPCA and two patients with dominant OPCA. Platelet GDH activity in patients and controls was inactivated by guanosine-5′-triphosphate (GTP) and was stimulated by adensoine-5′-diphosphate (ADP). The activating effect of ADP was enhanced in the presence of Triton X-100. In one unaffected member of another family, with the dominant-type OPCA, GDH activity was in the control range and was not activated by ADP in the presence or absence of Triton. From these results, the authors suggested that there might be two alterations of GDH in patients with OPCA: one that decreases the maximum catalytic activity and another that impairs the regulatory properties of the enzyme, with the latter occurring in the dominantly inherited forms.

Finocchiaro et al. (105) also reported decreased GDH activities in leukocytes of 11 patients with dominant OPCA and 4 patients with sporadic-recessive form. As can be seen from the foregoing findings, different authors have reported decrease in GDH activity in the peripheral tissues, but the mode of inheritance differs widely.

There are contrasting views among different authors whether the changes in GDH have any role in the pathogenesis of OPCA. Grossman et al. (106) compared activities of brain GDH at necropsy in patients with autosomal dominant OPCA and controls and found no significant reduction in brain GDH activity, and Rosenberg and Banner (107) found normal GDH activity in cerebellar homogenates from a patient with dominant OPCA. More recently, Chokroverty et al. (108) reported neuropathological findings in a patient with antemortem diagnosis of OPCA and reduced leukocytic GDH activity. They found that brain GDH activity was not reduced and brain GDH mRNA was normal.

Kish et al. (109) examined autopsied brains of ten patients with dominantly inherited OPCA and measured the concentration of glycerophosphoethanolamine (GPEA), a membrane breakdown product, and found that mean GPEA levels were significantly elevated over controls in 11 of the 15 brain areas examined, including extracellular brain regions in which no neuronal cell loss could be detected by semiquantitative estimation. They raised the possibility that altered membrane phospholipid metabolism could be a contributing factor in neuronal cell death. Other neurotransmitters, such as aspartate, might be playing a similar role in the pathogenesis of other types of multisystem atrophies (110).

3. *Striatonigral Degeneration*

First described in 1961 by Adams and colleagues (111), the signs and symptoms of striatonigral degeneration (SND) are those of an akinetic–rigid syndrome very similar to Parkinson's disease (PD), although tremor is usually not a feature. If tremor is present, it is not a prominent sign. Severe akinesia, rigidity, and postural instability occur as SND progresses. Speech and swallowing difficulties may be present early on, and corticospinal tract signs may eventually be evident. These symptoms do not respond to levodopa therapy, which clearly distinguishes SND from PD. The pathological changes consist of marked neuronal degeneration in the striatum (putamen more involved than caudate). The involvement of the substantia nigra is variable. The pathological changes of this disorder may occur in combination with changes seen in OPCA; hence, some authors prefer to use the term multiple-system atrophy (MSA) when describing it.

The etiology of SND is unknown. It is unlikely that SND is due to a viral agent or a form of postencephalitic disease. Cerebellar ataxia and autonomic dysfunction that is seen in this disease has never been reported in postencephalitic parkinsonism. The disorder does not respond to levodopa therapy, but postencephalitic parkinsonism nearly always has a good initial response to levodopa. Adams et al. (112) raised the possibility that the degeneration occurred possibly secondary to an exogenous agent.

4. Shy–Drager Syndrome

Shy–Drager syndrome combines progressive autonomic failure and other CNS findings, particularly basal ganglia and cerebellar signs. Autonomic nervous system dysfunction is common in PD; however, the severity (e.g., postural hypotension, causing syncope) is much less than that which occurs in Shy–Drager syndrome. The signs and symptoms of autonomic nervous system dysfunction (hypotension, urinary difficulty, bowel complaints, loss of thermoregulation, and so forth) are often the earliest symptoms in Shy–Drager syndrome. Other common features are parkinsonian signs, such as bradykinesia and rigidity. Tremor is usually not a prominent feature. These symptoms respond poorly to levodopa therapy. Cerebellar disturbances (dysarthria, ataxia of gait and limbs, oculomotor dysfunction) may be dominant features. Respiratory abnormalities are not uncommon. Pyramidal tract, anterior horn cell, and peripheral nerve dysfunction complete the variable clinical picture. Degeneration of the intermediolateral column in the spinal cord is responsible for the autonomic nervous system dysfunction. Neuronal loss and gliosis can occur in many other brain areas, similar to those described for the OPCAs (e.g., striatum, cerebellum, and midbrain).

Similar to other neurodegenerative syndromes, the etiology of Shy–Drager syndrome is unknown. No inheritance or toxic cause has been identified. In 1983, Bannister et al. (113) studied 16 patients with progressive autonomic failure and found that the frequency of HLA-Aw32 was 13 times more common in these patients than in controls. They suggested that a genetic defect might cause defects in catecholamine metabolism in brain or might affect the immune response to a virus, leading to autonomic failure. However, when Nee et al. (114) studied 30 patients with progressive autonomic failure and multisystem atrophy, they did not find any clearly defined inheritance pattern for any neurological disease, and only one of their patients with progressive autonomic failure had HLA-A32 phenotype. Iwasaki et al. (115) and Kano et al. (116) reported patients with human T-lymphotrophic virus type-I associated with myelopathy, progressive cerebellar syndrome, and with Shy–Drager syndrome, respectively. However, when Yokota et al. (117) investigated 21 patients with Shy–Drager syndrome, they did not find a single patient with elevated HTLV-I titers. Although it is possible that a few cases of Shy–Drager syndrome might be associated with HTLV-I, no conclusive evidence is yet available.

C. Amyotrophic Lateral Sclerosis–Parkinsonism–Dementia Complex of Guam

Parkinsonism with dementia and amyotrophic lateral sclerosis (ALS) is endemic in certain parts of the western Pacific, including Guam, west New Guinea, and the Kii Peninsula of Japan. This syndrome of parkinsonism, dementia, and motor neuron disease (ALS) has been called the ALS–parkinsonism–dementia complex of Guam.

There are several theories on the cause of ALS–parkinsonism–dementia. One of the hypotheses is that it is caused by an exogenous toxin. A number of studies have shown that there is an unusually low concentration of calcium and magnesium in garden soil and drinking water in Guam and other endemic areas, such as west New Guinea. (118–123). Yanagihara et al. (124) reported that there were disturbances in calcium and vitamin D metabolism in Guamanian patients with ALS and Parkinson's disease. There have also been reports of cortical bone loss in Guamanian children and adults (125,126) and of intraneuronal accumulation of calcium and aluminum in brain tissues from patients with ALS–parkinsonism–dementia (127,128). From these observations, Rodgers-Johnson et al. (129) postulated that secondary hyperparathyroidism, induced by chronic deficiencies of calcium, lead to increased intestinal absorption of toxic metals and deposition of metals in the central nervous system (127,128,130–133). However, Reed et al. (134) reviewed the epidemiological data on ALS–parkinsonism–dementia and did not find evidence for the hypothesis that a chronic nutritional deficiency of calcium was the cause.

Koerner (135) and Kurland and Mulder (136) have reported that about 40% of the Guamanian patients have a family history of the disease. Although there were some reports of dominant inheritance, for the most part, no definite pattern could be established. Plato et al. (137) reported similar findings that 23% of the cases had one or more first-degree relatives with ALS–PD. They also reported male relatives had a much higher risk of developing the disease. Yanagihara et al. (122) conducted a epidemiological surveillance of ALS–PD in the Northern Mariana Islands. They found that, although the origin and genotypic composition of Chamorros on all the Mariana Islands was indistinguishable, there was a strikingly lower mortality rate of ALS and Parkinson's disease on Saipan, suggesting that environmental factors were also important in the etiology of the disease. Furthermore, in 1985, the results of a 25-year prospective case–control study (138) showed that there was a increased risk among spouses of patients and a lack of increase among their offspring, suggesting that exogenous factors are playing a role. Genetic studies that have included pedigree analysis of villages with high incidence of the disease, formation of prospective patient–control registries, search for specific gene markers, such as histocompatibility antigens (HLA-A and HLA-B), serum proteins, red blood cell enzymes, and immunoglobulin allogroup systems have not resulted in a satisfactory genetic explanation (139,140). However, the possibility of genetic susceptibility, with an environmental trigger remains a possibility (141).

Maurizi (142) drew similarities between ALS–parkinsonism–dementia and postencephalitic parkinsonism. He claimed that both had a hereditary component, linkage to 1920, peak incidence in 1960s, and a significant decline in the incidence starting in 1960s. From these observations he suggested that ALS–parkinsonism–dementia could be the result of an unusual complication of a neurovirulent influenza virus in a population that had a concentration of vulnerable individuals. Although there are no new cases of postencephalitic parkinsonism, new cases of ALS–parkinsonism–dementia continue to appear. Attempts to link viruses with this disorder have been unsuccessful (143,144). Gibbs and Gajdusek (145) failed to transmit the disease to primates and nonprimates.

It has been suggested that cycad nuts, which are used as a source of food starch in the island, might represent the source of an environmental toxin that could cause the disease. Reed et al. (134) conducted an epidemiological study and found that preference for traditional Chamorro food was the only one of the 23 tested variables significantly associated with an increased risk for ALS–parkinsonism–dementia. Spencer et al. (146) have reviewed the data on the cycad hypothesis and found that there was evidence that there might be a causal relation with ALS–parkinsonism–dementia. In Guam, the cycad flour used for food preparation is believed to contain residual plant chemicals with neurotoxic properties, namely cycasin (147) and β-*N*-methylamino-L-alanine (BMAA; 147,148). In contrast, in the Ryukyu Islands of southern Japan, where cycad foodstuffs are now rarely consumed, and where cycasin is eliminated in the processing of cycad flour, ALS–parkinsonism–dementia is absent (146,149). Similarly, ALS–parkinsonism–dementia is unknown among the South Fore people of Papua, New Guinea (150). It has been suggested that this absence of ALS–PD is because these people do not use cycad seed to dress large skin sores, which is commonly practiced by the Chamorro people (151). Finally, in the past, cycad seed was used to prepare tonic and folk medicines (118), but in the present era, the medicinal use of the cycad seed has declined, and the younger population has decreased the consumption of cycad-containing food, all of which may have played a part in the apparent decline of the disease in the affected regions (129).

There are reasons to believe that ALS–parkinsonism–dementia might be a long-latency neurodegenerative disease (152). There have been various studies that have shown that patients who migrate from endemic areas do not develop the disease for 15–45 years (153,154).

β-*N*-methylamino-L-alanine and cycasin are the two neurotoxins in the cycad seed that have been identified. BMAA has weak glutamate-like excitotoxin properties (155–158). It has been reported that the potency of the excitotoxin properties can be increased by bicarbonate (159) and decreased by glutamate receptor antagonists (155–159). BMAA can be rapidly taken up by CNS tissue, both in culture and in situ and is sodium-dependently transported into synaptosomes, where the agent concentrates (158). Seawright et al. (160) demonstrated that BMAA caused selective degeneration of cerebellar cortical neurons in rats. However, Perry et al. (161), after prolonged oral administration of BMAA, could not demonstrate any neurotoxicity in mice. In primates, there were some clinical and neuropathological features reminiscent of ALS–parkinsonism–dementia, but it lacked the Alzheimer-like neurofibrillary pathology, and the disease fails to progress once the exposure to the neurotoxin ceases (162). Recently, Duncan et al. (148) conducted an investigation on the levels of BMAA in the cycad flour. They found that 87% of the total BMAA processed from cycad seeds was removed during processing and, in half the samples, more than 99% was removed. They concluded that processed cycad flour contained extremely low levels of BMAA and was unlikely to be a source of the disease.

Cycasin is the other neurotoxin found in the cycad seed, and it might be involved in the etiology of ALS–parkinsonism–dementia. Cycasin is also known to be carcinogenic (163,164). Shimizu et al. (165) studied the drug in goats and found that it caused ataxia, followed by hind limb weakness, muscle wasting, and damage to long tracts. In rodents, cycasin disrupts cerebral and cerebellar development (166–168). Dastur and his associates showed that it caused leg weakness and bradykinesia in rats and caused motor neuron degeneration in primates (169–171). In rodents, large doses of cycasin or methylazoxymethanol (MAM), which is a metabolite of cycasin, have caused an increased incidence of liver, intestinal, and renal tumors (163,164).

However, when rodents are fed cycad flour, they fail to develop these tumors (172). As there have been no studies that have shown an increased incidence of tumors in the western Pacific area (173), Spencer et al. (146) have suggested that the human susceptibility to the carcinogenic properties may not be as strong as in rodents, whereas, humans may develop neuromuscular disease more similar to ruminants (165). There is the possibility that the toxins from the cycad are airborne from trees and could have a role in the etiology of the disease (Kurland L, personal communication).

In conclusion, at this stage, there is not enough evidence to conclude that cycad is responsible for ALS–parkinsonism–dementia. On the other hand, there has been no association with exposure to coffee, tea, cocoa, petrochemicals, paints, soaps, insecticides, fertilizers, manufactured medicines, textiles, or ceramics with ALS–parkinsonism–dementia. This disorder has sparked such major attention because it is the only geographically defined and isolated population seen with a disease with parkinsonian features. It is hoped that clues to the etiology of this disorder will help in the understanding of the etiology of PD. For additional discussion of ALS–PD see Chapter 12.

D. Hereditary Diseases

1. Wilson's Disease

Wilson's disease is a rare disorder that is inherited as an autosomal recessive trait and results in degeneration of the basal ganglia and cirrhosis of the liver owing to an inborn error of copper metabolism (174). The onset is usually in adolescence, and the symptoms begin insidiously and are slowly progressive, with a fluctuating course. Tremor is common, but it is usually postural or kinetic, rather than resting. Other symptoms may include behavioral changes, drooling, choreoathetosis, incoordination, rigidity, akinesia, loss of postural reflexes, dystonia, dementia, and seizurevs.

2. Huntington's Chorea

Huntington's disease is an autosomal dominantly inherited disease of the nervous system characterized by mental disturbances and hyperkinesias (175). Although this condition is predominantly a hyperkinetic disorder, close examination may reveal mild parkinsonian signs, such as rigidity, akinesia, and gait disturbances, typical of Parkinson's disease (176). A variant of Huntington's disease that has its onset in childhood or young adults is the rigid–akinetic form (177). Juvenile Huntington's disease is characterized by mental disturbances and a high incidence of seizures. Tremor may be present, but it is more often action, rather than resting.

3. Hallervorden–Spatz Disease

Hallervorden–Spatz disease is a rare hereditary disorder that typically begins between the ages of 5 and 15 years (178). Clinical features of this disease include optic atrophy, rigidity, dystonia, choreoathetosis, akinesia, or resting tremor. Infrequently, parkinsonism is the presenting feature.

The etiology of this condition is unknown. There is excessive iron and pigment deposition in the basal ganglia. It has been proposed that these pigments are formed by a metal-catalyzed pseudoperoxidation of lipofuscin, involving an increased amount of iron and copper in the affected regions. Similarly, there might be accumulation of lipid peroxides during fatty acid oxidation of myelin (179), leading to free oxygen radicals and cell death.

Another proposal, by Perry et al. (180), suggests that there is excessive cysteine in the globus pallidus owing to an enzymatic block in the metabolic pathway from cysteine to taurine. Accumulated cysteine may chelate iron, accounting for the local increase in the iron content. The excess of cysteine and ferrous iron may generate free radicals that might damage neuronal membranes to cause typical morphological changes.

E. Other Central Nervous System Diseases That May Manifest Variable Degrees of Parkinsonism

Patients with Alzheimer's (AD) and Pick's disease usually have normal motor function early in the illness (181). With disease progression, some of the more commonly observed motor signs may include hypokinesia, rigidity, and an expressionless face (182). The diagnosis in differentiating AD from Parkinson's disease is made difficult when dementia occurs in Parkinson's disease. One group has suggested that the dementia of Parkinson's disease may differ from that of AD in that patients have less difficulty with memory, language, and orientation, but more problems with speed of information processing and mood changes (183). This is likely to vary depending on the pathological substrate of the dementia (see previous discussion).

Parkinsonism may be present in some patients with Creutzfeldt–Jakob disease (CJD), but it typically occurs late in the illness, often in association with multiple other neurological signs. Creutzfeldt–Jakob is an infective illness caused by an atypical agent; prions (small proteinaceous infectious particles that are devoid of nucleic acid) have been implicated as a possible cause for the disease (184). Parkinsonism may also occur in late stages of Gerstmann–Straussler–Scheinker (GSS) disease, which presents in midlife with ataxia, pyramidal signs, and dementia (185) and is thought to be caused by prions.

Nondegenerative diseases of the CNS can also cause a parkinsonian syndrome. Normal pressure hydrocephalus (NPH) is characterized by progressive dementia, gait difficulty, and urinary incontinence (186). The gait at times may resemble the gait of Parkinson's disease (187). Occasionally, tremor may be present (188). Rigidity and hypokinesia may be present in NPH. Parkinsonism has also been reported secondary to hydrocephalus, cause by mass lesions and aqueductal stenosis (189,190). These conditions can usually be distinguished from Parkinson's disease by brain imaging.

In 1929, Critchley (191) introduced the concept of a vascular form of parkinsonism, reporting that a flexed attitude, slowness of movement, and a festinating gait developed in the course of "cerebral arteriosclerosis." The onset is insidious and occurs late in life. Tremor does not occur, but emotional lability; dementia; pyramidal, cerebellar, and pseudobulbar signs are often present, indicating extensive cerebrovascular disease. Cerebral infarction is a rare cause of parkinsonism. There have been cases of parkinsonism reported with multiple infarcts in the basal ganglia (192).

There have been numerous reports of parkinsonism secondary to brain tumors (193–195). Clinically, there is contralateral tremor and rigidity associated with signs of increased intracranial pressure. Pyramidal and sensory changes may also be present; however, parkinsonism is usually not the main clinical feature.

Posttraumatic parkinsonism is a parkinsonian syndrome that occurs as the result of significant head trauma. This parkinsonian syndrome is often progressive and includes mental status changes and cerebellar and pyramidal tract changes (196). Posttraumatic parkinsonism can result from acute trauma or after mild constant trauma for many years (dementia pugilistica, pugilistic parkinsonism, chronic encephalopathy of boxers). Neuropathological findings include minute areas of tissue necrosis in the putamen, pallidum, thalamus, and midbrain; a decrease in pigmented neurons in the substantia nigra; along with changes in the pons, cerebellum, dentate nucleus, and olives (197–199).

A few studies have shown that head trauma may be a risk factor for the development of Parkinson's disease (200–203). However, Factor and colleagues (204), in 1988, reviewed the literature on trauma as an etiology for Parkinson's disease and did not find an association between an episode of trauma and pathologically proved Parkinson's disease. Epidemiological studies on head trauma need cautious interpretation because they tend to be retrospective, and one of the main flaws is recall bias.

Before leaving the category of CNS disorders, it should also be mentioned that elderly individuals often have mild parkinsonian features, such as stooped posture, uncertainty and stiffness in turning, gait problems, and generalized slowing (205). Although, these features are similar to Parkinson's disease, they do not seem to respond to levodopa (206).

F. Infection

Parkinsonism secondary to infectious and postinfectious causes are now uncommon (see Chapter 14). Postencephalitic parkinsonism which occurred after the pandemic in the United States in the early 1920s is now mainly of historical interest (207). The latency between the infection and the development of neurological symptoms could be as long as 10 years. Epidemiological studies have revealed that among the patients who developed parkinsonism, symptoms occurred in 33 % by 3 years, 50% by 5 years, and 80% by 10 years (207,208). The features that separate this entity from Parkinson's disease include very slow or no progression, dyskinetic movements, oculogyric crisis, presence of behavioral changes, focal neurological deficits, including ophthalmoplegia, pupillary abnormalities, hemiparesis, bulbar palsies, and a much younger age of patients at the time of onset (209,210). Most patients with postencephalitic parkinsonism have since died as a result of natural causes, and there have been no new major outbreaks.

Parkinsonism is rare with other encephalitides. It typically occurs during convalescence phases (211,212). Nath et al. (213). reported parkinsonism associated with human immunodeficiency virus (HIV) infection. With the increasing incidence of HIV-related diseases, it is possible more cases might be seen in the future.

There is minimal evidence to suggest that Parkinson's disease is caused by a viral agent. Although viruses, such as measles, varicella, poliovirus, coxsackievirus, western equine encephalitis, and Japanese B encephalitis, can infect the CNS and produce transient tremor, rigidity, and masking of facial expression, none of them has been shown to produce progressive parkinsonian deficits (29). There have been speculations that Parkinson's disease may be caused by latent viral infections. However, despite extensive investigations of serum and cerebrospinal fluid viral antibodies, no definite association has been identified (29,214–216). The alternative explanation of an unconventional or slow virus is also unlikely, as it is not possible to transmit Parkinson's disease from the brain of patients to any other species (71). An interesting hypothesis is put forward by Mattock et al. (217). They raised the possibility that influenza virus exposure in utero may increase the likelihood of developing Parkinson's disease by decreasing the number of nigral neurons. They analyzed birth years of Parkinson's disease cases born between 1900 and 1930. They found that 4 out of the 6 years in which Parkinson's disease births were most common, coincided with influenza pandemics. Although this is an interesting hypothesis, more studies are needed to further define the role of viral agents in utero.

Nocardia asteroides is a soil-contained pathogen that has been reported to cause a clinical syndrome resembling Parkinson's disease in the murine model (218). *Nocardia* species affect the brain primarily in immunocompromised humans; hence, it seems unlikely it would produce Parkinson's disease. Hubble et al. (219) raised the possibility that subclinical or minor infections with nocardia could produce Parkinson's disease. However, they did not find any increased incidence of positive nocardial serology in Parkinson's disease patients, when compared with controls.

G. Toxins

Parkinsonism can be caused by various toxins. Workers exposed to manganese may develop neuropsychiatric symptoms along with parkinsonism (220,221). However, the mental status changes, cerebellar dysfunction, postural, and kinetic tremors help to differentiate it from Parkinson's disease. Manganese-induced parkinsonism has been reported in almost all mining regions of the world, including South America, India, Africa, and the United States. Manganese-induced parkinsonism can also be seen in persons exposed to pesticides containing manganese (222). The concentration of manganese needed to produce symptoms is 5 mg/m^3, and the duration of exposure is about 2 years (221). Manganese intoxication, in some animal studies has affected brain catecholamine concentrations (223,224).

Parkinsonism has also been reported following exposure to carbon monoxide, carbon disulfide, and cyanide (225–230). The neurological sequelae with carbon monoxide could consist of pure parkinsonism, or it could be associated with seizures, cortical blindness, ataxia, cognitive impairment, and other neurological symptoms. Carbon monoxide and cyanide act by producing anoxic damage in vulnerable brain regions. The inhibition of the cytochrome oxidase mitochondrial enzyme system possibly leads to the anoxia in cyanide poisoning (230). For a more complete discussion see Chapter 12.

It is unlikely that any of the aforementioned toxins play a role in the etiology of Parkinson's disease, as the neuropathological changes are different from Parkinson's disease. 1-Methyl-4-phenyl-1,2,3,6-tetrahydropyridine (MPTP) is the only toxin that consistently produces a clinical syndrome similar to Parkinson's disease (231,232). The MPTP-induced parkinsonism reproduces all the major features of Parkinson's disease, and the condition is responsive to levodopa therapy. (MPTP-induced parkinsonism is discussed in detail in Chapter 13). The similarities between MPTP-induced parkinsonism and Parkinson's disease led to the hypothesis that it might be the result of exposure to a compound similar to MPTP (29). Exposure to such an agent might arise through work, residence, life-style, or hobbies. The toxin has to be uncommon, as the prevalence of Parkinson's disease is relatively low. Although there are agents resembling MPTP in the environment, such as paraquat and diquat, except for occasional case reports, there is as yet no direct evidence that these compounds cause Parkinson's disease (233–234). However, epidemiological studies have suggested toxins associated with industrialization (235) or with use of chemicals (235–238), and early use of well water for drinking might play a role (239–241). However, these factors have been inconsistently present, and true clusters of Parkinson's disease appear to be extremely rare. This evidence makes it unlikely that a toxin is solely responsible for Parkinson's disease.

H. Pharmacologic Cases of Parkinsonism

There are a numerous drugs that can cause a parkinsonian syndrome (Table 4). Neuroleptics (dopamine blockers) are the leading cause of drug-induced parkinsonism. Psychiatric illness is the primary reason for the use of these agents. Other uses include gastrointestinal disorders; namely, nausea, vomiting, hiatal hernia, diabetic gastroparesis, peptic ulcer and gastric ulcers, and diverticulitis (242). The reported incidence of neuroleptic-induced parkinsonism varies from 15 to 60% (242–245). However, it has been suggested that the prevalence of drug-induced parkinsonism is grossly underestimated (246). Drug-induced parkinsonism is more common in women and in the elderly (242,244,245).

Table 4 Pharmacological Causes of Parkinsonism

Neuroleptics
Phenothiazines
Butyrophenones
Thioxanthines
Benzamides
Reserpine, tetrabenazine
Miscellaneous
α-Methyldopa
Lithium
Cinnarizine, flunarizine, diltiazem
Phenelzine
Meperidine

Drug-induced parkinsonism is said to occur more commonly with potent piperazine phenothiazines, or with butyrophenones (244). Miller et al. (242) reported haloperidol and a combination of amitriptyline—perphenazine as the most common drugs responsible for drug-induced parkinsonism. The other drugs included thioridazine, chlorpromazine, thiothixene, trifluoperazine, fluphenazine, metoclopramide, prochlorperazine, perphenazine, and loxapine.

Higher doses of neuroleptics were thought to be associated with greater incidence of drug-induced parkinsonism; however, attempts to correlate total drug dose with the incidence of parkinsonism have failed to show a clear relation (247). In patients who develop parkinsonism, the signs usually begin within a few days of treatment with neuroleptics, with a gradual increase in incidence so that 50–70% of cases appear by 1 month and 90% of cases within 3 months (248). Some patients develop parkinsonism on a small dose of phenothiazines after a few days of treatment, some only after larger doses, and some never do, irrespective of the dose or duration. Certain factors that have been suggested to increase the likelihood of a patient developing parkinsonism are advanced age, female gender, higher doses, coexisting brain damage, genetic predisposition, and the use of piperazine side chain phenothiazines, plus the important, but unidentifiable, individual sensitivity (see Ref. 6, pp. 599–644). The mechanism determining individual susceptibility is unclear.

A genetic predisposition may explain why only some patients taking neuroleptics develop parkinsonism. Myrianthopoulous et al. (49) compared the incidence of drug-induced parkinsonism in 728 relatives of 59 white patients, who were susceptible to drug-induced parkinsonian syndrome, with the incidence of Parkinson's disease among 777 relatives of 67 white controls, who were free from drug-induced symptoms. Among relatives of the patients taking neuroleptic medication who developed parkinsonism, they found 13 cases of Parkinson's disease, whereas in the control group they only found 3 cases of Parkinson's disease. The observed incidence of Parkinson's disease among relatives of the patients who developed parkinsonism was higher than the observed incidence among the controls, as well as higher than the expected incidence in the general population. They repeated a similar study and included both black and white patients (250). The increased incidence was present only among whites, which appears to be what is expected in the general population. These studies did suggest a hereditary susceptibility to parkinsonism produced by phenothiazine drugs, but they could not demonstrate a specific genetic pattern.

The possibility that preclinical Parkinson's disease might predispose to drug-induced parkinsonism has been suggested by several groups (251,252). The report by Rajput et al. (253) is perhaps the most convincing. These investigators described two patients with drug-induced parkinsonism whose symptoms resolved after drug withdrawal. Postmortem examination, however, revealed findings consistent with Parkinson's disease.

Reserpine and tetrabenazine, dopamine depletors, are often reported to cause parkinsonism (245). Parkinsonian symptoms caused by these drugs are often milder, and a prolonged exposure is needed to cause parkinsonism. Ethanol withdrawal may occasionally cause a parkinsonian syndrome (254,255). It has been suggested that alcohol can facilitate the emergence of drug-induced parkinsonism and lower the tolerance to neuroleptic medication. However, studies by Lang (256) and Koller (257) have not been able to substantiate this concept.

Flunarizine and cinnarizine, calcium-entry blockers, can also cause parkinsonism (258–263) Gimenez-Roldan et al. (263) studied a group of patients with cinnarizine-induced parkinsonism and found that it occurred at an older age than Parkinson's disease, and these patients had a family history of essential tremor. Similarly, there have been reports of parkinsonism with diltiazem (264), another calcium channel antagonist.

The mechanism of action of calcium channel blockers may relate to an altered sensitivity in the aging brain to the pharmacological effects of calcium entry blockers (265). It is also possible that the density of calcium channel receptors may be decreased in the brains of Parkinson's disease patients (266,267). Giminez-Roldan et al. (263) suggest that drugs with calcium antagonistic properties may act presynaptically by decreasing the content of dopamine-β-hydroxylase, the activity of which appears to be regulated by protein-bound calcium calmodulin (268) and by inhibiting depolarization-induced calcium uptake (269).

Ross (270) reported six patients who consumed large amounts of common drugs for many years and developed parkinsonism. These drugs included antihistamines—diphenhydramine, chlorpheniramine, dimenhydrinate—and anorexiants, *dextro*-amphetamine and diethylpropion. One patient used a combination of trimethoprim–sulfamethoxazole for 7 years. Whether these drugs were causally related to the development of parkinsonism is unclear.

Lithium can cause postural tremor; however, its role in producing parkinsonism is debatable. A small percentage of patients taking lithium have been reported to have developed cogwheel rigidity (271). Two patients reported to have developed parkinsonian syndrome, had a history of previous exposure to neuroleptics (272). Lutz (273) has described a patient who developed parkinsonian features with lithium toxicity.

Mclean et al. (274) described two survivors of methanol poisoning who developed blindness, parkinsonian symptoms, and dementia. The CT scans in both patients demonstrated bilateral infarction in the frontocentral white matter and putamen. Levodopa administration in one patient had no effect on the parkinsonian features. However, the parkinsonian features described in these two patients may have been secondary to putamenal damage caused by hypoxia or hypotension.

There has been a single case report of an elderly man, who developed ataxia, dizziness, masked facies, generalized muscle weakness with rigidity, and fine tremor of all extremities when receiving 5-fluorouracil (275). All signs and symptoms cleared on cessation of this drug. The mechanism by which this could occur is unknown.

Amiodarone has been reported to cause parkinsonian syndrome (276). Palakurthy et al. (277) described 102 patients taking amiodarone and reported that 45 developed neurotoxic reactions, with tremor being the most common (44 patients). They described "a peculiar" coarse rotatory jaw tremor in two patients. None of their patients had bradykinesia, rigidity, or postural instability. Werner et al. (276) described a patient who developed reversible dose-related coarse, resting tremor of his left leg, which was abolished with active or passive movement of either leg.

Phenelzine, a monoamine oxygenase (MAO) inhibitor, has been reported to cause rigidity, shuffling gait, tremor, and masked facies in an elderly woman (278). All the signs resolved on discontinuation of the drug. The possible mechanisms suggested included (a) increase in brain epinephrine, leading to an increase in central acetylcholine activity; (b) increase in serotonergic activity, causing inhibition of the dopamine neurons in the striatum; and (c) increased dopamine autoreceptor activity, leading to shutdown of dopamine transmission as the accumulated dopamine at the presynaptic site causes excessive feedback, which causes inhibition of dopamine neuron firing.

Recently, Armon et al. (279) reported that 33 of their 36 patients receiving therapeutic doses of valproate for at least 12 months developed parkinsonism. The findings ranged from minimal to mild personality changes and cognitive impairment, combined with mild parkinsonism, to a severe parkinsonism–dementia syndrome. However, considering the widespread use of valproate, one would have expected previous reports of valproate-induced parkinsonism. This association, therefore will, need to be confirmed or refuted by future studies.

A patient who received procaine intramuscularly developed parkinsonian features (280). However, this patient had received chlorpromazine 2 days before evaluation. There have been cases of parkinsonism reported with the use of meperidine (267,281). It was postulated that the patient's parkinsonism resulted from the metabolism of meperidine by a pathway resulting in the production of an MPTP-like substance, which was responsible for the parkinsonism. As with valproate, if one considers the widespread use of meperidine, it is noteworthy that other cases of drug-induced parkinsonism have not been reported with meperidine. There have been cases of parkinsonism reported with combination of vincristine and doxorubicin and (Adriamycin) (282) amphotericin B (283), and cephaloridine (284).

The mechanism of drug-induced parkinsonism appears to be related to functional deficiency of the striatal dopaminergic system (248). Phenothiazines and butyrophenones cause postsynaptic dopamine receptor blockage. Reserpine and its derivatives deplete dopamine and other amines from the brain and adrenal medulla by interfering with presynaptic storage mechanism, thereby permitting increase in degradation by monamine oxidase (285). Tetrabenazine, a synthetic analogue of reserpine, also depletes amines, but may also block postsynaptic dopamine receptors (286).

Methyldopa has been reported to cause parkinsonism. It does so by competing for sites on the enzyme dopa decarboxylase with dihydroxyphenyl alanine, the precursor of norepinephrine and dopamine (297). Methyldopa has been reported to exacerbate Parkinson's disease (288,289), even though it has been employed in treatment of this disorder (290).

Jurna et al. (291) produced drug-induced parkinsonism in rats by injecting tremorine and oxotremorine. They then studied the effects of various drugs; namely, methixine (metixene), atropine, beperiden, propranolol, pronetalol (pronethalol), azapetine, haloperidol, and phentolamine. Their studies demonstrated that drugs that depressed tremor activity also antagonized the effect of oxotremorine on α- and γ-motor activity, whereas those drugs that only decreased tremor activity, depressed the increased α-reflex discharge, without reducing spontaneous γ-activity. When the α-reflex discharge was normalized, rigidity disappeared. They concluded that experimental rigidity may be due to a disturbance in the balance between monoaminergic and cholinergic mechanisms in the brain.

Metzer et al. (292) investigated the human leukocyte antigen (HLA) prevalence in patients with neuroleptic-induced parkinsonism. All patients used in the study were white men, with chronic schizophrenia. They found that HLA-B44 was significantly more prevalent in the group with parkinsonism than in the group without parkinsonism. However, additional studies have not be done to confirm this finding, nor is its significance clear.

Although there a numerous drugs that can cause parkinsonian features, none of these drugs has been shown to cause Parkinson's disease. Drug-induced parkinsonism may favor a toxin theory for the etiology of Parkinson's disease, but the lack of a history in Parkinson's disease patients and that most of the present-day drugs were not available 175 years ago, make drugs an unlikely cause of Parkinson's disease. It is possible that some commonly used drugs are involved in some manner in the causation of Parkinson's disease. However, currently, there is little data to support this hypothesis.

I. Metabolic Causes

Rarely, metabolic conditions can cause parkinsonism. Calcium metabolism disorders can result in basal ganglia calcification and sometimes cause parkinsonism (293). Pseudohypoparathyroidism, idiopathic hypoparathyroidism, and postoperative hypoparathyroidism can be associated with parkinsonian features (294,295). Dyskinesias, parkinsonism, mental changes, cerebellar dysfunction, seizures, and corticospinal symptoms are possible signs that can result from basal ganglia calcification (295). A chronic progressive neurological syndrome that may include resting tremor, rigidity, akinesia, and dysarthria is seen in some patients with repeated episodes of hepatic coma (296). Other associated indications include dementia, intention tremor, ataxia, dyskinesia, weakness, and upper motor neuron signs. Sustained hepatic encephalopathy can produce changes in the brain and microcavitation in the pallidum, caudate, putamen, and the subthalamus have been reported (297).

IV. DIAGNOSING PARKINSON'S DISEASE

Given the large number of conditions that can cause parkinsonism, it is not surprising that accurately diagnosing the disease with consistency has proved to be very difficult. As can be seen from the preceding section, some of these conditions, particularly the neurodegenerative diseases that cause atypical parkinsonism, can be extremely difficult to differentiate from Parkinson's disease during life. Adding to this problem is the subtlety of early signs and symptoms and the variability of disease expression, even when it is fully developed.

A. Clinical Heterogeneity

One of the major difficulties in diagnosing Parkinson's disease is the marked diversity of clinical expression of the disorder, even when there is relative uniformity of the pathological changes. A report by Sage and colleagues (298) highlights this problem. They described six patients with pathologically typical

Lewy body parkinsonism with widely divergent clinical manifestations. Atypical clinical features included juvenile onset, retrocollis, strong family history, absence of tremor, lack of flexed posture, and lack of levodopa response. The authors suggest that these cases provide evidence that the pathological features of Parkinson's disease are associated with a broader spectrum of clinical findings than has been previously thought. Similarly, Quinn and colleagues (299) reported a case of pathologically typical Parkinson's disease, with akinesia and freezing of gait, without tremor or rigidity (pure akinesia), indicating that this disorder, which usually has other causes, can be a part of the clinical spectrum of Parkinson's disease.

B. Laboratory Procedures

Adding to the problem of diagnosis is that there are no laboratory tests available that can be used to confirm the presence of Parkinson's disease. Neuroimaging studies, such as MRI may yield some useful information. Moderate to severe putamenal hypointensity relative to pallidal hypointensity is seen more frequently in the atypical forms of parkinsonism, particularly striatonigral degeneration (300). The MRI in progressive supranuclear atrophy may show atrophy of the midbrain, with concurrent dilation of the aqueduct, quadrigeminal plate, and posterior portion of the third ventricle (301). Olivopontocerebellar atrophy patients may demonstrate focal atrophy of the olives, pons, brachium pontis, medulla, and cerebellum (301). Another important imaging technique is using high-field MRI of brain iron. In normal subjects and Parkinson's disease patients, there is decreased signal intensity in the globus pallidus, reticular substantia nigra, red nucleus, and dentate nucleus (302). These areas correlate with sites of accumulation of ferric iron. In multiple system atrophy syndromes, there are abnormally increased concentrations of iron in the putamen and less prominent increases in the caudate nucleus and lateral pars compacta of the substantia nigra (302).

Fluorodopa positron emission tomography (PET) is capable of assessing the integrity of the dopaminergic nigrostriatal system (303). Typically, there is a reduction in fluorodopa uptake, which is greater in the putamen than in caudate nucleus (303). The observation that the putamen is affected more than the caudate is consistent with neurochemical data concerning the distribution of dopamine depletion in Parkinson's disease (304). A more equal involvement of the caudate and putamen is observed in progressive supranuclear palsy. Other laboratory tests may reveal other possible causes of parkinsonism e.g., serum ceruloplasmin levels for Wilson's disease on disorders of calcium metabolism.

C. Response to Dopaminergic Drugs

Parkinson's disease generally responds well to levodopa, whereas other neurodegenerative processes that cause atypical parkinsonism syndromes tend to show a transient and only limited response, or no responsiveness. Apomorphine, a potent direct-acting dopamine agonist, with affinity for both D_1 and D_2 dopamine receptors, can be used to help assess dopaminergic responsiveness (305,306). Given subcutaneously, apomorphine has an antiparkinsonian effect within 10 min. The apomorphine test has a high predictive rate for responsiveness to sustained oral levodopa treatment. However, some patients have tested negative to apomorphine and have experienced a good or partial response to long-term levodopa treatment (307,308). Bonuccelli et al. (309) tested the predictivity of apomorphine in distinguishing between idiopathic Parkinson's disease and other parkinsonisms in previously untreated patients with parkinsonian features. He found that, of 30 patients with a clinical diagnosis of Parkinson's disease, 26 had a positive response to the apomorphine test. Of 7 patients who were thought to have some other form of parkinsonism, 1 had a positive apomorphine test. Although the apomorphine test showed a high predictivity (86.4% in this study) in distinguishing Parkinson's disease from other parkinsonian syndromes, both false-positive and false-negative responses can occur.

D. Other Diagnostic Considerations

Asymmetry of clinical signs may be helpful in distinguishing Parkinson's disease from other parkinsonian syndromes. Almost all Parkinson's disease patients will present with unilateral complaints. Therefore, a symmetrical onset is considered, by many, to be highly suggestive of atypical disease. The diagnosis of Parkinson's disease is thought to be questionable if dementia is an early and dominant feature of the illness. Other clinical features may be helpful in establishing the diagnosis of Parkinson's disease, such as the presence of a resting tremor. Finally, failure to manifest evidence of progression constitutes strong evidence against the disease.

E. Accuracy of Diagnosis: Current Status

Given the importance of establishing a correct diagnosis for clinical and epidemiological investigations of the cause of Parkinson's disease, there have been surprisingly few clinicopathological studies aimed at assessing the accuracy of clinical diagnosis. Rajput and colleagues (310) reported their 22-year experience of 65 parkinsonian patients who came to autopsy. Parkinson's disease was diagnosed in 43 of these patients when initially seen by a neurologist; of these only 65% had typical Lewy body lesions at the time of autopsy. After a mean duration of 12 years, the final clinical diagnosis was Parkinson's disease in 41 cases (the remaining 24 were thought to have other forms of parkinsonism) However, only 31 (76%) of the 41 patients had Parkinson's disease when examined pathologically. The remaining 10 cases were found to have the following conditions: striatonigral degeneration (4 subjects), profound substantia nigra cell loss without

Lewy bodies (2 subjects), neurofibrillary tangles (2 subjects), a lack of abnormalities (probable drug-induced parkinsonism; 1 subject), and Alzheimer's disease (1 subject). With the exception of these 10 cases, the authors found that the correct clinical diagnosis was possible within 5 years of disease onset in most cases of parkinsonism. Therefore, they recommended that studies aimed at including only Parkinson's disease cases restrict their enrollment to those patients who have had parkinsonian motor manifestations for at least 5 years.

Hughes and colleagues (311) examined 100 brains of patients with a clinical diagnosis of Parkinson's disease by neurologists and found pathological evidence of Parkinson's disease in only 76%. In the 24 cases without Lewy bodies, diagnoses included progressive supranuclear palsy, multiple system atrophy, Alzheimer's disease, Alzheimer's-type pathology, and basal ganglia vascular disease. An unexpected finding was the high incidence of Alzheimer's disease lesions in patients with the clinical diagnosis of Parkinson's disease. The authors suggest that their observations challenge the current concepts of Parkinson's disease as a single distinct morbid entity.

The same investigators (312) assessed the clinical features of these patients diagnosed prospectively by neurologists as having Parkinson's disease confirming the pathologic findings. The majority of cases had at least two of the four conventional features of Parkinson's disease, demonstrating the general use of the broad clinical definition of this disorder. However, the positive predictive value of these criteria was not remarkable, as the specificity was low, since other conditions mimicking Parkinson's disease also shared these features. By using selected criteria, such as asymmetrical onset, no clinically atypical features, and no known cause for other forms of parkinsonism, the proportion of true Parkinson's disease cases identified was increased from 79 to 93%; however, 32% of pathologically confirmed cases were rejected on this basis. The authors concluded that using the standard diagnostic criteria, by the presence of three of four motor criteria, will include cases other than Parkinson's disease, which could distort results. The strict use of additional criteria could reduce misdiagnosis. However, a significant number of cases with Parkinson's disease are likely to be excluded.

F. Diagnostic Criteria:

Most studies of Parkinson's disease simply diagnose the disease in the presence of two of the three cardinal motor signs (tremor, rigidity, or bradykinesia), or by the presence of three of the four motor signs (tremor, rigidity, bradykinesia, or postural instability). However, the clinicopathological studies cited in the preceding section highlight the need for better diagnostic criteria. Although several groups have attempted to develop such criteria, most of those that have been suggested have yet to be tested for reliability (degree of agreement among investigators) or validity (comparison with another standard, e.g., pathological examination of the brain). Some of those that have been suggested to date are described in this section.

Gibb (313) suggests that the clinical diagnosis of Parkinson's disease should rely on excluding patients with clinical manifestations of other parkinsonian syndromes or those patients who respond poorly to levodopa (L-dopa) and offer the following exclusion criteria:

- More than one affected relative
- Remitting course
- History of definite encephalitis lethargica
- Oculogyric crises
- Neuroleptic therapy within the previous year
- Supranuclear down or lateral gaze palsy
- Cerebellar signs
- Autonomic neuropathy
- Alzheimer-type dementia from onset of symptoms
- Pyramidal signs not explained by discrete strokes
- Cerebrovascular disease (implied by ataxic gait, stroke at onset, incontinence in the first year, or early severe dementia; or (two or the following three) hypertension, emotional incontinence, or spastic gait).

Koller (314) suggests the following inclusion criteria: (a) the presence for 1 year or more of two of three of the cardinal motor signs of Parkinson's disease (resting or postural tremor, bradykinesia, rigidity), and (b) responsiveness to levodopa therapy (at least 1000 mg/day for 1 month), given that the degree of improvement is moderate to marked, and duration of improvement is 1 year or more. He raised concerns about some of the exclusion criteria of Gibb and proposed the following list of exclusion criteria:

- Abrupt onset of symptoms
- Remitting course
- Stepwise progression
- Neuroleptic therapy within previous year of onset of symptoms or exposure to any drug or toxin reported to cause parkinsonism
- History of encephalitis
- Oculogyric crises
- Supranuclear downward or lateral gaze palsy
- Cerebellar signs
- Unexplained pyramidal signs
- Lower motor neuron signs
- Severe autonomic failure, causing repeated syncope
- Dementia from the onset of the disease
- Postural instability, with falling early in the course of the disease

- Evidence of cerebrovascular disease
- Unilateral dystonia associated with apraxia, cortical sensory loss.

In an effort to provide more stringent criteria for research purposes, Ward and Gibb (315) have proposed the following "research criteria for probable Parkinson's disease":

1. Evidence of disease progression
2. The presence of at least two of the three cardinal features of parkinsonism: tremor, rigidity, or bradykinesia
3. The presence of at least two of the following:
   a. Marked response to levodopa (functional improvement or dyskinesia)
   b. Asymmetry of signs
   c. Asymmetry at onset
4. The absence of clinical features of alternative diagnosis
5. The absence of etiology known to cause similar features

Because of the lack of agreement on a set of clinical criteria for diagnosis, and the difficulties in validating those that have been proposed, Calne et al. (326) suggest a less rigid approach, preferring a probabilistic classification scheme using the following categories of diagnosis:

1. Clinically possible: The presence of any one of the salient features: tremor, rigidity, or bradykinesia. Impairment of postural reflexes is not included because it is too nonspecific. The tremor must be of recent onset, but may be postural or resting.
2. Clinically probable: A combination of any two of the cardinal features: resting tremor, rigidity, bradykinesia, or impaired postural reflexes. Alternatively, asymmetrical resting tremor, asymmetrical rigidity, or asymmetrical bradykinesia are sufficient.
3. Clinically definite: Any combination of three of the features: resting tremor, rigidity, bradykinesia, or impairment of postural reflexes. Alternatively sufficient are two of these features, with one of the first three displaying asymmetry.

These attempts to more carefully define diagnostic criteria for Parkinson's disease are important steps in the right direction. Unfortunately, until there is a biomarker for the disease, validating each of the criteria will not be easily done because of the need for pathological confirmation.

V. CONCLUSIONS

In this chapter, we have attempted to provide a comprehensive description of Parkinson's disease as a clinicopathological entity, as well as to review the many disorders that can cause signs and symptoms similar to the disease (parkinsonism). A better understanding of the many forms of parkinsonism may well provide clues to the etiology of Parkinson's disease. Although there are now no toxins or drugs that replicate all of the clinical and pathological features of Parkinson's disease, it remains possible that one or more of these or, alternatively, a yet to be identified toxin or drug, may either cause or trigger the disease. It is also possible that the etiologic agents that produce other neurodegenerative conditions might also cause Parkinson's disease. There are multiple metabolic conditions that cause parkinsonism; however, none of the currently detected metabolic abnormalities appear to be involved in the etiology of Parkinson's disease.

It has been stressed that diverse entities can produce a clinical syndrome nearly indistinguishable from Parkinson's disease and that the clinical picture of Parkinson's disease can vary considerably, making diagnosis a challenging proposition. In some instances, making a correct diagnosis will have therapeutic indications quite different from the initiation of traditional antiparkinsonian therapy (e.g., drug-induced parkinsonism, hypothyroidism, brain tumor, and Wilson's disease), but in most instances, these conditions will not be confused with Parkinson's disease. When it comes to other neurodegenerative conditions that cause atypical parkinsonism, distinguishing the different conditions can be very difficult. However, for the most part, the therapeutic approach will be similar, although the atypical disorders are usually far less responsive to medications.

On the other hand, diagnostic accuracy is critical to research on the treatment, pathogenesis, etiology, and epidemiology of Parkinson's disease. Better diagnostic criteria are needed, but the situation is not likely to improve dramatically until a biomarker for the disease is found. Indeed, this currently represents one of the greatest needs in the field of Parkinson's disease research. Until such a marker is found, however, it will be necessary to rely on clinical observation. One can only hope that, in the future, more carefully designed studies aimed at developing improved diagnostic criteria will be carried out, with an emphasis on clinical, radiologic, and pathological correlations to validate our best attempts at deciding which patients with parkinsonism have Parkinson's disease and which do not.

REFERENCES

1. Parkinson J. An essay on the shaking palsy. London: Whittingham and Rowland for Sherwood, Neely, Jones, 1817.
2. Charcot JM, Vulpian A. De la paralysie agitante. Gaz Hebdom Med Chir 1861; 8:765–767.
3. Gowers WR. A manual of diseases of the nervous system, vol. 2. Philadelphia: Blakiston, 1893:636–657.

4. Schwab R, England A, Peterson A. Akinesia in Parkinson's disease. Neurology 1959; 9:65–72.
5. Yahr MD. Parkinson's disease—overview of its current status. Mt Sinai J Med 1977; 44:183–191.
6. Weiner WJ, Lang AE. Movement disorders: a comprehensive survey. Mount Kisco, NY: Futura Publishing, 1989.
7. Snider S, Sandyk N. Sensory dysfunction. In: Koller W, ed. Handbook of Parkinson's disease. New York: Marcel Dekker, 1987:171–180.
8. Doty RL, Deems D, Stellar S. Olfactory dysfunction in parkinsonism: A general deficit unrelated to neurologic signs, disease stage, or disease duration. Neurology 1988; 38:1237–1244.
9. Ward CD, Hess WA, Calne DB. Olfactory impairment in Parkinson's disease. Neurology 1983; 33:943–946.
10. Shipley MT. Transport of molecules from nose to brain: transneuronal anterograde and retrograde labeling in the rat olfactory system by wheat germ agglutinin–horseradish peroxidase applied to the nasal epithelium. Brain Res Bull 1985; 15:129–142.
11. Tomlinson AH, Esiri MM. Herpes simplex encephalitis. Immunohistological demonstration of spread of virus via olfactory pathways in mice. J Neurol Sci 1983; 60:473–484.
12. Pollock M, Hornabrook RW. The prevalence, natural history and dementia of Parkinson's disease. Brain 1966; 89:429–448.
13. Lieberman A, Dziatolowski M, Kupersmith M. Dementia in Parkinson's disease. Ann Neurol 1979; 6:355–359.
14. Pirozzolo FJ, Swihart A, Rey G, Jankovic J, Mortimer JA. Cognitive impairments associated with Parkinson's disease and other movement disorders. In: Jankovic J, Tolosa E, eds. Baltimore: Urban & Schwarzenberg, 1988:425–440.
15. Marder K, Leary D, Tang M. Are demented patients with Parkinson's disease accurately reflected in prevalence surveys? A survival analysis. Neurology 1991; 41:1240–1243.
16. Rajput AH, Rozdilsky B. Parkinsonism and dementia: effects of levodopa. Lancet 1975; 1:1084.
17. Marttila RJ, Rinne UK. Dementia in Parkinson's disease. Acta Neurol Scand 1976; 54:431–441.
18. Mindham RH, Ahmed SW, Clough CG. A controlled study of dementia in Parkinson's disease. J Neurol Neurosurg Psychiatry 1982; 45:969–974.
19. Mayeux R, Stern Y, Rosenstein R, et al. An estimate of the prevalence of dementia in idiopathic Parkinson's disease. Arch Neurol 1988; 45:260–262.
20. Mayeux R, Stern Y, Rosenstein R, et al. An estimate of the prevalence of dementia in idiopathic Parkinson's disease. Arch Neurol 1988; 45:260–262.
21. Huber SJ, Shuttleworth EC, Christy JA, Chakeres DW, Curtin A, Paulson GW. Magnetic resonance imaging in dementia of Parkinson's disease. J Neurol Neurosurg Psychiatry 1989; 52:1221–1227.
22. Marder K, Flood P, Cote L, Mayeux R. A pilot study of risk factors for dementia in Parkinson's disease. Mov Disord 1990; 5:156–161.

23. Glatt SL, Hubble JP, Karst A, et al. Risk factors for dementia in Parkinson's disease [abstract]. Mov Disord 1993; 8:408.
24. Mindham RHS. Psychiatric symptoms in parkinsonism. J Neurol Neurosurg Psychiatry 1970; 33:188–191.
25. Celesia G, Wanamaker W. Psychiatric disturbances in Parkinson's disease. Dis Nerv Syst 1972; 33:577–583.
26. Santamaria J, Tolosa E, Valles A. Parkinson's disease with depression: a possible subgroup of idiopathic parkinsonism. Neurology 1986; 36:1130–1133.
27. Tanner C, Goetz C, Klawans H. Autonomic nervous system disorders. In: Koller W, ed. Handbook of Parkinson's disease. New York: Marcel Dekker, 1987:145–170.
28. Koller WC, Langston JW, Hubble JP, et al. Does a long pre-clinical period occur in parkinson's disease? Neurology 1991; 41(suppl 2):8–13.
29. Calne DB, Duvoisin RC, McGeer E. Speculations on the etiology of Parkinson's disease. In: Hassler RG, Christ JF, eds. Parkinson-specific motor and mental disorders, role of the pallidum: pathophysiological, biochemical, and therapeutic aspects. Adv Neurol, 1984; 40:353–360.
30. Koller WC. When does Parkinson's disease begin? Neurology 1992; 42(suppl 4):27–31.
31. Snider SR, Fahn S, Isgreen WP, Cote LJ. Primary sensory symptoms in parkinsonism. Neurology 1976; 26: 423–429.
32. Koller WC. Sensory symptoms in Parkinson's disease. Neurology 1984; 34:957–959.
33. Marttila RJ, Rinne UK. Disability and progression in Parkinson's disease. Acta Neurol Scand 1977; 56:159–169.
34. Hoehn MM, Yahr MD. Parkinsonism: onset, progression and mortality. Neurology 1967; 17:427–442.
35. Tetrud JW, Langston JW. The effect of Deprenyl (selegiline) on the natural history of Parkinson's disease. Science 1989; 245:519–522.
36. The Parkinson Study Group. Effect of Deprenyl on the progression of disability in early Parkinson's disease. N Engl J Med 1989; 321:1364–1371.
37. Diamond SG, Markham CH, Treciokas LJ. Long-term experience with L-dopa: efficacy, progression and mortality. In: Birkmayer W, Hornykiewicz O, eds. Advances in parkinsonism. Basel: Roche, 1976:444–455.
38. Hoehn MM. Parkinsonism treated with levodopa: progression and mortality. J Neural Transm [Suppl] 1983; 19:253–264.
39. Hoehn MM. Result of chronic levodopa therapy and its modification by bromocriptine in Parkinson's disease. Acta Neurol Scand 1985; 71:97–106.
40. Hoehn MM. Parkinson's disease: progression and mortality. In: Yahr MD, Bergmann KJ, eds. Parkinson's disease. Adv Neurol 1986; 45:457–461.
41. Hoehn MM. Natural history of the untreated pre-levodopa disease. In: Stern G, ed. Parkinson's disease. London: Chapman & Hall Medical, 1990:307–314.
42. Birkmayer W. Distinction between benign and malignant type of Parkinson's disease. Clin Neurol Neurosurg 1979; 81:158–164.

43. Goetz CG, Tanner CM, Stebbins GT, Buchman AS. Risk factors for progression in Parkinson's disease. Neurology 1988; 38:1841–1844.
44. Zetusky W, Jankovic J, Pirozzolo F. The heterogenicity of Parkinson's disease. Clinical and prognostic implications. Neurology 1985; 35:522–526.
45. Narabayashi H, Yokochi M, Iizuka R, Nagatsu T. Juvenile parkinsonism. In: Vinken PJ, Bruyn GW, Klawans HL, eds. Handbook of clinical neurology, vol. 5: extrapyramidal disorders. Amsterdam: Elsevier Science, 1986:153–165.
46. Furukawa Y, Nishi K, Kondo T, Mizuno Y, Narabayashi H. Juvenile parkinsonism: ventricular CSF biopterin levels and clinical features. J Neurol Sci 1992; 108:207–213.
47. Yokochi M. Juvenile Parkinson's disease—part I. Clinical aspects. Adv Neurol Sci 1979; 23:1048–1059.
48. Yokochi M, Narabayashi H, Iizuka R, Nagatsu T. Juvenile parkinsonism: some clinical, pharmacological, and neuropathological aspects. In: Hassler RG, Christ JF, eds. Parkinson-specific motor and mental disorders, role of pallidum: pathological, biochemical, and therapeutic aspects. Adv Neurol 1984; 40:407–413.
49. Greenfield JG, Bosanquet PD. The brainstem lesion in parkinsonism. J Neurol Neurosurg Psychiatry 1953; 16:213–226.
50. Ross GW, Mahler ME, Cummings JL. The dementia syndromes of Parkinson's disease: cortical and subcortical features. In: Huber SJ, Cummings JL, eds. Parkinson's disease: neurobehavioral aspects. New York: Oxford University Press, 1992:132–148.
51. Sudarsky L, Morris J, Romero J, Walshe TM. Dementia in Parkinson's disease: the problem of clinicopathological correlation. J Neuropsychiatry Clin Neurosci 1989; 1:159–166.
52. Kosaka K. Diffuse Lewy body disease in Japan. J Neurol 1990; 237:197–204.
53. Lennox G, Lowe J, Landon M, Byrne EJ, Mayer RJ, Godwin-Austen RB. Diffuse Lewy body disease: correlative neuropathology using anti-ubiquitin immunocytochemistry. J Neurol Neurosurg Psychiatry 1989; 52:1236–1247.
54. Sage JI, Mark MA. Diffuse Lewy body disease. In: Stern MB, Koller WC, eds. Parkinsonian syndromes. New York: Marcel Dekker, 1993:393–411.
55. Joachim CL, Morris JH, Selkoe DJ. Clinically diagnosed Alzheimer's disease: autopsy results in 110 cases. Ann Neurol 1988; 24:50–56.
56. Qualman SJ, Haupt KM, Yang P., Hamilton SR. Esophageal Lewy bodies associated with ganglion cell loss in achalasia: similarity to Parkinson's disease. Gastroenterology 1984; 87:848–856.
57. Wakabayashi K, Takahashi H, Takeda S, Ohama E, Ikuta F. Parkinson's disease: the presence of Lewy bodies in Auberbach's and Meissner's plexuses. Acta Neuropathol 1988; 76:217–221.
58. Scherman D, Desnos C, Darchen F, Pollak P, Javoy-Agid F, Agid Y. Striatal dopamine deficiency in Parkinson's disease: role of aging. Ann Neurol 1989; 26:551–557.
59. Agid Y, Cervera P, Hirsch E, et al. Biochemistry of Parkinson's disease 28 years later: a critical review. Mov Disord 1989; 4:S126–S144.
60. Calne DB, Peppard RF. Aging of the nigrostriatal pathway in humans. Can J Neurol Sci 1987; 14:424–427.

61. Carlsson A, Winblad B. Influence of age and time interval between death and autopsy on dopamine and 3-methoxytyramine levels in human basal ganglia. J Neural Transm 1976; 38:271–276.
62. Carlsson A, Nyberg P, Winblad B. The influence of age and other factors on concentrations of monoamines in the human brain. In: Nyberg P, ed. Brain monoamines in normal aging and dementia. Sweden: Umea University medical dissertations, 1984:53–84.
63. Severson JA, Marcusson J, Winblad B, Finch CE. Age-correlated loss of dopaminergic binding sites in human basal ganglia. J Neurochem 1982; 39:1623–1631.
64. McGeer PL, McGeer EG, Suzuki JS. Aging and extrapyramidal function. Neurology 1977; 34:33–35.
65. Mann DMA, Yates PO. Possible role of neuromelanin in the pathogenesis of Parkinson's disease. Mech Age Dev 1983; 21:193–203.
66. Mann DMA. Dopamine neurones of the vertebrate brain: some aspects of anatomy and pathology. In: Winlow W, Markstein R, eds. The neurobiology of dopamine systems. Manchester: Manchester University Press, 1984:87–103.
67. Langston JW. Predicting Parkinson's disease. Neurology 1990; 40 (suppl):70–74.
68. Gibb WRG, Lees AJ. A comparison of clinical and pathological features of young- and old-onset Parkinson's disease. Neurology 1988; 38:1402–1406.
69. McGeer PL, Itagaki S, Akiyama H, NcGeer G. Rate of cell death in parkinsonism indicates active neuropathological process. Ann Neurol 1988; 24:574–576.
70. Fearnley JM, Lees AJ. Ageing and Parkinson's disease; substantia nigra regional selectivity. Brain 1991; 114:2283–2301.
71. Calne DB, Langston JW. Aetiology of Parkinson's disease. Lancet 1983; 2:1457–1459.
72. Stern MB, Koller WC. Parkinson's disease. In: Stern MB, Koller WC, eds. Parkinsonian syndromes. New York: Marcel Dekker, 1993:3–29.
73. Quinn NP. Classification of multiple system atrophy (MSA). Presented at the 11th International Symposium on Parkinson's Disease, Rome, Italy; March 26–30, 1994:29.
74. Richardson J, Steele J, Olszewski J. Supranuclear ophthalmoplegia, pseudobulbar palsy, nuchal dystonia and dementia. Trans Am Neurol Assoc 1963; 88:25–29.
75. Steele JC, Richardson J, Olszewski J. Progressive supranuclear palsy; a heterogenous degeneration involving the brainstem, basal ganglia and cerebellum with vertical gaze and pseudobulbar palsy, nuchal dystonia, and dementia. Arch Neurol 1964; 10:333–359.
76. Messert B, Van Nuis C. A syndrome of paralysis of downward gaze, dysarthria, pseudobulbar palsy, axial rigidity of neck and trunk and dementia. J Nerv Ment Dis 1966; 143:47–54.
77. Anzil A. Progressive supranuclear palsy: case report with pathological findings. Acta Neuropathol (Berlin) 1969; 14:72–76.
78. Behrman S, Carroll J, Mathews W. Progressive supranuclear palsy: clinico-pathological study of four cases. Brain 1969; 92:663–678.
79. Steele JC. Progressive supranuclear palsy. Brain 1972; 95:693–704.
80. Steele JC. Progressive supranuclear palsy. In: Vinken P, Bruyn G, eds. Handbook

of clinical neurology: system disorders and atrophies. Amsterdam: Elsevier 1975:217-229.
81. Weinmann R. Heterogenous system degeneration of the central nervous system associated with peripheral neuropathy. Neurology 1967; 17:597–603.
82. Ishino H, Higashi H, Kuroda S, Yabuki S, Hayahara T, Otsuki S. Motor nuclear involvement in progressive supranuclear palsy. J Neurol Sci 1974; 22:235–244.
83. Kurihara T, Landau W, Torack R. Progressive supranuclear palsy with action myoclonus seizures. Neurology 1974; 24:219–223.
84. Tellez-Nagel I, Wisniewski H. Ultrastructure of neurofibrillary tangles in Steele–Richardson–Olszewski syndrome. Arch Neurol 1973; 29:324–327.
85. Powell H, London G, Lampert P. Neurofibrillary tangles in progressive supranuclear palsy: electron microscopic observations. J Neuropathol Exp Neurol 1974; 33:98–106.
86. Roy S, Datta C, Hirano A, Ghatak N, Zimmerman H. Electron microscopic study of neurofibrillary tangles in Steele–Richardson–Olszewski syndrome. Acta Neuropathol (Berl) 1974; 29:175–179.
87. Dubinsky R, Jankovic J. Progressive supranuclear palsy and a multi-infarct state. Neurology 1987; 37:570–576.
88. David N, Mackey E, Smith J. Further observations in progressive supranuclear palsy. Neurology 1968; 18:349–356.
89. Ishino H, Otsuki S. Contribution to clinical pathology of progressive supranuclear palsy: subcortical argyrophilic dystrophy. J Neurol Sci 1975; 24:471–481.
90. Perkin G, Lees A, Stern G, Kocen R. Problems in the diagnosis of progressive supranuclear palsy. Can J Neurol Sci 1978; 5:167–173.
91. Davis PH, Golbe LI, Duvoisin RC, Schoenberg BS. Risk factors for progressive supranuclear palsy. Neurology 1988; 38:1546–1552.
92. Dejerine J, Thomas A. L'atrophie olivo-ponto-cerebelleuse. Nouv Iconogr Salpet 1900; 13:330–370.
93. Berciano J. Olivopontocerebellar atrophy. In: Jankovic J, Tolosa E, eds. Parkinson's disease and movement disorders. Baltimore: Urban & Schwarzenberg, 1988:131–151.
94. Destunis G. Olivopontocerebellar atrophy. Neurol Psychiatry 1944; 188:683–699.
95. Yakura H, Wakisaka A, Fujimoto S, Itakura K. Hereditary ataxia and HLA genotypes. N Engl J Med 1974; 291:154–155.
96. Currier R, Glover G, Jackson J, Tipton A. Spinocerebellar ataxia, study of a large kindred. Part 1 (general information and genetics). Neurology 1972; 22:1040–1043.
97. Schut J, Haymaker W. Hereditary ataxia. A pathological study of five cases of common ancestry. J Neuropathol Clin Neurol 1951; 1:183–213.
98. Koningsmark B, Weiner J. The olivopontocerebellar atrophies. A review. Medicine 1970; 49:227–241.
99. Plaitakis A, Nicklas W, Desnick R. Glutamate dehydrogenase deficiency in three patients with spinocerebellar syndrome. Ann Neurol 1980; 7:297–303.
100 Yamaguchi T, Hayaski K, Murakami H. Glutamate dehydrogenase deficiency in spinocerebellar degeneration. Neurochem Res 1982; 7:627–636.

101. Duvoisin RC, Chokroverty S, Lepore F. Glutamate dehydrogenase in patients with olivopontocerebellar atrophy. Neurology 1983; 33:1322–1326.
102. Plaitakis A, Berl L, Yahr M. Neurological disorders associated with deficiency of glutamate dehydrogenase. Ann Neurol 1984; 15:144–153.
103. Plaitakis A, Berl S, Yahr M. Abnormal glutamate metabolism in an adult onset degenerative neurological disorder. Science 1982; 216:193–196.
104. Sorbi S, Tonini S, Giannini E, Piacentini S, Marini P, Amaducci L. Abnormal platelet glutamate dehydrogenase activity and activation in dominant and nondominant olivopontocerebellar atrophy. Ann Neurol 1986; 19:239–245.
105. Finocchiaro G, Taroni F, DiDonato S. Glutamate dehydrogenase in olivopontocerebellar atrophies: leukocytes, fibroblasts and muscle mitochondria. Neurology 1986; 36:550–553.
106. Grossman A, Rosenberg R, Warmoth L. Glutamate and malate dehydrogenase activities in Joseph disease and olivopontocerebellar atrophy. Neurology 1987; 37:106–111.
107. Rosenberg R, Banner C. Normal cerebellar glutamate dehydrogenase protein in spinocerebellar degeneration. J Neurol Sci 1989; 52:666–668.
108. Chokroverty S, Nicklas W, Miller D, et al. Multiple system degeneration with glutamate dehydrogenase deficiency: pathology and biochemistry. J Neurol Sci 1990; 53:1099–1101.
109. Kish SJ, Robitaille Y, Ball M, et al. Glycerophosphoethanolamine concentration is elevated in brain of patients with dominantly inherited olivopontocerebellar atrophy. Neurosci Lett 1990; 120:209–211.
110. Plaitakis A. Abnormal metabolism of neuroexcitatory amino acids in olivopontocerebellar atrophy. In: Duvoisin RC, Plaitakis A, eds. The olivopontocerebellar atrophies. Adv Neurol 1984; 41:225–243.
111. Adams RD, Van Bogaert L, Vandereecken H. Dégénerescence nigro-striées et cérébello-nigro-striée. Psychiatr Neurol 1961; 142:219–259.
112. Adams RD, Adam MJ. Striatonigral degeneration. In: Vinken P, Bruyn G, Klawans H, eds. Handbook of clinical Neurology, vol 49, extrapyamidal disorders. Amsterdam: Elsevier, 1986: 205–212.
113. Bannister R, Mowbray J, Sidgwick A. Genetic control of progressive autonomic failure: evidence for association with an HLA antigen. Lancet 1983; 1:1017.
114. Nee L, Brown R, Polinsky R. HLA in autonomic failure. Arch Neurol 1989; 46:758–759.
115. Iwasaki Y, Kinoshita M, Ikeda K, Takamiya K. Human T-lymphotrophic virus type-I associated myleopathy presenting as spinocerebellar syndrome. Ann Neurol 1989; 25:419–420.
116. Kano M, Mitsuhata Y, Kishida S, Yano Y, Muro T. Shy–Drager syndrome and human T-lymphyotrophic virus type I infection. Ann Neurol 1989; 25:420–421.
117. Yokota T, Tanabe H. Serum antibodies to HTLV-I in autonomic failure with multisystem atrophy. Ann Neurol 1990; 27:110–111.
118. Spencer PS, Ohta M, Palmer VS. Cycad use and motor neurone disease in Kii Peninsula of Japan. Lancet 1987; 2:1462–1463.
119. Anderson F, Richardson E, Okazaki H. Neurofibrillary degeneration of Guam:

frequency in Chamorros and non-Chamorros with no known neurologic disease. Brain 1975; 102:65–77.

120. Garruto RM, Yanagihara R, Gajdusek DC. Cycads and amyotrophic lateral sclerosis/parkinsonism–dementia. Lancet 1988; 2:1079.
121. Duncan M, Kopin IJ, Lavine L, Garruto R, Markey S. The putative neurotoxin BMAA in cycad-derived foods is an unlikely cause of ALS–PD. Lancet 1988; 2:631-632.
122. Yanagihara RT, Garruto RM, Gajdusek DC. Epidemiological surveillance of amyotrophic lateral sclerosis and parkinsonism–dementia in the commonwealth of the Northern Mariana Islands. Ann Neurol 1983; 13:79–86.
123. Plato CC, Garruto R, Fox K. Familial and epidemiological studies of amyotrophic lateral sclerosis and parkinsonism–dementia of Guam: a twenty-five year prospective patient control study. Am J Epidemiol 1984; 120:478.
124. Yanagihara R, Garruto R, Gajdusek D, Tomita A, Uchikawa T. Calcium and vitamin D metabolism in Guamanian Chammorros with amyotrophic lateral sclerosis and parkinsonism–dementia. Ann Neurol 1984; 15:42–48.
125. Plato CC, Garruto R, Yanagihara R, Chen K, Wood J. Cortical bone loss and measurements of the second metacarpal bone. I. Comparisons between adult Guamanian Chamorros and American Caucasians. Am J Phys Anthropol 1982; 59:461–465.
126. Plato CC, Grelich W, Garruto R, Yanagihara R. Cortical bone loss and measurements of the second metacarpal bone. II. Hypodense bone in post-war Guamanian children. Am J Phys Anthropol 1984; 63:57–63.
127. Garruto RM, Fukatsu R, Yanagihara R. Imaging of calcium and aluminum in neurofibrillary tangle-bearing neurons in parkinsonism–dementia of Guam. Proc Natl Acad Sci USA 1984; 81:1875–1879.
128. Perl DP, Gajdusek DC, Garruto RM, Yanagihara RT, Gibbs CT Jr. Intraneuronal aluminum accumulation in amyotrophic lateral sclerosis and parkinsonism–dementia of Guam. Science 1982; 217:1053–1055.
129. Rodgers-Johnson P, Garruto R, Yanagihara R. Amyotrophic lateral sclerosis and parkinsonism–dementia on Guam: a 30 year evaluation of clinical and neuropathological trends. Neurology 1986; 36:7–13.
130. Gajdusek DC. Environmental factors provoking physiological changes which induce motor neuron disease and early neuronal aging in high incidence foci in the western Pacific: calcium deficiency-induced secondary hyperparathyroidism and resultant CNS deposition of calcium and other metallic cations as the cause of ALS and PD in high incidence foci. In: Rose F, ed. Progress in motor neuron disease. Kent: Pitman Books, 1984:44–69.
131. Yanagihara R. Heavy metals and essential minerals in motor neuron disease. In: Rowland L, ed. Human motor neuron diseases. Adv Neurol 1982; 36:233–247.
132. Yase Y. The pathogenesis of amyotrophic lateral sclerosis. Lancet 1972; 2:292–296.
133. Yase Y. The role of aluminum in CNS degeneration with interaction of calcium. Neurotoxicology 1980; 1:101–109.
134. Reed D, Labarthe D, Chen KM, Stallones R. A cohort study of amyotrophic

lateral sclerosis and parkinsonism–dementia on Guam and Rota. Am J Epidemiol 1987; 125:92–100.
135. Koerner D. Amyotrophic lateral sclerosis on Guam. Ann Intern Med 1952; 37:1204.
136. Kurland LT, Mulder D. Epidemiologic investigations of amyotrophic lateral sclerosis. 2. Familial aggregations indicative of dominant inheritance. Neurology 1955; 5:182–196.
137. Plato CC, Reed DM, Elizan TS, Kurland LT. Amyotrophic lateral sclerosis–parkinsonism–dementia complex of Guam. IV. Familial and genetic investigations. Am J Hum Genet 1967; 19:617–632.
138. Plato CC, Garruto RM, Fox KM, Gajdusek DC. Amyotrophic lateral sclerosis and parkinsonism–dementia on Guam: a 25-year prospective case–control study. Am J Epidemiol 1986; 124:643–656.
139. Plato CC, Cruz MT, Kurland LT. Amyotrophic lateral sclerosis–parkinsonism–dementia complex of Guam: further genetic investigations. Am J Hum Genet 1969; 21:133–141.
140. Shiraki H, Yase Y. Amyotrophic lateral sclerosis. In: Vinken P, Bruyn G, eds. Handbook of clinical neurology, vol. 22. System disorders and atrophies. Part II. Amsterdam: Elsevier, 1975:353–419.
141. Garruto RM, Yase Y. Neurodegenerative disorders of the western Pacific: the search for mechanisms of pathogenesis. Trends Neurosci 1986; 9:368–374.
142. Maurizi CP. Was a neurovirulent influenza virus the cause of amyotrophic lateral sclerosis and parkinsonism–dementia on Guam. Med Hypotheses 1987; 23:325–326.
143. Viola M, Myers J, Gibbs C Jr, Roos R. Failure to detect poliovirus genetic information in amyotrophic lateral sclerosis. Ann Neurol 1979; 5:402–403.
144. Viola M, Frazier M, White L, Brody JA, Spiegelman S. RNA-instructed DNA polymerase activity in a cytoplasmic particulate fraction in brain from Guamanian patients. J Exp Med 1975; 142:483–494.
145. Gibbs CJ Jr, Gajdusek DC. An update on long-term in vivo and in vitro studies designed to identify a virus as the cause of amyotrophic lateral sclerosis, parkinsonism dementia and Parkinson's disease. In: Rowland L, ed. Human motor neuron diseases. Adv Neurol 1982; 36: 343–353.
146. Spencer PS, Kisby G, Ludolph A. Slow toxins, biologic markers, and long-latency neurodegenerative disease in the western Pacific region. Neurology 1991; 41(suppl 2):62–66.
147. Kisby G, Gold B, Spencer P. Neurotoxic effects of cycasin in murine organotypic cultures. Soc Neurosci Abstr 1990; 16:1113.
148. Duncan MW, Steele JC, Kopin IJ, Markey SP. 2-Amino-3-(methylamino)propionic acid (BMAA) in cycad flour: An unlikely cause of amyotrophic lateral sclerosis and parkinsonism–dementia of Guam. Neurology 1990; 40:767–772.
149. Kobayashi A. Cycasin in cycad materials used in Japan. Fed Proc 1972; 31:1476–1477.
150. Spencer PS, Allen C, Kisby G. Lathyrism and western Pacific ALS: etiology of short- and long-latency motor-system disorders. In: Rowland L, ed. Proceedings of ALS conference. New York: Raven Press, 1991:287–299.

151. Spencer PS, Palmer VS, Herman A, Asmedi A. Cycad use and motor neurone disease in Irian Jaya. Lancet 1987; 2:1273–1274.
152. Spencer PS. Guam ALS/parkinsonism–dementia: a long-latency neurotoxic disorder caused by "slow toxin(s)" in food. Can J Neurol Sci 1987; 14:347–357.
153. Eldridge R, Ryan E, Rosario J, Brody JA. Amyotrophic lateral sclerosis and parkinsonism dementia in a migrant population from Guam. Neurology 1969; 19:1029–1037.
154. Garruto RM, Gajdusek DC, Chen KM. Amyotrophic lateral sclerosis among Chamorro migrants from Guam. Ann Neurol 1980; 8:612–619.
155. Spencer PS, Nunn PB, Hugon J, et al. Guam amyotrophic lateral sclerosis–parkinsonism–dementia linked to a plant excitant neurotoxin. Science 1987; 237:517–522.
156. Ross SM, Seelig M, Spencer PS. Specific antagonism of excitotoxic action of "uncommon" amino acids assayed by organotypic mouse cortical cultures. Brain Res 1987; 425:120–127.
157. Ross S, Spencer P. Specific antagonism of behavioral action of "uncommon" amino acids linked to motor-system disease. Synapse 1987; 1:248–253.
158. Weiss J, Koh J, Choi D. Neurotoxicity of β-*N*-methylamino-L-alanine (BMAA) and β-*N*-oxalylamino-L-alanine (BOAA) on cultured cortical neurons. Brain Res 1989; 497:64–71.
159. Weiss JH, Choi DW. beta-*N*-Methylamino-L-alanine neurotoxicity: requirement for bicarbonate as a cofactor. Science 1988; 241:973–975.
160. Seawright A, Brown A, Nolan C. Selective degeneration of cerebellar cortical neurons caused by cycad neurotoxin, L-β-methylaminoalanine (1-BMAA), in rats. Neuropathol Appl Neurobiol 1990; 16:153–169.
161. Perry TL, Bergeron C, Biro A, Hansen S. β-*N*-Methylamino-L-alanine—chronic oral administration is not neurotoxic to mice. J Neurol Sci 1989; 94:173–180.
162. Spencer PS, Ross S, Kisby G. Western Pacific amyotrophic lateral sclerosis: putative role of cycad toxins. In: Hudson A, ed. Amyotrophic lateral sclerosis: concepts in pathogenesis and etiology. Toronto: University of Toronto Press, 1990:263–295.
163. Spatz H, Laqueur G. Transplacental induction of tumors in Sprague–Dawley rats with crude cycad material. JNCI 1967; 38:233.
164. Laqueur G, Michelsen O, Whiting M, Kurland L. Carcinogenic properties of nuts from *Cycas circinalis* L. indigenous to Guam. JNCI 1963; 31:919–933.
165. Shimizu T, Yasuda N, Kono I. Hepatic and spinal lesions in goats chronically intoxicated with cycasin. Jpn J Vet Sci 1986; 8:1291–1295.
166. Jones M, Yang M, Michelsen O. Effects of methylazoxymethanol glucoside and methylazoxymethanol acetate on the cerebellum of the postnatal Swiss albino mouse. Fed Proc 1972; 31:1508–1511.
167. Haddad R, Rabe A, Dumas R. Comparison of the effects of methylazoxymethanol on brain development in different species. Fed Proc 1972; 31:1520–1523.
168. Haddad R, Rabe A, Dumas R. Neuroteratogenicity of methylazoxymethanol acetate: behavioral deficits of ferrets with transplacentally induced lissencephaly. Neurotoxicity 1979; 1:171–189.

169. Dastur D, Palekar R. The experimental pathology of cycad toxicity with special reference to oncogenic effects. Indian J Cancer 1974; 2:33–49.
170. Dastur DK. Cycad toxicity in monkeys: clinical, pathological, and biochemical aspects. Fed Proc 1964; 23:1368–1369.
171. Dastur DK, Palekar RS, Manhani DK. Toxicity of various forms of *Cycas circinalis* in rhesus monkeys. Pathology of brain, spinal cord and liver. In: Rose C, Norris F, eds. ALS: new advances in toxicology and epidemiology. London: Smith-Gordon, 1990:129–141.
172. Yang M, Michelsen O, Campbell M. Cycad flour used by Guamanians: effect produced in rats by long term feeding. J Nutr 1966; 90:153–156.
173. Kurland LT. An appraisal of the neurotoxicity of cycad and the etiology of amyotrophic lateral sclerosis on Guam. Fed Proc 1972; 31:1540–1542.
174. Walshe J. Wilson's disease. In: Vinken P, Bruyn G, eds. Handbook of clinical neurology. Amsterdam: North-Holland Publishing, 1976:379–414.
175. Shoulson I, Chase T. Huntington's disease. Annu Rev Med 1975; 26:419–426.
176. Koller WC, Trimble J. The gait abnormality of Huntington's disease. Neurology 1985; 35:1450–1455.
177. Bird M, Paulson G. The rigid form of Huntington's chorea. Neurology 1971; 21:271–276.
178. Hallervorden J, Spatz H. Eigenartige erkiankung in extrapyramidalen System mit besonderer Beteilgung des Globus Pallidus and der Substantia Nigra. Z Ges Neurol Psychiatry 1922; 79:259–268.
179. Park BE, Netsky MG, Betsill WL. Pathogenesis of pigment and spheriod formation in Hallervorden–Spatz syndrome and related disorders. Neurology .1975; 25:1172–1178.
180. Perry TL, Norman MG, Yong VW, et al. Hallervorden–Spatz disease: cysteine accumulation and cysteine dioxygenase deficiency in the globus pallidus. Ann Neurol 1985; 18:482–489.
181. Koller WC, Glatt S, Wilson R, Fox J. Motor signs are infrequent in dementia—Alzheimer type. Ann Neurol 1984; 16:514–516.
182. Mölsä PK, Marttila RJ, Rinne UK. Extrapyramidal signs in Alzheimer's disease. Neurology 1984; 34:1114–1116.
183. Huber S, Shuttleworth E, Freidenberg D. Neuropsychological differences in the dementia of Alzheimer's and Parkinson's disease. Arch Neurol 1989; 46:1287–1291.
184. Prusiner SB. Prions and neurodegenerative diseases. N Engl J Med 1987; 317:1571–1581.
185. Farlow M, Yee R, Clouhy S, Conneally P, Azzarelli B, Ghetti B. Gerstmann–Sträussler–Scheinker disease. 1. Extending the clinical spectrum. Neurology 1989; 39:1446–1452.
186. Hakim S, Adams RD. The special clinical problem of symptomatic hydrocephalus with normal cerebrospinal fluid pressure. J Neurol Sci 1963; 2:307–327.
187. Messert B, Wanamaker B. Reappraisal of the adult occult hydrocephalus syndrome. Neurology 1974; 24:224–231.
188. Sorensen P, Jansen E, Gjerris F. Motor disturbances in normal-pressure hydrocephalus. Arch Neurol 1986; 43:34–38.

189. de Vera Reyes JA. Parkinsonian-like syndrome caused by posterior fossa tumor. Case report. J Neurosurg 1970; 33:599–601.
190. Jankovic J, Newmark M, Peter P. Case report. Parkinsonism and acquired hydrocephalus. Mov Disord 1986; 1:59–64.
191. Critchley M. Arteriosclerotic parkinsonism. Brain 1929; 52:23–83.
192. Murrow R, Schweiger G, Kepes J, Koller W. Parkinsonism due to a basal ganglia lacunar state: clinicopathologic correlation. Neurology 1990; 40:897–900.
193. Oliver L. Parkinsonism due to midbrain compression. Lancet 1959; 2:817–819.
194. Sciarra D, Sprofkin B. Symptoms and signs referable to the basal ganglia in brain tumor. Arch Neurol Psychiatry 1953; 69:450–461.
195. Polyzoidis KS, McQueen JD, Rajput AH, MacFadyen DJ. Parkinsonism as a manifestation of brain tumor. Surg Neurol 1985; 23:59–63.
196. Factor SA. Posttraumatic parkinsonism. In: Stern MB, Koller WC, eds. Parkinsonian syndromes. New York: Marcel Dekker, 1993:95–110.
197. Bruetsch WL, DeArmond M. The parkinsonian syndrome due to trauma. J Nerv Ment Dis 1935; 81:531–541.
198. Jordan BD. Neurologic aspects of boxing. Arch Neurol 1987; 44:453–459.
199. Lampert PW, Hardman JM. Morphological changes in brains of boxers. JAMA 1984; 251:2676–2679.
200. Ward CD, Duvoisin RC, Ince SE, Nutt JD, Eldridge R, Calne DB. Parkinson's disease in 65 pairs of twins and in a set of quadruplets. Neurology 1983; 33:815–824.
201. Corsellis JAN, Bruton CJ, Freeman-Browne D. The aftermath of boxing. Psychol Med 1973; 3:270–303.
202. Factor SA, Weiner WJ. Prior history of head trauma in Parkinson's disease. Mov Disord 1991; 6:225–229.
203. Stern M, Dulaney E, Gruber S, et al. The epidemiology of Parkinson's disease: a case–control study of young-onset and old-onset patients. Arch Neurol 1991; 48:903–907.
204. Factor SA, Sanchez-Ramos J, Weiner WJ. Trauma as an etiology of parkinsonism: a historical review of the concept. Mov Disord 1988; 3:30–36.
205. Jenkyn C, Reeves A. Neurologic signs in uncomplicated aging (senescence). Semin Neurol 1981; 7:21–30.
206. Koller WC. The diagnosis of Parkinson's disease. Arch Intern Med 1984; 144:2146–2147.
207. Duvoisin RC, Yahr MD. Encephalitis and parkinsonism. Arch Neurol 1965; 12:227–239.
208. Ziegler L. Follow-up studies on persons who have had epidemic encephalitis. JAMA 1928; July 21:138–141.
209. Weiner W, Lang A. Parkinson's disease. In: Weiner W, Lang A, eds. Movement disorders: a comprehensive survey. Mount Kisco, NY: Futura Publishing, 1989:23–117.
210. Duvoisin RC, Yahr MD, Schweitzer MR, Merritte HH. Parkinsonism before and since the epidemic of encephalitis lethargica. Arch Neurol 1963; 9:232–236.
211. Finley KH. Postencephalitic manifestations of viral encephalitides. In: Field, WS,

ed. Pathogenesis and treatment of parkinsonism. Springfield: Charles C Thomas, 1958:69–93.
212. Mulder D, Parrott M, Thaler M. Sequelae of western equine encephalitis. Neurology 1951; 1:318–327.
213. Nath A, Jankovic J, Pettigrew L. Movement disorders and AIDS. Neurology 1987; 37:37–41.
214. Marttila RJ, Arstila P, Nikoskelaimen J, Halonen PE, Rinne UK. Viral antibodies in the sera from patients with Parkinson's disease. Eur Neurol 1977; 15:25–33.
215. Wetmur JG, Schwartz J, Elizan TS. Nucleic acid homology studies of viral nucleic acids in idiopathic Parkinson's disease. Arch Neurol 1979; 36:462–464.
216. Elizan TS, Casals J. The viral hypothesis in parkinsonism. J Neural Transm 1983; 19:75–88.
217. Mattock CH, Marmot M, Stern G. Could Parkinson's disease follow intra-uterine influenza? A speculative hypothesis. J Neurol Neurosurg Psychiatry 1988; 51:753–756.
218. Kohbata S, Beaman BL. L-Dopa-responsive movement disorder caused by *Nocardia asteroides* localized in the brains of mice. Infect Immunol 1991; 59:181–191.
219. Hubble J, Kjelstrom J, Beaman B, Koller W. Nocardia serology in Parkinson's disease [abstract]. Mov Disord 1992; 7:292–293.
220. Cotzias GC. Manganese in health and disease. Physiol Rev 1958; 38:503–529.
221. Mena I, Marin O, Fuenzalida S, Cotzias G. Chronic manganese poisoning. Clinical picture and manganese turnover. Neurology 1967; 17:128–136.
222. Ferraz HB, Betolucci PH, Pereira JS, Lima JG, Andrade LA. Chronic exposure to the fungicide maneb may produce symptoms and signs of CNS manganese intoxication. Neurology 1988; 38:550–553.
223. Neff NH, Barrett RE, Costa E. Selective depletion of caudate nucleus dopamine and serotonin during chronic manganese dioxide administration to squirrel monkeys. Experientia 1969; 25:1140–1114.
224. Inoue N, Tsukada Y, Barbeau A. Behavioral effects in rats following intrastriatal microinjection of manganese. Brain Res 1975; 95:103–124.
225. Ringel S, Klawans H. Carbon monoxide induced parkinsonism. J Neurol Sci 1972; 16:245–251.
226. Klawans HL, Stein RW, Tanner CM, Goetz CG. A pure parkinsonian syndrome following acute carbon monoxide intoxication. Arch Neurol 1982; 39:302–304.
227. Richter R. Degeneration of the basal ganglia in monkeys from chronic carbon disulfide poisoning. J Neuropathol Exp Neurol 1945; 4:324–353.
228. Peters HA, Levin RL, Matthews CG, Chapman LJ. Extrapyramidal and other neurologic manifestations associated with carbon disulfide fumigant exposure. Arch Neurol 1988; 45:537–540.
229. Rosenberg NL, Myers JA, Martin WR. Cyanide-induced parkinsonism: clinical, MRI, and 6-fluorodopa PET studies. Neurology 1989; 39:142–144.
230. Uitti RJ, Rajput A, Ashenhurst E, Rozdilsky B. Cyanide-induced parkinsonism. A clinicopathologic report. Neurology 1985; 35:921–925.
231. Ballard PA, Tetrud JW, Langston JW. Permanent human parkinsonism due to 1-

methyl-4-phenyl-1,2,3,6-tetrahydropyridine (MPTP): seven cases. Neurology 1985; 35:949–956.
232. Burns RS, LeWitt PA, Ebert MH, Pakkenberg H, Kopin IJ. The clinical syndrome of striatal dopamine deficiency: parkinsonism induced by 1-methyl-4-phenyl-1,2,3,6-tetrahydropyridine (MPTP). N Engl J Med 1985; 312:1418–1421.
233. Grcevic N, Jardro-Santel D, Jukic S. Cerebral changes in paraquat poisoning. In: Roizin L, Shiraki H, Grcevic N, eds. Neurotoxicology. New York: Raven Press, 1977:469–484.
234. Sechi GP, Agnetti V, Piredda M, et al. Acute and persistent parkinsonism after use of diquat. Neurology 1992; 42:261–263.
235. Tanner CM, Chen B, Wang WZ, et al. Environmental factors and Parkinson's disease: a case–control study in China. Neurology 1989; 39:660–664.
236. Ho SC, Woo J, Lee CM. Epidemiologic study of Parkinson's disease in Hong Kong. Neurology 1989; 39:1314–1318.
237. Golbe LI, Farrell TM, Davis PH. Follow-up study of early-life protective and risk factors in Parkinson's disease. Mov Disord 1990; 5:66–70.
238. Hertzman C, Wiens M, Bowering D, Snow B, Calne DB. Parkinson's disease: a case–control study of occupational and environmental risk factors. Am J Ind Med 1990; 17:349–355.
239. Rajput AH, Uitti RJ, Stern W, et al. Geography, drinking water chemistry, pesticides and herbicides and the etiology of Parkinson's disease. Can J Neurol Sci 1987; 14:414–418.
240. Koller W, Vetere-Overfield B, Gray C, et al. Environmental risk factors in Parkinson's disease. Neurology 1990; 40:1218–1221.
241. Wong GF, Gray CS, Hassanein RS, Koller WC. Environmental risk factors in siblings with Parkinson's disease. Arch Neurol 1991; 48:287–289.
242. Miller L, Jankovic J. Neurologic approach to drug-induced movement disorders: a study of 125 patients. South Med J 1990; 83:525–532.
243. Kurland AA. Genetic determinats of extrapyramidal motor effects from psychotropic drugs. In: Brill, ed. Int Congr neuro-psycho pharmacol 1990:616–618.
244. Koller WC, Hubble JP. Classification of parkinsonism. In: Koller WC, ed. Handbook of Parkinson's disease. Marcel Dekker, 1992:59–104.
245. Ayd F. A survey of drug-induced extrapyramidal reactions. JAMA 1961; 175:1054–1060.
246. McClelland H. Discussion on assessment of drug-induced extrapyramidal reactions. Br J Clin Pharmacol 1976; 3:401–403.
247. Hall R, Jackson R, Swan J. Neurotoxic reactions resulting from chlorpromazine administration. JAMA 1956; 161:214–218.
248. Marsden C, Tarsy D, Baldessarini RJ. Spontaneous and drug-induced movement disorders. In: Benson D, Blumer D, eds. Psychiatric aspects of neurologic disease. New York: Grune & Stratton, 1975:219–266.
249. Myrianthopoulos N, Kurland A, Kurland L. Hereditary predisposition in drug-induced parkinsonism. Arch Neurol 1962; 6:5.
250. Myrianthopoulos NC, Waldrop IN, Vincent BL. A repeat study of hereditary predisposition in drug-induced parkinsonism. In: Barbeau A, Brunette JB, eds. Progress in neurogenetics. Amsterdam: Excerpta Medica, 1969:486–491.

251. Delay J, Deniker P. Drug-induced extrapyramidal syndromes. In: Vinken P, Bruyn G, eds. Handbook of clinical neurology. Amsterdam: North-Holland Publishers, 1968:248–266.
252. Duvoisin RC. Problems in the treatment of parkinsonism. Adv Exp Med Biol 1977; 90:131–135.
253. Rajput AH, Rozdilsky B, Hornykiewicz O. Reversible drug-induced parkinsonism. Arch Neurol 1982; 39:644–646.
254. Neiman J, Borg S, Wahlund LO. Parkinsonism and dyskinesias during ethanol withdrawal. Br J Addict 1988; 83:437–439.
255. Carlen PL, Lee MA, Jacob M. Parkinsonism provoked by alcoholism. Ann Neurol 1981; 9:84–86.
256. Lang A, Marsden C, Obeso J. Alcohol and Parkinson's disease. Ann Neurol 1982; 12:254–256.
257. Koller WC. Alcohol and Parkinson's disease [letter]. Ann Neurol 1983; 13:467.
258. Chouza C, Caamano J, Aljanati R, Scaramelli A, DeMedina O, Romero S. Parkinsonism, tardive dyskinesia, akathisia, and depression induced by flunarizine. Lancet 1986; 1:1303–1304.
259. Meyboom R, Ferrari M, Dieleman P. Parkinsonism, tardive dyskinesia, akathisia, and depression induced by flunarizine. Lancet 1986; 2:292.
260. D'Alessandro R, Bennassi G, Morganti G. Side-effects of flunarizine. Lancet 1986; 1:463.
261. Micheli F, Fernandez-Pardal M, Giannaula R. Movement disorders and depression due to flunarizine and cinnarizine. Mov Disord 1989; 4:139–146.
262. Melo-Souza S, Ragazzo P. Neurologic side-effects of flunarizine. Neurology 1989; 39 (suppl 1):390.
263. Gimenez-Roldan S, Mateo D. Cinnarizine-induced parkinsonism. Susceptibility to aging and essential tremor. Clin Neuropharmacol 1991; 14:156–164.
264. Dick RS, Barold SS. Diltiazem-induced parkinsonism. Am J Med 1989; 87:95–96.
265. Govoni S, Battaini F, Magnoni M, Trabucchi M. Non-vascular central nervous system effects of calcium entry blockers. Cephalalgia 1985; 5(supp 2):115–118.
266. Nishino N, Noguchi-Kuno S, Sugiyama T, Tanaka C. [^{3}H] + Nitrendipine binding sites are decreased in the substantia nigra and striatum of the brain from patients with Parkinson's disease. Brain Res 1986; 377:186–189.
267. Watson D, Carpenter C, Marks S, Greenberg D. Striatal calcium channel antagonist receptors in Huntington's disease. Ann Neurol 1988; 23:303–305.
268. Pileblad E, Cardenas A. The Ca^{2+}-antagonist nimodipine decreases and the Ca^{2+}-agonist Bay K 8644 increases catecholamine synthesis in mouse brain. Neuropharmacology 1987; 26:101–105.
269. Cohan S, Redmond D. Flunarizine inhibits depolarization-induced calcium uptake by gerbil synaptosomes. Neurology 1990; 40(suppl 1):384.
270. Ross RT. Young age parkinsonism and common drugs [letter]. Can J Neurol Sci 1989; 16:366–367.
271. Kane J, Rifkin A, Quitkin F, Klein D. Extrapyramidal side effects with lithium treatment. Am J Psychiatry 1978; 135:851–853.
272. Tyrer P, Alexander M, Regan A, Lee I. An extrapyramidal syndrome after lithium therapy. Br J Psychiatry 1980; 136:191–194.

273. Lutz E. Acute lithium-induced parkinsonism precipitated by liquid protein diet. J Med Soc MJ 1978; 75:165–166.
274. McLean D, Jacobs H, Mielke B. Methanol poisoning: a clinical and pathological study. Ann Neurol 1980; 8:161–167.
275. Bergevin P, Patwardhan V, Weissman J. Neurotoxicity of 5-fluorouracil. Lancet 1975; 1:410.
276. Werner E, Olanow C. Parkinsonism and amiodarone therapy. Ann Neurol 1989; 25:630–632.
277. Palakurthy P, Iyer V, Meckler R. Unusual neurotoxicity associated with amiodarone therapy. Arch Intern Med 1987; 147:881–884.
278. Teusink JP, Alexopoulos GS, Shamoian CA. Parkinsonian side effects induced by a monamine oxidase inhibitor. Am J Psychiatry 1984; 141:118–119.
279. Armon C, Miller P, Carwile S, et al. Valproate-induced parkinsonism–dementia syndrome: a potential model for acquired chronic degenerative diseases. Ann Neurol 1991; 30:41–42.
280. Gjerris F. Transitory procaine-induced parkinsonism. J Neurol Neurosurg Psychiatry 1971; 34:20–22.
281. Lieberman A, Goldstein M. Reversible parkinsonism related to meperidine. N Engl J Med 1985; 8:509.
282. Boranic M, Raci F. A parkinson-like syndrome as side effect of chemotherapy with vincristine and Adriamcycin in a child with acute leukaemia. Biomedicine 1979; 31:124–125.
283. Fisher J, Dewald J. Parkinsonism associated with intraventricular amphotericin B. J Antimicrob Ther 1983; 12:97–99.
284. Mintz U, Lieberman U, Vries A. Parkinsonian syndrome due to cephaloridine. JAMA 1971; 216:1200.
285. Ross RT. Drug-induced parkinsonism and other movement disorders. Can J Neurol Sci 1990; 17:155–162.
286. Reches A, Burk R, Kuhn C, Fahn S. Tetrabenazine, an amine-depleting drug, also blocks dopamine receptors in rat brain. J Pharmacol Exp Ther 1983; 225:515–521.
287. Schwab RS, England AC. Parkinson syndromes due to various specific causes. In: Vinken PJ, Bruyn GW, eds. Handbook of clinical neurology. Amsterdam: North-Holland Publishers, 1968:227–247.
288. Rosenblum A, Montgomery E. Exacerbation of parkinsonism by methyldopa. JAMA 1980; 224:2727–2728.
289. Gillman M, Sandyk R. Parkinsonism induced by methyldopa. S Afr Med J 1984; 65:194.
290. Fermaglich J, Chase T. Methyldopa or methyldopahydrazine as levodopa synergists. Lancet 1973; 1:1261–1262.
291. Jurna I, Nell T, Schreyer I. Motor disturbance induced by tremorine and oxotremorine. Naunyn Schmiedebergs Arch Pharmacol 1970; 267:80–98.
292. Metzer WS, Newton JEO, Steele RW, et al. HLA antigens in drug-induced parkinsonism. Mov Disord 1989; 4:121–128.
293. Koller WC, Cochran JW, Klawans HL. Calcification of the basal ganglia: computerized tomography and clinical correlation. Neurology 1979; 29:328–333.

294. Moskowitz M, Winickoff R, Heinz E. Familial calcification of the basal ganglion. A metabolic and genetic study. N Engl J Med 1971; 280:72–77.
295. Muenter M, Whisnant J. Basal ganglia calcifications, hypoparathyroidism, and extrapyramidal motor manifestations. Neurology 1968; 18:1075–1083.
296. Victor M, Adams RD, Cole M. The acquired (non-Wilsonian) type of chronic hepatocerebral degeneration. Medicine 1965; 44:345–396.
297. Finlayson MH, Superville B. Distribution of cerebral lesions in acquired hepatocerebral degeneration. Brain 1981; 104:79–95.
298. Sage JI, Miller DC, Golbe LI, Walters A, Duvoisin RC. Clinically atypical expression of pathologically typical Lewy-body parkinsonism. Clin Neuropharmacol 1990; 13:36–47.
299. Quinn NP, Luthert P, Honavar M, Marsden CD. Pure akinesia due to Lewy body Parkinson's disease: a case with pathology. Mov Disord 1989; 4:85–89.
300. Stern MB, Braffman BH, Skolnick BE, Hurtig HI, Grossman RI. Magnetic resonance imaging in Parkinson's disease and parkinsonian syndromes. Neurology 1989; 39:1524–1526.
301. Rutledge JN. Magnetic resonance of movement disorders. In: Jankovic J, Tolosa E, eds. Parkinson's disease and movement disorders. Baltimore: Urban & Schwartzenberg, 1988:441–460.
302. Drayer BP, Olanow W, Burger P, Johnson GA, Herfkens R, Riederer S. Parkinson plus syndrome: diagnosis using high field MR imaging of brain iron. Radiology 1986; 159:493–498.
303. Martin WRW. Parkinson's disease and aging: presynaptic nigrostriatal function. In: Martin WRW, ed. Functional imaging in movement disorders. Boca Raton: CRC Press, 1990:103–113.
304. Kish SJ, Shannak K, Hornykiewicz O. Uneven pattern of dopamine loss in the striatum of patients with idiopathic Parkinson's disease: pathophysiologic and clinical implications. N Engl J Med 1988; 318:876–880.
305. Oertel WH, Gasser T, Ippisch R, Trenkwalker C, Poewe W. Apomorphine test for dopaminergic responsiveness. Lancet 1989; 1:1262–1263.
306. Hughes AJ, Lees AJ, Stern GM. Apomorphine in the diagnosis and treatment of parkinsonian tremor. Clin Neuropharmacol 1990; 13:312–317.
307. Gasser T, Schwarz J, Arnold G, Trenkwalder C, Oertel WH. Apomorphine test for dopaminergic responsiveness in patients with previously untreated Parkinson's disease. Arch Neurol 1992; 49:1131–1134.
308. Hughes AJ, Lees AJ, Stern GM. Challenge tests to predict the dopaminergic response in untreated Parkinson's disease. Neurology 1991; 41:1723–1725.
309. Bonuccelli O, Piccini P, Del Dotto P, Rossi G, Corsini GU, Muratorio A. Apomorphine test for dopaminergic responsiveness: a dose assessment study. Mov Disord 1993; 8:158–164.
310. Rajput AH, Rozdilsky B, Rajput A. Accuracy of clinical diagnosis in parkinsonism—a prospective study. Can J Neurol Sci 1991; 18:275–278.
311. Hughes AJ, Daniel SE, Kilford L, Lees AJ. Accuracy of the clinical diagnosis of idopathic Parkinson's disease: a clinicopathological study of 100 cases. J Neurol Neurosurg Psychiatry 1992; 55:181–184.

312. Hughes AJ, Ben-Shlomo Y, Daniel SE, Lees AJ. What features improve the accuracy of clinical diagnosis in Parkinson's disease: a clinicopathologic study [published erratum appears in Neurology 1992;42:1436]. Neurology 1992; 42:1142–1146.
313. Gibb WRG. The neuropathology of Parkinson's disease. In: Jankovic J, Tolosa E, eds. Parkinson's disease and movement disorders. Baltimore: Urban and Schwarzenberg, 1988:205–223.
314. Koller WC. How accurately can Parkinson's disease be diagnosed? Neurology 1992; 42(suppl 1):6–16.
315. Ward CD, Gibb WR. Research diagnostic criteria for Parkinson's disease. In: Streifler MB, Korczyn AD, Melamed E, Youdim MBH, eds. Parkinson's disease: anatomy, pathology and therapy. Adv Neurol, 1990; 53:245–247.
316. Calne DB, Snow BJ, Lee C. Criteria for diagnosing Parkinson's disease. Ann Neurol 1992; 32(suppl):125–127.

2

Is Parkinson's Disease a Single Entity with a Single Cause? A Cautionary Note

Matthew M. Zack

Centers for Disease Control and Prevention, Atlanta, Georgia

J. William Langston

The Parkinson's Institute, Sunnyvale, California

I. INTRODUCTION

At first glance, there are few reasons to question the proposition that Parkinson's disease is a single entity. As described in Chapters 1 and 3, the disease has been well characterized over the last century both clinically and pathologically. Furthermore, its neurochemical substrate has been elucidated over the last few decades, and appears to be equally well defined—with a striatal dopamine deficiency as the sina qua none of the disease. Standard neurology text books betray little evidence of controversy concerning Parkinson's disease as a single disease entity. Most of the discussions that can be found in the rest of this volume are based (at least to some degree) on the proposition that Parkinson's disease is a unitary clinicopathological entity, with a cause that can be identified through epidemiological or laboratory techniques. Yet the cause of Parkinson's disease remains unknown some 175 years since James Parkinson first described the disease (1).

The purpose of this chapter is to explore the possibility that the failure to identify the cause is due to the acceptance of one or both of the following assumptions: (a) that Parkinson's disease is a single disease, or (b) that Parkinson's disease results from a single cause. If what we call Parkinson's disease is, in fact, a conglomerate of different entities, with similar clinical and pathological features, then it is likely that the cause of each of the different disorders may be different. Furthermore, each cause may account for only one of these component diseases. Then, unless the cause of one of these component diseases represents a substantial fraction of all of the cases, it will be difficult to relate that cause to the disease. A similar problem arises if Parkinson's disease is a single disease, but results from many different causes. Unless one of those causes accounts for a substantial fraction of all Parkinson's disease cases, it will also be difficult to relate that cause to the disease. If Parkinson's disease is both many different diseases and results from many different causes, then determining these causes will be very difficult, making the task that lies ahead of us enormously complex.

II. PARKINSONISM VERSUS PARKINSON'S DISEASE

As described in Chapter 1, the term *parkinsonism* is used to denote a group of symptoms—resting tremor, bradykinesia, rigidity, and impaired postural reflexes—that result from striatal dopamine deficiency (2,3). Damage to the dopaminergic neurons in the nigrostriatal pathway, loss of striatal dopamine, blockade of striatal dopamine receptors, or damage to the striatal neurons bearing dopamine receptors may cause parkinsonism (4–6). Damage to specific areas in the extrapyramidal system has been related to each of the symptoms of parkinsonism: bradykinesia, to damage of the nigrostriatal pathway; rigidity, to the release from inhibition (excitation) of the globus pallidus and the ventral lateral and the ventral anterior thalamic nuclei; and resting tremor, to disruptions in the connections between the cerebellum and both the mesencephalon and the latter thalamic nuclei that release from inhibition thalamic and cortical effects on α-motor neurons (4). If another disease, toxin, or medication can act through any of these mechanisms, then parkinsonism can result (2). Part of the progress in Parkinson's disease research has occurred as the result of recognizing other causes of parkinsonism and distinguishing them from what is left, presumably the clinicopathological entity known as idiopathic Parkinson's disease.

The problem of differentiating parkinsonism from Parkinson's disease is not an easy one. Parkinsonism can result from infections (encephalitis lethargica, viral encephalitides), exposure to toxins [manganese, carbon disulfide, carbon monoxide, cyanide, methanol, 1-methyl-4-phenyl-1,2,3,6-tetrahydropyridine (MPTP)], the use of medications (neuroleptics, reserpine, α-methyldopa, lithium), a variety of central nervous system disorders (normal pressure hydrocephalus, tumor, subdural hematoma, stroke, trauma), metabolic disturbances (hypoparathyroidism with basal ganglia calcification, hepatic coma), and other hereditary nervous system disorders (Wilson's disease, Huntington's disease, Hallervorden–Spatz disease). Other symptoms and signs, however, often accompany and distinguish these causes of secondary parkinsonism from Parkinson's disease (for a more detailed description, see Chapter 1). If a patient with parkinsonism that is due to a secondary cause presents without that cause being obvious, or if a patient with a neurodegenerative form of atypical parkinsonism (see Chapter 1 for a more detailed description of these diseases) presents with relatively pure parkinsonism, then that patient may be difficult to distinguish from a patient with Parkinson's disease (2,3,7,8). Until a biological marker for Parkinson's disease is found, any research that rests on clinical diagnosis will have to deal with this problem, regardless of whether it is a large population-based epidemiological study, or a small, highly focused trial of a new therapeutic agent for the disease.

Most clinicians (and many of the authors contributing to this volume, for that matter) believe that both the other neurodegenerative diseases that cause atypical parkinsonism (the so-called parkinson-plus syndromes), as well as all forms of clearly defined secondary parkinsonism, are different from Parkinson's disease. For example, patients with Parkinson's disease do not have the gaze paralysis of progressive supranuclear palsy, the cerebellar dysfunction of olivopontocerebellar atrophy, nor the severe autonomic dysfunction of Shy–Drager syndrome. Parkinson's disease usually has a slower course and a better response to levodopa therapy (2,9). The pattern and extent of neuronal damage in Parkinson's disease and the occurrence of Lewy bodies in the damaged areas typically differ from those in other degenerative diseases that cause parkinsonism (2,3,8; see also Chapters 1 and 3). For these reasons, most clinicians and neuropathologists accept Parkinson's to be a disease on its own and more than a residual syndrome (that is, parkinsonism without a known secondary cause and without the additional symptoms of the atypical or parkinsonism-plus syndromes). Yet because there are so many forms of parkinsonism, some of which are quite similar to the idiopathic disease, at least raises the question of whether or not what we call Parkinson's disease may harbor multiple entities.

III. THE PROBLEM OF DISEASE VARIABILITY

Another line of evidence that suggests we are dealing with multiple diseases under the rubric of Parkinson's disease relates to the problem of disease variability. It has been suggested repeatedly that variations in disease expression may be providing clues to diverse diseases or etiologies within the diagnostic category of what we call Parkinson's disease. For example, patients often differ in their clinical characteristics—their presenting symptom, the presence or absence of dementia, the age at onset, and the clinical course (2). These differences hint that even classically defined Parkinson's disease is not a single disease, but a group of related diseases, each with a different cause. Each presenting symptom or the presence of dementia may reflect different sites of damage and a different extent of damage (4,5); this could imply either selective vulnerability (or accessibility) of neurons at different sites to the same cause, or the effects of different causes. Differences in age at onset may suggest differences in dopamine levels at birth (constitutional or inherited causes), environmental insults that reduce dopamine levels after birth, accelerated loss of dopamine with aging, or processes unrelated to aging that cause dopamine loss (10,11). Those with more rapid courses may be more highly exposed, more recently exposed, or more continually exposed to these causes.

The preponderant presenting symptom—tremor, bradykinesia, or rigidity—may distinguish several subgroups of Parkinson's disease patients relative to ancillary symptoms, prior risk factors, and clinical course (12–14). Different presenting symptoms are likely to reflect different sites of damage. In one study, for example, severe bradykinesia was associated with impaired visual–spatial abilities and psychomotor speed; on the other hand, severe tremor was associated with better memory for spatial orientation (12). In another study (13), Parkinson's disease patients with rigidity or bradykinesia at onset before aged 40 were more likely than those with tremor at onset to have a more severe clinical course and were less likely to have relatives with tremor. Those with a first-degree relative who had Parkinson's disease were more likely to present with rigidity or bradykinesia, but less likely to have had gray hair before aged 35 or a history of hyperthyroidism. It has also been reported that those with predominant bradykinesia, postural instability, and gait difficulty were more likely than those with tremor to have had a worse mental status, a worse clinical course, and a later age at onset, but less likely to have had a family history of parkinsonism (14).

In autopsy studies of Parkinson's disease, patients with dementia were reported to have been more likely than those without dementia to be younger at onset of Parkinson's disease and to have a shorter clinical course (15). The former group also had a higher proportion of siblings with Parkinson's disease than expected. In another study, patients with impairment of verbal memory only were younger at onset and less likely to have bradykinesia than those with impairments of both verbal and visual–spatial memory (16).

Finally, age at onset may affect the clinical course of disease, although the reported effect varies in different studies. In one study, patients with onset of Parkinson's disease before aged 40 had a shorter, more severe course than those with later onset (17). However, another study found the reverse to be true (18). Differences between the studies in diagnostic accuracy or in the prevalence of potential confounding factors, such as the predominant symptom at onset or the presence of dementia, may account for these differences in the effect of age at onset on the course of disease. Overall, the occurrence of the different mosaics within the broader definition of Parkinson's disease raises the question of multiple disease subtypes, and could be signaling the presence of multiple diseases, rather than a single entity.

IV. ONE DISEASE, MANY CAUSES?

An alternative possibility is that Parkinson's disease is a final outcome for multiple etiopathogenic agents. If the disease actually results from different causes, these causes may either (a) act through the same common pathway, or (b) add small increments of damage until some threshold is exceeded that leads to neuronal death. Both alternatives have been called "multifactorial." An example of the former alternative is the free radical hypothesis of the pathogenesis of Parkinson's disease (19). Free radicals are unstable atoms or molecules with at least one orbital containing a single, unpaired electron (see Chapter 4 for a detailed discussion). They react almost instantaneously with adjacent proteins, lipids, and DNA to obtain an electron to complete their orbitals. This oxidation reaction may damage cell membranes and kill the cell.

The brain may be more vulnerable to these reactions than other tissues because it has more oxygen, more polyunsaturated lipids that react with free radicals, and fewer protective agents (e.g., glutathione, catalase, tocopherol) against these reactions. Certain regions within the brain, including the substantia nigra, have increased levels of iron that can donate electrons to enhance oxidation. The substantia nigra in patients with Parkinson's disease has increased levels of iron and lipid peroxidation products, but decreased levels of ferritin which binds iron, and of glutathione and glutathione peroxidase, which remove the hydrogen peroxide that is formed during oxidation reactions and that generate free radicals. Either excesses of factors that promote oxidation or deficiencies of factors that limit oxidation may work through this common pathway that leads to Parkinson's disease.

Another meaning of *multifactorial causation* is that many genetic and environmental causes, the individual effects of which may be too small to be detectable, act together to exceed a threshold of risk that distinguishes those with and without disease (20–24). The application of this kind of causation to Parkinson's disease arose from studies of familial associations among cases from Rochester, Minnesota, and from nine Swedish neurology clinics (21). These observed associations were more compatible with multifactorial causation than with rare single-gene (X-linked or autosomal dominant or recessive) inheritance. These observations also suggested that genetic causes contributed more (79–91%) than environmental causes to Parkinson's disease. In the Swedish data, the ratio of affected to all siblings and the proportion of affected parents decreased with increasing age at onset of the proband; this is consistent with another prediction of multifactorial causation: the risk for relatives is inversely related to age at disease onset. The importance of heredity and the possibility of multifactorial causation in Parkinson's disease suggested by the Minnesota and the Swedish studies are being evaluated through linkage-mapping studies of affected sib and relative pairs to identify the gene loci that confer susceptibility to Parkinson's disease (22).

Other observations hinting at the possibility of more than one cause for Parkinson's disease include the following: (a) It has proved difficult to identify one specific and predominant risk factor for a sizable proportion of Parkinson's disease cases (23), and (b) the risk for Parkinson's disease is greater for those who have more than one risk factor than for those who have a single risk factor (24). It should be emphasized that, although none of the observations cited in this chapter provide definitive evidence for more than one cause, they serve to remind us that it would be premature to close the book on this possibility.

V. FUTURE DIRECTIONS

After secondary and the atypical neurodegenerative forms of parkinsonism are excluded (and at the current time this may require postmortem examination, thus limiting the accuracy of clinical studies), the question remains of whether Parkinson's disease is one disease or more than one disease (26). Does Parkinson's disease have one preponderant cause, or more than one cause? As discussed earlier, the observed clinical heterogeneity of patients with Parkinson's disease relative to preponderant presenting clinical symptom(s), presence of dementia, age at onset, and clinical course, at least raise the possibility that Parkinson's disease may be more than one disease. The evidence for multifactorial causation, the attempts at linkage mapping, and the difficulty in identifying a specific, preponderant cause that affects a sizable proportion of patients further highlight this possibility. Therefore, until the cause or causes of the disease are found, anyone carrying out research in this area must be constantly aware that failure to recognize these possibilities could represent a major pitfall.

What can be done to sort these questions out, given our current state of knowledge and technical capabilities? Conducting new studies or reanalyses of previous studies to ascertain and define meaningful subgroups represents one avenue for future research. Several investigators have already used multivariate statistical techniques, such as cluster analysis and logistic regression, to do this (16,24). The purpose of cluster analysis would be to assign patients with Parkinson's disease into subgroups based on their characteristics so that those in a subgroup tend to resemble one another (have similar characteristics), and those in different subgroups do not (27); each of these homogeneous subgroups may then define patients whose disease resulted from a single cause. The purpose of logistic regression would be to determine the relative importance of different presumed causes of Parkinson's disease (28).

Because the conclusions from the previous studies were occasionally inconsistent and based on small numbers, new studies based on larger numbers of newly diagnosed cases from a defined population may corroborate or refute previous subgroup analyses. These studies should categorize patients on the basis not only of age at onset, presenting symptoms, and clinical course, but also on the basis of possible risk factors (e.g., rural upbringing, family history of Parkinson's disease), proposed preventive factors (e.g., cigarette smoking—see Chapter 11), or biomarkers, if and when they become available. If certain patient subgroups have particular risk factors, preventive factors, biomarkers, or clinical factors in common, this may spark a creative search for what links them together.

Because the incidence of Parkinson's disease increases with age, as does the incidence of other diseases such as cancer, the study of the causes of Parkinson's disease may benefit from the application of concepts used in the study of the causes of cancer. The multistage model of carcinogenesis represents one such model (29). In the multistage model, a cell moves from being normal at the initial precancerous stage, through several stages until, after the transition to the last stage, it becomes cancerous. If the carcinogen affects mainly early stages, and if the exposure to the carcinogen is continual, then this model predicts that the relative risk of exposure to a carcinogen decreases with increasing age at first exposure after adjustment for duration of exposure. If the carcinogen affects mainly early stages, and if the exposure to the carcinogen stops, then the relative risk of exposure to the carcinogen increases after the exposure stops, then remains at a plateau. If the carcinogen affects mainly later stages, and if the exposure to the carcinogen is continual, then the relative risk of exposure to the carcinogen is unchanged with increasing age at first exposure, after adjustment for duration of exposure. If the carcinogen affects mainly later stages, and if the exposure to the carcinogen stops, then the relative risk of exposure to the carcinogen decreases rapidly after the exposure stops.

Analogously, cells in the substantia nigra may move through several stages before they die. Perhaps the results of old studies of Parkinson's disease could be reanalyzed, or new studies planned, to determine patterns of how the relative risk for a putative cause of Parkinson's disease change with age at first exposure and duration of exposure. These patterns may then explain when it acts during these stages. Focusing on that period may provide insight into how that cause may be acting and what other causes may be acting at the same time.

Epigenesis theory is another approach with application to the cause(s) of Parkinson's disease (30). This theory attempts to determine how two or more causal variables interact in the pathogenesis of disease. It predicts what their expected effects might be if they are related to the same causal action, if only one pathogenic process leads to disease, and if they contribute to the same pathogenic process. If, for example, only oxidative reactions can cause Parkinson's disease, then two factors that act at different points in this pathogenic process would be expected to have multiplicative effects: The relative risk of Parkinson's disease for persons exposed to both causes would be the product of the relative risk of Parkinson's disease for persons exposed to only the first cause times that for persons exposed to only the second cause. If the two causes acted in separate pathogenic processes, they would be expected to have additive effects: The relative risk of Parkinson's disease for persons exposed to both causes would be the sum of the relative risk of Parkinson's disease for persons exposed to only the first cause plus that for persons exposed to only the second cause minus 1.

If more than one factor causes Parkinson's disease, the extent to which these factors all operate through one common pathway and the effectiveness of available means in changing that pathway will determine the extent to which the disease can be prevented. The search for other factors and other pathways will have to continue if changing the presumed pathway does not prevent a substantial proportion of cases.

VI. SUMMARY

We began with the premise that part of the progress in Parkinson's disease research since Parkinson's time has occurred in recognizing other causes of parkinsonism and distinguishing them from what is left, presumably a unitary disease entity. This process of continual refinement in diagnosis yields a more homogeneous disease that presumably has one or at least fewer causes. But the cause(s) of Parkinson's disease(s) have remained elusive. Perhaps we should shift our thinking about Parkinson's disease from a single disease, with a single cause, to the study of the different subtypes of Parkinson's disease, with a long-term goal of identifying different contributing factors, and even different causes.

In the future, studies directed at finding the cause of the disease should examine the distinction between Parkinson's disease and parkinsonism (including the many disorders that may mimic Parkinson's disease) and the attempt to distinguish different subtypes of Parkinson's disease. In general, the latter distinctions will be made based on more detailed assessment of the neuropathological and neurochemical differences, as well as the clinical variants considered in Chapter 1. Finally, anyone carrying out research in this area should constantly keep in mind the possibility that different causes may work together or interact to produce Parkinson's disease.

REFERENCES

1. Parkinson J. An essay on the shaking palsy. London: Whittingham and Rowland for Sherwood, Neely, Jones, 1817.
2. Koller WC, Hubble JP. Classification of parkinsonism. In: Koller WC, ed. Handbook of Parkinson's disease. New York: Marcel Dekker, 1992:59–104.
3. Duvoisin RC. Etiology of Parkinson's disease: current concepts. Clin Neuropharmacol 1986; 9:S3–21.
4. Papeschi R. Dopamine, extrapyramidal system, and psychomotor function. Psychiatr Neurol Neurochir 1972; 75:13–48.
5. Marsden CD. Basal ganglia disease. Lancet 1982; 2:1141–1147.
6. Yurek DM, Sladek JR Jr. Dopamine cell replacement: Parkinson's disease. Annu Rev Neurosci 1990; 13:415–440.
7. Sima AA, Hoag G, Rozdilsky B. Shy–Drager syndrome: the transitional variant. Clin Neuropathol 1987; 6:49–54.

8. Gibb WRG, Lees AJ. The significance of the Lewy body in the diagnosis of idiopathic parkinson's disease. Neuropathol Appl Neurobiol 1989; 15:27–44.
9. Quinn N. Disproportionate antecollis in multiple system atrophy [letter]. Lancet 1989; 1:844.
10. Savoiardo M, Strada L, Girotti F, et al. Olivopontocerebellar atrophy: MR diagnosis and relationship to multisystem atrophy. Radiology 1990; 174:693–696.
11. Duvoisin RC, Golbe L, Lepore F. Progressive supranuclear palsy. Can J Neurol Sci 1987; 14:547–554.
12. Mortimer JA, Pirozzolo FJ, Hansch EC, Webster DD. Relationship of motor symptoms to intellectual deficits in Parkinson disease. Neurology 1982; 32:133–137.
13. Barbeau A, Pourcher E. Genetics of early onset Parkinson's disease. Amsterdam: Excerpta Medica, 1983:1–16.
14. Zetusky W, Jankovic J, Pirozzolo F. The heterogenicity of Parkinson's disease. Clinical and prognostic implications. Neurology 1985; 35:522–526.
15. Heston LL. Dementia associated with Parkinson's disease: a genetic study. J Neurol Neurosurg Psychiatry 1980; 43:846–848.
16. Mortimer JA, June SP, Kuskowski MA, Webster R. Sybtypes of Parkinson's disease defined by intellectual impairment. J Neural Transm 1987; 24:101–104.
17. Mjönes H. Paralysis agitans: a clinical and genetic study. Acta Psychiatr Neurol 1949; 54:1–195.
18. Birkmayer W. Distinction between benign and malignant type of Parkinson's disease. Clin Neurol Neurosurg 1979; 81:158–164.
19. Olanow CW. Oxidation reactions in Parkinson's disease. Neurology 1990; 40 (suppl):32–37.
20. Falconer DC. The inheritance of liability to certain diseases, estimated from the incidence among relatives. Am J Hum Genet 1965; 29:51–76.
21. Kondo K, Kurland LT, Schull WJ. Parkinson's disease. Genetic analysis and evidence of a multifactorial etiology. Mayo Clin Proc 1973; 48:465–475.
22. Johnson W, Davidson M, Yoshidome H, Lustenberger A, Stenroos S. Genetics of Parkinson's disease (PD), the multifactorial/threshold (MF/T) model [abstract]. Mov Disord 1990; 5:92.
23. Kondo K. Epidemiological clues for the etiology of Parkinson's disease. Adv Neurol 1984; 40:345–351.
24. Kondo K. Epidemiological evaluations of risk factors in Parkinson's disease. In: Parkinson's disease. Adv Neurol, 1986; 45:289–293.
25. Olanow CW, Calne D. Does selegiline monotherapy in Parkinson's disease act by symptomatic or protective mechanisms? Neurology 1991; 42 (supp 4):13–26.
26. Parkinson's disease: one illness or many syndromes? Lancet 1992; 339:1263–1264.
27. Hartigan JA. Clustering algorithms. New York: John Wiley & Sons, 1975.
28. Lemeshow S, Hosmer DW Jr, Klar J, Lwanga SK. Applied logistic regression. New York: John Wiley & Sons, 1898.
29. Breslow NE, Day NE. Statistical methods in cancer research, vol 2. The design and analysis of cohort studies. New York: Oxford University Press, 1987:256–262.
30. Koopman JS, Weed DL. Epigenesis theory: a mathematical model relating causal concepts of pathogenesis in individuals to disease patterns in populations. Am J Epidemiol 1990; 132:366–390.

3

Pathological Considerations in the Etiology of Parkinson's Disease

Lysia S. Forno

Department of Veterans Affairs Medical Center and Stanford University School of Medicine, Palo Alto, California

I. INTRODUCTION

A. Background and Historical Note

Although neuropathological studies rarely reveal the etiology of a disease, the character of the structural abnormalities and the location of the lesions frequently yield important clues to the etiology and pathogenesis. This is also true for Parkinson's disease (PD).

When James Parkinson, in 1817, described the syndrome we now call PD, he had no autopsy studies to support his suggestions concerning the pathological site of the disorder. Attempts at establishing the pathological substrate for PD were unsuccessful for many years, although in Charcot's time there already were hints that the substantia nigra (SN) might be involved. This suspicion, first mentioned by Brissaud (1) was based on three reports of tuberculomas in the SN or adjacent cerebral peduncle in individuals with contralateral parkinsonism (see also Ref. 2). It was not until Ehringer and Hornykiewicz (3) had established the dopamine deficiency in the striatum, and the nigrostriatal dopaminergic pathway had been documented (4) that the nerve cell degeneration in the SN became accepted as a critical part of the pathology of PD.

The credit for attributing a key role to the nerve cell degeneration in SN must be shared between Tretiakoff (5), Hassler (6), and Greenfield and Bosanquet (7). Without yet knowing why the SN was important for PD, they maintained their belief in the validity of their personal observations. In the United States, only

Freeman (8) emphasized the abnormalities in the SN, not only in postencephalitic parkinsonism, but also in PD. Although Lewy (9,10) described the neuronal inclusion bodies (Lewy bodies), which now appear to be an important part of the disease process in PD, he did not believe that involvement of the SN was important. The inclusions he described were found mainly in the innominate substance, the hypothalamus, and the dorsal motor nucleus of the vagus.

The foregoing contributions demonstrate how pathological observations can pave the way for insights later obtained from other disciplines. Knowledge of the pathological substrate for a disease is a useful, and perhaps necessary, basis for any hypothesis.

Cotzias et al (11) strengthened the concept of dopamine deficiency as the main biochemical defect in PD, when they succeeded in reversing parkinsonian symptoms by giving a protracted regimen of large oral doses of the precursor to dopamine, D,L-dihydroxyphenylalanine (dopa), to PD patients. The study was prompted by their interest not only in the decrease in catecholamines in the basal ganglia in PD, but also in the role of dopa in melanogenesis. They found, however, that administration of β-melanocyte-stimulating hormone intramuscularly actually made the parkinsonism worse.

Bernheimer et al. (12) confirmed the intimate relation between nerve cell loss in the zona compacta of the SN and the decrease in dopamine and its metabolite, homovanillic acid (HVA), in a combined biochemical and neuropathological study. Their large study included 69 cases of various forms of parkinsonism: 12 with postencephalitic parkinsonism; 39 with idiopathic parkinsonism (paralysis agitans); 7 with "arteriosclerotic"–senile parkinsonism; and 11 atypical or unclassified cases. Biochemical examination was performed in 28 brains from the parkinsonism group, along with 28 neurologically normal controls and 14 Huntington's disease brains. The dopamine decrease in the striatum showed a positive correlation with the degree of nerve cell loss in the SN. There was some overlap between the generally severely affected postencephalitic patients (with the severest reduction in dopamine) and those patients with paralysis agitans, who exhibited the most marked cell loss.

Another important finding in this study was that the dopamine depletion in the idiopathic cases was more severe in the putamen than in the caudate, a result later confirmed by the authors (13). This was interpreted as being because the relatively spared medial rostral cell group of the SN projects mainly to the caudate.

B. Parkinson's Disease and Parkinsonism

For this chapter *Parkinson's disease* has been defined clinically as a distinctive progressive disorder, affecting mainly persons in middle age or older, with tremor, rigidity, and bradykinesia as the cardinal features. For pathological confirmation, nerve cell loss in the SN and Lewy body inclusions have been required. However, several other movement disorders may be difficult to distinguish from PD in the living patient. Their different neuropathological substrate might be also expected to yield insights into the etiology and pathogenesis of PD, as happened when postencephalitic parkinsonism drew attention to the SN.

Bernheimer et al. (12) also made the diagnosis of idiopathic parkinsonism in the absence of Lewy bodies, but these inclusions were present in 36 of their 39 cases (92%). In addition 3 of the 7 cases with arteriosclerotic parkinsonism and 1 of the 12 with postencephalitic parkinsonism had Lewy bodies. The authors felt that "the occurrence of Lewy bodies in idiopathic parkinsonism or of neurofibrillary changes in the postencephalitic condition appears to be of minor importance, since they are considered as non-specific sequelae of disorders of cytoplasmic protein synthesis." Twenty years later the accuracy of this statement is still being debated.

Lewy bodies have occasionally been found in parkinsonian syndromes other than PD, for example, in rare cases of progressive supranuclear palsy (PSP; 14), striatonigral degeneration (SND; 15,16), and the amyotrophic lateral sclerosis–parkinsonism–dementia of Guam (ALS–PD; 17–21). The significance of the Lewy inclusions in these disorders is unclear. Possibilities include (a) Lewy bodies as an age-related phenomenon, (b) nonspecificity of this cytoskeletal abnormality, or (c) coincidence of PD and the particular disease. These syndromes share with PD the cardinal feature of a substantial loss of nerve cells in the SN, but differ in other respects (Table 1).

In PSP (14), degeneration of nerve cells in the globus pallidus, subthalamic nucleus, tegmentum of the midbrain, and rostral pons is accompanied by neurofibrillary tangles, often with a characteristic ultrastructure that differs from the paired helical filaments of Alzheimer's disease (AD). The inferior olive and the dentate nucleus in the cerebellum may also be affected, and cortical lesions with Alzheimer like changes are present to a variable degree. In SND (15), changes in the striatum resemble those of Huntington's disease, but the putamen is always more severely damaged than the caudate, and SN degeneration can be severe. The globus pallidus may be moderately affected. The focality of the process, with involvement frequently restricted to a portion (often the dorsolateral part) of the putamen, is another distinguishing feature of this syndrome. Moreover, SND is rarely an isolated finding, since it is often part of a multisystem atrophy (MSA; 16), such as olivopontocerebellar degeneration (OPC) or Shy–Drager syndrome (with autonomic failure). The parkinsonism–dementia complex of Guam (17,21–24) forms a link to ALS, since it usually has lesions also in cranial nerve nuclei and anterior horn cells and may display symptoms of ALS. It differs from other forms of ALS in having neurofibrillary tangles (NFT) in its degenerating nerve cells, including those in the SN and cerebral cortex, especially the basal forebrain and limbic areas.

Table 1 Location of Pathology in Some Neurodegenerative Disorders

	Neurodegenerative disorder[c]						
Location[a,b]	PD	PSP	SND	MSA	AD/LB	AD	HD
SN	A	A	A	F	F	R	R
LC	A	F	S	F	A	A	R
CP	NV	S	A	F	S	S	A
GP	NV	A	F	F	N	N	F
NBM	F	S	N	N	A	A	N
Hth	F	R	N	N	F	F	R
Ctx	S	S	N	R	A	A	A
E–W	F	R	N	R	S	S	N
Rph	F	F	N	S	F	F	N
DMVg	F	R	N	F	F	S	N
Cord	S	S	S	A	S	N	R
Symp	F	N	R	S	F	N	N

[a]A, always; F, frequently; S, sometimes; R, rarely; N, not present; NV, not visible.
[b]SN, substantia nigra; LC, locus coeruleus; CP, neostriatum; GP, globus pallidus; NBM, nucleus basalis of Meynert; Hth, hypothalamus; Ctx, cortex; E–W, Edinger–Westphal nucleus; Rph, raphe nuclei; DMVg, dorsal motor nucleus of the vagus; Cord, spinal cord; Symp, sympathetic ganglia.
[c]PD, Parkinson's disease; PSP, progressive supranuclear palsy; SND, striatonigral degeneration; MSA, multisystem atrophy; AD, Alzheimer's disease; LB, Lewy body; HD, Huntington's disease.

Another form of parkinsonism with neurofibrillary tangles can be seen in prize-fighters (25). It has features in common with AD, but there are fewer neuritic plaques and there is nerve cell loss in the SN with NFT.

Klawans et al. (26) described calcification of the basal ganglia as a cause of levodopa-resistant parkinsonism. The causal effect of the calcifications for the parkinsonism in this patient is unproved, since this is not a pathologically confirmed case, and mineral deposits of varying severity are common in the basal ganglia in routine autopsy material.

Although this selection does not in any way do justice to the large number of syndromes associated with parkinsonism, it covers those most likely to present difficulties for the clinician in differential diagnosis from PD. Striatonigral degeneration and PSP, along with the Shy–Drager syndrome, are particularly difficult in the initial stages of the disease. The different neuropathological substrate of these disorders might then be expected to be of some help when considering the etiology of PD, but except for the confirmation of the importance of SN degeneration, no significant insights have yet been achieved. This is probably because we know even less about the etiology of PSP, SND, and Shy–Drager syndrome than we do about PD, for which hypotheses about extrinsic and intrinsic toxins have been put forward and for which treatment prospects are more advanced.

Practically all the parkinsonian syndromes have dopamine deficiency, but in PD, the situation is relatively simple. The nerve cells in the neostriatum that contain the dopamine receptors are largely intact, whereas in SND, a considerable, though variable, number of striatal projection neurons are lost. In PSP, Agid (27) has emphasized the marked involvement of the cholinergic system. This is, however, more marked biochemically than morphologically, since the nerve cells in the cholinergic nucleus basalis of Meynert may be relatively preserved. Attention has recently focused on the role of the subthalamic nucleus and its glutamatergic projection to the globus pallidus and the SN in PD, but although the subthalamic nucleus is morphologically intact in PD, it is severely affected in PSP. How this influences the parkinsonism in PSP is unknown.

Shy–Drager syndrome may be misdiagnosed in cases of PD with autonomic failure, since both involve very similar anatomical sites, especially the sympathetic intermediolateral column in the spinal cord (28). In PD, hypothalamic autonomic nuclei, as well as sympathetic ganglia, may contain Lewy body inclusions, suggesting a pathogenesis different from that for Shy–Drager syndrome in which these bodies are absent.

The Guamanian ALS–PD syndrome may yet yield important insights into this particular form of parkinsonism, but the etiology of this disorder is still controversial, and we must await further developments. However, the evidence that this is an environmentally determined condition is very strong and adds to the expectation that exogenous harmful substances may play a role in PD.

II. CLUES FROM NEUROPATHOLOGY OF PARKINSON'S DISEASE TO ITS PATHOGENESIS

The cardinal pathological features of PD are the degeneration of the SN and the nigrostriatal pathway and the formation of characteristic intraneuronal inclusion bodies, called Lewy bodies. Although this apparently simple structural correlate of the disease process may be the logical starting point for a search for etiologic factors, the neuropathology of PD is not limited to the nigrostriatal tract and dopamine deficiency. A selective involvement of other nerve cell nuclei and other neurotransmitters can be found in most PD brains. The noradrenergic locus coeruleus (LC) and the cholinergic nucleus basalis of Meynert are the most conspicuous sites of the disease process, but a more complete list is given in Table 2. Not all of these anatomical areas are involved in every case of PD, but the SN is practically never the only one of the cell groups affected.

The widespread affection of these selected nuclei is such an integral part of the disease process that it deserves to be considered in relation to the etiology of the disorder. Lewy bodies, more than nerve cell loss, are the main morphological

Table 2 Nerve Cell Nuclei and Neurotransmitter Systems Involved in PD

Neurotransmitter	Nerve cell group	Lewy bodies	Nerve cell loss
Dopamine	Substantia nigra	+	+
	Ventral tegmental area	+	Sometimes present
Norepinephrine	Locus coeruleus	+	Usually present
	Sympathetic ganglion	+	Not documented
Acetylcholine	Nucleus basalis Meynert	+	+
	Peripeduncular nucleus	+	+
	Edinger–Westphal nucleus	+	?
	Intermediosacral nucleus	+	?
	Intestinal autonomic ganglion (Auerbach's and Meissner's plexus)	+	?
Serotonin	Dorsal raphe nucleus	+	?
	Superior central nucleus	+	?
?	Hypothalamus (esp. posterior and lateral cell groups)	+	?
?	Amygdala, hippocampal–parahippocampal region		
?	Cingulate gyrus, insula		
?	Tuberculum olfactorium	+	Sometimes present
?	Spinal cord (mainly intermediolateral, but also other nerve cells)		

abnormality in several of these nuclei. The Lewy bodies (see Section III. B) may form part of a spectrum of Lewy body disorders (29). A distribution of Lewy bodies, similar to that in PD, is found in AD with Lewy bodies (Lewy body variant of AD; 30) and in Lewy body dementia (31). The difficulty in evaluating the effect of the involvement of these extranigral nuclei in the disease process in PD lies in (a) the slight alterations in nondopaminergic neurotransmitter systems and (b) the paucity of clearly documented clinical–pathological correlation. However, in PD with dementia, nerve cell loss in the nucleus basalis of Meynert and the presence of cortical Lewy bodies appear to be the rule; autonomical symptoms may be explained by the involvement of hypothalamic nuclei and of sympathetic ganglia. The lesson from this widespread abnormality is that whatever the noxious influence that causes PD turns out to be, it is not a local phenomenon, and the common denominator is not one neurotransmitter, but because the insult is particularly severe in SN, and SN is the source of dopamine, the result is parkinsonism.

The crucial questions for PD, as for most neurodegenerative disorders, concern the nerve cell death (why and how?) and the selectivity of the process. In PD, certain features, such as the site of the disease process, the anatomical connections, the neuromelanin, the inclusion bodies, and other special characteristics of the metabolism of the affected nerve cells, are promising subjects for etiologic and pathogenetic considerations.

Over the years, many possible causes for PD have been suggested. An incomplete list is given in Table 3. Most of the causes suggested fall into the categories of either exogenous or endogenous exposure to potentially harmful agents. Some combine exogenous and endogenous influences. Since many persons who do not develop PD are exposed to the same potentially harmful substances as those who do, the individual variation in susceptibility has to be accounted for. This will often mean that a certain genetic predisposition is required. A multifactorial pathogenesis of PD, rather than one neurotoxin or one genetic defect, appears to be the most plausible hypothesis. Barbeau (32) described a "global hypothesis." He thought that there was a genetically determined susceptibility that was reflected in all cells, and that PD was the combined result of a general cell-aging process that was accelerated in susceptible individuals by various trigger factors. Such factors were thought to cause a transient increase in catecholamine turnover, resulting in accumulations of free radicals and neuromelanin in the neurons. When this accumulation exceeded the coping mechanisms of the nerve cells, damage to organelles and membranes resulted. Lewy bodies were formed from damaged filaments, and cell death ensued. This resulted in further stress, with repetition of the destructive process, leading to an imbalance of neurotransmitters in the basal ganglia, explaining the PD symptoms.

Some of these hypotheses are discussed in other chapters in this volume (see Chapters 5–7 and 12–14). Neuromelanin, Lewy bodies, and certain other factors that can be studied by morphological methods will be addressed.

Table 3 Main Hypotheses for Etiology of Parkinson's Disease

Aging
(accelerated or superimposed on previous insult)
Infections
(cohort hypothesis now abandoned)
Environmental toxins
(tetrahydropyridines; heavy metals; pesticides; others)
Metabolic and genetic
(free radicals; mitochondrial toxins; excitotoxins; neuromelanin, and other harmful metabolites of catecholamines; lack of growth factors; others)
Andre Barbeau's "global hypothesis"
("compatible with all previously proposed hypotheses")

Lewy body inclusions are important because they appear to be linked to the nerve cell degeneration. Therefore, they can be expected to provide a tangible clue to the faulty metabolism of the affected nerve cells. Lewy body inclusions are not pathognomonic for PD (29,33). On rare occasions, they are present in other neurodegenerative disorders, but they also occur in a certain percentage (approximately 10%, depending on age; 29,34,35) of older individuals without manifest parkinsonism. The discovery of the existence of a syndrome of Lewy body dementia or diffuse Lewy body disease has added to the interest in this particular disorder of the neuronal cytoskeleton. If it can be established what biochemical and molecular derangements lead to the formation of the Lewy body and how this body is related to the nerve cell death, this knowledge may also contribute to the understanding of the etiologic factors that cause PD. The close association between Lewy bodies and PD is confirmed, in Lewy body dementia cases, by the circumstance that the SN and locus coeruleus (LC) also contain Lewy bodies and often show nerve cell loss. When the Lewy body phenomenon is present in older persons without overt parkinsonism, it has been suggested that such individuals may have preclinical PD (29,34) or a forme fruste of the disease (35).

The most recent hypotheses for the etiology of PD (see Table 3) have focused on exogenous or endogenous toxins (especially their effect on mitochondria), on excitotoxins, and on damage caused by free radicals (see Chapters 7 and 12–14). It will be important to look at how these hypotheses fit either known pathological changes or special morphological characteristics that might be appreciated, once it is known what to look for. These hypotheses will not be taken up separately, but in the context of the pathological features under discussion, especially the nerve cell degeneration.

III. THE SUBSTANTIA NIGRA

A. The Vulnerable Nerve Cells

This discussion will also be relevant to other nerve cell groups vulnerable to the disease process in PD, but certain characteristics of neurons in SN, such as their content of neuromelanin, may be particularly important for the degenerative process in PD.

1. Neuromelanin Content

The presence of neuromelanin in the human brain (Fig. 1) is the visible evidence that catecholamines have been present or are active in a nerve cell, but the role played by this pigment is still a debated issue (36; see also Ref. 37, pp. 196–200 for review). Briefly, neuromelanin is generally considered to be a waste product of catecholamine metabolism. Graham (38,39) has described its derivation from

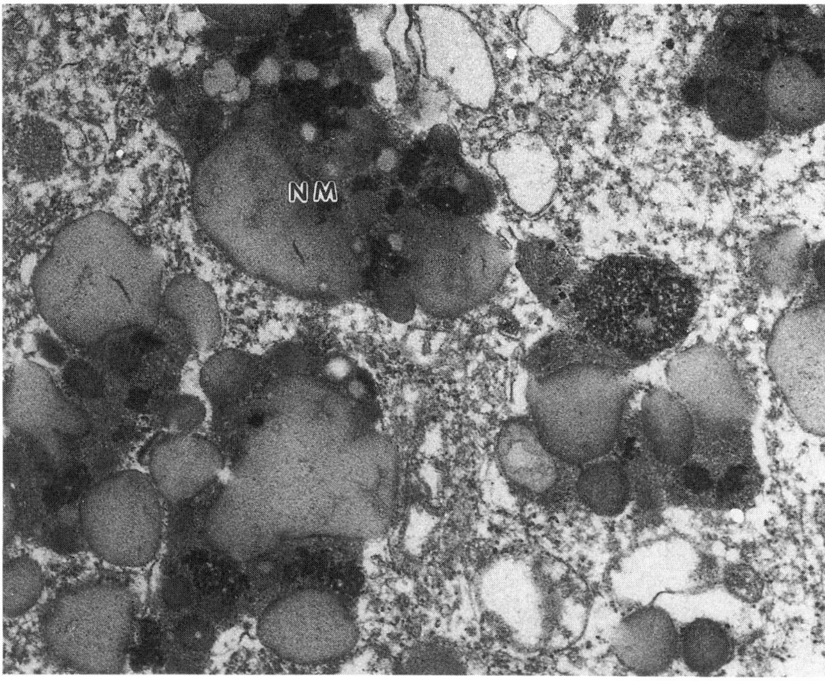

Figure 1 Neuromelanin pigment (NM) in the cytoplasm of nerve cell in the substantia nigra in Parkinson's disease. Note that the pigment granules have three components: the pale and the moderately dense components are similar to the composition of lipofuscin, whereas the third, extremely dense and granular constituent is characteristic of neuromelanin (× 27,500).

oxidation of dopamine, norepinephrine, and compounds related to quinones. Details of its biochemistry and arguments for and against a harmful effect of this compound are given in Chapter 7.

Since this residue is sequestered in phagolysosomes as a melanized lipofuscin, the formation of neuromelanin may act as a protective device to shield the nerve cell from harmful effects caused by the neurotransmitter it produces. At the same time, there is a suspicion that free radicals, as well as harmful quinones, are generated in the process, or that neuromelanin may bind toxic substances that it later releases (40,41). It has been suggested that such a process may take place in 1-methyl-4-phenyl-1,2,3,6-tetrahydropyridine (MPTP)-induced parkinsonism (40,41). D. Graham has postulated (39) that the accumulation of neuromelanin itself does not result in nerve cell degeneration, but that catecholamine neurons may degenerate because of lifelong injury from the by-products of catecholamine oxidation. He found that potentially toxic quinones were likely to form more readily in the SN than in the LC, because autoxidation occurs more rapidly for dopamine than for norepinephrine (38).

Carstam et al. (42) examined neuromelanin from the human substantia nigra after extraction of lipids and proteins (this method would presumably remove most of the lipofuscin component). They suggested that neuromelanin formation would occur when the glutathione–cysteine protective system was exhausted, and that neuromelanin might be a marker for such exhaustion. This appears unlikely, since neuromelanin is present from early childhood and does not seem to interfere with nerve cell function in normal individuals without parkinsonism.

In 1974, Mann and Yates (43) suggested that the nerve cells would die when neuromelanin had accumulated to the extent that it interfered with the normal function of the cell. Later (44), they added the presence of cytotoxic metabolites in the cell to this scenario.

The presence of neuromelanin in the nerve cells that degenerate in PD raises several other questions, such as why nerve cells in the SN of rodents do not contain neuromelanin. Are these cells under less stress than similar cells in humans? One might also ask, what happens in dopamine terminals in the striatum? No neuromelanin is formed here. Carstam et al. (42) have concluded that, since dopamine and its oxidation products are also abundant in the striatum, the mere presence of catecholic compounds is not sufficient for neuromelanin to be formed. They believe that free radicals, such as the superoxide anion, must be involved.

To put forward a personal speculation, given the hypothetical assumption that neuromelanin is protective, rather than harmful, is it possible that dopamine terminals are especially vulnerable because they do not have the ability to generate the protective neuromelanin? In that event, the nerve cell degeneration in the nigrostriatal pathway might start in the terminals and reach the parent cell bodies in the SN only when the protective mechanisms there are exhausted.

Many questions about the role of neuromelanin in PD remain to be resolved. Because neuromelanin is found in combination with lipofuscin, the formation of this age-related pigment may also have relevance to neuromelanin and PD. In a recent review, Porta (45) discussed two hypotheses of lipofuscinogenesis—the lipid peroxidative theory, and the proteolytic decline theory—but found objections to both. In the free radical theory of aging, he felt that it had not been proved that the tissue levels of nonenzymatic antioxidants decrease with age. In proteolysis, the reasons for the decline of intracellular protein synthesis and degradation with age were unclear, since it is not known if the lysosomal thiol proteases of normal animals decline with age. He argued that more research into the process of autophagocytosis and lysosomal protein degradation during development and aging is needed to better understand the aging process.

In the previous discussion, it has been taken for granted that the neuromelanin-containing nerve cells are the ones especially at risk in PD. This concept has been suggested by several authors (44,46,47). Mann and Yates (44) found that in aging, and to a much greater degree in PD, nerve cells remaining in the SN and LC contained less neuromelanin pigment than those in the SN and LC of normal adult brains. They interpreted this to mean that the nerve cells with the higher content of neuromelanin were the first to die. Hirsch and associates (46,47) have also come to the conclusion that neuromelanin-containing nerve cells are particularly vulnerable in the PD disease process.

However, although not denying the general vulnerability of the nerve cells in the compact zone of the SN, Gibb et al. (48) have found that the nerve cells that are most severely affected in PD contain less neuromelanin pigment than the relatively resistant, more dorsally situated, nerve cell groups in the SN. The vulnerability of the more lateral cell groups in the SN, and especially the ventral lateral group, was noted in 1938 by Hassler (6) and is not generally disputed. German et al. (49), using computer visualization techniques, also found the most severe nerve cell loss in the ventral portion of SN compacta when comparing five PD brains with three controls.

Because PD is an age-related disease, and often thought of as an accelerated-aging process in selected neuronal populations, it might have been expected that the cell groups most vulnerable in PD, would also be those most likely to succumb to the aging process, but Fearnley and Lees (50) have reported that nerve cell loss in the SN in human aging tended to spare the least pigmented ventral lateral tier. Hirsch et al. (46) found that neuromelanin-containing nerve cells were most vulnerable to the disease process in PD, but they compared SN compacta pigmented nerve cells with largely unpigmented catecholaminergic cells in the periaqueductal region and in the retrorubral (A8) area. They did not compare individual nerve cell groups within the SN compacta. Therefore, their findings do not necessarily contradict those of Gibb et al. (48). Nerve cells that do not harbor the neuromelanin pigment can be severely affected in PD; For example, this is true for the nucleus basalis of Meynert, and also for the dorsal motor nucleus of the vagus, in which mainly it is the unpigmented nerve cells that contain Lewy bodies and undergo nerve cell loss (see Ref. 51). The question whether neuromelanin provides protection or vulnerability in the disease processes of PD and aging must be answered if we are to understand the role played by neuromelanin in the etiology of PD. Therefore, the findings by Gibb et al. (48) and by Fearnley and Lees (50) need to be confirmed.

2. *Other Factors of Importance for Nerve Cell Vulnerability*

Calcium-Binding Proteins. The story of nerve cell degeneration has only just begun to unfold. Insights into the role played by calcium-binding proteins, such as calbindin and parvalbumin, are important developments. Yamada and associates (52) found that calbindin-positive nerve cells, located in the mediodorsal portion of the SN compacta, were relatively spared in PD, and suggested that calbindin might offer some protection against the disease process. These nerve cell groups are among those found by Gibb et al. (48) to be relatively preserved in PD. Similarly, German et al. (53), using computer-imaging techniques to map and quantify the distribution of dopamine and calbindin neurons in human controls and PD midbrains, demonstrated that calbindin-positive nerve cells, present in mainly the dorsal SN compacta, the retrorubral area (A8), and the ventral tegmental area, were relatively spared in PD, compared with the calbindin-negative ventral portion of the SN compacta.

The results in the study by Hirsch et al. (54) were slightly different, since these authors, by their methods, found very little calbindin immunoreactivity in the SN compacta, in contrast with the calbindin-rich catecholaminergic nerve cells in the ventral tegmental area, retrorubral area, and periaqueductal gray matter. Although they concluded that the calbindin-rich nerve cells appeared less vulnerable, they also pointed out that a number of calbindin-negative nerve cells in the SN compacta still survived, suggesting the role of other factors also in determining the degree and rate of death in these vulnerable neurons. Although proteins active in regulation of calcium and calcium channels might be expected to be particularly important, it is likely that any number of other substances in nerve cells contribute in either a positive or a negative direction to the health of the nerve cell.

Heavy Metals, Especially Iron. Many reports discuss the role played by iron accumulation in the SN (55–62). This is a controversial subject, with conflicting data. Iron has been increased in SN of PD brains in all the reports except one (62). These authors used atomic absorption and atomic emission spectroscopy and found no significant difference when comparing 9 PD brains with 12 control brains and 15 brains from patients with other neurological diseases. Sofic et al. (56) reported that mainly ferric iron was increased, with a higher ferric/ferrous ratio of iron than in control SN, and they suggested that this reversal may indicate that iron is present in a free state and, therefore, might participate in auto-oxidation of dopamine, with generation of hydrogen peroxide and free radicals. Disagreement exists over the iron-binding protein ferritin, which Jellinger et al. (60,63) and Sofic et al. (56) found to be increased in PD, whereas Dexter et al. (64) found it to be decreased.

Other controversies concern the location of the iron within the SN. Jellinger et al. (60,63), in studies of histological sections, found the increased iron in the SN compacta in astrocytes, macrophages, and reactive microglia; in nonpigmented neurons; and in areas with nerve cell loss. Sofic et al. (56) suggested that glia might play a role in PD. Hirsch et al. (59), on the other hand, using X-ray microanalysis, found high levels of iron in neuromelanin aggregates and in Lewy bodies, but in this study, as in studies on neuromelanin content (46) and calbindin(54), comparison was made between mainly periaqueductal gray and SN compacta. They were unable to state if the iron was actually located in or attached to the melanin pigment. The exact location of the metal is important for the etiology of PD because of the propensity of iron to generate free radicals and to bind to neuromelanin. Therefore, the question about the role of iron in the etiology of PD still needs clarification.

Neuropathologists, such as Jellinger, are well aware of the common finding of iron deposits in the SN, in older control brains, and in excessive amounts in Hallervorden–Spatz disease, but Jellinger points out that the increased iron in PD is located in the compact zone, and not in the reticulata where age-related iron tends to become deposited. Unfortunately, computed tomography (CT) scans and magnetic resonance imaging (MRI) are not of much help, since they would not be able to detect the cellular location of the metal.

However, two recent studies, (63,65) have convincingly shown that iron accumulates in neuromelanin in PD. Jellinger et al.(63), using an energy dispersive X-ray microanalysis, found increase in ferric iron in neuromelanin of PD patients, but not in controls. Lewy bodies did not contain iron. Good et al. (65) used the laser microprobe mass analyzer (LAMMA) and demonstrated accumulation of iron and aluminum in neuromelanin granules. It is still unclear if this accumulation is primary or secondary. Dexter et al. (66) not only found increased iron in other neurodegenerative disorders (e.g., MSA and PSP), but in PD, the accumulation of iron appeared not to be an early event, since no increase was found in brains from patients with presumed presymptomatic PD (they had Lewy bodies and slight SN nerve cell loss). Since the brain very readily accumulates heavy metals under pathological circumstances, one explanation for the accumulation of iron in neuromelanin would be the uptake of iron by ailing nerve cells, which would sequester the metal in phagolysosomes, which is where neuromelanin is found. Considerable skepticism about the role of iron in PD is still warranted.

Mitochondrial Toxins, Monoamine Oxidase, Free Radicals, and Such. This topic cannot be clearly separated from what has already been discussed concerning iron, but since most of the factors in question are difficult to evaluate in autopsy tissue sections, neuropathological studies have not as yet made important contributions. The subject has been discussed in detail in other chapters (see Chapters 4,6,7). Mizuno et al. (67,68) and Hattori et al. (69) did, however, use postmortem human tissue to examine mitochondrial enzymes in the striatum and in the SN. With immunocytochemistry and antibodies against complex I–IV they found complex I decrease in PD, with minor changes in complex II. The interest in complex I in PD partly derives from what has been learned from the study of the MPTP animal model for PD (70–76). The 1-methyl-4-phenylpyridinium ion (MPP^+), which is the active neurotoxin at work in this model, is a mitochondrial toxin, and becomes concentrated in the mitochondrion, where it disrupts the respiratory chain by its effect on complex I. Because the formation of MPP^+ is mediated by monoamine oxidase (MAO) B, present mainly in astrocytes, the conversion of MPTP to MPP^+ can be prevented by administration of MAO inhibitors. The attempt at slowing down the progression of human PD by using the MAO inhibitor selegiline is based partly on an analogy with MPTP-induced parkinsonism, but also on the ability of drugs such as selegiline to inhibit formation of free radicals. Free radicals may also have a deleterious effect on mitochondria.

Aging. It is well established that PD is a disease that mainly affects middle-aged and older persons. The average age of onset is usually given as 58–62 (77), but onset after aged 70 is not uncommon. Almost one-third of the PD patients in the study by Riederer and Wuketich (78) had an average age of onset of 73 years. Most patients develop PD between 50 and 79 years of age (77), and a great number of patients with PD are older than 70, but there is controversy over the incidence of PD in very old age, especially older than 90 (77). Mutch et al. (79) examined 267 community-based PD patients, with ages ranging from 40–92, and with average duration of the illness for 7 years. Eighty-three percent were older than 65 and, therefore, are likely to have developed the disease late in life, although age of onset was not given for this group. Reviews discussing the hypotheses for the etiology and pathogenesis of PD have multiplied as progress has been made in understanding and treating the disorder. Most of these articles include considerations given to the role of aging (78,80–90).

Aging and the nerve cell loss in SN expected with age is often seen only as the added element that pushes an already ailing dopaminergic nigrostriatal system beyond the threshold at which it produces overt parkinsonism (83,88). Fearnley and Lees (50) consider the aging process and the degenerative process in SN in PD as different and possibly unrelated events, because the nerve cell populations most vulnerable in PD appear to be relatively resistant to the effect of aging. This viewpoint, even if confirmed, does not deal with the issue: Why is PD mainly a disease of older individuals?

B. The Lewy Body

The Lewy body inclusion is a characteristic structure that appears to be closely linked to the nerve cell degeneration. If the molecular and biochemical events and the cytoskeletal changes that precede and accompany its formation can be unraveled, it may have implications for the pathogenesis of the nerve cell degeneration in PD.

1. Lewy Bodies and Aging: Lewy Body Disorders

When Lewy (9,10) described and illustrated inclusion bodies in the nucleus basalis of Meynert, the hypothalamus, and the dorsal motor nucleus of the vagus, he stated that he had seen these bodies only in PD; inexplicably, he did not attribute a great deal of importance to their presence. Since then, it has been amply documented (see Refs.29,33, and 91 for review) that Lewy bodies can occasionally be found in other neurodegenerative disorders, usually in connection with nerve cell loss in the SN, and in a percentage of aging individuals. Most remarkable are cases in whom Lewy bodies have been present in quite young individuals, for example, in a 17-year old-girl with neuroaxonal dystrophy (92), and in a case of subacute sclerosing panencephalitis (93), in whom no parkinsonism appears to have been present. Other recently published examples documenting the occurrence of Lewy bodies at a young age have had some parkinsonian symptomatology; for example, a 28-year-old man with dementia (94) and a 23-year-old woman with dopa-responsive dystonia (95). In most other situations Lewy bodies have been closely linked to age (34,35). Lewy bodies are frequently found in the brains of individuals without overt parkinsonism during life. Forno and Langston (35) found that Lewy bodies were present in 8% of persons older than 50. This percentage increased to 12.8% of those older than 70, and to 15.9% in those older than 80. It has been suggested (29,34,91) that in the elderly, the presence of Lewy bodies represents subclinical or presymptomatic PD. Since "incidental" Lewy body cases are much more common in routine autopsy material than PD cases with Lewy bodies, this suggests that a large percentage of the elderly population may be at risk for developing PD. Whether the presence of Lewy bodies always indicates a progressive nerve cell degeneration, such as in PD, is unknown.

In cases of clinically typical PD, in spite of this lack of specificity Lewy bodies are sufficiently common that they can be considered highly characteristic for the disorder. Recently, the status of the Lewy body and its importance as a marker for PD has been questioned, after the discovery that Lewy bodies are sometimes present, not only outside the brainstem in the nucleus basalis of Meynert and hypothalamus, where Lewy described them, but in the cerebral cortex, especially in limbic cortical areas. Such cases, which have been called diffuse Lewy body disease or Lewy body dementia (96), have been associated with varying degrees of SN degeneration, on one hand, and Alzheimer-like lesions on the other. Clinically, dementia is usually the prominent feature. Although parkinsonism is not always present in Lewy body dementia (97) there is a close connection to PD abnormalities, since Lewy bodies are always present in the SN or LC. The discovery of the frequent association of AD and Lewy bodies, especially cortical Lewy bodies, has been a result of the recently heightened interest and awareness of AD and of Lewy bodies. In many studies (98,99), the percentage of AD cases with Lewy bodies has been 25% or more, and the term *Lewy body variant of AD* has been coined for such cases (30). An even higher proportion of AD brains with Lewy bodies (57% for the substantia nigra and 66% for the locus coeruleus) was recently reported by Jellinger (100) in a very large series of more than 500 AD brains.

The use of the term *diffuse Lewy body disease* has given rise to some confusion, since some authors include AD with Lewy bodies as part of diffuse Lewy body disease, whereas others confine the term to cases without overt PD and without sufficient Alzheimer-like lesions for a diagnosis of AD (101). The discovery of a spectrum of Lewy body disorders has made some of us suspect a closer relation between AD and PD, and between Lewy bodies and Alzheimer is disease than previously thought possible (102). This may be of importance for studies of the etiology of these two diseases. A connection between Lewy bodies and AD is also suggested by the contribution AD cases make to incidental Lewy body statistics (35,101). The relation between AD and PD has been addressed from a neurochemical viewpoint by Whitehouse (103), who found similar reductions in nicotinic cholinergic receptors and in corticotropin-releasing factor and neuropeptide Y immunoreactivity in the two diseases.

2. *Morphology, Including Immunocytochemistry and Ultrastructure of Lewy Bodies*

Although it is not known how often formation of Lewy bodies precede the nerve cell degeneration in PD, studies of the composition and the mechanism of formation of Lewy bodies are relevant to the etiology of PD. Greenfield and Bosanquet (7), described the morphology and general staining reactions. Bethlem and den Hartog Jager (104) performed various histochemical procedures on Lewy body-containing tissues and demonstrated that the inclusions were composed of mainly protein and did not contain DNA or RNA. They (105) also described Lewy bodies in sympathetic ganglia in five of six cases of PD with Lewy bodies in the brainstem. Similar to the Lewy bodies first illustrated and described by Lewy (9,10), many of the inclusions in the sympathetic ganglia were elongated sausage-shaped structures, which seemed to be located extracellularly, but actually were within nerve cell processes.

Duffy and Tennyson (106) first examined Lewy bodies in SN and LC from PD brains by electron microscopy. They found a composition of filamentous material, 7–20 nm wide, radiating out from a denser central core and ending, without a membrane, among the neuromelanin granules. A more variable ultrastructure was later found to be present in Lewy bodies in sympathetic ganglia (107). In 1983, Goldman et al.(108) demonstrated that antibodies to neurofilaments had antigenic sites in common with Lewy bodies. Subsequently, Lewy bodies have also been shown to react strongly with antibodies to ubiquitin, a 76-amino acid protein that is involved in ATP-dependent proteolysis. Newer data on neuronal cytoskeletal abnormalities of Lewy bodies have been reviewed by Jellinger (109). He emphasized pathological phosphorylation of neurofilaments along with ubiquitination, but cautioned that the relation of Lewy bodies to neuromelanin and to nerve cell degeneration is still unknown. Gibb et al.(110) have also reviewed our present knowledge on Lewy bodies.

To summarize some of the characteristics of the Lewy body: this inclusion is a spherical or sometimes oblong or elongated structure, consisting of mainly cytoskeletal proteins in the form of filaments. In the classic Lewy body, which is the most common form in the SN and LC, the filaments radiate out from an electron-dense core (Fig. 2). In some locations, including the cerebral cortex, the filamentous material is randomly oriented, and other cell constituents may be included or perhaps trapped within the inclusion. The Lewy body may be located not only in the perikaryon of nerve cells, but also in nerve cell processes. The perikaryal site is most common in the SN and LC, the raphe nuclei, and the cerebral cortex, whereas elongated forms in nerve cell processes are more often seen in the nucleus basalis of Meynert, hypothalamus, dorsal motor nucleus of the vagus, and sympathetic ganglia.

The Lewy body is easily recognized in routine hematoxylin and eosin-stained sections, where it presents as a pink or slightly polychromatophilic body, with a more intensely staining core and a peripheral halo. Lewy bodies are rarely

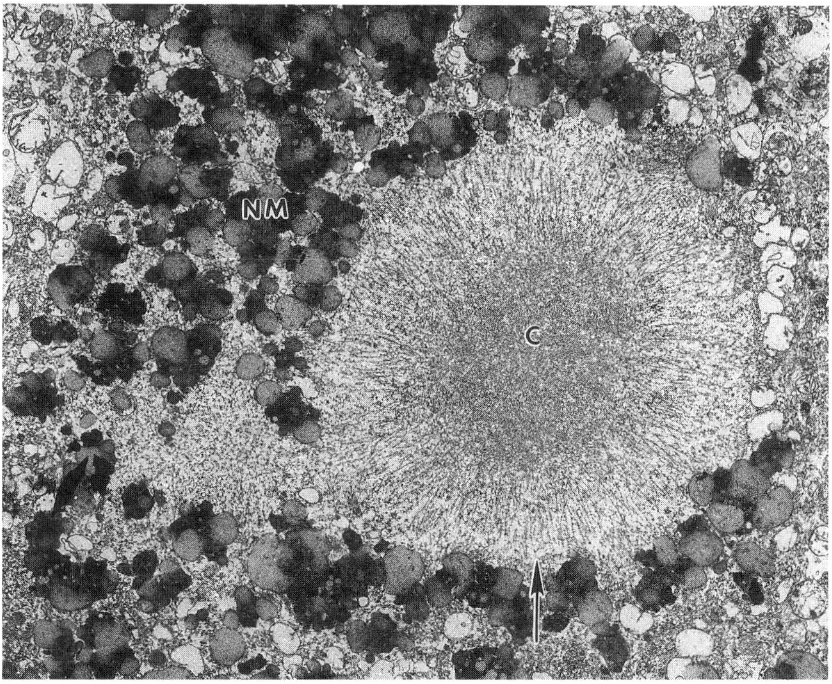

Figure 2 Ultrastructure of a Lewy body in the substantia nigra. It has a dense core (C), has radiating filaments (arrow), and is surrounded by neuromelanin (× 5500).

plentiful enough for isolation and direct biochemical analysis, but numerous attempts at analyzing the inclusion with immunocytochemical and ultrastructural, including immunoelectron microscopic, methods have been made, especially during the last decade. Only those papers that promise insights into the molecular events responsible for the formation of the Lewy body and may lead to dissection of the mechanism involved in the death of the nerve cell will be discussed.

The immunocytochemical studies have continued to emphasize the significant contribution of cytoskeletal elements and, especially, neurofilaments, to the formation of the Lewy body (see Refs. 109 and 111 for review). One important finding has been that the microtubule associated protein (MAP) *tau*, an important component of neurofibrillary tangles and Pick bodies, usually does not react with Lewy bodies. This negative reaction has been thought to be helpful in separating globose tangles, for example, in the amygdala, from Lewy bodies, but there is now some evidence that this distinction is less absolute than originally thought (112,113).

An animal model for producing Lewy bodies would be helpful (73). The inclusions that have been produced in aging MPTP-treated squirrel monkeys (114) usually lack a central core, and only one inclusion per nerve cell is present, in contrast with the frequent multiplicity of Lewy bodies in PD. The MPTP-induced inclusions are probably stress-related and may be reversible. Although their relation to Lewy bodies is as yet uncertain, there is some evidence that the formation of Lewy bodies may also be an active process. Lewy bodies tend to be more numerous in recently diagnosed PD cases, and in some of the AD brains with Lewy bodies, than in long-standing, slowly progressive cases (unpublished personal observation). Lowe et al.(115) have made the same suggestion, based on studies with ubiquitin hydrolases.

The work done on the relation between normal neurofilaments and the filaments in the Lewy bodies, on one hand, and on the role of ubiquitin and ubiquitin hydrolases on the other, can be viewed as some of the more important recent developments in Lewy body research. Duffy and Tennyson (106), who first examined Lewy bodies by electron microscopy, remarked on the similarity between neurofilaments and the filamentous material in the Lewy body. This association was strengthened when antibodies to neurofilaments became available and were found to react with epitopes in Lewy bodies (108).

Because the fixatives used are important for the reaction of many antibodies, not all antibodies to neurofilaments will react with routinely processed, formalin-fixed and paraffin-embedded material. The most detailed examination yet of neurofilaments and Lewy bodies has been performed by Hill et al.(116). They used 37 well-characterized antibodies to neurofilaments and determined to what extent the three subunits were represented by epitopes in the Lewy body. They found that all 37 antibodies reacted with the Lewy body, but that they differed in the site of the reaction within the inclusion. Their conclusion was that the entire extent of each neurofilament subunit appears to be represented in the Lewy body, but that some alterations of the subunits might take place in the course of the formation of the inclusion. However, it is, puzzling that the *tau*-positive cytoskeletal elements in Pick bodies, inclusions characteristically present in Pick's disease, a rare dementia with lobar atrophy, react much more intensely with antibodies to phosphorylated neurofilaments than do Lewy bodies (117).

Equally exciting have been the developments resulting from studies of ubiquitin, a 76-amino acid protein, that is highly conserved during evolution and that has epitopes on several intraneuronal inclusions, such as neurofibrillary tangles, Pick bodies, and especially, Lewy bodies (see Refs. 109,118, and 119 for review). Ubiquitin is conjugated with short-lived proteins that are earmarked for destruction, but it is also a stress (heat-shock) protein, which might have a protective function in the nerve cell. Therefore, there may be more than one explanation for its role in formation of Lewy bodies.

Lowe and associates have reported (115) that a ubiquitin hydrolase (PGP 9.5) reacts differently with Lewy bodies than with neurofibrillary tangles; they reasoned that the positive reaction in the Lewy body points to a more active process than the one in the neurofibrillary tangles. Kwak et al.(120), working with a multicatalytic protease, which also is involved in ATP–ubiquitin-mediated proteolysis, have come to a very similar conclusion, since their antibody reacts with Lewy bodies and loosely arranged globose tangles, but not with compact neurofibrillary tangles. These authors feel, as does Lowe et al., that studies of the biological role of these proteases may help us understand how inclusions, such as Lewy bodies, are formed. Iwatsubo et al.(121) have found a positive immunoreaction with a protein kinase (Ca^{2+}–calmodulin-dependent protein kinase II), which can phosphorylate neurofilaments and other cytoskeletal proteins. Since phosphorylation of proteins is a widespread tool for modulation of protein function (122) and may contribute to the distribution and conformation of proteins, this might also have implications for the formation of inclusions, such as the Lewy body.

Further developments have involved direct analysis of Lewy body fibrils (summarized in Ref. 123). In an ultrastructural and biochemical analysis of Lewy bodies in the SN and LC (124), the filaments, but not the core, of Lewy bodies were insoluble to ionic detergents such as sodium dodecyl sulfate (SDS). This is in contrast to the SDS-soluble normal neurofilaments, but similar to the neurofibrillary tangles of AD. The possibility that Lewy body filaments might be composed of markedly altered neurofilaments was mentioned. Pollanen et al.(125) used a different approach. They isolated Lewy body fibrils from cortical Lewy bodies, taking advantage of the insolubility of these fibrils. They found that the main component of the cortical Lewy body was a 68-kDa species that reacted with polyclonal antibody to both *tau* and neurofilament, and was thought to contain proteolytic fragments of neurofilaments. They speculated that the

68-kDa neurofilament might be a truncated and altered form of the 170-kDa neurofilament. Pollanen et al.(123) have proposed that Lewy bodies form in three overlapping steps, involving, first, self-assembly and aggregation of protein, followed by posttranslational phosphorylation and, last, proteolysis. They suggested that the ubiquitination of Lewy bodies is a late stage, and that the colocalization of neurofilament and ubiquitin epitopes in the Lewy bodies indicates that the insoluble Lewy body neurofilaments are the proteins destined for proteolysis.

This is a rapidly evolving field of study with more intriguing information to be expected in the near future.

A final note with possible relevance to the discussion of the relation between PD and AD can be added. This is the finding that an antibody to a gelsolin variant reacts with Lewy bodies (126). Antibodies to the actin-modulating protein gelsolin, which differs from the variant by a single amino acid substitution, does not react with Lewy bodies. The gelsolin variant is of interest because it is the amyloid protein found in familial amyloidosis, Finnish type, an age-associated form of amyloidosis. Nevertheless, although different from the β-amyloid of AD, there might be unexpected connections to this amyloid. The patient in whom this was first found was demented and had β-amyloid plaques in the brain.

IV. THE STRIATUM

The various agents so far discussed have been chosen mainly because of their potential for damage to nerve cells in the SN, leaving out of the discussion not only the important noradrenergic locus coeruleus (127) and the cholinergic nucleus basalis of Meynert, but also the striatum, the destination for the dopaminergic nigrostriatal nerve fibers. Although several studies have contributed to our understanding of the chemical neuroanatomy of the striatum, they have not as yet given us an important clue to the etiology of PD; therefore, most of them are not discussed in this chapter. This should not be taken to detract from the important advances that have been made in understanding the neurophysiology and the connections of the basal ganglia, the role of neuropeptides, or the striatal mosaic.

We do not as yet know enough about what happens in dopaminergic terminals and their targets in the human disease. For the neuropathologist, whose routine diagnostic methods do not reveal the exciting events in the striatum, the SN, with its obvious nerve cell loss and inclusion bodies in PD, is a more tempting target to aim at for clues to the etiology of PD, but it is still a possibility that the disease process might originate in the terminals of the nigrostriatal tract, as recently suggested by Hornykiewicz (128). He pointed to a mismatch between striatal and SN dopamine loss in PD, with the decrease in striatum more marked than in SN, and a similar discrepancy between striatal dopamine loss and nerve cell loss in SN.

If the dopamine terminals in the basal ganglia are the main target of the disease process, the death of the nerve cell bodies might then be caused by (a) retrograde degeneration; (b) retrograde transport of an extrinsic or intrinsic neurotoxin; or (c) deprivation of a growth factor or other vital element. The loss of such a factor, perhaps derived from postsynaptic structures, might send a signal to the nerve cell perikaryon and initiate a death program. If there is clear evidence that terminals are first affected, the events in the striatum in PD will need more detailed scrutiny, also from the neuropathologist. The old hypothesis for several neuropathies and other neurodegenerative diseases of a "dying-back" process, assumed that the nerve cell body somehow was unable to supply the terminals with the necessary metabolites, although the nerve cell perikaryon might be morphologically intact. Nowadays, other explanations are also possible and, perhaps, equally plausible.

If we assume for a moment that the disease process responsible for PD attacks the dopamine terminals in the neostriatum before the cell bodies, it becomes important to be able to recognize the dopamine terminal. The character of the dopaminergic synaptic terminal in the striatum has for many years been controversial. For a time, it was thought that the dopamine innervation exerted a rather nonspecific modulation of the activity of striatal neurons. There is now convincing evidence (see Ref. 129 for review), that medium spiny output neurons in the striatum receive symmetrical inputs on their distal dendritic spines and shafts from dopaminergic terminals. Since the same dendritic spines also receive an asymmetrical (excitatory) input from the cortex, this arrangement may permit important interactions between these two afferent systems. Major difficulties will have to be overcome before it becomes possible to study the disease process in the terminals and in their postsynaptic receptors in the human brain. It may, however, be feasible in experimental MPTP-induced parkinsonism, for which dopamine terminals are generally thought to be involved before nerve cell bodies (130). The morphological changes in the dopamine terminals in PD are of interest, regardless of where the disease process starts.

Recent advances in the understanding of the circuits involved in information processing and control of movement in the basal ganglia may also be relevant to the etiology of PD. In a recent review Parent and Hazrati (131) emphasized the complexity of the circuitry of the primate basal ganglia. They felt that the organization cannot be reduced to either multiple, functionally segregated, parallel circuits, or to a convergence of functionally distinct inputs within the striatopallidonigral projection system. The current ideas about the influence of the subthalamic nucleus on the movement disorder in PD are largely based on the concept of a direct and an indirect striatopallidal pathway to the SN, with loss of dopamine neurons in the SN, resulting in an increase in the excitatory output from the subthalamic nucleus.

The important biochemical observation by Hornykiewicz and associates (13,132) that the putamen is more affected by the dopamine deficiency than the caudate nucleus, has a structural correlate in the MPTP-treated squirrel monkey. Moratella et al. (133) used radioautographic labeling of monoamine uptake sites and found greater loss of uptake sites in the putamen than in the striatum. In human PD, the special vulnerability of ventral SN neurons, which project to the putamen, is consistent with the greater importance of the putamen for PD than that of the caudate nucleus. The affinity of the disease process in PD for the putamen also has implications for the selection of the most favorable site for transplantation of tissue for dopamine cell replacement in PD (134).

Scherman et al. (85) have published an interesting study on the role of aging on striatal dopamine deficiency in PD, which used PD and control autopsy material. They found that a specific ligand of the vesicular monoamine transporter was reduced in the striatum with age, as well as in PD. The reduction was greater in PD than with age, but the authors concluded that aging did not play a major role in the process of nigrostriatal neuron degeneration, since the reduction in ligand binding was not increased in late-, compared with early-onset, PD. These findings may be open to different interpretations.

Excitotoxic mechanisms in the etiology of PD have briefly been mentioned in connection with the organization of the circuits in the basal ganglia and the role played by the excitatory output (glutamatergic) of the subthalamic nucleus. Excitotoxins have most often been discussed in connection with Huntington's disease and with ischemic brain disease. Beal (135) has reviewed the role of impairment of energy metabolism in excitotoxic neuronal death in neurodegenerative disease. He pointed out that impaired ATP, induced by a toxin such as MPP^+, in experimental parkinsonism, might result in excitotoxic neuronal death caused by partial membrane depolarization and relief of the block on the *N*-methy-D-aspartate (NMDA) receptor. Although Turski et al. (136) were able to prevent MPTP-induced neuronal death by administration of NMDA antagonists, it is unclear as yet what role excitotoxicity plays in nerve cell death in the SN in the slowly progressive human disease.

V. DIRECTIONS FOR FUTURE RESEARCH

Most likely, the greatest progress in our understanding of the etiology of PD will be coming from molecular neurobiology, for which many new techniques are now available. For neuropathology, much remains to be learned about the way nerve cells die and how the formation of inclusion bodies is involved in this process. The methods used in the recent studies described in the section on morphology (including immunocytochemistry and ultrastructure) involving protein kinases active in phosphorylation of neurofilaments and other proteins, and the various other factors responsible for protein folding (stress proteins, chaperonins, and others) appear to provide the most promising avenues to follow. Since immunocytochemistry, including immunoelectron microscopy, will play a role in such studies, this will also leave room for those neuropathologists who are not molecular neurobiologists to contribute their share.

There are considerable limitations for what routine neuropathological examination will be able to contribute to an understanding of the etiology of PD, but most biochemical and molecular events have structural correlates that can be demonstrated, once the right tools are in place. In situ hybridization and polymerase chain reaction (PCR) are methods increasingly being used, and since they usually require tissue samples, the neuropathologist is in an ideal position to take advantage of these new methods, in the same way light and electron microscopic immunocytochemistry have been put to use. Hill and associates (137) recently used in situ hybridization immunocytochemistry in postmortem tissue from PD and control brains for semiquantitative studies of neurofilament mRNA: it was diminished in the SN compacta in PD brains, especially in Lewy body-containing neurons. Although often neuropathologists will be able to examine structural alterations after a biochemical or molecular finding has pointed to their existence, there are also situations during which pathological studies have led to a search for the underlying molecular events. This has been true for amyloid in the neuritic plaques and for neurofibrillary tangles and now also for the Lewy body. The fact that it has become possible to propose a scheme for the stages in the development of Lewy bodies (123) shows how far we have come by morphological methods. Neuropathology cannot provide the full explanation of the etiology of PD, but the riddle of this disorder is not likely to be solved without some help from neuropathology.

ACKNOWLEGMENTS

This chapter is based on work supported by the Veterans Affairs Medical Research Program.

REFERENCES

1. Brissaud E. Lecons sur les maladies nerveuses. Paris: Masson et Cie, 1895.
2. Stern G. The effects of lesions in the substantia nigra. Brain 1966; 89:449–478.
3. Ehringer H, Hornykiewicz O. Verteilung von Noradrenalin und Dopamin (3-Hydroxytyramin) in Gehirn des Menschen und ihr Verhalten bei Erkrankungen des extrapyramidalen Systems. Klin Wochenschr 1960; 38:1236–1239.
4. Anden NE, Carlsson A, Dahlstrom A, Fuxe K, Hillarp NA, Larsson K. Demonstration and mapping out of nigro-neostriatal dopamine neurons. Life Sci 1964; 3:523–530.

5. Trétiakoff C. Contribution a l'etude de l'anatomie pathologique du locus niger de Soemmering avec quelques deductions relatives a la pathogenie des troubles du tonus musculaire et de la maladie de Parkinson. 1919.
6. Hassler R. Zur Pathologie der Paralysis agitans und des postenzephalitischen Parkinsonismus. J Psychol Neurol 1938; 48:387–476.
7. Greenfield JG, Bosanquet PD. The brainstem lesion in parkinsonism. J Neurol Neurosurg Psychiatry 1953; 16:213–226.
8. Freeman W. The pathology of paralysis agitans. Ann Clin Med 1925; 4:106–116.
9. Lewy FH. Paralysis agitans. I Pathologische anatomie. In: Lewandowsky M, ed. Handbuch der Neurologie. Berlin: Springer, 1912:920–933.
10. Lewy FH. Die Lehre vom Tonus und der Bewegung. Berlin: Springer, 1923.
11. Cotzias GC, Van Woert MH, Schiffer LM. Aromatic amino acids and modification of Parkinsonism. N Engl J Med 1967; 276:374–379.
12. Bernheimer H, Birkmayer W, Hornykiewicz O, Jellinger K, Seitelberger F. Brain dopamine and the syndromes of Parkinson and Huntington. J Neurol Sci 1973; 20:415–455.
13. Kish SJ, Shannak K, Hornykiewicz O. Uneven pattern of dopamine loss in the striatum of patients with idiopathic Parkinson's disease: pathophysiologic and clinical implications. N Engl J Med 1988; 318:876–880.
14. Jellinger KA, Bancher C. Neuropathology. In: Litvan I, Agid Y, eds. Progressive supranuclear palsy. Clinical and research approaches. New York: Oxford University Press, 1992:44–88.
15. Fearnley JM, Lees AJ. Striatonigral degeneration. A clinicopathological study. Brain 1990; 113:1823–1842.
16. Quinn N. Disproportionate antecollis in multiple system atrophy. Lancet 1989; 1:844.
17. Kurland LT. Amyotrophic lateral sclerosis and Parkinson's disease complex on Guam linked to an environmental neurotoxin. Trends V Neurosci 1988; 11:51–54.
18. Kurtzke JF, Murphy FM. The changing patterns of death rates in parkinsonism. Neurology 1990; 40:42–49.
19. Poskanzer DC, Schwab RS. Cohort analysis of Parkinson's syndrome. Evidence for a single etiology related to subclinical infection about 1920. J Chronic Dis 1963; 16:961–973.
20. Spencer PS, Ross SM, Kisby G, Roy DN, Nunn PB. Western Pacific parkinsonism–dementia complex: role of plant neurotoxic factors. Ninth international symposium on Parkinson's disease, 1988:10.
21. Spencer PS, Nunn PB, Hugon J, et al. Guam amyotrophic lateral sclerosis–parkinsonism–dementia linked to a plant excitant neurotoxin. Science 1987; 237:517–522.
22. Hirano A, Malamud N, Kurland LT. Parkinsonism–dementia complex, an endemic disease on the island of Guam. II. Pathological features. Brain 1961; 84:662–679.
23. Elizan TS, Hirano A, Abrams BM, Need RL, Van Nuis C, Kurland LT. Amyotrophic lateral sclerosis and parkinsonism–dementia complex of Guam. Neurological reevaluation. Arch Neurol 1966; 14:356–368.
24. Hirano A, Malamud N, Elizan TS, Kurland LT. Amyotrophic lateral sclerosis and

parkinsonism–dementia complex of Guam: further pathologic studies. Arch Neurol 1966; 15:35–51.
25. Corsellis JAN, Bruton CJ, Freeman-Browne D. The aftermath of boxing. Psychol Med 1973; 3:270–303.
26. Klawans HL, Lupton M, Simon L. Calcification of the basal ganglia as a cause of levodopa-resistant parkinsonism. Neurology 1976; 26:221–225.
27. Agid Y. Conclusions. In: Litvan I, Agid Y, eds. Progressive supranuclear palsy. Clinical and research approaches. New York: Oxford University Press, 1992:270–273.
28. Bannister R, Oppenheimer DR. Degenerative disease of the nervous system associated with autonomic failure. Brain 1972; 95:457–474.
29. Gibb WRG, Lees AJ. The relevance of the Lewy body to the pathogenesis of idiopathic Parkinson's disease. J Neurol Neurosurg Psychiatry 1988; 51:745–752.
30. Hansen L, Salmon D, Galasko D, et al. The Lewy body variant of Alzheimer's disease: A clinical and pathological entity. Neurology 1990; 40:1–8.
31. Gibb WRG, Esiri MM, Lees AJ. Clinical and pathological features of diffuse cortical Lewy body disease (Lewy body dementia). Brain 1985; 110:1131–1153.
32. Barbeau A. Parkinson's disease: clinical features and etiopanthology. In: Vinken PJ, Bruyn GW, Klawans HL, eds. Handbook of clinical neurology, vol. 5. Extrapyramidal disorders. Amsterdam: Elsevier Science Publishers, 1986:87–152.
33. Forno LS. The Lewy body in Parkinson's disease. In: Parkinson's disease. Adv Neurol 1986; 45:35–43.
34. Forno LS. Concentric hyalin intraneuronal inclusions of Lewy type in the brains of elderly persons (50 incidental cases): relationship to parkinsonism. J Am Geriatr Soc 1969; 17:557–575.
35. Forno LS, Langston JW. Lewy bodies and aging: relation to Alzheimer's and Parkinson's diseases. Neurodegeneration 1993; 2:19–24.
36. Marsden CD. Neuromelanin and Parkinson's disease. J Neural Transm [Suppl] 1983; 19:121–141.
37. Forno LS. Pathology of Parkinson's disease, the importance of the substantia nigra and the Lewy bodies. In: Stern G, ed. Parkinson's disease. London: Chapman & Hall, 1990:185–238.
38. Graham DG. Oxidative pathways for catecholamines in the genesis of neuromelanin and cytotoxic quinones. Mol Pharmacol 1978; 14:633–643.
39. Graham DG. On the origin and significance of neuromelanin. Arch Pathol Lab Med 1979; 103:359–362.
40. D'Amato RJ, Lipman ZP, Snyder SH. Selectivity of the parkinsonian neurotoxin MPTP: toxic metabolite MPP^+ binds to neuromelanin. Science 1986; 231:987–989.
41. Snyder SH, D'Amato RJ. MPTP: a neurotoxin relevant to the pathophysiology of Parkinson's disease. Neurology 1986; 36:250–258.
42. Carstam R, Brinck C, Hindemith-Augustsson A, Rorsman H, Rosengren E. The neuromelanin of the human substantia nigra. Biochim Biophys Acta 1991; 1097:152–160.
43. Mann DMA, Yates PO. Lipoprotein pigments—their relationship to ageing in the

human nervous system—II. The melanin content of pigmented nerve cells. Brain 1974; 97:489–498.
44. Mann DMA, Yates PO. Pathological basis for neurotransmitter changes in Parkinson's disease. Neuropathol Appl Neurobiol 1983; 8:3–19.
45. Porta EA. Advances in pigment research. Arch Gerontol Geriatr 1991; 12:303–320.
46. Hirsch EC, Graybiel AM, Agid Y. Selective vulnerability of pigmented dopaminergic neurons in Parkinson's disease. Acta Neurol Scand [Suppl] 1989; 126:19–22.
47. Graybiel AM, Hirsch EC, Agid Y. The nigrostriatal system in Parkinson's disease. In: Streifler MD, Korczyn AD, Melamed E, Youdim MBH, eds. Parkinson's disease: anatomy, pathology and therapy. Adv Neurol 1990; 53:17–29.
48. Gibb WRG, Fearnley JM, Lees AJ. The anatomy and pigmentation of the human substantia nigra in relation to selective neuronal vulnerability. In: Streifler MB, Korczyn AD, Melamed E, Youdim MBH, eds. Parkinson's disease: antomy, pathology and therapy. Adv Neurol 1990; 53:31–34.
49. German DC, Manaye K, Smith WK, Woodward DJ, Saper CB. Midbrain dopaminergic cell loss in Parkinson's disease: computer visualization. Ann Neurol 1989; 26:507–514.
50. Fearnley JM, Lees AJ. Ageing and Parkinson's disease; substantia nigra regional selectivity. Brain 1991; 114:2283–2301.
51. Eadie MJ. Pathology of certain medullary nuclei in parkinsonism. Brain 1963; 86:781–792.
52. Yamada T, McGeer PL, Baimbridge KG, McGeer EG. Relative sparing in Parkinson's disease of substantia nigra dopamine neurons containing calbindin-D28K. Brain Res 1990; 526:303–307.
53. German DC, Manaye KF, Sonsalla PK, Brooks BA. Midbrain dopaminergic cell loss in Parkinson's disease and MPTP-induced parkinsonism. Sparing of calbindin D28K-containing cells. Ann NY Acad Sci 1992; 648:42–62.
54. Hirsch EC, Mouatt A, Thomasset M, Javoy-Agid F, Agid Y, Graybiel AM. Expression of calbindin D28K-like immunoreactivity in catecholaminergic cell groups in the human midbrain. Normal distribution and distribution in Parkinson's disease. Neurodegeneration 1992; 1:83–93.
55. Youdim MB, Ben-Shachar D, Riederer P. Is Parkinson's disease a progressive siderosis of substantia nigra resulting in iron and melanin induced neurodegeneration. Acta Neurol Scand [Suppl] 1989; 126:47–54.
56. Sofic E, Paulus W, Jellinger K, Riederer P, Youdim MB. Selective increase of iron in substantia nigra zona compacta of parkinsonian brains. J Neurochem 1991; 56:978–982.
57. Dexter DT, Wells FR, Lees AJ, et al. Increased nigral iron content and alterations in other metal ions occurring in brain in Parkinson's disease. J Neurochem 1989; 52:1830–1836.
58. Riederer P, Sofic E, Rausch WD, et al. Transition metals, ferritin, glutathione, and ascorbic acid in parkinsonian brains. J Neurochem 1989; 52:515–520.
59. Hirsch EC, Brandel JP, Galle P, Javoy-Agid F, Agid Y. Iron and aluminum increase in the substantia nigra of patients with Parkinson's disease: an X-ray microanalysis. J Neurochem 1991; 56:446–451.

60. Jellinger K, Paulus W, Grundke-Iqbal I, Riederer P, Youdim MB. Brain iron and ferritin in Parkinson's and Alzheimer's diseases. J Neural Transm Park Dis Dement Sect 1990; 2:327–340.
61. Olanow CW. Oxidation reactions in Parkinson's disease. Neurology 1990; 40(suppl):32–37.
62. Uitti RJ, Rajput AH, Rozdilsky B, Bickis M, Wollin T, Yuen WK. Regional metal concentration in Parkinson's diseases other chronic neurological diseases, and control brains. Can J Neurol Sci 1989; 16:310–314.
63. Jellinger KA, Kienzl E, Rumpelmaier G, et al. Iron and ferritin in substantia nigra in Parkinson's disease. In: Narabayashi H, Nagatsu T, Yanagisawa N, Mizuno Y, eds. Parkinson's disease: from basic research to treatment. Adv Neurol 1993; 60:267–272.
64. Dexter DT, Carayon A, Vidailhet M, et al. Decreased ferritin levels in Parkinson's disease. J Neurochem 1990; 55:16–20.
65. Good PF, Olanow CW, Perl DP. Neuromelanin-containing neurons of the substantia nigra accumulate iron and aluminum in Parkinson's disease: a LAMMA study. Brain Res 1992; 593:343–346.
66. Dexter DT, Sian J, Jenner P, Marsden CD. Implications of alterations in trace element levels in brain in Parkinson's disease and other neurological disorders affecting the basal ganglia. In: Narabayashi H, Nagatsu T, Yanagisawa N, Mizuno Y, eds. Parkinson's disease: from basic research to treatment. Adv Neurol 1993; 60:273–281.
67. Mizuno Y, Suzuki K, Ohta S. Postmortem changes in mitochondrial respiratory enzymes in brain and a preliminary observation in Parkinson's disease. J Neurol Sci 1990; 96:49–57.
68. Mizuno Y, Ohta S, Tanaka M, et al. Mitochondrial complex I deficiency in Parkinson's disease and MPTP-induced Parkinsonism [abstract]. Mov Disord 1990; 5:30.
69. Hattori N, Tanaka M, Ozawa T, Mizuno Y. Immunohistochemical studies on complexes I, II, III, and IV of mitochondria in Parkinson's disease. Ann Neurol 1991; 30:563–571.
70. Koller WC. Paraquat and Parkinson's disease [letter]. Neurology 1986; 36:1147.
71. Langston JW. Mechanisms underlying neuronal degeneration in Parkinson's disease: an experimental and theoretical treatise. Mov Disord 1989; 4:S15–S25.
72. Lewin R. Environmental hypothesis for brain diseases strengthened by new data. Science 1987; 237:483–484.
73. Forno LS, Langston JW, DeLanney LE, Irwin I, Ricaurte GA. Locus ceruleus lesions and eosinophilic inclusions in MPTP-treated monkeys. Ann Neurol 1986; 20:449–455.
74. Sandyk R, Iacono RP. The neurotoxicity of MPTP and its relationship to the pathophysiology of Parkinson's disease. Int J Neurosci 1989; 44:165–167.
75. Stern Y. MPTP-induced parkinsonism. Prog Neurobiol 1990; 34:107–114.
76. McCrodden JM, Tipton KF, Sullivan JP. The neurotoxicity of MPTP and the relevance to Parkinson's disease. Pharmacol Toxicol 1990; 67:8–13.
77. Marttila RJ. Epidemiology. In: Koller WC, ed. Handbook of Parkinson's disease. New York: Marcell Dekker, 1992:35–57.

78. Riederer P, Wuketich S. Time course of nigrostriatal degeneration in Parkinson's disease. J Neural Transm 1976; 38:277–301.
79. Mutch WJ, Strudwick A, Roy SK, Downie AW. Parkinson's disease: disability, review, and management. Br Med J 1986; 293:675–677.
80. Calne DB, Duvoisin RC, McGeer E. Speculations on the etiology of Parkinson's disease. In: Hassler RG, Christ JF, eds. Parkinson-specific motor and mental disorders, role of the pallidum: pathophysiological, biochemical, and therapeutic aspects. 1984;40:353–360.
81. Calne DB, Langston JW. Aetiology of Parkinson's disease. Lancet 1983; 2:1457–1459.
82. Calne DB, Peppard RF. Aging of the nigrostriatal pathway in humans. Can J Neurol Sci 1987; 14:424–427.
83. Calne DB. Current concepts on the etiology of Parkinson's disease. Mov Disord 1989; 4:S11–S14.
84. Calne S, Schoenberg BS, Martin W, Uitti RJ, Spencer P, Calne DB. Familial Parkinson's disease: possible role of environmental factors. Can J Neurol Sci 1987; 14:303–305.
85. Scherman D, Desnos C, Darchen F, Pollak P, Javoy-Agid F, Agid Y. Striatal dopamine deficiency in Parkinson's disease: role of aging. Ann Neurol 1989; 26:551–557.
86. Langston JW. Parkinson's disease: current view. Am Fam Physician 1987; 35:201–206.
87. Langston JW. Current theories on the cause of Parkinson's disease. J Neurol Neurosurg Psychiatry 1989; 52(Special Suppl):13–17.
88. Thiessen B, Rajput AH, Laverty W, Desai H. Age, environments, and the number of substantia nigra neurons. In: Parkinson's disease: anatomy, pathology and therapy. Neurol 1990; 50:201–206.
89. Burton K, Calne DB. Aetiology of Parkinson's disease. In: Stern GM, ed. Parkinson's disease. Baltimore: Johns Hopkins University Press, 1990:269–293.
90. Duvoisin RC. Etiology of Parkinson's disease: current concepts. Clin Neuropharmacol 1986; 9:S3–21.
91. Gibb WRG, Lees AJ. The significance of the Lewy body in the diagnosis of idiopathic Parkinson's disease. Neuropathol Appl Neurobiol 1989; 15:27–44.
92. Defendini R, Markesbery WR, Mastri AR, Duffy PE. Hallervorden–Spatz disease and infantile neuroaxonal dystrophy. J Neurol Sci 1973; 20:7–23.
93. Cobb WA, Marshall J, Scaravilli F. Long survival in subacute sclerosing panencephalitis. J Neurol Neurosurg Psychiatry 1984; 47:176–183.
94. Popovitch ER, Wisniewski HM, Kaufman MA, Grundke-Iqbal I, Wen GY. Young adult-form of dementia with neurofibrillary changes and Lewy bodies. Acta Neuropathol (Berl) 1987; 74:97–104.
95. Olsson JE, Brunk U, Lindvall B, Eeg-Olofsson O. Dopa-responsive dystonia with depigmentation of the substantia nigra and formation of Lewy bodies. J Neurol Sci 1992; 112:90–95.
96. Kosaka K, Yoshimura M, Ikeda K, Budka H. Diffuse type of Lewy body disease: progressive dementia with abundant cortical Lewy bodies and senile changes of varying degree—a new disease? Clin Neuropathol 1984; 3:185–192.

97. Sage JI, Miller DC, Golbe LI, Walters A, Duvoisin RC. Clinically atypical expression of pathologically typical Lewy-body parkinsonism. Clin Neuropharmacol 1990; 13:36–47.
98. Jellinger K, Riederer P. Dementia in Parkinson's disease and (pre) senile dementia of Alzheimer type: morphological aspects and changes in intracerebral MAO activity. In: Hassler RG, Christ JF, eds. Parkinson-specific motor and mental disorders. Role of the pallidum: pathophysiological, biochemical and therapeutic aspects. 1984; 40:199–210.
99. Bergeron C, Pollanen M. Lewy bodies in Alzheimer disease—one or two diseases. Alzheimer Dis Assoc Disord 1989; 3:197–204.
100. Jellinger K. Morphology of Alzheimer's disease and related disorders. In: Maurer K, Riederer P, Beckman H, eds. Epidemiology, neuropathology, neurochemistry, and clinics. New York: Springer Verlag, 1990:61–77.
101. Forno LS. Neuropathological features of Parkinson's Huntington's, and Alzheimer's diseases. Ann NY Acad Sci 1992; 648:6–16.
102. Rinne JO, Rummukainen J, Paljarvi L, Sako E, Molsa P, Rinne UK. Neuronal loss in the substantia nigra in patients with Alzheimer's disease and Parkinson's disease in relation to extrapyramidal symptoms and dementia. Prog Clin Biol Res 1989; 317:325–332.
103. Whitehouse PJ. Parkinson's disease and Alzheimer's disease: new neurochemical parallels. Mov Disord 1989; 4:S57–S62.
104. Bethlem J, den Hartog Jager WA. The incidence and characteristics of Lewy bodies in idiopathic paralysis agitans (Parkinson's disease). J Neurol Neurosurg Psychiatry 1960; 23:74–80.
105. den Hartog Jager WA, Bethlem J. The distribution of Lewy bodies in the central and autonomic nervous systems in idiopathic paralysis agitans. J Neurol Neurosurg Psychiatry 1960; 23:283–290.
106. Duffy PE, Tennyson VM. Phase and electron microscopic observations of Lewy bodies and melanin granules in the substantia nigra and locus coeruleus in Parkinson's disease. J Neuropathol Exp Neurol 1965; 24:398–414.
107. Forno LS, Norville RL. Ultrastructure of Lewy bodies in the stellate ganglion. Acta Neuropathol (Berl) 1976; 34:183–197.
108. Goldman JE, Yen SH, Chiu FC, Peress NS. Lewy bodies of Parkinson's disease contain neurofilament antigen. Science 1983; 221:1082–1084.
109. Jellinger K. New developments in the pathology of Parkinson's disease. In: Parkinson's disease: anatomy, pathology and therapy. Adv Neurol 1990; 53:1–16.
110. Gibb WRG, Scott T, Lees AJ. Neuronal inclusions of Parkinson's disease. Mov Disord 1991; 6:2–11.
111. Alvord EC, Forno LS. Pathology. In: Koller WC, ed. Handbook of Parkinson's disease. 2nd ed. New York: Marcel Dekker, 1992:255–284.
112. Galloway PG, Bergeron C, Perry G. The presence of *tau* distinguishes Lewy bodies of diffuse Lewy body disease from those of idiopathic Parkinson's disease. Neurosci Lett 1989; 100:6–10.
113. Forno LS, Murphy GM, Eng LF. Immunocytochemical study of Lewy bodies in sympathetic ganglia. Neurodegeneration 1992; 1:135–144.
114. Forno LS, DeLanney LE, Irwin I, Langston JW. Similarities and differences

between MPTP-induced parkinsonism and Parkinson's disease. In: Narabayashi H, Nagatsu T, Yanagisawa N, Mizuno Y, eds. Parkinson's disease: from basic research to treatment. Tenth international symposium on Parkinson's disease. Adv Neurol 1993; 60:600–608.
115. Lowe J, McDermott H, Landon M, Mayer J, Wilkinson KD. Ubiquitin carboxyl-terminal hydrolase (PGP 9.5) is selectively present in ubiquitinated inclusion bodies characteristic of human neurodegenerative diseases. J Pathol 1992; 161:153–160.
116. Hill WD, Lee VM-Y, Hurting HI, Murray JM, Trojanowski JQ. Epitopes located in spatially separate domains of each neurofilament subunit are present in Parkinson's disease Lewy bodies. J Comp Neurol 1991; 309:150–160.
117. Tiller-Borcich JK, Forno LS. Parkinson's disease and dementia with neuronal inclusions in the cerebral cortex: Lewy bodies or Pick bodies. J Neuropathol Exp Neurol 1988; 47:526–535.
118. Mayer RJ, Lowe J, Lennox G, Landon M, MacLennan K, Doherty FJ. Intermediate filament—ubiquitin diseases: implications for cell sanitization. Biochem Soc Symp 1989; 193–201.
119. Lennox G, Lowe J, Morrell K, Landon M, Mayer RJ. Anti-ubiquitin immunocytochemistry is more sensitive than conventional techniques in the detection of diffuse Lewy body disease. J Neurol Neurosurg Psychiatry 1989; 52:67–71.
120. Kwak S, Masaki T, Ishiura S, Sugita H. Multicatalytic proteinase is present in Lewy bodies and neurofibrillary tangles in diffuse Lewy body disease brain. Neurosci Lett 1991; 128:21–24.
121. Iwatsubo T, Nakano I, Fukunaga K, Miyamoto E. CA^{2+}/calmodulin-dependent protein kinase II immunoreactivity in Lewy bodies. Acta Neuropathol 1991; 82:159–163.
122. Kemp BE, Pearson RB. Protein kinase recognition sequence motifs. Trends Biochem Sci 1990; 15:342–346.
123. Pollanen MS, Dickson DW, Bergeron C. Pathology and biology of the Lewy body. J Neuropathol Exp Neurol 1993; 52:183–191.
124. Galloway PG, Mulvihill P, Perry G. Filaments of Lewy bodies contain insoluble cytoskeletal elements. Am J Pathol 1992; 140:809–822.
125. Pollanen MS, Bergeron C, Weyer L. Detergent-insoluble cortical Lewy body fibrils share epitopes with neurofilament and *tau*. J Neurochem 1992; 58:1953–1956.
126. Wisniewski T, Haltia M, Ghiso J, Frangione B. Lewy bodies are immunoreactive with antibodies raised to gelsolin related amyloid—Finnish type. Am J Pathol 1991; 138:1077–1083.
127. Sandyk R, Iacono RP. Early versus late-onset Parkinson's disease: the role of the locus coeruleus [letter]. Int J Neurosci 1990; 52:243–247.
128. Hornykiewicz O. The primary site of dopamine neuron damage in Parkinson's disease: substantia nigra or striatum. Mov Disord 1992; 7:288.
129. Smith AD, Bolam JP. The neural network of the basal ganglia as revealed by the study of synaptic connections of identified neurones. Trends Neurosci 1990; 13:259–265.
130. Herkenham M, Little MD, Bankiewicz K, Yang SC, Markey SP, Johannessen JN. Selective retention of MPP^+ within the monoaminergic systems of the primate

brain following MPTP administration: an in vivo autoradiographic study. Neuroscience 1991; 40:133–158.

131. Parent A, Hazrati LN. Anatomical aspects of information processing in primate basal ganglia. Trends Neurosci 1993; 16:111–116.
132. Kish SJ, Rajput A, Gilbert J, et al. Elevated gamma-aminobutyric acid level in striatal but not extrastriatal brain regions in Parkinson's disease: correlation with striatal dopamine loss. Ann Neurol 1986; 20:26–31.
133. Moratalla R, Quinn B, DeLanney LE, Langston JW, Graybiel AM. Differential vulnerability of primate caudate–putamen and striosome–matrix dopamine systems to the neurotoxic effect of MPTP. Proc Natl Acad Sci USA 1992; 89:3859–3863.
134. Yurek DM, Sladek JR, Jr. Dopamine cell replacement: Parkinson's disease. Annu Rev Neurosci 1990; 13:415–440.
135. Beal MF. Does impairment of energy metabolism result in excitotoxic neuronal death in neurodegenerative illnesses? Ann Neurol 1992; 31:119–130.
136. Turski L, Bressler K, Rettig K-J, Löschmann P-A, Wachtel H. Protection of substantia nigra from MPP^+ neurotoxicity by *N*-methyl-D-aspartate antagonists. Nature 1991; 349:414–418.
137. Hill WD, Arai M, Cohen JA, Trojanowski JQ. Neurofilament mRNA is reduced in Parkinson's disease substantia nigra pars compacta neurons. J Comp Neurol 1993; 329:328–336.

4

Mechanism of Cell Death

Ian Irwin and J. William Langston

The Parkinson's Institute, Sunnyvale, California

I. INTRODUCTION

Parkinson's disease is one of the major neurodegenerative disease of aging. As such, its core feature is the death of neurons, particularly dopaminergic neurons of the nigrostriatal system. Any attempt to explore the cause of the disease must ultimately deal with this fact. Consequently, it is important to try to understand the different ways that cells are known to die. In this chapter, we will first review some of the general mechanisms of cell death, with particular reference to how they might be involved in the process of neuronal degeneration in Parkinson's disease. Chemically induced mechanisms will be emphasized, since these are likely to be at play if either an endogenous or exogenous toxin is involved. If the disease proves to be genetic, it will still be important to define the neurochemical sequence of events that orchestrate the process of cell degeneration. Even if the disease is eventually discovered to have an infectious origin, it is still likely that understanding the way that an infectious agent actually kills the cell will be important. For these reasons, we will cover, in some depth, what is known about the actual mechanisms that mediate cell death.

II. REDUCED OXYGEN SPECIES AND OXIDATIVE STRESS

Oxygen is a major constituent in the cells of most higher animals. The stepwise reduction of molecular oxygen is the basis of all aerobic life. Reduced oxygen species are essential intermediates in the production of cellular energy, a process that is mediated by the action of the mitochondrial electron transport proteins. Many other enzymes, including tyrosine hydroxylase, monoamine oxidase, NADPH-cytochrome P-450 reductase, and xanthine oxidase, also produce or utilize reactive oxygen intermediates. In addition, reduced oxygen species are generated by the action of several endogenous and exogenously administered chemical agents.

Although reduced oxygen species have a definite role in many ordered biological processes (1), when formed in excessive amounts, they may also be associated with cytotoxicity, a condition that is generally referred to as "oxidative stress." In this setting, active oxygen species are thought to be the ultimate mediators of cell damage through the peroxidation of lipid membranes (2), the oxidation of protein sulfhydryl and other groups, and by direct damage to DNA (3–5).

The mechanism of oxygen radical formation involves the transfer of electrons from a chemical substrate to molecular oxygen. Several possible oxygen radical species arise by the stepwise reduction of molecular oxygen and by the interaction of reduced oxygen species with each other (Fig. 1).

The single-electron reduction of oxygen results in the superoxide anion radical, which contains one unpaired electron (I). Superoxide itself is highly unstable and can take part in a number of metabolic and chemical reactions, including

I. $$\underset{\text{Oxygen}}{O_2} + 1e^- \longrightarrow \underset{\text{Superoxide anion radical}}{O_2^{-\cdot}}$$

II. $$O_2^{-\cdot} + 1e^- \longrightarrow \underset{\text{Peroxide ion}}{O_2^{2-}}$$

III. $$O_2^{-\cdot} + H_2O_2 \longrightarrow O_2 + \underset{\text{Hydroxyl radical}}{OH^{\cdot}}$$

IV. $$H_2O_2 + Fe^{2+} \longrightarrow OH^- + OH^{\cdot} + Fe^{3+}$$

Figure 1 Production of reduced oxygen radical species. (I). Single electron reduction of molecular oxygen to yield superoxide radical anion. (II) Reduction of superoxide to peroxide ion. Peroxide anion exists as a combination of hydrogen peroxide and the hydroperoxide ion. (III) Haber–Weiss reaction of superoxide and hydrogen peroxide to yield hydroxide radical. (IV) Fenton reaction showing the production of hydroxyl radical from hydrogen peroxide in the presence of an oxidizable transition metal ion (ferrous iron shown).

protonation to hydroperoxy radical and dismutation to hydrogen peroxide (6). Further reduction of superoxide anion radical results in the formation of peroxide ion (II), which at physiological pH exists as an equilibrium mixture of hydrogen peroxide (H_2O_2) and hydroperoxyl anion (HO_2^-). Once formed, superoxide and peroxide can further interact to generate the hydroxyl radical through the Haber–Weiss (7) reaction (III). The hydroxyl radical is an extremely reactive species that can participate in radical-induced chain reactions to generate other radical species, such as singlet oxygen or lipid hydroperoxides. Many investigations have suggested that the generation of a hydroxyl radical may be the critical step in cytotoxicity, because the hydroxyl radical may be the ultimate oxygen species that damages cells (8). Under laboratory conditions, in highly purified water, the rate of formation of a hydroxyl radical by the Haber–Weiss reaction is extremely slow, but even traces of transition metal ions, such as copper, iron, or manganese, can catalyze the reaction and greatly accelerate the formation of hydroxyl radicals. The hydroxyl radical may also be produced directly by the interaction of reduced metal ions with hydrogen peroxide (Fenton reaction; IV).

Given the production of oxygen radicals in the normal course of cellular life and the potentially damaging effects of these agents, it is not surprising that cells possess several biochemical mechanisms to detoxify these agents and to protect against and repair damage caused by these reactive oxygen species. The enzyme superoxide dismutase (SOD) reduces superoxide anion to hydrogen peroxide and oxygen. This enzyme exists both in a cellular (Cu-Zn) and a mitochondrial form (Mn). The cellular burden of hydrogen peroxide is handled, in part, by the enzyme catalase, which converts it to oxygen and water. The detoxification of cytosolic and mitochondrial hydrogen peroxide is handled primarily by the enzyme glutathione peroxidase. Glutathione peroxidase is a selenoprotein that catalyzes the reduction of hydrogen peroxide to water. The enzyme can also reduce organic peroxides and has an absolute requirement for reduced glutathione (GSH), which is oxidized to its disulfide (GSSG) in the process. Although neurons may contain lower levels of reduced glutathione (9–11), maintenance of high levels of GSH is a critical line of defense against the effects of reactive oxygen species. Typical cellular ratios of GSH/GSSG are on the order of 100:1 (12).

High GSH/GSSG ratios are maintained by the action of the NADPH-dependent enzyme glutathione (GSSG) reductase, which converts GSSG to GSH. The GSH functions in a protective capacity, not only by decomposing hydrogen peroxide, but also by reacting directly with oxygen radicals and other oxidizing species, such as the products of lipid peroxidation. Glutathione also protects against damage induced by reactive oxygen intermediates through the repair of oxidized proteins (reduction of protein dithiols) with glutathione-*S*-transferase activity found within cells. These protective actions are potentially so important that it has been suggested that many of the features of oxidative stress (e.g., lipid peroxidation) are the consequence not of enhanced production of reactive oxygen intermediates, but of exhausted stores of reduced glutathione (13).

Alternate cellular lines of defense against reactive oxygen intermediates consist of other small molecules, such as vitamin E or vitamin C, that can react directly with oxygen radicals either by undergoing oxidation or by forming covalent adducts. These are known as free radical scavengers, and they may also represent an important line of defense against potentially damaging oxygen species.

Various chemical agents interfere with the homeostatic balance between oxygen radical production and the process of detoxification, thereby inducing oxidative stress. For example, chemically induced oxidative stress can occur by enhancing the production of oxygen radicals sufficiently to exceed cellular defense capabilities or by depleting or disabling cellular defenses against oxygen radicals. Alternatively, certain chemical agents and their metabolites can react directly with molecular oxygen to generate one or more of the reduced oxygen species described earlier. Examples of toxicants that are thought to generate oxygen radicals include 6-hydroxydopamine (14,15) alloxan (16), and paraquat (17).

Although the quantity of oxygen radical species produced can be dependent on the amount of the precipitating chemical agent present (this is known as stoichiometric production), in certain cases, the production of oxygen radicals is greatly amplified by the phenomenon of redox cycling. Probably the best known example of redox cycling is to be found in the mechanism of action of dipyridyl herbicides, such as paraquat and diquat. These toxins undergo a single electron reduction, mediated by enzymes such as NADPH-cytochrome P-450 reductase, to form a dipyridyl radical. The dipyridyl radical quickly reacts with molecular oxygen to form superoxide and to regenerate the original dipyridyl compound. The dipyridyl is again reduced to the radical and again reacts with molecular oxygen to form a second molecule of superoxide. With each cycle of oxidation and reduction another molecule of superoxide is formed. Thus, a single molecule of dipyridyl can generate large amounts of active oxygen species. Redox cycling can lead not only to overproduction of reactive oxygen species, but also to the exhaustion of cofactors, such as pyridine nucleotides, and the complete consumption of reduced glutathione.

A. Implications for Parkinson's Disease

A careful review of enzyme systems that play a role in defending against free radical damage suggests that the nigrostriatal system may be especially prone to oxidative stress. The levels of SOD activity are 40–50% greater in the substantia nigra than in areas such as cortex or cerebellum (18). Ceballos and colleagues (19) have reported that the pigmented cells of the substantia nigra, thought by some to be the most vulnerable to degeneration in Parkinson's disease (20), express high amounts of mRNA for Cu–Zn SOD (21), suggesting localization of SOD within these nigral neurons and indicating the presence of high amounts of superoxide in these cells.

High levels of SOD activity in nigral neurons might be expected to promote the formation of greater amounts of peroxide. Recent evidence suggests that nigral neurons may be exceptionally vulnerable to these high fluxes of peroxide. For example, catalase activity in the substantia nigra is similar to, or slightly lower than, that found in other brain regions, including the cortex and cerebellum (18,22). Measurements of glutathione peroxidase (18,23) suggest that the activity of this enzyme shows no marked regionalization in normal brain, although "generalized peroxidase activity" appeared to be slightly higher in the substantia nigra, when using an older, nonspecific technique (22). If the more recent studies are correct, they indicate that potential increases in substantia nigra peroxide are not compensated for by a corresponding increase in levels of glutathione peroxidase. Furthermore, there is no significant regionalization of glutathione reductase activity in the normal brain (18). Levels of total glutathione (GSSG + GSH) are slightly lower in substantia nigra, and reduced glutathione (GSH) concentrations are much lower in the substantia nigra than in other brain areas (24,25). Thus, this system would seem to be in a precarious situation when it comes to risk for oxidative stress, with an apparent disparity in the substantia nigra between the potential to produce hydrogen peroxide by SOD and its ability to detoxify peroxide by catalase and glutathione peroxidase.

In Parkinson's disease, this gap may have widened even further. Cytosolic (18) and particulate (26) fractions of SOD in substantia nigra from Parkinson's brain are increased relative to controls. Levels of catalase (18,23), glutathione peroxidase activity (18,23), and nonspecific peroxidase activity (23) are reduced or unchanged, whereas levels of reduced glutathione appear to be dramatically lowered in the substantia nigra (24,25,27).

More direct evidence that reactive oxygen-mediated damage occurs in the substantia nigra in Parkinson's disease comes from a recent study comparing eight brain areas obtained from autopsy tissue from parkinsonian patients with age-matched controls (28,29). The results of these studies demonstrated a selective reduction (about 15%) in nigral polyunsaturated fatty acid concentrations. Polyunsaturated fatty acids, present in lipid membranes, represent a prime target for oxygen radical damage, and the reported reductions are suggestive of loss by this means. These same investigators reported increases of approximately 30% in nigral levels of malondialdehyde, an intermediate in the lipid peroxidation process. These changes were reported to be statistically significant ($p < 0.05$) only in the substantia nigra, although examination of these data suggests that the observations in the substantia nigra would not have reached statistical significance had multiple comparisons techniques been employed to account for the numerous comparisons made.

In summary, there are several theoretical considerations that raise the possibility that oxidative stress may play a role in Parkinson's disease. This possibility is now supported by a substantial body of evidence. However, proving this hypothesis still remains a formidable task.

III. COVALENT BONDING

Another mechanism by which endogenous compounds cause cellular damage is by reacting directly with nucleophilic cellular constituents to form covalent bonds. Free radicals can participate in this process, as can other chemically reactive, electrophilic species, such as epoxides. Targets of reactive intermediates include macromolecules (e.g., proteins and DNA) and small constituent cellular molecules (e.g., glutathione). Covalent bonding compromises cellular function by various mechanisms, including enzyme inactivation, inactivation of transport pumps, and disruption of the cytoskeleton. Covalent bonding correlates with the toxicity of a variety of toxins (30). For example, *n*-hexane is metabolized to a 2,5-diketone intermediate, which is believed to act by forming covalent bonds with free amino groups (lysine residues) to form pyroles. This process leads to the formation of covalent cross-linking between adjacent neurofilaments, impeding axoplasmic flow, which is an essential feature of *n*-hexane-induced peripheral neuropathy (31).

In contrast with the variety of mechanisms for protecting against and repairing damage caused by reactive oxygen intermediates described earlier, the known defenses against alkylation or arylation by reactive intermediates are limited. The primary defense against such agents is reduced glutathione. The cisteinal sulfhydryl group of glutathione functions as a generalized nucleophile, combining directly with electrophilic metabolites and intermediates, thereby protecting cellular elements.

The reaction between a reactive electrophilic species and glutathione may occur directly, or by enzymatic catalysis by glutathione-S-transferase (12). Glutathione conjugates are transported out of the cell and are substrates for γ-glutamyl transpeptidases. By a series of extracellular reactions these GSH conjugates are cleaved to *S*-cysteinyl-conjugates. These are acetylated and ultimately excreted in the urine or feces as mercapturic acids. Such conjugation–detoxification reactions have been amply demonstrated for a variety of exogenous and endogenous agents that form reactive intermediates and, again, illustrate the pivotal role of GSH in detoxification processes. The GSH conjugation–detoxification pathway is very efficient and, for at least some compounds, completely prevents the formation of covalent bonds to critical cellular nucleophiles.

The drug acetaminophen clearly illustrates this principle. About 4% of the administered dose is metabolized by the cytochrome P-450 mixed function oxidases to a very reactive intermediate NABQI, which is a potent electrophile that modifies sulfhydryl residues in proteins. The widespread use of this over-the-counter drug with few side effects attests to the efficiency of this detoxification pathway. At higher doses, however, the increased formation of NABQI leads to the exhaustion of GSH, and the reactive metabolite attacks tissue proteins, primarily in the liver, causing widespread hepatic necrosis. Individuals with deficiencies of GSH demonstrate an enhanced sensitivity to acetaminophen hepatotoxicity (32,33).

A. Implications for Parkinson's Disease

There is a plausible basis to believe that covalent bond-forming reactive intermediates might be involved in Parkinson's disease. The presence of neuromelanin, a complex polymer that includes covalently bound dopamine and cysteine, in the substantia nigra (34–36) and locus ceruleus indicates the existence of reactive catecholamine intermediates in these regions. Furthermore, the recent isolation of 5-*S*-cysteinyl dopamine from brain and cerebrospinal fluid, and the suggestion that high levels of this metabolite may correlate with the extent of nigral degeneration, implicate a possible role for covalent bonding as a mechanism in Parkinson's disease (37). As will be seen, covalent bonding may play a role in the toxic effects of several of the compounds to be discussed in this chapter.

IV. ENERGY DEPLETION

Adenosine triphosphate (ATP) is the basic energy currency of cells. It is required for the vast majority of cellular reactions, including maintenance of the cytoarchitecture, the operation of myriad transport pumps and uptake systems, and the synthesis of proteins and DNA. Thus, any event or agent that interferes with ATP production is likely to have disastrous consequences for cellular function and, ultimately, for survival.

Mitochondria produce ATP by the oxidation of substrates with molecular oxygen. The pathways are complex, involving various sequential reactions, which together constitute what is known as the mitochondrial respiratory chain. Each step is controlled by specific enzyme complexes, called electron transport proteins. There are four such complexes, labeled I–IV. Several toxins, including rotenone (38–40), piericidin (38) and, most notably, the toxic metabolite of MPTP, 1-methyl-4-phenylpyridinium ion (MPP^+; 41–43: for review, see Ref. 44), are known to act at this level of the mitochondrial respiratory chain, directly interfering with the production of ATP. Generally, such toxins bind specifically to one of the proteins that make up the complexes of the transport chain which, in turn, inhibits the flow of electrons through this chain, blocking ATP production.

A. Implications for Parkinson's Disease

One of the surprises of the last decade is that impaired mitochondrial ATP production appears to be a feature of idiopathic Parkinson's disease. A reduction of complex I activity had been found in a variety of tissues, including substantia nigra, striatum, muscle, and platelets (45–63). Although the sheer number of studies constitute a convincing case that there is an abnormality in mitochondrial function in Parkinson's disease, there have been several inconsistencies in the results reported to date. For example, Schapira and colleagues (47,53,64) have found the deficit only in the substantia nigra. At least three separate groups have reported a deficiency in muscle, but two other groups have been unable to confirm these results. Although most of the studies to date have identified complex I as the primary site of dysfunction, a few have found abnormalities in other mitochondrial complexes as well (57).

There are at least two possible explanations for these observed mitochondrial defects. First there could be an inherited abnormality in the DNA (mitochondrial) that encodes subunits for one or more of the electron transport proteins. However, in spite of a rapidly increasing number of studies, no clear pattern has emerged on defects in mitochondrial DNA (mtDNA) that might orchestrate such an abnormality (49,50,65–70). In perhaps the most definitive study yet, Ikebe et al. (71) have sequenced mtDNA in 5 patients and 35 controls, and found no common abnormalities within the patient group. The failure to identify definite abnormalities in DNA coding for complex I proteins points toward the possibility that the observed mitochondrial defects in Parkinson's disease could be the consequence of an "on-board" mitochondrial toxin. If these mitochondrial deficits stand the test of time as a feature of Parkinson's disease, the implications could be profound, since they would represent the first confirmation that a failure of energy production may be important in human neurodegenerative disease.

V. INCREASES IN CYTOSOLIC CALCIUM

Cytosolic free calcium concentrations are maintained at very low levels relative to extracellular concentrations (0.1 μM vs. >1000 μM). This intra- versus extracellular calcium gradient is maintained by the active extrusion of calcium from the cell and by the energy-dependent compartmentalization of calcium within the mitochondria and the endoplasmic reticulum. The movement of calcium is controlled by specific calcium-transporting enzymes (Ca^{2+}, Mg^{2+}-ATPase).

Disruption of calcium homeostasis and sustained increases in cytosolic free calcium have grave consequences for cellular integrity and survival. Elevated free calcium activates several specific degradative enzymes, including phospholipases (enzymes that can degrade the cell membrane) and calcium-activated proteases, which degrade both the cytoskeleton and integral membrane proteins. Increased cytosolic calcium can also interact directly with cytoskeletal elements, producing a dissociation of actin microfilaments (72). Either independently or in concert, these calcium-dependent events are capable of destroying cell integrity, producing disruption of the cytoarchitecture and plasma membrane rupture, which are fatal events for the cell.

Such calcium-dependent changes are thought to underlie the mechanism of action of several toxins. Most notably, calcium influx is a key mediator of excitatory amino acid toxicity mediated by *N*-methyl-D-aspartate (NMDA) receptors (73,74). A sustained rise in cytosolic free calcium is also an early response to, and is highly correlated with, the toxicity of several toxic compounds, including hydroperoxides, diquat, cytotoxic quinones, and carbon tetrachloride (75). Further evidence for the involvement of calcium in cell death comes from the observation that, under certain circumstances, inhibitors of some of the calcium-activated degradative enzymes described can prevent or delay the effects of toxins (67,76–79) and ischemia (80). The role of calcium in apoptosis (see Section VI) also supports its possible involvement in cell death.

A. Implications for Parkinson's Disease

The neurotoxin MPTP has also been reported to produce increases in cytosolic free calcium (81). However, with the possible exception of this observation, there is as yet little evidence to suggest that there are alterations in calcium homeostasis in Parkinson's disease. On the other hand, techniques for investigating alterations in calcium in situ are just being developed. Strategies in such a search for calcium-mediated effects in Parkinson's disease would be expected to involve adaptation of the methods used in cell culture to measure intracellular calcium distribution and the further identification and measurement of specific proteins that are involved in calcium-mediated cell death.

Indeed, such evidence may already be emerging. It has recently been reported that neurons in the substantia nigra that contain the calcium-binding protein, calbindin, are relatively preserved in comparison with calbindin-negative neurons (82–84). Such neurons are also spared in MPTP-induced parkinsonism in nonhuman primates (83). These observations appear to open up an entirely new avenue of research in Parkinson's disease; it will be very interesting to see where it leads in the future.

VI. APOPTOSIS

Apoptosis is a process by which cells die in a specific manner, according to a controlled and presumably genetically coded program; the process may occur in response to specific stimuli (85). Apoptosis is thought to occur in the natural course of development (86) and governs the senescence of certain tissues, such as neutrophils (87); it may also occur in response to the removal of specific growth factors (88–90). Apoptosis is also reported to occur under the influence of specific chemical agents such as 2,3,7,8-tetrachlorodibenzo-*p*-dioxin (TCDD; 91) and tributyltin (92).

The hallmark of apoptosis is the condensation and fragmentation of nuclear material (93). Cytoplasmic organelles, with the exception of mitochondria, become compacted together. The fragmentation of nuclear material into oligonucleotides precipitates cell death (94) and is linked to an endonuclease activity (93). Endonuclease activity, in turn, appears to be linked to both an increase in cytosolic calcium and the de novo synthesis of one or more proteins (see Ref. 95). The involvement of increased cytosolic free calcium is suggested by the successful prevention of apoptosis by calcium chelators.

The requirement for protein synthesis appears to be more complex. Inhibitors of protein synthesis, such as cycloheximide or dactmomycin (actinomycin D), prevent the induction of apoptosis by glucocorticoids (96) and tetrachlorodibenzo-*p*-dioxin (TCDD). Because this suggests that de novo protein synthesis is a requirement for apoptotic cell death, it has been speculated that apoptosis involves either the new synthesis of a protein that promotes calcium influx, or that activation of endonuclease activity requires the presence of a rapidly turning over protein. Of interest is a recent report (97), that inhibitors of protein synthesis prevent damage in serotonergic neurons induced by methamphetamine. These findings raise the possibility of chemically induced apoptotic cell death in the CNS and point to the possible involvement of apoptosis in other neurotoxicological processes as well.

Recently, there has been increasing interest in apoptosis as a mechanism that might underlie chronic neurogenerative disease. Relative to Parkinson's disease, there is as yet little evidence that such a process may be at play, although some interesting evidence is accumulating from work done with MPTP.

Ultrastructural features of apoptosis have been observed in cerebellar tissue culture after MPP^+ exposure (98), and we have recently seen similar changes in the substantia nigra of primates exposed to MPTP (unpublished observations). Although it is to early to tell where this type of study is going, it opens up an entirely new avenue of investigation for those who are interested in the study of neurodegnerative diseases, such as Parkinson's disease.

A. Implications for Parkinson's Disease

Chemically induced apoptosis is a relatively new concept in toxicology; however, it is emerging as an important one. Although we could find no studies in Parkinson's disease investigating the involvement of apoptosis in neurodegeneration, we believe that it should be considered as yet another possible mechanism that might be involved in the toxic hypothesis of the disease. This is because many of the current theories on the cause of neuronal degeneration in Parkinson's disease involve similar mechanisms. Hypotheses invoking apoptosis would be consistent with the involvement of neuronal growth factors in the degenerative process and the emerging evidence concerning these agents (99,100).

VII. SUMMARY

There are relatively few clearly defined mechanisms by which cytotoxic agents are thought to kill cells. However, considerable overlap may exist among these mechanisms. The mitochondrial story provides an excellent opportunity to illustrate how these different mechanisms all may be interrelated. A deficiency in mitochondrial energy production could enhance the susceptibility to oxidative stress, either directly or by exhaustion of cellular stores of glutathione as a consequence of ATP depletions. A decline in glutathione would, in turn, lead to enhanced covalent bonding, assuming such a process is at play in the parkinsonian brain. Reductions in cellular ATP concentrations might also lead to a failure of calcium sequestration mechanisms, precipitating increases in cytosolic calcium and the likelihood of calcium-mediated cell damage. Thus, one could envision a wide array of cellulotoxic mechanisms snowballing into a rather formidable neurodegenerative process.

As we survey the sites of injury and degeneration in Parkinson's disease and find clues suggestive of an etiological toxin, these will have to be placed in the context of developing data and theories of chemically induced cell death. Doing so will serve both as a methodological resource on which to draw for techniques to adapt and apply to the investigation and, also, as a theoretical framework in which to interpret the results. If a toxin eventually proves to be an etiological factor in the disease, it can be hoped that current and yet to be developed techniques for identifying and monitoring these processes will allow us to identify the elusive agent(s) causing this mysterious disease.

REFERENCES

1. Brunori M, Rotilio G. Biochemistry of oxygen radical systems. In: Packer L, ed. Oxygen radicals in biological systems. Methods Enzymol 1984; 105:22–31.
2. McBrien DCH, Slater TF. Free radicals, lipid peroxidation and cancer. London: Academic Press, 1982.

3. Fridovich I. Oxygen free radicals and tissue damage. Amsterdam: Excerpta Medica, 1979.
4. Halliwell B, Gutteridge JMC. Oxygen radicals and the nervous sytem. Trends Neurosci 1985; 7:22–26.
5. Halliwell B, Gutteridge JMC. Free radicals in biology and medicine. Oxford: Clarendon Press, 1985.
6. Green MJ, Hill HAO. Chemistry of dioxygen. In: Packer L, ed. Oxygen radicals in biological systems. Methods Enzymol, 1984;105:3–21.
7. Haber F, Weiss J. Uber die katalyse des hydroperoxydes. Naturwissenschaften 1932; 20:948–950.
8. Dormandy TL. An approach to free radicals. Lancet 1983; 2:1010–1014.
9. Di Monte DA, Chan P, Sandy MS. Glutathione in Parkinson's disease: a link between oxidative stress and mitochondrial damage. Ann Neurol 1992; 32 (suppl): S111–S115.
10. Slivka A, Mytilineou C, Cohen G. Histochemical evaluation of glutathione in brain. Brain Res 1987; 409:275–284.
11. Raps SP, Lai JCK, Hertz L, Cooper AJL. Glutathione is present in high concentrations in cultured astrocytes, but not in cultured neurons. Brain Res 1989; 493:398–401.
12. Meister A. Selective modification of glutathione metabolism. Science 1983; 220:472–477.
13. Starke PE, Farber JL. Ferric iron and superoxide ions are required for the killing of cultured hepatocytes by hydrogen peroxide. Evidence for the participation of hydroxyl radicals formed by an iron-catalyzed Haber–Weiss reaction. J Biol Chem 1985; 260:10099–10104.
14. Cohen G, Heikkila RE. Mechanisms of action of hydroxylated phenylethylamine and indoleamine neurotoxins. Ann NY Acad Sci 1978; 305:74–84.
15. Cohen G, Heikkila RE. The generation of hydrogen peroxide, superoxide radical, and hydroxyradical of 6-hydroxydopamine, dialuric acid, and related cytotoxic agents. J Biol Chem 1974; 249:2447–2452.
16. Heikkila RE, Winston B, Cohen G, Barden H. Alloxan-induced diabetes—evidence for hydroxyl radical as a cytotoxic intermediate. Biochem Pharmacol 1976; 25:1085–1092.
17. Bus JS, Aust SD, Gibson JE. Paraquat: model for oxidant-initiated toxicity. Environ Health Perspect 1984; 55:37–46.
18. Marttila RJ, Lorentz H, Rinne UK. Oxygen toxicity protecting enzymes in Parkinson's disease: increase of superoxide dismutase-like activity in the substantia nigra and basal nucleus. J Neurol Sci 1988; 86:321–331.
19. Ceballos I, Javoy-Agid F, Delacourte A. Neuronal localization of copper–zinc superoxide dismutase protein and mRNA within the human hippocampus from control and Alzheimer's disease brains. Free Radical Res Commun 1991; 12–13 (pt 2):571–580.
20. Hirsch EC, Graybiel AM, Agid Y. Selective vulnerability of pigmented dopaminergic neurons in Parkinson's disease. Acta Neurol Scand [Suppl] 1989; 126:19–22.
21. Ceballos I, Lafon M, Javoy-Agid F, et al. Superoxide dismutase and Parkinson's disease [letter]. Lancet 1990; 335:1035–1036.

22. Ambani LM, Van Woert MH, Murphy S. Brain peroxidase and catalase in Parkinson's disease. Arch Neurol 1975; 32:114–118.
23. Kish SJ, Morito C, Hornykiewicz O. Glutathione peroxidase activity in Parkinson's disease brain. Neurosci Lett 1985; 58:343–346.
24. Perry TL, Godin DV, Hansen, S. Parkinson's disease: a disorder due to nigral glutathione deficiency. Neurosci Lett 1982; 33:305–310.
25. Perry TL, Young VW, Jones K, Wright JM. Manipulation of glutathione contents fails to alter dopaminergic nigrostriatal neurotoxicity of *N*-methyl-4-phenyl-1,2,3,6-tetrahydropyridine (MPTP) in the mouse. Neurosci Lett 1986; 70:261–265.
26. Saggu H, Cooksey J, Dexter DT. A selective increase in particulate superoxide dismutase activity in parkinsonian substantia nigra. J Neurochem 1989; 53:692–697.
27. Riederer P, Sofic E, Rausch WD, et al. Transition metals, ferritin, glutathione, and ascorbic acid in parkinsonian brains. J Neurochem 1989; 52:515–520.
28. Dexter D, Carter C, Agid F, et al. Lipid peroxidation as cause of nigral cell death in Parkinson's disease [letter]. Lancet 1986; 2:639–640.
29. Dexter DT, Carter CJ, Wells FR, et al. Basal lipid peroxidation in substantia nigra is increased in Parkinson's disease. J Neurochem 1989; 52:381–389.
30. Gillette JR. A perspective on the role of chemically reactive metabolites of foreign compounds in toxicity—I. Correlation of changes in covalent binding of reactivity metabolites with changes in the incidence and severity of toxicity. Biochem Pharmacol 1974; 23:2785–2794.
31. Graham DG, Szakal-Quin GY, Priest JW, Anthony DC. In vitro evidence that covalent cross-linking of neurofilament occurs in gamma-diketone neuropathy. Proc Natl Acad Sci USA 1984; 81:4979–4982.
32. Lauterburg BH, Smith CV, Hughes H, Mitchell JR. Determinants of hepatic glutathione turnover: toxicological significance. Trends Pharmaco/Sci 1982; 3:245–248.
33. Mitchell JR, Jollow DJ. Metabolic activation of drugs to toxic substances. Gastroenterology 1975; 68:392–410.
34. Graham DG. Oxidative pathways for catecholamines in the genesis of neuromelanin and cytotoxic quinones. Mol Pharmacol 1978; 14:633–643.
35. Van Woert MH, Prasad KN Borg DC. Spectroscopic studies of substantia nigra pigment in human subjects. J Neurochem 1967; 14:707–716.
36. Carstam R, Brinck C, Hindemith-Augustsson A, Rorsman H, Rosengren E. The neuromelanin of the human substantia nigra. Biochim Biophys Acta 1991; 1097:152–160.
37. Carlsson A, Fornstedt B. Catechol metabolites in the cerebrospinal fluid as possible markers in the early diagnosis of Parkinson's disease. Neurology 1991; 40 (suppl 2):50–52.
38. Ramsay RR, Krueger MJ, Youngster SK, Gluck MR, Casida JE, Singer TP. Interaction of 1-methyl-4-phenylpyridinium ion (MPP^+) and its analogs with the rotenone/piericidin binding site of NADH dehydrogenase. J Neurochem 1991; 56:1184–1190.
39. Greenamyre JT, Higgins DS, Eller RV. Quantitative autoradiography of dihydroro-

tenone binding to complex I of the electron transport chain. J Neurochem 1992; 59:746–749.
40. Windholx M, Budavari S, Blumetti RF, Otterbein ES. The Merck index. Rahway, NJ: Merck & Company, 1983: 1191.
41. Nicklas WJ, Vyas I, Heikkila RE. Inhibition of NADH-linked oxidation in brain mitochondria by 1-methyl-4-phenyl-1,2,3,6-tetrahydropyridine. Life Sci 1985; 36:2503–2508.
42. Ramsay RR, Youngster SK, Nicklas WJ. Structural dependence of the inhibition of mitochondrial respiration and of NADH oxidase by 1-methyl-4-phenylpyridinium (MPP^+) analogs and their energized accumulation by mitochondria. Proc Natl Acad Sci USA 1989; 86:9168–9172.
43. Sayre LM, Singh MP, Arora PK, Wang F, McPeak RJ, Hoppel CL. Inhibition of mitochondrial respiration by analogues of the dopaminergic neurotoxin 1-methyl-4-phenylpyridinium: structural requirements for accumulation-dependent enhanced inhibitory potency on intact mitochondria. Arch Biochem Biophys 1990; 280:274–283.
44. Di Monte DA. Mitochondrial DNA and Parkinson's disease. Neurology 1991; 41(suppl. 2):38–42.
45. Bindoff LA, Birch-Machin MA, Cartlidge NEF, Parker WD Jr, Turnbull DM. Mitochondrial function in Parkinson's disease. Lancet 1989; 2:49.
46. Hornsby PJ. Parkinson's disease, vitamin E, and mitochondrial energy metabolism [letter]. Arch Neurol 1989; 46:840–841.
47. Schapira AHV, Cooper JM, Dexter D, Jenner P, Clark JB, Marsden CD. Mitochondrial complex I deficiency in Parkinson's disease. Lancet 1989; 1:1269.
48. Parker WD, Boyson SJ, Parks JK. Abnormalities of the electron transport chain in idiopathic Parkinson's disease. Ann Neurol 1989; 26:719–723.
49. Mizuno Y, Ohta S, Tanaka M, et al. Deficiencies in complex I subunits of the respiratory chain in Parkinson's disease. Biochem Biophys Res Commun 1989; 163:1450–1455.
50. Ikebe S, Tanaka M, Ohno K, et al. Increase of deleted mitochondrial DNA in the striatum in Parkinson's disease and senescence. Biochem Biophys Res Commun 1990; 170:1044–1048.
51. Schapira AHV, Mann VM, Cooper JM, et al. Anatomic and disease specificity of NADHCoQ1 reductase (complex I) deficiency in Parkinson's disease. J Neurochem 1990; 55:2142–2145.
52. Mizuno Y, Suzuki K,Ohta S. Postmortem changes in mitochondrial respiratory enzymes in brain and a preliminary observation in Parkinson's disease. J Neurol Sci 1990; 96:49–57.
53. Schapira AHV, Cooper JM, Dexter D, Clark JB, Jenner P, Marsden CD. Mitochondrial complex I deficiency in Parkinson's disease. J Neurochem 1990; 54:823–827.
54. Hattori N, Tanaka M, Ozawa T, Mizuno Y. Immunohistochemical studies on complexes I, II, III, and IV of mitochondria in Parkinson's disease. Ann Neurol 1991; 30:563–571.
55. Boyson SJ. Parkinson's disease and the electron transport chain. Ann Neurol 1991; 30:330–331.

56. Parker WD. Preclinical detection of Parkinson's disease: biochemical approaches. Neurology 1991; 41 (suppl 2):34–37.
57. Shoffner JM, Watts RL, Juncos JL, Torroni A, Wallace DC. Mitochondrial oxidative phosphorylation defects in Parkinson's disease. Ann Neurol 1991; 30:332–339.
58. Dagani F, Anderson JJ, Chase TN. Mitochondrial function in Parkinson's disease. Ann Neurol 1992; 32:226–227.
59. Mann VM, Cooper JM, Schapira AHV. Quantitation of a mitochondrial DNA deletion in Parkinson's disease. FEBS Lett 1992; 299:218–222.
60. Mizuno Y, Ikebe S, Hattori N, Nakagawa-Hattori Y, Tanaka M, Ozawa T. Mitochondrial abnormalities in Parkinson's disease. Mov Disord 1992; 7 (suppl 1):11.
61. Shoffner JM, Watts RL, Juncos JL, Torroni A, Wallace DC. Mitochondrial function in Parkinson's disease. Ann Neurol 1992; 32:227.
62. Wallace DC. Mitochondrial genetics: a paradigm for aging and neurodegenerative diseases. Science 1992; 256:628–632.
63. Yoshino H, Nakagawa-Hattori Y, Kondo T, Mizuno Y. Mitochondrial complex I and II activities of lymphocytes and platelets in Parkinson's disease. J Neural Transm 1992; 4:27–34.
64. Schapira AHV, Mann VM, Cooper JM, Krige D, Jenner PJ, Marsden CD. Mitochondrial function in Parkinson's disease. Ann Neurol 1992; 32 (suppl):S116-S124.
65. Lestienne P, Nelson J, Riederer P, Jellinger K, Reichmann H. Normal mitochondrial genome in brain from patients with Parkinson's disease and complex I defect. J Neurochem 1990; 55:1810–1812.
66. Schapira AH, Holt IJ, Sweeney M, Harding AE, Jenner P, Marsden CD. Mitochondrial DNA analysis in Parkinson's disease. Mov Disord 1990; 5:294–297.
67. Cortopassi GA, Arnheim N. Detection of a specific mitochondrial DNA deletion in tissues of older humans. Nucleic Acids Res 1990; 18:6927–6933.
68. Ozawa T, Tanaka M, Ino H, et al. Distinct clustering of point mutations in mitochondrial DNA among patients with mitochondrial encephalomyopathies and with Parkinson's disease. Biochem Biophys Res Commun 1991; 176:938–946.
69. Ozawa T, Tanaka M, Sugiyama S, et al. Patients with idiopathic cardiomyopathy belong to the same mitochondrial DNA gene family of Parkinson's disease and mitochondrial encephalomyopathy. Biochem Biophys Res Commun 1991; 177:518–525.
70. Wallace DC, Shoffner JM, Watts RL, Juncos JL, Torroni A. Mitochondrial oxidative phosphorylation defects in Parkinson's disease. Ann Neurol 1992; 32:113–114.
71. Ikebe S, Hattori N, Mizuno Y, Tanaka M, Ozawa T. Point mutation of mitochondrial DNA in Parkinson's disease. Mov Disord 1992; 7 (suppl 1):71.
72. Mirabelli F, Salis A, Marinoni V. Menadione-induced bleb formation in hepatocytes is associated with the oxidation of thiol groups in actin. Arch Biochem Biophys 1988; 264:261–269.
73. Cotman CW, Iversen LL. Excitatory amino acids in the brain—focus on NMDA receptors. Trends Neurosci 1987; 10:263–265.

74. Choi DW. Calcium-mediated neurotoxicity: relationship to specific channel types and role in ischemic damage. Trends Neurosci 1988; 11 (10):465–469.
75. Orrenius S, McConkey DJ, Jones DP, Nicotera P. CA^{2+}-activated mechanisms in toxicity and programmed cell death. ISI Atlas Sci Pharmacol 1988; 2:319–324.
76. Kosower NS, Glaser T, Kosower EM. Membrane-motility agent-promoted fusion of erythrocytes: fusibility is correlated with attack by calcium-activated cytoplasmic proteases on membrane proteins. Proc Natl Acad Sci USA 1983; 80:7542–7546.
77. Nicotera P, Hartzell P, Davis G, Orrenius S. The formation of plasma membrane blebs in hepatocytes exposed to agents that increase cytosolic Ca^{2+} is mediated by the activation of a non-lysomal proteolytic system. FEBS Lett 1986; 209:139–144.
78. Nicotera P, Hartzell P, Baldi C, Svensson SA, Bellomo G, Orrenius S. Cystamine induces toxicity in hepatocytes through the elevation of cytosolic Ca^{2+} and the stimulation of a nonlysosomal proteolytic system. J Biol Chem 1986; 261:14628–14635.
79. Mirabelli F, Salis A, Viaretti M, Bellomo G, Thor H, Orrenius S. Cytoskeletal alterations in human platelets exposed to oxidative stress are mediated by oxidative and Ca^{2+}-dependent mechanisms. Arch Biochem Biophys 1989; 270:478-488.
80. Chien KR, Pfau RG, Farber JL. Ischemic myocardial cell injury. Prevention by chlorpromazine of an accelerated phospholipid degradation and associated membrane dysfunction. Am J Pathol 1979; 97:505-530.
81. Kass GEN, Wright JM, Nicotera P, Orrenius S. The mechanism of 1-methyl-4-phenyl-1,2,3,6-tetrahydropyridine toxicity: role of intracellular calcium. Arch Biochem Biophys 1988; 260:789-797.
82. Yamada T, McGeer PL, Baimbridge KG, McGeer EG. Relative sparing in Parkinson's disease of substantia nigra dopamine neurons containing calbindin-D28K. Brain Res 1990; 526:303-307.
83. German DC, Manaye KF, Sonsalla PK, Brooks BA. Midbrain dopaminergic cell loss in Parkinson's disease and MPTP-induced parkinsonism: sparing of calbindin-D28k-containing cells. Ann NY Acad Sci 1992; 648:42-62.
84. Hirsch EC, Mouatt A, Thomasset M, Javoy-Agid F, Agid Y, Graybiel AM. Expression of calbindin D28K-like immunoreactivity in catecholaminergic cell groups in the human midbrain. Normal distribution and distribution in Parkinson's disease. Neurodegeneration 1992; 1:83-93.
85. Kerr JFR, Wyllie AH, Currie AR. Apoptosis: a basic biological phenomenon with wide-ranging implications in tissue kinetics. Br J Cancer 1972; 26:239-257.
86. Hinchliffe JR. Cell death in embryogenesis. In: Bowen ID, Lockshin RA, eds. Cell death in biology and pathology. London: Chapman and Hall, 1981:35-78.
87. Savill JS, Wyllie AH, Hensen JE, Walport MJ, Hensen PM, Haslett C. Macrophage phagocytosis of ageing neutrophils in inflammation: programmed cell death in the neutrophil leads to its recognition by macrophage. J Clin Invest 1989; 83:865-875.
88. Sandow BA, West NB, Norman RJ Brenner RM. Hormonal control of apoptosis in hamster uterine luminal epithelium. Am J Anat 1979; 156:15-35.
89. Duke RC, Cohen JJ. IL-2 addiction: withdrawal of growth factor activates a suicide program in dependent T cells. Lymphokine Res 1986; 5:289-299.

90. Nieto MA, Lopez-Rivas A. IL-2 protects T lymphocytes from glucocorticoid-induced DNA fragmentation and cell death. J Immunol 1989; 143:4166-4170.
91. McConkey DJ, Hartzell P, Duddy SK, Hakansson H, Orrenius S. 2,3,7,8-tetra-chlorodibenzo-*p*-dioxin kills immature thymocytes by Ca^{2+}-mediated endonuclease activation. Science 1988; 242:256-259.
92. Aw TY, Nicotera N, Manzo L, Orrenius S. Tributyltin stimulates apoptosis in rat thymocytes. Arch Biochem Biophys 1990; 283:46-50.
93. Wyllie AH. Glucocorticoid-induced thymocyte apoptosis is associated with endogenous endonuclease activation. Nature 1980; 284:555-556.
94. McConkey DJ, Hartzell P, Nicotera P, Orrenius S. Calcium-activated DNA fragmentation kills immature thymocytes. FASEB J 1989; 3:1843-1849.
95. Fawthrop DJ, Boobis AR, Davies DS. Mechanisms of cell death. Arch Toxicol 1991; 65:437-444.
96. McConkey DJ, Nicotera P, Hartzell P, Bellomo G, Wyllie AH, Orrenius S. Glucocorticoids activate a suicide process in thymocytes through an elevation of cytosolic CA^{2+} concentration. Arch Biochem Biophys 1989; 269:365-370.
97. Finnegan KT, Karler R. Protein synthesis inhibition blocks the neurotoxic effects of methamphetamine in rats [abstract]. Soc Neurosci 1991; 17:1277.
98. Dipasquale B, Marini AM, Youle RJ. Apoptosis and DNA degradation induced by 1-methyl-4-phenylpyridinium in neurons. Biochem Biophys Res Commun 1991; 181:1442-1448.
99. Stewart SS, Appel SH. Trophic factors in neurologic disease. Annu Rev Med 1988; 39:193-201.
100. Hyman C, Hofer M, Barde YA, et al. BDNF is a neurotrophic factor for dopaminergic neurons of the substantia nigra. Nature 1991; 350:230-232.

5

Genetics of Parkinson's Disease

Lawrence I. Golbe

University of Medicine and Dentistry of New Jersey–
Robert Wood Johnson Medical School,
New Brunswick, New Jersey

I. INTRODUCTION

The collaboration of this volume's authors as the Parkinson's Epidemiology Research Committee arose, in part, as a call to arms following the 1983 description of 1-methyl-4-phenyl-1,2,3,6- tetrahydropyridine (MPTP)-induced parkinsonism by Langston et al.(1). Much of this volume reviews our progress to date in the search for an exogenous MPTP analogue or other toxin as the cause of Parkinson's disease (PD). The emergence of the "environmental hypothesis" provided welcome outlet for those of us searching for the meaning of Gowers' century-old concept of *abiotrophy*, the notion that neuronal degeneration is determined by an unspecified intrinsic cellular defect. The likelihood of an extrinsic, nonheritable factor as the cause of PD was enhanced by a publication, also in 1983, by Ward et al., showing a very low concordance rate for PD among monozygotic twins(2). Indeed, the papers of Langston et al. and of Ward et al. continue as the principal buttresses of the environmental hypothesis and are among the most frequently cited publications in basal ganglia disease.

More recent developments, however, have prompted some to reexamine the possibility that an intrinsic, inherited cellular defect is a necessary part of the cause of PD:

(a) First is the understanding that what we call PD is an etiologically and clinically heterogeneous group of entities, some of which may be inherited (3,4). (b) Next is the hypothesis that PD has a long preclinical phase and that a large subclinical (or preclinical) population may have, in the past, produced falsely low estimates of familial occurrence (5). (c) Next, the statistical and biological interpretation of the twin data cited earlier has come under criticism by Duvoisin (the principal investigator of that twin study) and colleagues (6). A principal difficulty with the twin studies has been insensitive definitions of PD in cotwins. (d) Widespread rejection of a genetic hypothesis has been based, in large part, on the skeptical interpretation of autopsyless "PD kindreds" as olivopontocerebellar atrophy or familial tremor. Recently, however, several kindreds, some that are quite large, with autopsy-proved PD (or other Lewy body diseases) have come to light (7–13; Table 1). These provide precedent for the notion that an apparently genetic defect can produce parkinsonian pathology. (e) Finally, recent advances in the understanding of mitochondrial genetics and observations of defects in mitochondrial enzymes and DNA have provided a fresh set of genetic hypotheses that fit some of the data better than do traditional mendelian mechanisms.

This chapter summarizes the early clinical genetic investigations of PD and the recent diverse set of advances that have reopened the question.

II. KINDRED DESCRIPTIONS

Until 1949, most investigation on the genetics of PD took the form of anecdotal reports of kindreds, with little clinical detail and no autopsy confirmation. Bell and Clark (14) reviewed the ten such reports up to 1926 and added an 11th. Allan, in 1937 (15), reported an additional 25 selected kindreds, mostly referred to his practice in western North Carolina. Inspection of most of the pedigree charts in both papers reveals a pattern highly consistent with autosomal dominant inheritance. A few are too small to draw any useful inference on genetic mechanisms, but none suggests an autosomal recessive, X-linked, or mitochondrial mechanism. In fact, among Allan's 25 kindreds, the illness occurred in almost exactly half (146 of 290) of persons surviving to age 50 and having an affected parent, as an autosomal dominant model would predict. All 25 kindreds included affected individuals in a least two successive generations. In 18 kindreds, at least three successive generations were affected, despite apparent absence of consanguinity. This would not occur for a recessive trait with low allelic frequency in the population. The kindreds were referred from many areas of the southeastern United States, lessening the probability of their reflecting a locally prevalent recessive trait.

Referral of kindreds to Allan's series was probably biased in favor of families with a high percentage of members affected. The series may thereby be biased in favor of a conclusion of dominant inheritance. Furthermore, there is little statistical data (such as symptom onset age) and no autopsy data. The diagnostic criteria and the number of secondary cases the author examined are unspecified. Allan's sparse descriptions do not allow the modern reader to exclude autosomal dominant spinocerebellar atrophy with parkinsonism, or even familial essential tremor.

The next major contribution to our inventory of PD kindreds, and a landmark development in the modern history of the genetics of PD, was a large 1949 study by Mjönes (16). The material included several large kindreds. The largest, the Lister family, with 15 affected persons in three generations, showed a probable autosomal recessive pattern, with each affected individual the product of a consanguineous marriage. However, the other pedigrees were closely compatible with autosomal dominant inheritance. Mjönes found the frequency of consanguinity among these kindreds to be similar to that in Sweden in general, and not nearly enough to posit pseudodominance of a recessive trait.

Mjönes' lone familial case with microscopical autopsy data was a 63-year-old man who died in 1946 after a 6-year symptomatic course. Also affected were his father and grandfather, but none of his four siblings who reached age 50. The brain showed neuronal loss and gliosis that was severe in the substantia nigra and moderate in the globus pallidus. Lewy bodies are not mentioned, but these were not widely considered important to the diagnosis of PD at that time. The pallidal lesions casts doubt, however, on the diagnosis of PD, at least in that individual, if not in his kindred.

The first PD kindred with typical findings of PD on autopsy was published only recently (7,17). This Italian and American family originated in a town in Salerno province and includes, as of 1993, 45 known affected members in four generations. The clinical picture is atypical only for relative infrequency of tremor, early onset (mean age 46.5), and rapid course (mean of 9.7 years), despite dopa responsiveness. Autopsy of two individuals shows typical PD with Lewy bodies.

There are at least two other kindreds with pathologically typical PD. One includes eight affected individuals in six generations, with a somewhat atypical clinical picture (18). The mean onset age was only 17, dopa response was usually only fair, and the course was very long and benign. The other (12) includes two living clinically typical members. Autopsy of a third member with atypical parkinsonism showed lesions typical of PD.

Most other parkinsonian kindreds for which postmortem data exist are both clinically and pathologically very different from "sporadic" PD. For example, Joseph disease is an autosomal dominant form of clinically atypical multiple system atrophy or spinocerebellar degeneration(19). Muenter et al., in 1986 (10), reported a kindred with 12 members having parkinsonism and severe dementia, with Lewy bodies and neuronal loss not only in the "typical" areas, but also in the limbic system. The same kindred had been reported without autopsy data in 1962 by Spellman (20). Even more recently, Wszolek et al. (21) presented a large kindred with parkinsonism and dementia with degeneration in nigra, pontine tegmentum, and globus pallidus, without Lewy bodies. Apparently autosomal dominant diffuse Lewy body disease has also been described recently (8,22–24).

Table 1 Anecdotally Reported Kindreds With Proved or Presumptive Adult-Onset PD

Ref. (first author)	Yr	Kindreds	Number affected	Generations affected	Mean onset age	Dopa responsive?	Autopsy
Allan (15)	1937	25	258	2–5	?	?	
Bhatia (34)	1993	1	8	3	40s	yes	Cell loss in SN and locus coeruleus, gliosis of caudate and pallidum, "scarce" LBs
Bell (14)	1926	1	5–7	3	38	?	
Carlier (25)	1979	1	4	1	14	Yes	
Degl'Innocenti (26)	1989	1	8	2	56	Yes	
de Yebenes (27)	1989	8	19	1	?	?	
Dwork (110)	1993	1	14	3	20s	Yes	Neuronal loss only in SN; no LBs
Golbe (7,93)	1990, 1993	1	45	4	46	Yes	Typical PD
Golbe (18)	1993	1	8	6	20s	Yes	Typical PD
Hussels (28)	1967	1	5	4	?	?	
Inose (8)	1988	1	4	3	37	±	Diffuse LB disease
Mark (12)	1992	3	9	1–2	18, 57, 72	Yes	Diffuse LB disease
Mauri (29)	1990	1	10	2	67	Yes	
Mizutani (24)	1991	1	2	2	37	?	Diffuse LB disease

Mjönes (16)	1949	46	159	2–4	Range: 10–83	?	
Muenter[a] (10)	1986	1	12	4	20s,30s	?	Typical PD plus limbic involvement
Nair (31)	1986	1	3	1	30	±	
Nukuda (30)	1978	1	36	5	39–69	Yes	
Ota (35)	1958	1	3	1	12	?	Cell loss typical of PD, but no LBs
Perry (11)	1990	1	10	3	53 at death	no	Cell loss typical of PD, with "rare" LBs
Roy (32)	1983	3	11	?	?	?	
Sandy (33)	1983	1	5	3	"Middle life"	?	
Sawle (56)	1992	1	4 (clinical) + 1 (by PET)	1	39	Yes	
Spellman[a] (20)	1962	1	8	3	29	?	
Takada (23)	1991	1	2	1	45	?	Diffuse LB disease
Waters (13)	1991	1	7	4	30s	±	Atypical LBs in typical PD distribution
Wszolek (21)	1992	1	32	8	40s	Usually no	Cell loss in pallidum, SN, pons, without LBs

[a]These kindreds are one and the same.
LB, Lewy body; SN, substantia nigra.

There have been many other reports of parkinsonian kindreds (see Table 1). In some (13–15,20,22–34), the clinical and (if available) pathological pictures differ from PD, and their relevance to the question of a genetic cause of PD is hypothetical. In others (7–11,16,35,36), the clinical picture is typical, or nearly so, but there is no autopsy confirmation of the diagnosis of PD in any member.

In theory, autopsy is critical in excluding such hereditary conditions as rigid-variant Huntington's disease, Joseph disease, dopa-responsive dystonia, or spinocerebellar atrophy, which are all autosomal dominant and can be confused clinically with PD. Importantly, however, there appears to be no report of clinically typical familial PD with an autopsy atypical of PD. Furthermore, there is no report of a kindred with solely maternal inheritance as would occur in a mitochondrial disease. (In fact, careful search for this inheritance pattern has been negative; 37,38.) Nor is there a kindred with a strong likelihood of sex linkage. There are only a few reports, besides the Lister family of Mjönes (16), of autosomal recessive patterns, and none of these had autopsy confirmation or careful biochemical analysis.

The "hereditary mental depression and parkinsonism with taurine deficiency," reported by Perry et al. (39) in 1975 and by Purdy (40) in 1978, seems, on my reading, to be clinically compatible with Parkinson's disease, except for early onset, similar to the large kindred of Golbe et al. (7,17). Perry et al., in a publication 15 years later (11), concluded that the taurine deficiency was an incidental finding and was absent from several more recently studied members of the kindred. The mental depression seems of a magnitude occasionally seen in PD, particularly familial PD (41).

At the very least, the significance of the autopsy-confirmed kindreds is as a demonstration of the possibility of an apparently single gene producing PD, including its distinctive pathological picture. More important, they provide an opportunity, using modern molecular genetic techniques, to isolate a PD gene (42) which, once its structure and function are understood, may reveal the etiology, or at least the pathogenesis, of "sporadic" PD. At the most, these kindreds may represent PD without the mask of factors, perhaps other genes, that confer some degree of protection on the relatives of most patients.

III. TWIN STUDIES

A special case of quantitative genetic studies are the twin studies, of which now there have been four (2,43–45). With the exception of the most recent, which has been reported only in preliminary form, the studies showed a concordance rate among monozygotic (MZ) twins that was far lower than predicted for a genetic illness. The summed data from all four studies showed that the MZ concordance rate, 5 of 82 pairs (6.1%), was no different from that of dizygotic (DZ) pairs, 3 of 66 pairs (4.6%) (Table 2). However, the data analysis of the

Table 2 Twin Studies

First author	Yr	Country	Concordance (MZ pairs)[a,b]	Concordance (DZ pairs)[a,b]
Marsden (43)	1987	UK	1/11	0/19
Marttila (44)	1988	Finland	0/18	1/14
Vieregge (45)	1991	Germany	3/10	2/14
Ward (2)	1983	US, Canada	1/43	0/19
Totals			5/82 (6.1%)	3/66 (4.6%)

[a]MZ, monozygotic; DZ, dizygotic
[b]The denominator refers to the number of twin pairs with at least one affected member.

large U.S.–Canadian twin study (2) and, by inference, that of the two smaller European studies then available (43,44), have recently been questioned in a paper of Johnson et al. (6), the senior author of which is Duvoisin, the U.S.–Canadian twin study's principal investigator.

The U.S.–Canadian twin study (2) advertised in patient newsletters and professional journals for patients with PD who had a living twin. The authors examined each patient and cotwin, finding only one of the 43 pairs of MZ twins and none of 19 pairs of DZ twins to be concordant for "definite" PD. Johnson et al. (6) argue that we should not accept this data at face value. First, since the time of the twin study, the notion of a long preclinical course of PD has gained favor (5), raising the possibility of a long interval between the onset of symptoms in the members of a twin pair (Table 3). In a concordant MZ twin pair, separately reported by Koller et al. (46), the interval between onset age was 6.5 years. In the one definitely concordant MZ pair in the twin study, the interval was 10 years (2). Follow-up of 20 of the original discordant MZ pairs a decade later revealed that one of the pairs had become clinically concordant after a discordance interval of 23 years(47,48). This suggests that additional MZ cotwins may have preclinical PD and, therefore, that the true concordance rate may be much higher than 1:43.

The U.S.–Canadian twin study (2) found several twin pairs concordant for an atypical parkinsonian syndrome and rejected these from the main analysis as not having PD. The wisdom of this policy depends on one's definition of PD, a definition that has not been widely agreed on (49). Two series have documented that the "typical" autopsy picture of PD correlates to a far-from-perfect degree with the typical premortem clinical state (4,50). This suggests that the clinical spectrum of the pathological picture is very wide. If one accepts this pathological picture as the more valid (albeit less practical) definition of "PD," then epidemiological studies, such as the twin studies, should recognize the possibility that, nevertheless, clinically atypical cases may be the genuine article. When Johnson

Table 3 Reports of Monozygotic Twin Pairs Concordant for PD

First author	Yr	Country	Ages at PD onset	Discordance interval	Atypical features
Jankovic (109)	1986	U.S., Israel	71, 71	0	None
Kissel (110)	1976	France	39, 39	0	Anosmia in both
Koller (46)	1986	U.S.	60, 66.5	6.5	None
Marsden (43)	1987	U.K.	69, 71	2	None
Pahwa (111)	1993	U.S.	62, 63	1	None
Vieregge (45)	1991	Germany	Not stated[a]	4, 7, 13	(No details)[a]
Ward (2)	1983	U.S., Canada	35, 45	10	Both alcoholics with multiple episodes of minor head trauma
Zimmerman (47)	1991	U.S., Canada	40, 63	23	(No details)[a]
Median				4	
Mean				6.7	

[a]These reports were abstracts with few clinical details.

et al. (6) applied the broadest possible definition of PD, the concordance rate for MZ twins in the U.S.–Canadian study was 6:50 and for DZ twins 1:19.

When Johnson et al. (6) applied a definition of intermediate restrictiveness to the twin data ("possible" PD, but not "atypical" PD or isolated dementia) the concordances were 2:43 and 0:19. The coefficient of genetic determination, G, a statistic based on a polygenic–threshold disease model, was 0.78. (A G of 1.00 indicates a wholly genetic cause, 0 a nongenetic cause.) However, for nearly any level of diagnostic restrictiveness, the 95% confidence intervals for G included both 0 and 1.00. Clearly, then, the U.S.–Canadian twin study (2) was too small to permit any firm conclusions concerning the heritability of PD.

A potential bias in the subject ascertainment method of the U.S.–Canadian twin study has been pointed out by Burton and Calne (51), the latter author, one of the twin study's coinvestigators. The twin study solicited only *living* pairs to allow personal examination of both twins. Inasmuch as PD increases mortality risk, both members of a concordant-affected pair are less likely to be alive at a given time than are both members of a discordant pair. Discordant pairs, therefore, were probably more likely to answer the appeal for living twin pairs. Furthermore, discordant pairs may be more likely to include one member who was able to respond to the query and arrange for the pair to participate in the study.

The other three twin studies (see Table 2) were much smaller, and two (43,45) are reported in only brief form. One (43) ascertained its cases by advertisements in the newsletter of the Parkinson's Disease Society of the United Kingdom, and cases were not examined by the author. Another, from Germany, does not specify its ascertainment methods in the preliminary communication, but found the highest concordance rates, 3:10 MZ and 2:14 DZ. The third (44), based on a linkage of the Finnish Twin Cohort with the Finnish Hospital Discharge Register, rather than on advertised appeals, is perhaps the strongest of the four from a methodological viewpoint, but suffers from small numbers.

An ambitious twin study that avoids all of the methodological pitfalls of the others (except the insufficient validity of clinical examination in diagnosing PD) is under way in the United States using a cohort of 8000 white male military veteran twin pairs (52).

The most important pitfall of the twin studies—clinical diagnostic insensitivity—may be avoided, to some extent, by use of positron emission tomography (PET) to detect reduction in uptake of [^{18}F]fluorodopa by the presynaptic dopamine uptake system in the striatum of patients with PD (53). The use of PET has also detected preclinical dopaminergic damage in persons exposed to MPTP (54), in Guamanians at risk of developing the amyotrophic lateral sclerosis–parkinsonism–dementia complex of Guam (55), and in asymptomatic at-risk members of kindreds with PD (56). Burn et al. (57) used PET to measure putaminal [^{18}F]fluorodopa uptake in asymptomatic cotwins of probands with PD. They found uptake reduced to more than 2 standard deviations below the control mean in four of ten MZ cotwins and in two of seven DZ cotwins. Two of the four MZ cotwins with abnormal scans had isolated postural tremor, without rest tremor or other sign of PD.

These PET results suggest two important conclusions. One is that the twin concordance rate is far higher than clinical history and examination alone indicate. The other is that isolated postural tremor, in at least some cases, may represent a dopamine-deficiency state, a "forme fruste" of PD.

IV. THE "PARKINSON'S DISEASE ICEBERG"

Additional reason to question the findings of any survey of familial PD comes from recent tabulations of autopsy findings in nonparkinsonian patients finding a surprisingly high prevalence of asymptomatic Lewy bodies (58–60). This pathological hallmark of PD is present in 5–6% of the autopsied population older than 40 and in over 10% of the population older than 70. (Nigral neuronal counts could not be easily performed for the large number required to generate this data.) Assuming that nigral Lewy bodies are equivalent to presymptomatic PD, we may conclude that far more people have PD (or its pathological substrate) than meets the eye.

Duvoisin (61) has estimated the magnitude of this "iceberg effect" as follows: Age-adjustment of the data of Gibb et al. (59,60) to the age structure of the living U. S. population suggests that 5.6% of persons older than 40 have Lewy bodies in their substantia nigra. The prevalence of clinically diagnosable PD in this population, as measured by the community-based Copiah County study (62), is 0.35%. Dividing 5.6% by this observed prevalence gives 16. Given the uncertainty of clinical diagnosis and the wide confidence limits of the data, we may conclude that the ratio of asymptomatic PD to clinically diagnosable PD is at least 10 or 20. Presumably, PET scanning with ^{18}F-dopa would reveal some of the submerged portion of the iceberg, as it did among the asymptomatic cotwins of Burn et al. (57).

Given the foregoing considerations, the PD prevalence of 5 cases among the 82 MZ cotwins and the 3 cases among the 66 DZ cotwins may then be augmented considerably, bringing the results much closer to what would be predicted by a purely genetic hypothesis of the cause of PD. However, in so elderly a population (the cotwins), the fraction of the iceberg remaining submerged must be smaller than the fraction calculated for the general population older than 40, which has a younger mean age than did the cotwins.

The concept of the PD iceberg (61) reduces the need to invoke hypothetical asymmetrical distribution of etiologic or protective factors between MZ fetuses in utero (63,64) or to posit the occurrence of a somatic mutation in one of the twins (65). However, both intrauterine factors and somatic mutation remain intriguing possibilities as a contribution to the cause of PD.

V. EPIDEMIOLOGIC INVESTIGATIONS OF FAMILIAL PARKINSON'S DISEASE

The frequency with which relatives of patients with PD suffer from the disease is unclear. Clinic-based surveys of familial prevalence of PD are difficult to interpret. One reason is that the investigator's interest in familial PD is often known among referring physicians. Another is the highly variable, and often unspecified criteria, used in identifying secondary cases. Usually, neither alleged secondary cases, nor allegedly unaffected relatives, were examined by the author. Even worse, the degree of relation used to define a "relative" is not always specified. Inasmuch as Kurland (66) calculated the lifetime incidence of parkinsonism (mostly PD) as 2.4%, if each patient with PD can supply data on only six or seven relatives reaching old age, 16% of the family histories will be positive. Clearly, then, the use of a control group will increase the quality of such epidemiological studies. One remaining pitfall, however, is the possibility of recall bias, wherein an ill person (and his or her relatives) may more carefully consider his or her family history in search of secondary cases and, in fact, have often done so even before that data was requested for research purposes. Finally, and most important, the question of preclinical PD subverts not only the twin studies, but any survey of PD prevalence, familial or otherwise.

The most useful surveys on the prevalence of familial PD, therefore, are those that use a control population as a reference. Unfortunately, there have been only seven such studies (67–73; Table 4). In only three of these (67,69,70) did the investigators examine the living secondary cases, and in only one (69), a study of patients' siblings, did the investigators examine the allegedly unaffected relatives. Even here, the authors examined only 69% of the living siblings of patients and controls and made no attempt to ascertain or examine affected parents of patients. In this study, Duvoisin et al. found a low prevalence of affected siblings of patients, similar to that of the siblings of their unaffected spouses, and to the prevalence of PD in the general population. When only those cases that Duvoisin et al. (69) defined as definite PD are considered, the prevalence of PD among

Table 4 Controlled Epidemiological Studies of Familial PD

First author	Yr	Country	Definite PD in first-degree relatives of: Probands	Controls	*p* value[a]
Alonso (67)	1986	Mexico	10/105 (9.5%)	1/100 (1%)	0.017 (chi-square) 0.0006 (Fisher's exact test)
Butterfield (68)	1993	U.S.	16/63 (25.4 %) (1st, 2nd and 3rd degree considered)	7/68 (10.3%) (1st, 2nd and 3rd degree considered)	0.037
Duvoisin (69)	1969	U.S.	3/146 sibs (2.1%)	1/145 sibs (0.7%)	NS
Martin (70)	1973	U.S.	22/130 (16.9%)	11/130 (8.5%)	0.062 (chi-square) 0.031 (Fisher's exact test)
Marttila (71)	1976	Finland	27/429 (6.3%)	19/443 (4.3%)	NS
Semchuk (72)	1993	U.S.	14/128 (10.9%)	13/255 (5.1%)	<0.05
Vieregge (73)	1992	Germany	(9.3%) of 1st- and 2nd-degree relatives	(1.0%) of 1st- and 2nd-degree relatives	<0.01

[a]NS, Not statistically significant

probands' siblings is three times that among their spouses' siblings (3:146 vs. 1:145), but the difference is nonsignificant.

A similar result emerged from the survey of Marttila and Rinne (71), in which 27 of 429 patients (6.3%) and 19 of 443 controls (4.3%) reported PD "in the family" (difference not statistically significant). There were no examinations of secondary cases.

Alonso et al. (67), by contrast, found 10 of 105 patients (9.5%) to have an affected first-degree relative, compared with only 1 of 105 (1%) for controls. The authors do not state how many affected secondary cases were, in fact, available for examination among each group, the ages of the at-risk relatives in each group, nor the diagnostic criteria for examined secondary cases.

Martin et al. (70) provided a highly detailed report of familial PD among 130 consecutive patients with PD seen for initial treatment with levodopa, also using their spouses as controls. The prevalence of allegedly affected first-degree relatives was twice as high among patients as among controls (16.9 vs. 8.5%), and the prevalence of PD among patients' parents who had reached age 25 was nearly three times as high as among controls (6.2 vs. 2.3%). Both comparisons were at the margin of statistical significance. The authors did not examine the allegedly affected relatives.

The ideal study of the question of the prevalence of familial PD would have to (a) establish a rigid definition of PD for probands and secondary cases, (b) specify how the probands were questioned concerning their family, (c) include an adequately motivated control group, (d) examine all alleged secondary cases, (e) specify the age structure of probands' and controls' families, and (f) examine at least a statistically valid sample of the allegedly unaffected relatives as a measure of the sensitivity of probands' allegations of PD in the family. No study has yet met this ideal, and despite the virtues of the four controlled studies, the magnitude of PD risk among relatives of PD patients remains uncertain.

A noncontrolled study, but one that, over four decades later, is unmatched in scope and ambition, is that of Mjönes (16; Table 5). Published as a thesis for Doctor of Medicine, in 1949, it surveyed hereditary and other clinical aspects of PD from nine large clinics in Sweden. In 46 of Mjönes' 79 cases alleging a secondary familial case, that secondary case was a parent. For 22 of the remaining 33, a sibling was affected. A first-degree relative, therefore, was affected in 68 of the 79 familial cases. The author examined about half of the probands and secondary cases, most of the remainder having died. He did not examine family members alleged to be unaffected.

Among his 115 nonfamilial cases and his 33 cases with a positive family history that spared the parents, Mjönes found that 24% of parents died before aged 60, whereas among affected parents of cases, only 9% died before 60. This suggests that the frequency of parental secondary cases may have been higher with greater longevity and opens the possibility that autosomal dominant

Table 5 Noncontrolled Epidemiological Studies of Familial PD

First author	Yr	Country	Definite PD in a 1st-degree relative[a]
Atazhanov (112)	1973	U.S.S.R.	15/32 (47%)
Barbeau (3)	1984	Canada	14/342 (4%)
Campanella (85)	1984	Italy	14/336 (4.2%)
Gudmundsson (113)	1967	Iceland	25/87 (23%)
Hart (114)	1904	U.S.	13/219 (5.9%)
Jenkins (115)	1966	Australia	9/70 (12.9%) had "positive family history"
Kondo (81, 82)	1973, 1978	U.S., Japan	(9.67%) Rochester, Minnesota (1.64%) Niigata, Japan
Lazzarini (38)	in press	U.S.	2.8% (sisters) to 8.5% (mothers)
Maraganore (84)	1991	U.K.	5/243 (2%) definite by exam; additional 20 (8.2%) "likely"
Mjönes (16)	1949	Sweden	68/194 (35.1%)
Osuntokun (116)	1979	Nigeria	2/83 (2.4%) had "positive family history"
Pollock (117)	1966	New Zealand	11/84 (14%) had a sib, parent, aunt, or uncle with PD
Ringwald (118)	1984	?	20/424 (4.7%) had "positive family history"
Vassilopoulos (119)	1988	Greece	20/806 (2.5%) of 1st-degree relatives older than 30 had PD

[a]Figures are prevalence of PD among first-degree relatives, unless otherwise specified.

heredity may be obscured, in many cases, by the death of at-risk individuals before the age of greatest disease incidence. Parenthetically, this mortality effect may profoundly influence all studies of the demographics and genetic epidemiology of PD.

Mjönes' study has been criticized for including persons with isolated tremor as secondary familial cases, inflating the measured familial tendency (70,74). Indeed, among 162 secondary cases in probands' families, tremor was the only known parkinsonian sign in 110. However, the only other signs Mjönes tabulated were cogwheeling, rigidity, and parkinsonian mask. Postural instability and bradykinesia, two of the four modern cardinal signs of PD, were not considered and could have been present in some secondary cases. Furthermore, for only 23 of the 110 cases of "isolated tremor" were the other three parkinsonian signs specifically denoted as absent. In the other 87, most of which were deceased antecedents, the only information the lay informants apparently recalled was presence of a tremor. Perhaps the most telling vindication of Mjönes' methods are the ^{18}F-dopa PET results of Burn et al. (57), showing that isolated postural tremor in twins of affected individuals may be a sign of PD.

Although this does not establish a diagnosis of PD for all of Mjönes' "secondary cases," it at least blunts the single major criticism of his work. One may reverse the argument and wonder how many nontremulous secondary cases Mjönes (and subsequent investigators) failed to ascertain solely because surviving informants mistook bradykinesia, anteroflexed posture, and shuffling for normal aging.

A very recent study that included no control group, but otherwise approached the ideal for a PD multifamily study, is that of Lazzarini et al. (38). They surveyed 211 consecutive patients with PD from the referral practice of one of the authors. Of the 40 families in whom there was full PD status data on all of the proband's first- and second-degree relatives, 53% had a probable or definite secondary familial case. The authors point out that previous studies reporting lower figures did not ascertain full family data. In fact, their 171 patients, providing less thorough family data, reported a much lower frequency of probable or definite secondary cases–23% for those providing full data only on first-degree relatives, and 7% for those providing full data on neither first- nor second-degree relatives. Although the absence of a control group obscures the meaning of these figures somewhat, the point is clear that more thorough inquiry increases the yield of positive family PD histories.

Lazzarini et al. (38) found that the frequency of secondary cases among first-degree relatives who were able to provide complete information on those relatives, ranged from 2.0% of patients' sisters to 7.1% of patients' mothers. When isolated tremor is included in the definition of PD, as the PET data suggest it should, these figures increased to 2.8 and 8.5%.

Another excellent recent study does include controls. Semchuk et al. (72) performed a case–control study of risk factors in 128 patients with PD in Alberta and 255 matched controls. The questionnaire covered many aspects of occupational and other environmental exposure and family history. After multivariate conditional logistic regression analysis, a family history of PD emerged as the strongest predictor of PD risk. The crude odds ratio (the frequency of a positive family among the cases divided by that among the controls) was 2.4 for having an affected first-degree relative, 3.7 for a first- or second-degree relative, and 5.8 for a first-, second-, or third-degree relative, all statistically significant. Other, less strong, predictors of PD risk were a history of serious head trauma and occupational herbicide use, in that order. The family history odds ratios were virtually unchanged after adjusting for the other two risk factors.

Butterfield et al. (68) performed a similar case–control study, but in patients whose PD started before aged 50. The odds ratio for a positive family history was 2.5 ($p = 0.037$). The authors, whose principal interest was environmental factors, did not adjust this figure for the effect of other risk factors.

The results of both studies (68,72) are weakened slightly by the absence of confirmatory examination of familial secondary cases, or review of their medical records. If we assume that the patients were familiar with the hypothesis that head trauma and herbicide exposure were also candidate PD risk factors, recall bias could also have affected reporting of those.

VI. OTHER FAMILY STUDIES

Several other careful studies examining the question of clinical genetics of PD from a variety of angles have appeared over the past 15 years. Most analyzed a relatively large number of small PD kindreds.

One approach was taken by Calne et al. (75), who compared the difference in age at onset of six affected parent–child pairs with the absolute time difference between onset in the two. The mean age interval was 25.2 years, and the mean time interval was only 4.6 years, supporting a common environmental cause acting at a discrete time, rather than a hereditary cause. This method may have been confounded by the increased vigilance for parkinsonian symptoms that one would exercise after seeing a parent affected. Also, the younger generation may have had access to more skilled neurological diagnosis than did their parents, thereby receiving a diagnosis at an earlier stage of disease.

The opposite result was obtained by de Yebenes et al. (27), who found the onset age to be relatively uniform within eight PD kindreds and for there to be no clustering of years of onset. That preliminary report also found no differences in environmental exposures between affected and unaffected members of sibships. The same group, in a full publication (29), found that patients with a family history of PD were less likely to have drunk well water and more likely to have consanguinity in the family than were controls with PD and no family history. This despite the similar frequency of rural living in the groups. These data support the hypothesis that both environmental and genetic factors are necessary for the development of PD.

Barbeau and colleagues, in a series of papers, report an association between familial PD and familial benign tremor (3,32,76,77). Their most important observation was that 34 of their 50 PD kindreds actually had "essential tremor (ET)-related" familial PD inherited as an autosomal dominant trait and that this variant of PD accounted for 10% of all PD in their clinic. However, 28 of the 34 kindreds included only one member with parkinsonism and 8 had only two members. These, therefore, could have represented coincidental occurrence of PD in ET kindreds. Moreover, their 50 patients with familial ET reported that only three of their 541 first-degree relatives had PD (0.6%) and the 50 control subjects reported that 2 of their 466 first-degree relatives had PD (0.4%).

VII. GENETIC MECHANISMS

A. Clinical Studies

A recurring issue is whether the inheritance of familial PD is more closely compatible with an autosomal dominant or a polygenic mode of transmission.

Some of these studies were performed before the possibility of an acquired, environmental etiologic contribution was seriously considered, and this adds an additional dimension of complexity to the issue. A majority of studies have concluded that hereditary PD does indeed exist and that its most common mechanism, by far, is autosomal dominance. However, there is a small body of literature that supports a polygenic mode of inheritance in these families.

Young et al. (78) attempted to distinguish an autosomal dominant from a polygenic cause in 12 families having a proband and at least two secondarily affected antecedent cases. A polygenic model of inheritance of any trait predicts that two-thirds of such pairings should be unilateral (that is, on the proband's paternal or maternal side, but not both), and that one-third should be bilateral (79). The result was that 25 of the 29 pairings were unilateral. The authors claim that this is not significantly different from the polygenic model's prediction, but Kehrer et al. (80) perform the calculation on the same data differently and obtain a significant result, supporting an autosomal dominant mechanism.

Mjönes (16) also concluded that the mechanism was autosomal dominance with reduced penetrance, similar to that in essential tremor. Martin (70) reached the opposite conclusion, because in his series (a) PD prevalence within a sibship correlated with the prevalence of PD among nonsib relatives, whereas an autosomal dominant model (with any given degree of penetrance) predicts a sib prevalence rate (50%, given full penetrance) independent of PD prevalence elsewhere in the family. (b) The age of PD onset among probands correlates inversely with the prevalence of PD among siblings, declining smoothly from 8.3% of sibs affected for proband onset age 35–44, to 1.4% affected for proband onset age 65–74; the mechanism being greater "genetic load" in families with young-onset. (c) The less frequently affected sex, females, had more affected relatives; the greater abnormal "genetic load" in such families produced PD in the sex with greater resistance and also caused greater overall PD prevalence in the family.

Kondo (81–83) reanalyzed Martin's and Mjönes' data and replicated Martin's conclusions. His support for a polygenic model is based on the observations that (a) the segregation ratio (the percentage of affected children of an affected parent) that he calculated as 19% for Martin's data and 16% for Mjönes' data, demands a reduction of penetrance that seems unacceptably large; (b) the "heritability" of PD in families with more than one affected member (90.8% for Mjönes' data, 79.2% for Martin's, and 67.4% in a Japanese city (81) is uniformly much greater than and independent of the frequencies of multicase sibships sib recurrence rates, which were 11.7,9.7, and 1.6%, respectively; (c) frequencies of multicase subships decreased in more remote relatives and increased in sibships with one affected parent, in sibships with more than one sib already affected, in sibships of whom the proband had young onset, and in geographic areas with higher general population PD prevalence.

The analysis by Maraganore et al. (84) supports an autosomal dominant mechanism. These authors admit that their "nonrandom ascertainment of small numbers of cases (20 probands) severely restricts testing for polygenicity." However, they tentatively exclude polygenicity because (a) the frequency of secondary cases among probands' siblings was similar in sibships with an affected parent (23% of sibs affected) and without one (21%) and not at least the 2.5:1 ratio predicted by a polygenic model; and (b) all antecedent cases were unilaterally (i.e., paternal or maternal, not both) distributed. They exclude a mitochondrial mechanism because maternal transmission was no more common than paternal transmission among their kindreds and among those from seven previous reports (15,26,70,75,85–87).

The study of Lazzarini et al. (38) addressed the question of an autosomal dominant versus a multifactorial (or coincidental) cause of the familial aggregation in their 80 multicase families. Diagnosis in about half of the alleged secondary cases was confirmed by personal examination by the authors or by autopsy. Cumulative calculated lifetime risk was 45% for parents and 42% for siblings. The similarity in these numbers supports the hypothesis that PD in these families is autosomal dominant and not multifactorial. Furthermore, the unilateral/bilateral ratio of multiple antecedent cases was 73:4, significantly greater than the 2:1 predicted by a multifactorial model. This is strong evidence against the hypothesis that PD occurs in these families as chance aggregations of a common disease. It also supports an autosomal dominant model at the expense of a polygenic model.

It must be emphasized that these genetic analyses considered only those patients with at least one secondary familial case. Their conclusions on genetic mechanisms, therefore, may not apply to the majority of patients with apparently "sporadic" PD.

B. Laboratory Studies

A more recent laboratory development provides a potential mechanism whereby a dominantly inherited gene could cause PD (or other neurodegenerative disease). Chalfie and Wolinsky (88) reported a dominantly inherited mutation in the nematode *Caenorhabditis elegans* causing late-onset death of a specific population of neurons. The cloned gene coded for a previously unknown protein that may impair membrane function. The neurons so affected had a pathological appearance different from that of neurons that degenerate as part of the worm's normal aging.

Two mechanisms that have been investigated in patients with sporadic PD are somatic mutation and a mitochondrial genetic defect. Robbins et al. (89) have found that cultured lymphoblastoid cell lines from patients with PD (without apparent family history) and Alzheimer's disease were especially sensitive to

DNA damage from X-rays. The resulting somatic mutation would not be inherited unless DNA, in at least some of the gonadal cells themselves, sustains damage. This intriguing finding awaits confirmation.

Another genetic model, one that has not been tested in PD, but can explain the low MZ twin concordance rate, is DNA rearrangement during development (90). This phenomenon is known to occur in lower animals and in human tumors and, if it occurs in one member of an MZ pair (or differently in each member) after the zygote divides, the pair will not be quite genetically identical.

A similar, recently observed molecular genetic phenomenon, postconceptional trinucleotide repeat expansion (91), may also help explain the low MZ twin pair concordance. (This phenomenon may provide a mechanism for the model outlined by Eldridge and Ince in 1984 (92). Strongly hereditary PD can exhibit anticipation, wherein successive generations suffer disease onset at progressive earlier ages (18,93). Other hereditary neurodegenerative diseases, such as Huntington's disease (HD), myotonic dystrophy, Kennedy's syndrome, spinocerebellar atrophy type 1 (SCA-1), and fragile X syndrome, are each associated with abnormal expansion of a trinucleotide repeat sequence. In the cases of HD, Kennedy's syndrome, and SCA-1, the length of the repeat varies inversely with onset age (94,95). With vertical transmission of the gene, the repeat often progressively lengthens and onset-age anticipation occurs. It has recently been shown that, at least for the fragile X syndrome, the trinucleotide repeat expands not at meiosis, but during mitosis in the very early postconceptional period (91). This, then, invites the hypothesis that repeat expansion may occur to different degrees in the two zygotes (or early embryos) and produce different PD onset ages or PD discordance in the two MZ twins.

Another important molecular genetic phenomenon, and one with better experimental support in PD, is that a large fraction of the mitochondrial genome is deleted from the striatum in PD (96–99). Part of the deleted section of genome codes for some of the subunits of complex I, a component of the mitochondrial respiratory chain. Indeed, activity of complex I has been deficient in striatum, muscle, and platelets of patients with PD (97,100,101). Adding to the appeal of this genetic mechanism is the confirmed observation (102) that the site of toxic action of the nigral toxin MPTP (see Chapter 13) is mitochondrial NADH–ubiquinone oxidoreductase, or complex I. The mitochondrial hypothesis, therefore, is compatible with much of the data from both environmental and familial studies of PD (103).

A disease with a mitochondrial mechanism is inherited only maternally, as the ovum, but not the spermatozoon, contains mitochondria. However, none of the large PD kindreds reported (see Table 1) shows this pattern. Nor are lone secondary cases more likely to be maternal than paternal (84). Still, the low MZ twin PD concordance rate may be explained by asymmetrical distribution in the dividing zygote of that fraction of mitochondria bearing a mutation. Also, lack of a protective histone coat on mitochondrial DNA renders it more vulnerable to somatic mutation, a genetic mechanism that can help explain the apparent low familial prevalence of PD (104).

One preliminary attempt to find the mitochondrial DNA deletion in platelets of patients with PD has failed (105), but a mitochondrial mechanism is an attractive one, especially for most of those patients with PD whose family history is poorly compatible with a mendelian, or any, genetic mechanism. As the physiology of dopamine and other neurotransmitters involved in PD is better understood and the genes controlling the production or function of enzymes, trophic factors, transport proteins and receptors in these systems are found, various candidates for a genetic basis of PD will arise. One prominent at present is the dopamine transporter (106). The gene for it and those for several other candidate proteins (tyrosine hydroxylase, brain-derived neurotrophic factor, debrisoquine hydroxylase, amyloid precursor protein, glutathione peroxidase, catalase, and superoxide dismutase) appear not to be linked to the PD gene in three families with atypical PD (107). These families did not have Lewy bodies at autopsy (21), so other families must be similarly tested.

Chapter 6 reviews the evidence that PD may be the result of an intrinsic, possibly genetically determined, defect in detoxification of exogenous substances. The principal candidates to date are the cytochrome P-450 system, monoamine oxidase B, *N*-methylation, *S*-oxidation, and *S*-methylation. These proposals, as enzyme deficiencies, lend themselves far more easily to an autosomal recessive model than to an autosomal dominant one, so would fail to explain PD in most of the families reported. However, a recessive pattern with low penetrance has not been excluded as an explanation of apparently sporadic PD. The philosophical question then arises: If the offending toxin is universal and ubiquitous, as Williams suggests (see Chapter 6), does it deserve to even be called a toxin, or is it part of "normal" human physiology? If the latter, how can we say that the cause of PD is anything but genetic?

VIII. Conclusions

Traditionally considered a sporadic disease, PD is now widely acknowledged to result, at least in part, from hereditary factors. This change in thinking is largely the result of increasing recognition of PD kindreds and of the possibility that a family pattern may be obscured by the long preclinical phase of PD or by failure of patients to reach medical attention. However, the degree to which the artifacts can explain the low frequency of familial cases remains unknown. "Negative" evidence of a genetic cause includes our failure as yet to discover an MPTP analogue in the environment that can explain PD, and the recent serious challenges to the methodology of the twin studies that concluded that the PD concordance rates in monozygotic pairs was very low. The use of PET with ^{18}F-dopa has found a much higher twin concordance rate than has clinical examination and has also informed us that isolated postural tremor in twins of PD probands is associated with dopaminergic dysfunction. The failure of clinical examination or PET to detect an important difference in the concordance rates of MZ and DZ twins remains an important obstacle to the genetic hypothesis.

Analysis of large and small families with multiple PD cases shows a nearly consistent autosomal dominant pattern. The highly asymmetrical distribution of multiple antecedent secondary cases is strong evidence against a multifactorial (including environmental) cause in those families. A major remaining question is whether PD occurring in families is the same disease at a molecular, etiologic, or pathogenetic level as PD occurring without apparent family history. The fact that autopsy in these families, in the handful of cases where it was obtained, usually shows a somewhat atypical pathological picture means that such differences may indeed exist.

The mechanism of the genetic component has only begun to come under investigation. There are many promising leads, and it is likely that more than one will exist in the parkinsonian population. The greatest reward will probably come from locating and cloning the culprit gene in large PD families. Multicenter cooperation, as yet lacking, will probably be crucial in this endeavor. Even if an elusive environmental factor is a necessary component to the cause of PD, assaying for the genetic defect could allow accurate diagnostic (even prenatal) testing and inactivating the gene or its product could arrest the progression of the disease.

REFERENCES

1. Langston JW, Ballard PA, Tetrud JW, Irwin I. Chronic parkinsonism in humans due to a product of meperidine-analog synthesis. Science 1983; 219:979–980.
2. Ward CD, Duvoisin RC, Ince SE, Nutt JD, Eldridge R, Calne DB. Parkinson's disease in 65 pairs of twins and in a set of quadruplets. Neurology 1983; 33:815–824.
3. Barbeau A, Roy M. Familial subsets in idiopathic Parkinson's disease. Can J Neurol Sci 1984; 11:144–150.
4. Sage JI, Miller DC, Golbe LI, Walters A, Duvoisin RC. Clinically atypical expression of pathologically typical Lewy-body parkinsonism. Clin Neuropharmacol 1990; 13:36–47.
5. Koller WC, Langston JW, Hubble JP, et al. Does a long pre-clinical period occur in Parkinson's disease? Neurology 1991; 41 (Suppl 2):8–13.
6. Johnson WG, Hodge SE, Duvoisin R. Twin studies and the genetics of Parkinson's disease—a reappraisal. Mov Disord 1990; 5:187–194.
7. Golbe LI, Di Iorio G, Bonavita V, Miller DC, Duvoisin RC. A large kindred with autosomal dominant Parkinson's disease. Ann Neurol 1990; 27:276–282.
8. Inose T, Miyakawa M, Miyakawa K, Mizushima S, Oyanagi S, Ando S. Clinical

and neuropathological study of a familial case of juvenile parkinsonism. Jpn J Psychiatry Neurol 1988; 42:265–276.
9. Golbe LI. A kindred with juvenile/young-onset Lewy body parkinsonism [abstract]. Neurology 1992; 42 (suppl 3):472.
10. Muenter M, Howard JF, Okazaki H, Forno L, Kish S, Hornykiewicz O. A familial Parkinson–dementia syndrome. Neurology 1986; 36:115.
11. Perry TL, Wright J, Berry K, Hansen S, Perry TL Jr. Dominantly inherited apathy, central hypoventilation, and Parkinson's syndrome: clinical, biochemical, and neuropathologic studies of 2 new cases. Neurology 1990; 40:1882–1887.
12. Mark MH, Dickson DW. The spectrum of Lewy body disease. Ann Clin Lab Sci 1992; 22:270.
13. Waters C, Miller C. Autosomal dominant transmission of Parkinson's disease in a four generation family. Ann Neurol 1994; 35:59–64.
14. Bell J, Clark AJ. A pedigree of paralysis agitans. Ann Eugen 1926; 455–462.
15. Allan W. Inheritance of the shaking palsy. Arch Intern Med 1937; 60:424–436.
16. Mjönes H. Paralysis agitans: a clinical and genetic study. Acta Psychiatr Neurol 1949; 54:1–195.
17. Golbe LI, Miller DC, Duvoisin RC. Autosomal dominant Lewy-body Parkinson's disease. In: Parkinson's disease: anatomy, pathology and therapy. Adv Neurol 1990; 53:287–292.
18. Golbe LI, Lazzarini AM, Schwarz KO, Mark MH, Dickson DW, Duvoisin RC. Autosomal dominant parkinsonism with benign course and typical Lewy-body pathology. Neurology 1993; 43:2222–2227.
19. Rosenberg RN, Nyhan WL, Bay C, Shore P. Autosomal dominant striatonigral degeneration. A clinical, pathologic, and biochemical study of a new genetic disorder. Neurology 1976; 26:703–714.
20. Spellman G. Report of familial cases of parkinsonism; evidence of a dominant trait in a patient's family. JAMA 1962; 179:372–374.
21. Wszolek ZK, Pfeiffer RF, Bhatt MH, et al. Rapidly progressive autosomal dominant parkinsonism and dementia with pallido-ponto-nigral degeneration. Ann Neurol 1992; 32:312–320.
22. Mark MH, Dickson DW, Schwarz KO. Familial diffuse Lewy body disease. In: Tenth international symposium on Parkinson's disease 1991:56.
23. Takada K, Nakamura H, Igo M. An autopsy case of diffuse Lewy body disease diagnosed as having familial PD [in Japanese]. In: 30th annual congress of neuropathologists in Japan, Tokyo, 1993:196.
24. Mizutani T, Inose T, Nakajima S, Gambetti P. Familial parkinsonism and dementia with "ballooned neurons." In: Narabayashi H, Nagatsu T, Yanagisawa N, Mizuno Y, eds. Parkinson's disease: from basic research to treatment. Adv Neurol 1993; 60:613–617.
25. Carlier G, Dubru JM. Familial juvenile parkinsonism. Acta Paediatr Belg 1979; 32:123–127.
26. Degl'Innocenti F, Maurello MT, Marini P. A parkinsonian kindred. Ital J Neurol Sci 1989; 10:307–310.
27. deYebenes JG, Jimenez A, Morales B, et al. Familial parkinsonism in Spain. Presented at meeting of the American Neurological Association 15.

28. Hussels I. [A family with sex-linked retinitis pigmentosa, Parkinson's disease and other neuro-psychiatric disorders]. J Genet Hum 1967; 16:106–155.
29. Mauri JA, Asensio M, Jimenez A, Huerta JR, Redondo MJ, del Villar V. [Familial Parkinson disease]. Neurologia 1990; 5:45–47.
30. Nukada H, Kowa H, Saitoh T, Tazaki Y, Miura S. [A big family of paralysis agitans (author's transl)]. Rinsho Shinkeigaku 1978; 18:627–634.
31. Rajasekhran Nair K, Bhaskaran R. Familial parkinsonism. Acta Neurol (Napoli) 1986; 8:633–638.
32. Roy M, Boyer L, Barbeau A. A prospective study of 50 cases of familial Parkinson's disease. Can J Neurol Sci 1983; 10:37–42.
33. Sandyk R. Parkinson's disease and thalassalmia in a South African family of Greek origin [letter]. S Afr Med J 1983; 63:141.
34. Bhatia KP, Daniel SE, Marsden CD. Familial parkinsonism with depression; a clinicopathological study. Ann Neurol 1993; 34:842–847.
35. Ota Y, Miyoshi S, Ueda O, Mukai T, Maeka A. Familial paralysis agitans juvenilis. A clinical anatomical and genetic study. Neurology 1958; 12:112–121.
36. Wszolek Z, Monsour H, Smith P, Pfeiffer R. Cryptococcal meningoencephalitis with parkinsonian features. Mov Disord 1988; 3:271–273.
37. Zweig RM, Singh A, Cardillo JE, Langston JW. The familial occurrence of Parkinson's disease—lack of evidence for maternal inheritance. Arch Neurol 1992; 49:1205–1207.
38. Lazzarini A, Myers RH, Zimmerman TR, et al. A clinical genetic study of Parkinson's disease: evidence for dominant transmission. Neurology 1994; 44:449–506.
39. Perry TL, Bratty P, Hansen S, Kennedy J, Urquhart N, Dolman C. Hereditary mental depression and parkinsonism with taurine deficiency. Arch Neurol 1975; 32:108–113.
40. Purdy A, Hahn A, Barnett HJM, et al. Familial fatal parkinsonism with alveolar hypoventilation and mental depression. Ann Neurol 1979; 6:523–531.
41. Santamaria J, Tolosa E, Valles A. Parkinson's disease with depression: a possible subgroup of idiopathic parkinsonism. Neurology 1986; 36:1130–1133.
42. Johnson W, Davidson M, Yoshidome H, Lustenberger A, Stenroos S. Genetics of Parkinson's disease (PD), The multifactorial/threshold (MF/T) model [abstract]. Mov Disord 1990; 5:92.
43. Marsden CD. Parkinson's disease in twins [letter]. J Neurol Neurosurg Psychiatry 1987; 50:105–106.
44. Marttila RJ, Kaprio J, Koskenvuo M, Rinne UK. Parkinson's disease in a nationwide twin cohort. Neurology 1988; 38:1217–1219.
45. Vieregge P, Schiffke A, Kompf D. Parkinson's disease in twins. Neurology 1991; 41(suppl 1):255.
46. Koller WC, O'Hara R, Nutt J, Young J, Rubino F. Monozygotic twins with Parkinson's disease. Ann Neurol 1986; 19:402–405.
47. Zimmerman TR, Bhatt MH, Calne DB, Duvoisin RC. Parkinson's disease in monozygotic twins: a follow-up. Neurology 1991; 41 (suppl 1):255.
48. Zimmerman TR. personal communication 1992.
49. Duvoisin RC, Golbe LI. Toward a definition of Parkinson's disease. Neurology 1989; 39:746.

50. Hughes AJ, Daniel SE, Blankson S, Lees AJ. A clinicopathologic study of 100 cases of Parkinson's disease. Arch Neurol 1993; 50:140–148.
51. Burton K, Calne DB. Aetiology of Parkinson's disease. In: Stern GM, ed. Parkinson's disease. Baltimore: Johns Hopkins University Press, 1990:269–293.
52. Ansley D. Aging twins offer clues to late-onset diseases. Science 1993; 259:1826–1828.
53. Brooks DJ, Ibanez V, Sawle GV, et al. Differing patterns of striatal ^{18}F-dopa uptake in Parkinson's disease, multiple system atrophy, and progressive supranuclear palsy. Ann Neurol 1990; 28:547–555.
54. Calne DB, Langston JW, Martin WR, et al. Positron emission tomography after MPTP: observations relating to the cause of Parkinson's disease. Nature 1985; 317:246–248.
55. Snow BJ, Peppard RF, Guttman M. Positron emission tomographic scanning demonstrates a presynaptic dopaminergic lesion in Lytico-Bodig, the amyotrophic lateral sclerosis parkinsonism dementia complex of Guam. Arch Neurol 1990; 47:870–874.
56. Sawle GV, Wroe SJ, Lees AJ, Brooks DJ, Frackowiak RSJ. The identification of presymptomatic parkinsonism: clinical and [^{18}F]-dopa positron emission tomography studies in an Irish kindred. Ann Neurol 1992; 32:609–617.
57. Burn DJ, Mark MH, Playford ED, et al. Parkinson's disease in twins studied with ^{18}F-dopa and positron emission tomography. Neurology 1992; 42:1894–1900.
58. Forno LS. Concentric hyalin intraneuronal inclusions of Lewy type in the brains of elderly persons (50 incidental cases): relationship to parkinsonism. J Am Geriatr Soc 1969; 17:557–575.
59. Gibb WRG, Lees AJ. The relevance of the Lewy body to the pathogenesis of idiopathic Parkinson's disease. J Neurol Neurosurg Psychiatry 1988; 51:745–752.
60. Gibb WRG, Lees AJ. The significance of the Lewy body in the diagnosis of idiopathic Parkinson's disease. Neuropathol Appl Neurobiol 1989; 15:27–44.
61. Duvoisin R. Epidemiological and genetic aspects of Parkinson's disease. In: Nappi C, ed. Focus on Parkinson's disease. Milan: 1991:79–93.
62. Schoenberg BS, Anderson DW, Haerer AF. Prevalence of Parkinson's disease in the biracial population of Copiah County, Mississippi. Neurology 1985; 35:841–845.
63. Eldridge R, Ince SE. The low concordance rate for Parkinson's disease in twins: a possible explanation. Neurology 1984; 34:1354–1356.
64. Eldridge R. Parkinson's disease in twins [reply from author]. Neurology 1984; 34:1399–1400.
65. Robbins JH. Parkinson's disease, twins, and the DNA-damage hypothesis [letter]. Ann Neurol 1987; 21:412.
66. Kurland LT. Epidemiology: incidence, geographic distribution and genetic considerations. In: Field WS, ed. Pathogenesis and treatment of parkinsonism. Springfield, IL: Charles C Thomas, 1958:5–49.
67. Alonso ME, Otero E, D'Regules R, Figueroa HH. Parkinson's disease: a genetic study. Can J Neurol Sci 1986; 13:248–251.
68. Butterfield PG, Valanis BG, Spencer PS, Lindeman CA, Nutt JG. Environmental antecedents of young-onset Parkinson's disease. Neurology 1993; 43:1150–1158.

69. Duvoisin RC, Gearing IR, Schweitzer MR, Yahr MD. A tamily study of parkinsonism. In: Barbeau A, Brunette JR, eds. Progress in neurogenetics. Amsterdam: Excerpta Medica Foundation, 1969:492–496.
70. Martin WE, Young WI, Anderson VE. Parkinson's disease. A genetic study. Brain 1973; 96:495–506.
71. Marttila RJ, Rinne UK. Arteriosclerosis, heredity, and some previous infections in the etiology of Parkinson's disease. A case–control study. Clin Neurol Neurosurg 1976; 79:46–56.
72. Semchuk KM, Love EJ, Lee RG. Parkinson's disease: a test of the multifactorial etiologic hypothesis. Neurology 1993; 43:1173–1180.
73. Vieregge P, Glaese A, Ulm G, Kompf D. Familial Parkinson's disease. Mov Disord 1992; 7(supp 1):23.
74. Duvoisin RC. Is Parkinson's disease acquired or inherited? Can J Neurol Sci 1984; 2:151–155.
75. Calne S, Schoenberg BS, Martin W, Uitti RJ, Spencer P, Calne DB. Familial Parkinson's disease: possible role of environmental factors. Can J Neurol Sci 1987; 14:303–305.
76. Barbeau A, Pourcher E. Genetics of early onset Parkinson's disease. Amsterdam: Excerpta Medica, 1983:1–16.
77. Barbeau A, Pourcher E. New data on the genetics of Parkinson's disease. Can J Neurol Sci 1982; 9:53–60.
78. Young WI, Martin WE, Anderson VE. The distribution of ancestral secondary cases in Parkinson's disease. Clin Genet 1977; 11:189–192.
79. Slater E. Expectation of abnormality on paternal and maternal sides: a computational model. J Med Genet 1966; 3:159–161.
80. Kahler SG, Riley E. Inherited parkinsonism [letter]. Clin Genet 1979; 15:110–111.
81. Kondo K. Motor neuron disease: changing population patterns and clues for etiology. In: Neurological epidemiology: principles and clinical applications. Adv Neurol 1978; 19:509–543.
82. Kondo K, Kurland LT, Schull WJ. Parkinson's disease. Genetic analysis and evidence of a multifactorial etiology. Mayo Clin Proc 1973; 48:465–475.
83. Kondo K. A genetic analysis of Parkinson's disease. Trans Am Neurol Assoc 1971; 96:261–262.
84. Maraganore D, Harding A, Marsden C. A clinical and genetic study of familial Parkinson's disease. Mov Disord 1991; 6:205–211.
85. Campanella G, Idone M, De Michele G, Filla A. Paternal preponderance in familial Parkinson's disease [letter]. Neurology 1984; 34:1398–1400.
86. Golbe LI, Duvoisin RC, Miller DC. A large kindred with autosomal dominanat Parkinson's disease. Ann Neurol 1988; 24:151–152.
87. Quinn N, Critchley P, Marsden C. Young onset Parkinson's disease. Mov Disord 1987; 2:73–91.
88. Chalfie M, Wolinsky E. The identification and suppression of inherited neurodegeneration in *Caenorhabditis elegans*. Nature 1990; 345:410–416.
89. Robbins JH, Otsuka F, Tarone RE, Polinsky RJ, Brumback RA, Nee LE. Parkinson's disease and Alzheimer's disease: hypersensitivity to X rays in cultured cell lines. J Neurol Neurosurg Psychiatry 1985; 48:916–923.

90. Johnson W. Genetic susceptibility to Parkinson's disease. Neurology 1991; 41(suppl 2):82–87.
91. Wöhrle D, Hennig I, Vogel W, Steinbach P. Mitotic stability of fragile X mutations in differentiated cells indicates early post-conceptional trinucleotide repeat expansion. Nature Genet 1993; 4:140–142.
92. Eldridge R, Ince S. The cause of parkinson's disease in twins. Am J Hum Genet 1983; 35:88A.
93. Golbe LI, Di Iorio G, Lazzarini AM, Bonavita V, Duvoisin RC. A large kindred with Parkinson's disease: onset age, segregation ratios, and anticipation. Mov Disord 1993; 8:406.
94. Caskey CT, Pizzuti A, Fu YH, Fenwick RG, Nelson DL. Triple repeat mutations in human disease. Science 1992; 256:784–789.
95. Ross CA, McInnis MG, Margolis RL, Li SH. Genes with triple repeats: candidate mediators of neuropsychiatric disorders. Trends Neurosci 1993; 16:254–260.
96. Ozawa T, Tanaka M, Ikebe S, Ohno K, Kondo T, Mizuno Y. Quantitative determination of deleted mitochondrial DNA relative to normal DNA in parkinsonian striatum by a kinetic PCR analysis. Biochem Biophys Res Commun 1990; 172:483–489.
97. Mizuno Y, Ohta S, Tanaka M, et al. Deficiencies in complex I subunits of the respiratory chain in Parkinson's disease. Biochem Biophys Res Commun 1989; 163:1450–1455.
98. Ikebe S, Tanaka M, Ohno K, et al. Increase of deleted mitochondrial DNA in the striatum in Parkinson's disease and senescence. Biochem Biophys Res Commun 1990; 170:1044–1048.
99. Schapira AH, Holt IJ, Sweeney M, Harding AE, Jenner P, Marsden CD. Mitochondrial DNA analysis in Parkinson's disease. Mov Disord 1990; 5:294–297.
100. Parker WD, Boyson SJ, Parks JK. Abnormalities of the electron transport chain in idiopathic Parkinson's disease. Ann Neurol 1989; 26:719–723.
101. Schapira AHV, Cooper JM, Dexter D, Clark JB, Jenner P, Marsden CD. Mitochondrial complex I deficiency in Parkinson's disease. J Neurochem 1990; 54:823–827.
102. Nicklas W, Vyas I, Heikkila E. Inhibition of NADH-linked oxidation in brain mitochondria by 1-methyl-4-phenyl-pyridine, a metabolite of the neurotoxin, 1-methyl-4-phenyl-1,2,5,6-tetrahydropyridine. Life Sci 1985; 36:2503–2508.
103. DiMonte D. Mitochondrial DNA and Parkinson's disease. Neurology 1991; 41(suppl 2):38–42.
104. Linnane AW, Marzuki S, Ozawa T, Tanaka M. Mitochondrial DNA mutations as an important contributor to ageing and degenerative diseases. Lancet 1989; 1:642–645.
105. Sandy MS, Smith J, Langston W, Di Monte D. Comparison of mitochondrial DNA from platelets of parkinsonian patients and controls. (Neurotoxins and their potential role in neurodegeneration) [abstract] NY Acad Sci 1991; May 6–9:PI-29.
106. Uhl GR, Kitayama S, Cerruti C, et al. Dopamine transporter: correlates with Parkinsonian pathogenesis. Mov Disord 1993; 8:403–404.
107. Gasser T, Wszolek Z, Trofatter J, et al. Genetic linkage studies in autosomal

dominantly inherited levodopa-responsive parkinsonism: evaluation of seven candidate genes. Mov Disord 1993; 8:408.
108. Dwork AJ, Balmaceda C, Fazzini EA, MacCollin M, Côtè L, Fahn S. Dominantly inherited, early-onset parkinsonism: neuropathology of a new form. Neurology 1993; 43:69–74.
109. Jankovic J, Reches A. Parkinson's disease in monozygotic twins. Ann Neurol 1986; 19:405–408.
110. Kissel P, Andre JM. [Parkinson's disease and anosmia in monozygotic twin sisters (author's transl)]. J Genet Hum 1976; 24:113–117.
111. Pahwa R, Busenbark K, Gray C, Koller WC. Identical twins with similar onset of Parkinson's disease: a case report. Neurology 1993; 43:1159–1161.
112. Atadzhanov M. [The role of heredity in Parkinson's disease]. Zh Nevropatol Psikhiatr 1973; 73:195–199.
113. Gudmundsson KR. A clinical survey of parkinsonism in Iceland. Acta Neurol Scand [Suppl] 1967; 33:1–61.
114. Hart TS. Paralysis agitans: some clinical observations based on the study of 219 cases seen at the clinic of Professor M. Allen Starr. J Nerv Ment Dis 1904; 31:177–188.
115. Jenkins AC. Epidemiology of parkinsonism in Victoria. Med J Aust 1966; 2:496–502.
116. Osuntokun BO, Bademosi O. Parkinsonism in the Nigerian African: a prospective study of 217 patients. East Afr Med J 1979; 56:597–607.
117. Pollock M, Hornabrook RW. The prevalence, natural history and dementia of Parkinson's disease. Brain 1966; 89:429–448.
118. Ringwald E. What causes Parkinson's disease? [letter]. Lancet 1984; 1:336.
119. Vassilopoulos D, Spengos M, Ilias A, Stamboulis E, Karabellas G. Morbidity risks for the relatives of patients with Parkinson's disease [abstract]. In: Ninth international symposium on Parkinson's disease, 1988:118.

6

Xenobiotics and Inherited Risk Factors

Adrian Williams

Queen Elizabeth Hospital, Edgbaston, Birmingham, England

I. INTRODUCTION

This chapter summarizes the conceptual arguments and preliminary data that support the proposition that the general population is exposed to chemicals that have toxic potential if either they or their metabolites are allowed to reach nigrostriatal dopaminergic neurons in sufficient quantity. Whether or not this potential for toxicity is then expressed and causes Parkinson's disease will depend on the innate ability of that individual's dopaminergic cells to withstand such attack (Fig. 1). For a given environmental exposure, the quantity of the toxin delivered to the vicinity of the cell will depend on several factors. These include its absorption, its ability to cross several physical barriers, and on the degree and type of metabolism that occurs. Normally, the metabolism of xenobiotics is mediated by a family of enzymes that are active preponderantly in liver, but also at the blood–brain barrier and in brain.

The degree of environmental exposure will be largely determined by circumstance, but it is important to realize that genetic factors may be involved, in that they may partly control the environment that individuals create for themselves—for instance, dietary preferences. Indeed, both genetic and acquired factors influence all the aforementioned variables, so there is enormous individual variation in response to drugs and chemicals. Polymorphisms in the proteins involved with xenobiotic biochemistry, their uptake pathways, and other defense mechanisms, form much of the genetic contribution of this variable response and the basis of individual hypersusceptibility (and resistance) to chemicals.

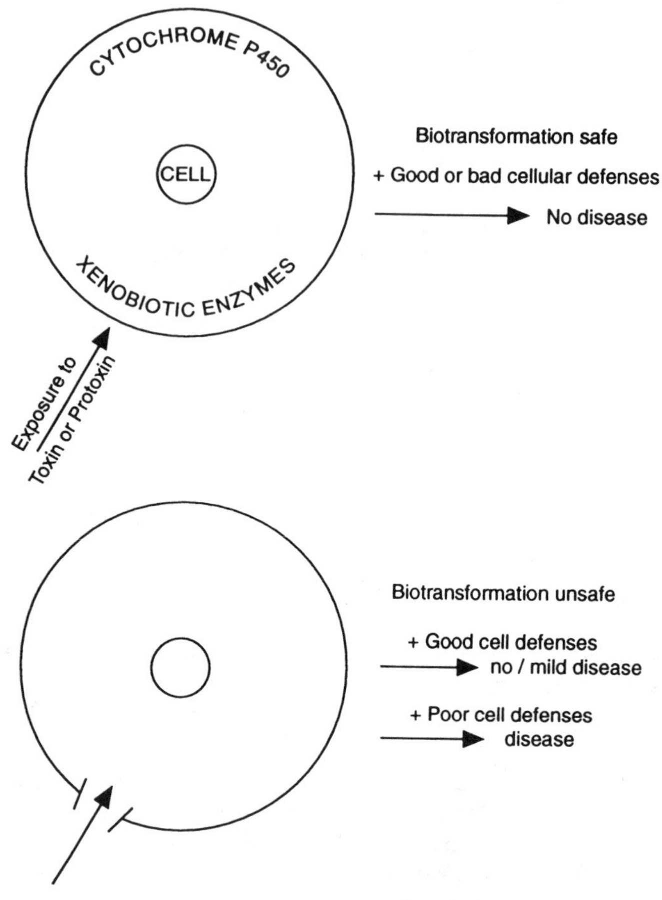

Figure 1 Interaction between safe and unsafe biotransformations and cellular defense systems. Currently topical defenses include uptake of chemical into cell or subcellular structures; ability to withstand oxygen and excitotoxic stress, including rises in intracellular calcium; and activation of proteolysis. The figure is diagrammatic and not anatomical, as important biotransformations can occur within neurons.

Hypersusceptibility to chemicals may prove to be an important risk factor for many "ecogenetic" diseases (1–4). Given that the 1-methyl-4-phenyl-1,2,3,6-tetrahydropyridine (MPTP) story has taught us that a relatively simple family of chemicals is capable of causing selective neuronal death within the nigrostriatal system (see Chapter 13) this may be true for Parkinson's disease (2,5–7). If so, there is probably no one "neurochemical assassin" in nonfamilial cases or in those who are not part of an epidemic, but a coaction of several risk factors

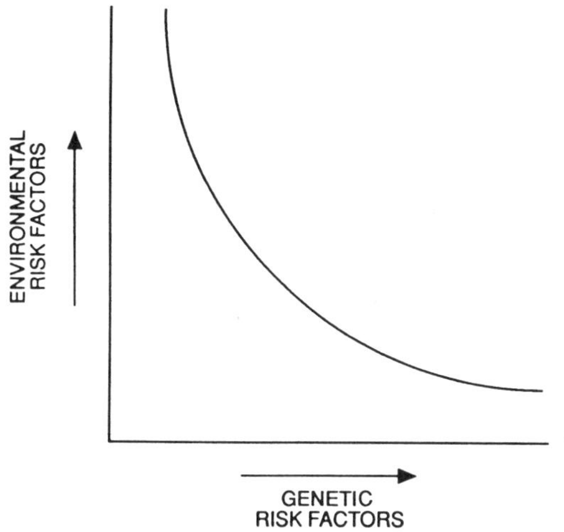

Figure 2 Relative contributions of environmental and genetic factors to neuronal cell death. At one extreme: An example of severe environmental risk factor is IV MPTP, for which little individual susceptibility is necessary. Or, at the other extreme: Apparent mendelian Parkinson's disease could be due to an inherited defect expressed within the cell, leading it to be defenseless against an ordinary unavoidable dose of a universal endogenous or exogenous chemical, or a severe defect in metabolism that leads to production of a dopaminergic toxin from a common substrate.

that, in an accumulative way, will lead to death of dopaminergic neurons. The exact contribution of different risk factors is likely to differ among individuals and so will the ratio between genetic and environmentally derived risk factors (Fig. 2). But in most cases, there may be a common theme and a final common pathway. If so, the potential for identifying at-risk groups and modifying the risk factors or protecting individuals, or the whole population, could have major therapeutic consequences.

This chapter will concentrate on possible abnormalities of xenobiotic enzyme biochemistry in Parkinson's disease. Other potential risk factors that might be expressed preponderantly within the cell destined to die, such as a genetically determined defect in mitochondrial function or antioxidant defenses, are discussed in detail elsewhere (see Chapter 4). The earliest changes so far described appear to be low glutathione levels (8,9) and then abnormal complex I activity (10,11); both could be secondary to toxic exposure. However, genetically determined defects in these pathways cannot as yet be excluded and may perhaps be present and sufficient to cause disease single handedly in some familial cases.

II. ASSESSMENT OF XENOBIOTIC ENZYME ACTIVITY

There are three main methods to study the activity of xenobiotic enzymes. The first is to use a probe compound, often a drug that is known to be safe and given by the oral route. Its metabolites can then be measured, usually in urine, although occasionally, in plasma. The compound is chosen because its pathway's metabolic conversion has already been identified and, usually, the enzymes concerned are known. This has been the classic method of pharmacogenetics from the first demonstration that there are rapid and slow metabolizers of drugs, such as isoniazid and debrisoquine (12,13). Polymorphisms were suspected on the basis of these studies and have subsequently been identified. The advantage of the method is that it is an in vivo assessment and, therefore, a test of function that permits the examination of enzymatic pathways concerned in a quasi-natural manner. Disadvantages usually include the need for large numbers of controls and patients, and the need to guard against confounding issues such as other drugs that a subject may be taking. Differences in technique for some of these assays can cause problems, as can difficulties in establishing quality control between laboratories.

The second method is to test the function of the enzyme in vitro. Although it might be possible to take a biopsy of the liver to measure the activity of these enzymes directly, for both practical and ethical reasons, red blood cells or platelets usually have to be used. A major disadvantage of this approach is that the enzyme is not functioning in its natural supramolecular state. Also, the same enzyme may have very different activity in different tissues, and such studies, although of interest, need to be backed up by other evidence, when possible, to be sure of biological relevance.

Third, the enzymes can be studied at the genomic level. Access to relevant tissue that is suitable for study, such as brain or liver, is a problem for mRNA–cDNA work although this is likely to become an active area of study. As with conventional biochemical techniques, there will be problems of interpretation when disease-damaged tissues are studied, and many proteins will be over- or underexpressed. At genomic DNA level, few of the relevant polymorphisms have yet been identified that include the debrisoquine mutations linked with slow metabolism of this agent (14). Nevertheless, this is an expanding area and has the enormous advantage that samples can be stored for multiple studies, patients need not be medication-free; and there is less of an issue concerning sample handling, storage, and methodological problems. On the other hand, some mutations will have no effect on enzyme activity or will have an unpredictable effect. Thus, tests of function at phenotypic level will still be required, in addition to their role in yielding important clues to which genes are candidates for important mutations.

III. CYTOCHROME P-450

The superfamily of enzymes known as cytochrome P-450 is the best known of the enzymes involved in drug metabolism. They have a crucial role in the metabolism of some endogenous compounds and many drugs and, also, one can safely assume, in a wide variety of environmental chemicals. These include several chemicals that have been mentioned as candidate toxins for Parkinson's disease, including the tetrahydroisoquinoles and MPTP itself (15). Early studies using the probe-drug approach with debrisoquine initially looked promising (5), but the results were largely retracted as being due to the effects of medication (16). Various studies followed, but patients receiving medication still interfered with the results and, overall, no clear-cut picture emerged (17–21). Our own study (22) had the advantages of using unmedicated, consecutively diagnosed patients, and comparing them with patients with motor neuron disease. We found no significant abnormality, although the study was open to the criticism that the number of normal controls was small. Nevertheless, at a phenotypic level, the results were not significant. Other studies that used phenytoin as a probe of cytochrome P-450 function showed changes, the importance of which was difficult to judge, as the numbers studied were small (23).

The cytochrome P-450 CYP2D6 polymorphism associated with the compromised metabolism of debrisoquine is an autosomal recessive defect found in 5–10% of the Caucasian population, and the defective metabolism in most persons is due to the absence of the CYP2D6 protein, which is attributed to at least three distinct mutations in poor metabolizers. By using DNA-based assays, up to 90% of poor metabolizers can be identified. With such assays, three separate studies, all of which are open to some criticism, have now suggested a 2.5-fold higher risk for developing Parkinson's disease among the poor metabolizers of debrisoquine (24–27).

It is somewhat surprising that phenotypic studies were so unimpressive, and alternative explanations have been suggested, including the possibility that CYP2D6 may be functionally related to the dopamine transporter. The absence of a transporter protein could affect neuronal response to neurotransmitters or to uptake of potential toxins. Alternatively, linkage of the *CYP2D6* locus to another gene that may or may not have anything to do with xenobiotic metabolism is a possibility. Although this finding of poor metabolizer genotypes has been upheld in several studies in different ethnic groups supports its validity, one reservation is that the recruitment of patients for these studies could be biased. Usually, subjects were entered through a Parkinson's disease clinic, which may attract unusual cases, perhaps of earlier onset, or that more patients are likely to have developed problems with their drug treatment. Further studies, therefore, are necessary to see if this abnormality is linked more closely with younger-onset patients or with familial cases, or to those in whom complications of therapy have developed at an early stage. The results also need to be replicated in a study for which recruitment from the population is more complete, with little or no referral bias.

IV. MONOAMINE OXIDASE B

Monoamine oxidase B (MAO-B) should be of interest in Parkinson's disease for several reasons. First, it is involved in the catabolism of dopamine; given that this pathway can produce oxygen free radicals, altered activity could put cells at risk of damage (see Chapter 4). Second, the neurotoxicity of MPTP depends on its oxidation to the 1-methyl-4-phenylpyridinium ion (MPP^+) (28), and so does the toxicity of many tetrahydroisoquinolines and β-carbolines that have been proposed as nigrostriatal toxins (see Chapters 7 and B). Third, blockade of MAO-B by selegiline has a symptomatically beneficial effect on Parkinson's disease and has been suggested to reduce disease progression (29,30).

In the brain, MAO-B activity tends to increase with age, although the reasons for this are unclear (31). Monoamine oxydase B is found in abundance in platelets, and there have now been several reports of differences in platelet MAO-B between controls and patients with Parkinson's disease (32–36). These are clearly in vitro tests using tissue that may not be directly relevant to brain activity or to the activity of MAO-B elsewhere, such as in liver. Nevertheless, there is some consistency between the reports that the rate of oxidation of either benzylamine or phenylethylamine is increased. The results using dopamine (35) showed an apparent decrease in activity, although this has not been replicated in a smaller study (37). In any event, before extrapolating that a change in dopamine metabolism occurs in vivo, further tests of function need to be developed. If a polymorphism is present, its storage characteristics between the time of collection and actual analysis might be different. Such a difference might provide one possible explanation for the discrepency in the published studies, because in the first study, the dopamine assay was done several weeks after the phenylethylamine assay. With MPTP as substrate, there does not appear to be any overall difference in activity, although there was a strong correlation between the activity with benzylamine and MPTP (38). However, MPTP is oxidized very slowly, compared with benzylamine, and is both a competitive and suicidal inhibitor of MAO-B; therefore, it remains possible that in vivo MPTP-like compounds may be metabolized more quickly to MPP^+-like compounds in the parkinsonian population. Recently, a polymorphism of MAO-B has been identified at the DNA level, and a twofold risk of Parkinson's disease was found with one allele (39).

V. *N*-METHYLATION

N-Methylation of pyridines is a well-established pathway and, indeed, was the first xenobiotic pathway discovered. There appear to be large interindividual differences in activity, although whether isoenzymes exist has never been established. There is interest in this pathway, as MPTP is an *N*-methylated compound. This appears to be a structural requirement for all toxic MPTP analogues and, for at least the more toxic variants, of the tetrahydroisoquinolines and β-carbolines that have been noted as potential dopaminergic neurotoxins and are known to be present in the natural environment (see Chapter 12). *N*-Methylase acts on several different substrates that include the substituted 4-phenyl pyridines that then produce MPP^+ itself (40). The same enzyme may metabolize nicotinamide to produce *N*-methy-1-nicotinamide as well as *N*-methyl-2-pyridone-5-carboxyamide. Further metabolism takes place that involves cytochrome P-450 and aldehyde oxidase in an apparently analogous way to the alternative pathway for the catabolism of MPTP, which is at least as active in liver tissue as the better known MAO-B pathway (15).

Our group has studied this pathway using nicotinamide as a probe compound. It initially appeared that there was considerable accumulation of *N*-methyl nicotinamide, compared with normal controls or in patients with amyotrophic lateral sclerosis (ALS; 41,42), although in a larger not yet completed study, the changes are less convincing. There is also doubt about whether or not nicotinamide is the most appropriate probe compound for the relevant *N*-methylase. Whether or not there might be an increase in methylation or a decrease in the catabolism of *N*-methyl compounds using enzymes such as cytochrome P-450 or aldehyde oxidase has yet to be elucidated. It remains a possibility that one or both could exist, with a final biochemical endophenotype that generates a rise in potentially toxic *N*-methyl pyridines (Fig. 3). This could provide a mechanism whereby there is individual hypersusceptibility to naturally occurring pyridines.

VI. SULFUR METABOLISM

An *S*-oxidation reaction has been studied in vivo using the compound *S*-carboxymethyl-cysteine as a probe and measuring sulfoxides in urine. Patients with Parkinson's disease, but also patients with amyotrophic lateral sclerosis and dementia, performed this reaction poorly (43–45). The enzyme involved appears to be cysteine dioxygenase, which converts cysteine to sulfate. To confirm this finding, plasma cysteine and sulfate levels in untreated patients with Parkinson's disease and ALS have been investigated. Relatively high levels of cysteine and low levels of sulfate were found (46).

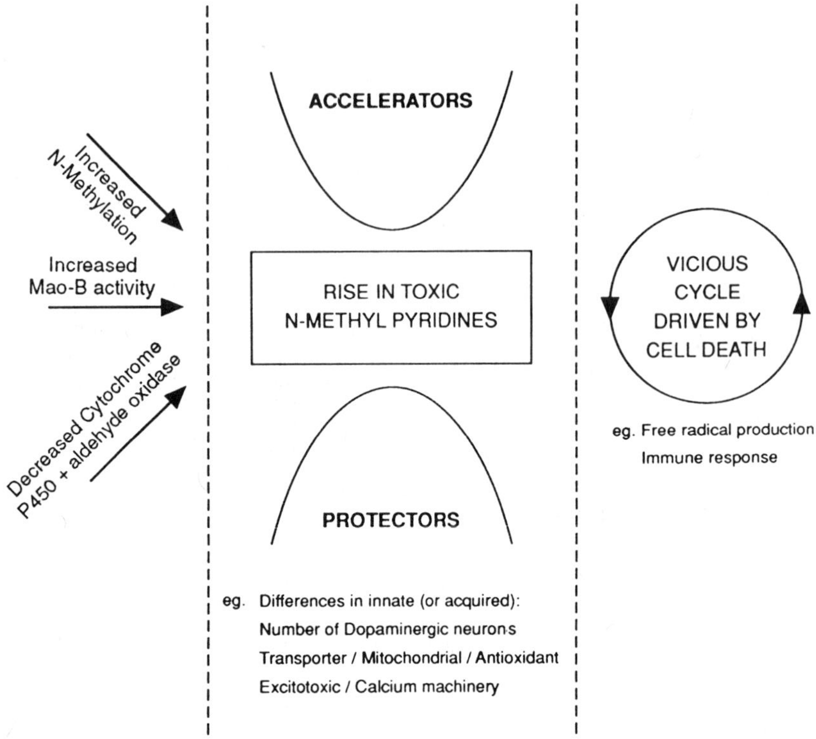

Figure 3 Interactive xenobiotic pathways that could lead to cell death in a multistage process.

Additionally, with acetaminophen (paracetamol) as a probe, we measured the sulfate conjugate of this compound as a method of measuring the amount of available sulfate in vivo. Low amounts of sulfate conjugate were seen (47). However, other groups have not confirmed all these findings (48,49) and, therefore, further studies appear warranted, paying careful attention to methodological problems with the measurement of cysteine and sulfate. For example, inclusion of treated patients may confound the results. If an abnormality of sulfur metabolism is confirmed, it will raise the possibility that individuals born with underactivity in this system are less capable of dealing with some sulfur compounds. There is a large sulfur load from the environment and, perhaps, some of it needs to be oxidized to reduce toxicity, or requires sulfate conjugation to reduce toxicity. The high cysteine levels, given that it has excitotoxic properties under certain conditions, may damage cells. Given that these findings were not specific to Parkinson's disease, but were also implicated in other neurodegenerative diseases (2), it is possible that this pathway acts as an exacerbating element to several disease processes. Clearly, other factors must be involved to define the specificity of neuronal death.

S-Methylation is another interesting detoxification reaction. The enzyme thiolmethyltransferase is best known for its role in the detoxification of hydrogen sulfide, which is metabolically convertible to carbon disulfide and to diethyldithiocarbamate, both of which have been linked with damage to the basal ganglia (50–52). In Parkinson's disease and in dementia patients, low values were recorded in vitro, using a red cell preparation (53). This has been confirmed from another laboratory (54). Overactivity was seen in amyotrophic lateral sclerosis.

VII. CONCLUSION

Hypersusceptibility to chemicals may be risk factors for several unexplained neurological diseases, including Parkinson's disease. These susceptibility factors could lie within the neuronal uptake mechanisms or chemical defense systems within neurons. An alternative and testable hypothesis is that they reside in xenobiotic pathways that handle the initial metabolism of such chemicals. These pathways have the capacity to detoxify or activate a protoxin. There is overlap between these two hypotheses, as some of the enzymes involved in xenobiotic metabolism are also present in the brain. Perhaps such risk factors are cumulative, with the need for a defect at both levels in most sporadic cases, although some extreme and pure examples may be found in some familial cases.

Pharmacogenetics is a growth area in general toxicology, and the application of lessons learned and techniques developed in that branch of science to Parkinson's disease could be rewarding. Once such risk factors are understood, epidemiology will enter a renaissance with combined studies that simultaneously measure the biochemical profile and estimated environmental exposure. Such studies will be far more incisive, as more relevant questions can be asked in surveys along with biochemical typing of Parkinson's disease patients. Individuals who appear biochemically to be at low risk, but who still develop clinical disease, simply may have a high load of environmentally derived risk factors, and this could be more prominent in an epidemiological survey.

REFERENCES

1. Williams AC, Steventon GB, Sturman SG, Waring RH. Hereditary variation of liver enzyme involved with detoxification and neurodegenerative disease. J Inherited Metab Dis 1991; 14:431–435.
2. Williams AC. Ecogenetics, xenobiotic biochemistry and neurological disease. J Neurol 1991; 238:187–190.
3. Williams AC. Ecogenetics. J R Coll Physicians Lond 1994; 28:2–3.

4. Williams A. Hypersusceptibility to chemicals: risk factors for neurological disease? Neurol Neurosurg Psychiatry, 1993; 56:943–946.
5. Barbeau A, Cloutier T, Roy M, Plasse L, Paris S, Poirier J. Ecogenetics of Parkinson's disease: 4-hydroxylation of debrisoquine. Lancet 1985; 2:1213–1216.
6. Barbeau A, Roy M, Bernier G, Campanella G, Paris S. Ecogenetics of Parkinson's disease: prevalence and environmental aspects in rural areas. Can J Neurol Sci 1987; 14:36–41.
7. Williams AC. Toxins, polymorphisms and Parkinson's disease. Focus Parkinson's Dis 1991; 3:12–15.
8. Marttila RJ, Rinne UK. Epidemiological approaches to the etiology of Parkinson's disease. Acta Neurol Scand 1989; 126:13–18.
9. Perry TL, Yong VW. Idiopathic Parkinson's disease, progressive supranuclear palsy and glutathione metabolism in the substantia nigra. Neurosci Lett 1986; 67:269–274.
10. Schapira AHV, Cooper JM, Dexter D, Jenner P, Clark JB, Marsden CD. Mitochondrial complex I deficiency in Parkinson's disease. Lancet 1989; 1:1269.
11. Schapira AHV, Mann VM, Cooper JM, et al. Anatomic and disease specificity of NADHCoQ1 reductase (complex I) deficiency in Parkinson's disease. J Neurochem 1990; 55:2142–2145.
12. Mahgoub A, Dring LG, Idle JR, Lancaster R, Smith RL. Polymorphic hydroxylation of debrisoquine in man. Lancet 1977; 1:584–586.
13. Weber WW, Hein DW. *N*-Acetylation pharmacogenetics. Pharmacol Rev 1985; 37:25–79.
14. Gonzalez FJ. The molecular biology of cytochrome P450s. Pharmacol Rev 1989; 40:243–288.
15. Wu E, Shinka T, Caldera-Munoz P, Yoshizumi H, Trevor A, Castagnoli N Jr. Metabolic studies on the nigrostriatal toxin MPTP and its MAO-B generated dihydropyridinium metabolite $MPDP^+$. Chem Res Toxicol 1988; 1:186–194.
16. Poirier J, Roy M, Campanella G, Cloutier T, Paris S. Debrisoquine metabolism in parkinsonian patients treated with antihistamine drugs. Lancet 1987; 2:386.
17. Benitez J, Ladero JM, Jiminez-Jiminez FJ, et al. Oxidative polymorphism of debrisoquine in Parkinson's disease. J Neurol Neurosurg Psychiatry 1990; 53:289–292.
18. Comella CL, Tanner CM, Goetz GC, Gans S, Rapp D, Fischer J. Debrisoquine metabolism in Parkinson's disease. Neurology 1987; 37:261–262.
19. Gudjonsson O, Sanz E, Alvan G, Aquilonius SM, Reviriego J. Poor hydroxylator phenotypes of debrisoquine and *S*-mephenytoin are not over-represented in a group of patients with Parkinson's disease [letter]. Br J Clin Pharmacol 1990; 30:301–302.
20. Kallio J, Marttila RM, Rinne UK, Sonninen V, Syvalahti E. Debrisoquine oxidation in Parkinson's disease. Acta Neurol Scand 1991; 83:194–197.
21. Steiger MJ, Lledo P, Quinn NP, Marsden CD, Turner P, Jenner PG. Debrisoquine hydroxylation in Parkinson's disease. Acta Neurol Scand 1992; 86:159–164.
22. Steventon GB, Heafield MTE, Sturman SG, Waring RH, Williams AC, Ellingham J. Degenerative neurological disease and debrisoquine-4-hydroxylation capacity. Med Sci Res 1989; 17:163–164.
23. Ferrari MD, Peeters EA, Haan J, et al. Cytochrome P450 and Parkinson's disease. Poor parahydroxylation of phenytoin. J Neurol Sci 1990; 96:153–157.

24. Kondo I, Kanazawa I. Association of *Xba I* allele (*Xba I* 44kb) of the human cytochrome P-450dbI (*CYP2D6*) gene in Japanese patients with idiopathic Parkinson's disease. In: Yoshida M, Nagatsu T, Narabayashi H, eds. Key topics in brain research: Parkinson's disease: from clinical aspects to molecular basis. New York: Springer-Verlag, 1991:111–117.
25. Kondo I, Kanazawa I. Debrisoquine hydroxylase and Parkinson's disease. In: Narabayashi H, Nagatsu T, Yanakisawa N, Mizuno Y, eds. Parkinson's disease: from basic research to treatment. Adv Neurol 1993; 60:338–342.
26. Smith CAD, Gough AC, Leigh PN, et al. Debrisoquine hydroxylase gene polymorphism and susceptibility to Parkinson's disease. Lancet 1992; 339:1375–1377.
27. Armstrong M, Daly AK, Cholerton S, Bateman DN, Idle JR. Mutant debrisoquine hydroxylation genes in Parkinson's disease. Lancet 1992; 339:1017–1018.
28. Chiba K, Trevor AJ, Castagnoli N Jr. Metabolism of the neurotoxic tertiary amine, MPTP, by brain monoamine oxidase. Biochem Biophys Res Commun 1984; 120:574–578.
29. Tetrud JW, Langston JW. The effect of Deprenyl (selegiline) on the natural history of Parkinson's disease. Science 1989; 245:519–522.
30. The Parkinson Study Group. Effect of Deprenyl on the progression of disability in early Parkinson's disease. N Engl J Med 1989; 321:1364–1371.
31. Jellinger K, Riederer P. Dementia in Parkinson's disease and (pre) senile dementia of Alzheimer type: morphological aspects and changes in intracerebral MAO activity. In: Hassler RG, Christ JF, eds. Parkinson-specific motor and mental disorders. Role of the pallidum: pathophysiological, biochemical and therapeutic aspects. Adv Neurol 1984; 40:199–210.
32. Bonuccelli U, Piccini P, Del Dotto P, Pacifici GM, Corsini GU, Muratorio A. Platelet monoamine oxidase B activity in parkinsonian patients. J Neurol Neurosurg Psychiatry 1990; 53:854–855.
33. Danielczyck W, Streifler M, Konradi C, Reiderer P, Moll G. Platelet MAO-B activity and the psychopathology of Parkinson's disease, senile dementia and multi-infarct dementia. Acta Psychiatr Scand 1988; 78:730–736.
34. Steventon GB, Sturman SG, Heafield MTE, Waring RH, Napier J, Williams AC. Platelet monoamine oxidase-B activity in Parkinson's disease. J Neural Transm 1989; 1:255–261.
35. Humfrey CDN, Steventon GB, Sturman SG, Waring RH, Griffiths B, Williams AC. Monoamine oxidase substrates in Parkinson's disease. Biochem Pharmacol 1990; 40:2562–2564.
36. Steventon GB, Humfrey C, Sturman SG, Williams AC, Waring RH. Monoamine oxidase-B and Parkinson's disease. Lancet 1990; 335:180.
37. Jarman J, Glover V, Sandler M, Turjanski N, Stern G. Platelet monoamine oxidase B activity in Parkinson's disease: a re-evaluation. J Neural Transm 1993; 5:1–4.
38. Sturman SG, Williams AC, Steventon GB, Waring RH. Metabolism of MPTP and benzylamine in Parkinson's disease. (in press)
39. Kurth JH, Kurth MC, Poduslo SE, Schwankhaus JD. Association of a monoamine oxidase B allele with Parkinson's disease. Ann Neurol 1993; 33:368–372.
40. Ansher SS, Cadet JL, Jakoby WB, Baker JK. Role of *N*-methyltransferases in the neurotoxicity associated with the metabolites of 1-methyl-4-phenyl-1,2,3,6-

tetrahydropyridine (MPTP) and other 4-substituted pyridines in the environment. Biochem Pharmacol 1986; 35:3359–3363.
41. Green S, Buttrum S, Molloy H, et al. *N*-Methylation of pyridines in Parkinson's disease. Lancet 1991; 338:120–121.
42. Williams AC, Pall HS, Steventon GB, et al. *N*-Methylation of pyridines and Parkinson's disease. Adv Neurol, 1993; 60:194–196.
43. Steventon GB, Heafield MTE, Waring RH, Williams AC. Xenobiotic metabolism in Parkinson's disease. Neurology 1989; 39:883–887.
44. Williams A, Sturman S, Steventon G. Metabolic biomarkers of Parkinson's disease. Acta Neurol Scand [suppl] 1991; 136:19–23.
45. Williams AC, Sturman SG, Steventon GB, Waring RH. Metabolic markers of Parkinson's disease. In: International workshop Berlin Parkinson's disease. How to proceed today in treatment; from basic research and early diagnosis to long-term treatment. Netherlands: Medicom, 1991:117–125.
46. Heafield MT, Fearn S, Steventon GB, Waring RH, Williams AC, Sturman SG. Plasma cysteine and sulphate levels in patients with motor neurone, Parkinson's and Alzheimer's disease. Neurosci Lett 1990; 110:216–220.
47. Steventon GB, Heafield MTE, Waring RH, Williams AC, Sturman SG, Green M. Metabolism of low-dose paracetamol in patients with chronic neurological disease. Xenobiotica 1990; 20:117–122.
48. Roos RAC, Steenvoorden JMC, Mulder GJ, Van Kempen GMJ. Acetaminophen sulfation in patients with Parkinson's disease or Huntington's disease is not impaired. Neurology 1993; 43:1373–1376.
49. Perry TL, Krieger C, Hansen S, Tabatabaei A. Amyotrophic lateral sclerosis: fasting plasma levels of cysteine and inorganic sulfate are normal, as are brain contents of cysteine. Neurology 1991; 41:487–490.
50. Fontan M, Petit H, Delahousse J, Ascher J, Decoulx-Poutignat M. Signes extrapyramidaux d'intoxications aigues ou subaigues par disulfiram ou disulfiram-alcool. Lille Med 1967; 12:814–817.
51. Hoogenraad TU. Dithiocarbamates and Parkinson's disease. Lancet 1988; 1:767.
52. Lidy C, Priollet P, Pepin B. Syndrome pyramidal et extra-pyramidal apparu au d'ecours d'une intoxication aiguee par le disulfiram. Nouv Presse Med 1979; 8:3561.
53. Waring RH, Sturman SG, Smith MCG, Steventon GB, Heafield MTE, Williams AC. *S*-Methylation in motor neurone disease and Parkinson's disease. Lancet 1989; 2:356–357.
54. Mircheva Y, Vidailhet M, Marconi R, Bonnet AM, Beaune P, Agid Y. Selective decrease in *S*-methylation in Parkinson's disease. Neurology 1993; 43(suppl):A154-A155.

7

Endogenous Toxins as Potential Etiologic Agents in Parkinson's Disease

Ian Irwin and J. William Langston

The Parkinson's Institute, Sunnyvale, California

I. INTRODUCTION

Aside from the general agreement that a loss of nigrostriatal dopamine represents the primary and most consistent neurochemical deficiency in Parkinson's disease (1,2), the importance of other biochemical agents, events, or deficiencies in causing this disorder has yet to be established. Nonetheless, the hypothesis that a toxic chemical may be responsible for the disease remains prominent in the thinking of many scientists who are interested in the cause of this disease. Not too surprisingly, several of the proponents of this hypothesis have come from the discipline of neurotoxicology.

The experimental tools of this discipline provide the means to search for offending neurochemical agents in a manner that is highly analogous to investigators arriving at the scene of the crime. Scattered about the scene are a variety of clues and other items that may or may not be related to the crime. These are carefully examined and evaluated, with the hope that they can be used to track down the perpetrator. In the case of Parkinson's disease, one can examine the affected brain regions (the crime scene) searching for chemical fingerprints and other markers of toxic injury, although many of the techniques to accomplish this are just emerging. Furthermore, neurotoxicologists also have considerable familiarity with some of the baser capacities and damaging activities of a number of noxious chemical agents. From such information, a surprisingly large number of compounds have been proposed as etiologic agents in the disease. As we obtain an increasingly clear picture of this "rogues gallery" of chemical suspects and a working knowledge of their toxic "modus operandi," it becomes more and more feasible to search for clues to their presence and possible roles in the neurodegenerative process.

If one or more neurotoxins do indeed play a role in Parkinson's disease, the first question that must be addressed is whether the offending agent exists in the external environment or is produced endogenously. Although there is currently great interest in both possibilities, the focus of this chapter will be on the "endogenous hypothesis." At first glance, this hypothesis is attractive because of its simplicity. This is in part because the task of isolating and identifying an environmental agent could be enormously complex. On the other hand, searching for an endogenous agent is limited to a much smaller universe, the human body. To return to our analogy, we might say that the criminal is likely to be found at the scene of the crime. This hypothesis is also attractive because the continual presence of such an agent could explain the insidious and ongoing nature of the disease. Finally, there is no shortage of suspects, as the normal brain is awash with potentially toxic endogenous agents. Transition metals, such as iron, manganese, or copper, although essential for the normal metabolism and housekeeping of neuronal cells, may cause the production of damaging reactive oxygen intermediates. Indeed, oxygen radicals are the routine products of many metabolic processes. Neurotransmitters that normally serve as faithful chemical messengers can, at least in theory, become cellular assassins under certain conditions.

In this chapter, a detailed discussion of endogenous compounds that have been implicated as potential causative agents in Parkinson's disease is presented. These compounds (a) have been implicated as possible offending agents in Parkinson's disease and (b) are known to exist endogenously in the brain. Many of the principles outlined in Chapter 4 are highly relevent to understanding the mechanism of action of the agents reviewed, and the reader may wish to read that chapter first. As will become apparent on reading this review, there is a remarkable abundance of chemical suspects lurking in the human brain, and the major problem is trying to sort out which of these agents is more suspect than the others.

II. DOPAMINE-RELATED NEUROTOXINS

The selective degeneration of the nigrostriatal dopaminergic neurons in idiopathic Parkinson's disease has led many investigators to seek answers to the question of etiology among the unique properties of these neurons. One of the most obvious and striking characteristics of the nigrostriatal system is the high concentration of dopamine found in its neurons. The concentration of dopamine in these neurons is several times greater than the concentrations of catecholamine neurotransmitters in other areas of the brain. Dopamine has been of interest as a possible causative agent for a variety of reasons, including (a) the production of hydrogen peroxide in the course of normal dopamine metabolism; (b) the tendency for dopamine to autoxidize, a process that could lead to the formation of potentially toxic dopamine analogs; and (c) the association of its chemical reactivity with the characteristic age-dependent accumulation of neuromelanin within the substantia nigra neurons.

A. The Role of Dopamine

1. Dopamine Metabolism and Hydrogen Peroxide

The first mechanism by which this neurotransmitter might damage neurons relates to its normal metabolic degradation. After release, dopamine is oxidatively deaminated by the enzyme monoamine oxidase (MAO) to yield 3,4-dihydroxyphenylacetaldehyde. The further oxidation of this aldehyde to 3,4-dihydroxyphenylacetic acid (DOPAC), a major metabolite of dopamine in the central nervous system, is rapid. The catabolism of dopamine uses molecular oxygen and, in the process, produces a single molecule of hydrogen peroxide for every molecule of dopamine that is oxidatively deaminated. The production of hydrogen peroxide is dependent on the levels of MAO and the rate of dopamine release.

Given the potential damaging effects of hydrogen peroxide, described in Chapter 4, it is not surprising that many investigators have singled out this pathway as one that could damage dopamine neurons, thereby linking the metabolism of dopamine to neuronal damage and loss in Parkinson's disease (3). A limited number of experimental studies have directly attempted to address the capacity of dopamine release in vivo to produce oxidative stress. The results suggest that increased dopamine release is accompanied by an increase in markers of oxidative stress such as oxidized glutathione and that MAO inhibitors partially block this increase (4,5).

2. A Vicious Cycle

If the continual release and metabolism of dopamine leads to peroxide-mediated damage and the eventual death of individual dopamine neurons, this process could become a vicious cycle. To maintain striatal dopaminergic output, the surviving neurons are likely to compensate by increasing the release of dopamine. However, increased release of dopamine would then lead to the enhanced production of hydrogen peroxide, in turn producing increased oxidative stress and further degeneration of dopaminergic neurons. Thus, a vicious cycle could be set in motion, leading to a continual process of neuronal degeneration. Eventually, this process may result in sufficient neuronal loss such that synaptic dopamine levels can no longer be maintained and symptoms of Parkinson's disease ensue.

3. Relation to Aging

Some investigators have extended these observations to suggest that this mechanism of oxidative stress may play a role in normal aging of the nigrostriatal system. Dopamine has been reported to decline with age (6,7), and age-dependent nigral cell loss has been observed by some investigators (8). These changes appear to be associated with an increase in the relative levels of DOPAC and homovanillic acid (HVA) (7) with age. In addition, an age-related increase in brain MAO-B activity has been reported in a variety of species, including humans (9,10).

The similarity between these age-related changes in the nigrostriatal dopamine system [i.e., dopamine decline, nigral cell loss, and increases in the indices of dopamine turnover (metabolite/DA ratios)] and those seen in Parkinson's disease, itself an age-related disorder, suggests an interaction between aging, monoamine oxidase, dopamine decline, and Parkinson's disease. However, such a relation may be very difficult to prove, particularly since the reason for these age-related changes in normal persons has yet to be elucidated. Thus, identification of an event that sets in motion, accelerates, or enhances normal age-related decline in the nigrostriatal dopamine system to produce Parkinson's disease has, as yet, not been demonstrated.

4. Experience With Levodopa Therapy

Further questions about the role of increased dopamine turnover in the human disease arise from clinical experience with levodopa (L-dihydroxyphenylamine, or L-dopa), the mainstay of treatment in Parkinson's disease. Levodopa treatment elevates nigrostriatal concentrations of dopamine and its metabolites severalfold (11). Therefore, it is logical to assume that these increases in turnover would also increase the availability of hydrogen peroxide and accelerate nigrostriatal degeneration. However, Quinn and colleagues (12) found no neuropathological evidence of nigrostriatal damage in a patient without Parkinson's disease who consumed more than 2 kg of L-dopa over a 4-year period. Although there are no reports of a prospective clinical trial of L-dopa verses placebo in patients with early Parkinson's disease, nearly 30 years of experience with this drug has failed to produce clear-cut evidence that L-dopa produces an acceleration of the underlying disease process in Parkinson's disease. Although it has been suggested that the incidence of L-dopa-induced complications correlate with the length of the period of L-dopa therapy (13), other recent evidence suggests that the complications of L-dopa therapy are more closely related to the severity of nigrostriatal loss (14,15). Indeed, several studies (16–19) suggest that early treatment with L-dopa improves survival of Parkinson's patients.

In light of the difficulties encountered in these human studies, it might be expected that experimental studies using animal or in vitro models would be more helpful in evaluating this hypothesis. Unfortunately, experimental studies have not greatly advanced our understanding of these issues. In rodents, discrete dopaminergic lesions induced by surgical means or with toxins such as 1-methyl-4-phenyl-1,2,3,6-tetrahydropyridine (MPTP) or 6-hydroxydopamine (6-OHDA) produce nigrostriatal damage and increased dopamine turnover (20,21). These lesions do not, however, set in motion the process of degeneration described in the foregoing. In fact, animals lesioned by chemical means frequently exhibit recovery with time (22,23).

Although the effects of long-term administration of L-dopa in these lesioned animals may be a better way to evaluate possible L-dopa-induced enhancement of degeneration in Parkinson's disease, such studies have not been reported. Prolonged L-dopa administration to normal adult mice (24) and rats (25), however, does not produce accelerated destruction of nigrostriatal neurons. In fact, just the opposite has been reported. Extended L-dopa treatment in rats is reported to ameliorate age-related motor impairment and produce a 50% increase in life span (26,27). On the other hand, L-dopa has been reported to reduce the effectiveness of neural grafts in promoting recovery in 6-OHDA lesioned rats (28,29). The relevance of these latter studies to survival of native dopaminergic neurons in Parkinson's disease, however, is unclear.

5. *Monoamine Oxidase Inhibitor Therapy*

Recent clinical studies with other pharmacological therapies in Parkinson's disease tend to support the idea that dopamine turnover may be involved in the progression of the disease and that reducing the release or metabolism of dopamine may be of some benefit in slowing the progression of the disease. The drug selegiline (deprenyl), a selective MAO inhibitor, appears to be effective in delaying the need for L-dopa therapy in patients with early, untreated disease (30–33). The question of whether these effects represent a true "neuroprotective" action of MAO-B inhibition, or if they are the consequence of a symptomatic effect, is an important one that has yet to be fully answered. One hopes that the results of additional, longer-term studies with selegiline and other MAO inhibitors will help resolve this important question.

Investigations into effects of MAO inhibitors on the aging process in animals also suggest that this drug may ameliorate age-related changes in brain function in rodents. Knoll and colleagues (34) have reported that selegiline extends the life span and raises the activity level and learning ability in older rats continuously administered this drug. No information on the levels of striatal dopamine or the numbers of nigral neurons between selegiline and control-treated animals was reported in these studies and, thus, unfortunately, the results of the "life-extending" effects of this drug do little to clarify the role of MAO in age-related degeneration of the nigrostriatal dopamine system.

6. *Studies with Pergolide*

The absence of observable clinical progression in some patients with Parkinson's disease has also been reported with the drug pergolide (35,36). Pergolide is a potent dopamine agonist, and by direct action at both postsynaptic and dendritic dopamine receptors reduces both the dosages of L-dopa required by patients and, presumably, the release and turnover of nigrostriatal dopamine (37).

The results of studies with pergolide in an animal model of aging (38,39) are also very provocative. Long-term administration (approximately 2 years) of dietary pergolide to Fischer 344 rats was reported to reduce the age-related reductions in the number of fluorescent DA cell bodies in the substantia nigra and terminals in the striatum. The significance of these age-related changes in fluorescence cytochemistry remain to be elucidated, however, since there were no differences in striatal dopamine in all groups of animals.

7. Summary

Although the results of clinical and basic studies have failed to conclusively establish a link between aging, dopamine turnover, hydrogen peroxide production, and Parkinson's disease, the very assumptions on which this hypothesis is based have recently been challenged. The age-related decrease in striatal dopamine in autopsied human brain has not been found by all investigators (40–42). One might expect that modern imaging techniques (positron emission tomography; PET) that allow the visualization and quantitation of striatal dopamine in living humans would clarify this question. Unfortunately, there appears to be disagreement among these studies as well. Calne and colleagues (43) noted an age-related decline in striatal dopamine using this technique, whereas Sawle et al. (44) found no relation between age and striatal ^{18}F-dopa uptake. The failure of these studies to clarify the extent of age-related dopamine decline in normal humans might be attributable to the difficulties in standardizing subject selection, as has been suggested (45).

Although one might expect animal models of aging to clarify these issues, the variability among different species used to study aging and nigrostriatal dopamine decline has tended to confound the interpretation of laboratory studies in humans. There is now increasing evidence that rats and mice, by far the most common models used for such studies, may be less than ideal to evaluate this hypothesis, because they do not consistently demonstrate an age-related decline in dopamine (23,46), or in cell numbers (47). If a normal age-related decline in striatal dopamine is a critical element in the pathophysiological process in Parkinson's disease, it may be necessary to extend laboratory studies to other species that more clearly exhibit this phenomenon if we are to make progress in unraveling these complex questions.

B. Dopamine Quinones

In addition to the production of hydrogen peroxide as a consequence of the ordered metabolic degradation of dopamine, a variety of other compounds arise from the spontaneous chemical reactions of which dopamine is capable. At least some of these compounds may be toxic. The spontaneous reactions that produce these potential etiologic agents are inherent in the chemistry of dopamine and do not require the participation of any biological or enzymatic machinery to elaborate an endogenous toxin.

The first family of such dopamine-derived compounds is the dopamine quinones. In the presence of oxygen, dopamine is rapidly and spontaneously converted through a semiquinone intermediate (dopamine semiquinone; DSQ) to an orthoquinone derivative (dopamine orthoquinone; DOQ). Oxygen is converted to superoxide or peroxide in the process (Fig. 1).

Dopamineorthoquinone appears to be an extremely unstable compound that undergoes a variety of chemical reactions, including further conversion to a number of other chemical species, described later in this section. Under laboratory conditions, activated forms of oxygen (i.e., hydrogen peroxide, superoxide anion, and hydroxyl radical) are both products (48) and promoters (49) of the formation of DSQ and DOQ from dopamine. The autoxidation of dopamine is enhanced in the presence of alkalai and is catalyzed by free metal cations, such as copper, manganese, and iron. Metal chelate complexes, in which the metal ion is adventitiously coordinated within an organic molecule, are even better at catalyzing the oxidation of dopamine than are the free metals themselves.

Both DSQ and DOQ are potentially cytotoxic compounds, and the toxicity of dopamine by the formation of these intermediates has been amply demonstrated in vitro. The toxicity of DSQ and DOQ involves two possible mechanisms that are discussed in detail in Chapter 4. The formation of DSQ and DOQ generates peroxide and superoxide (48,50,51) and, thus, may lead to free radical-mediated damage of cells. Because of their extreme reactivity, these quinones also rapidly form covalent adducts with nucleophilic agents (compounds with available electrons) and, thereby, may be toxic through covalent binding. Candidate biological nucleophiles include sulfhydryl compounds (glutathione, cysteine, protein thiols), amino compounds (amino acids), and water. The interaction of DSQ or DOQ with cellular nucleophiles in this way could inactivate important enzymes within nigral neurons or deplete these cells of necessary constituents, such as glutathione, thereby lowering the available pool of these protective elements.

Graham and colleagues (50,51) have carried out studies to determine which of these mechanisms was primary to the toxicity of dopamine; they also studied

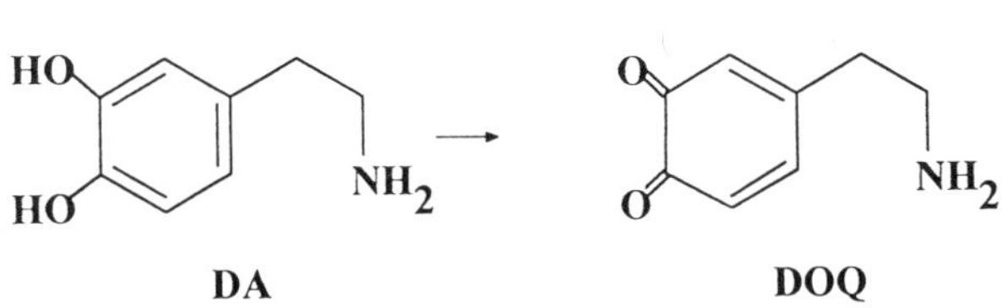

Figure 1 Oxidation of dopamine orthoquinone (DOQ).

a series of other polyphenols. To assess the role of oxygen radical-mediated damage these investigators (a) examined the relation between autoxidation and toxicity and (b) evaluated the ability of scavengers of superoxide, peroxide, and hydroxyl radical to protect against toxicity in C1300 neuroblastoma cells in vitro. They also investigated the ability of dopamine and its oxidized products to inhibit the activity of the sulfhydryl-containing DNA polymerase as a measure of the role played by covalent binding. Their results indicated that both oxidative stress and covalent binding contribute to the toxicity of dopamine in this culture system. These experimental results are interesting because they provide a mechanism that could lead to both free radical-mediated damage (through the direct effects of superoxide, peroxide, and hydroxyl radicals) *and*, in theory at least, to mitochondrial deficits.

The latter could occur, by a process of covalent binding, as a consequence of inactivation of mitochondrial sulfhydryl enzymes involved in energy production. Both oxygen radical-mediated damage and covalent binding could also contribute to deficits in glutathione observed in Parkinson's disease.

The ease of autoxidation of dopamine, which does not require any organized enzymatic process(es), but rather, occurs spontaneously, suggests that these reactions are also likely to occur in vivo. Indirect evidence for the existence of these oxidized intermediates in the human brain also comes from studies that demonstrate the likelihood that DSQ and DOQ are precursors in the formation of neuromelanin (50,52,53). Recent reports (54,55) of 5-*S*-cysteinyl dopamine in the brain of humans and other mammalian species also supports the occurrence of autoxidation of dopamine in vivo.

1. Implications for Parkinson's Disease

In spite of the attractiveness of these observations, there is little direct evidence that DOQ and DSQ are the endogenous toxins responsible for Parkinson's disease. Many of the issues raised in the previous section about the role of aging and observations with -dopa therapy also apply here. Levodopa would also be expected to increase the concentration of free dopamine and, thereby, increase products of its autoxidation. In addition, if the spontaneous oxidation of dopamine were responsible for nigrostriatal degeneration, MAO inhibition would be expected to exacerbate the damaging effects of dopamine on nigrostriatal neurons. This is exactly the opposite of what has been reported in experimental and clinical studies with MAO inhibitors.

Nonetheless, given the likely presence of these agents in the brain and their potential toxicity, it would seem an important focus of future investigations. Particular emphasis should be placed on isolating, identifying, and quantitating conjugates of dopamine from normal and parkinsonian brain and understanding the mechanism underlying the formation of the thiol conjugates of dopamine.

C. Leukochromes and Aminochromes

In the previous section, it was pointed out that residues of cellular macromolecules may be the ultimate targets of DOQ. Dopamine orthoquinones can also react with the amino nitrogen present within DOQ itself. This reaction (Fig. 2) occurs rapidly in the course of the autoxidation of dopamine.

Similar to the oxidation of DSQ to DOQ, the intermediate leukochrome is further oxidized to aminochrome. The chemical structure and biological effects of leukochromes and aminochromes have received considerable attention (for reviews, see Refs. 56 and 57).

Although the addition of an amino nitrogen to DOQ is much less favored than the addition of sulfhydryl groups, that DOQ itself contains an amino group increases the rate of the reaction. Pathways leading to the formation of leukochromes and aminochromes are potentially toxic by the same free radical-generating mechanism arising from DOQ (57). In the conversion of leukochrome to the aminochrome, an additional molecule of superoxide or peroxide would be generated.

In addition, the aminochrome formed from dopamine appears likely to undergo redox cycling (58). Under these circumstances, the potential production of oxygen radicals is greatly enhanced because, unlike the formation of DSQ or DOQ, which are likely to produce only stoichiometric amounts of superoxide (one molecule of superoxide per molecule of catechol oxidized), the more stable aminochrome can be reduced by flavoenzymes and subsequently reoxidize. This process is repeated until a source of reducing agent is exhausted. Thus, a continuous stream of free radicals can be produced, leading to extensive cellular damage. Aminochromes are also known to participate in a variety of addition and substitution reactions with sulfhydryl and other groups and, therefore, may exert toxicity by a covalent-binding mechanism (56,59–64).

1. *Implications for Parkinson's Disease*

A major problem with establishing a role for aminochromes in Parkinson's disease is the lack of studies demonstrating their formation in vivo. This may

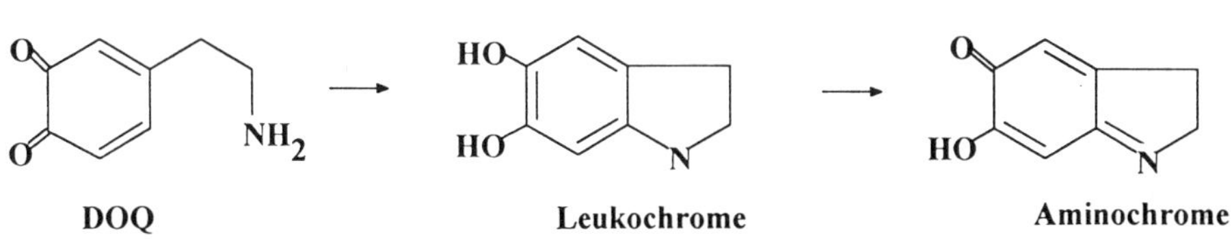

Figure 2 The cyclization of dopamine orthoquinone (DOQ) to form leukochrome. Leukochrome is subsequently oxidized to the aminochrome.

be because the reaction of DOQ with sulfhydryl-containing nucleophiles is more than three orders of magnitude greater than the internal cyclization (48); thus, only traces of aminochromes are formed. Given the high concentration of glutathione and cysteine present in the cellular compartment, any dopamine oxidized to DOQ would be expected to be converted to sulfhydryl conjugates. Nonetheless, the likely presence of aminochrome-derived subunits in neuromelanin has been established, and the production and participation of aminochromes in the formation of neuromelanin appears to be well accepted (53,65–67). It is plausible that the appearance of trace amounts of free aminochrome could have serious physiological consequences. Indeed, it has recently been argued that the presence of aminochrome-derived indole subunits in neuromelanin indicates the occurrence of periods of substantial glutathione and cysteine depletions and, therefore, represent markers of toxic events (53).

It is clear that additional work in this area will be needed to understand the possible role of aminochrome formation in Parkinson's disease. Such understanding awaits the development of animal models to study the effects of administered aminochrome and to characterize its neurochemical and neuropathological effects. In addition, any theory involving dopamine as the primary source of endogenous toxins will require an explanation for the previously discussed data on L-dopa and monoamine oxidase.

D. 6-Hydroxydopamine

Recognition of the selective toxicity of 6-OHDA for catecholaminergic neurons and the possibility for its spontaneous generation from dopamine led to the hypothesis that this compound might represent the endogenous toxin responsible for Parkinson's disease. In contrast with the lack of documentation of the effects of other putative dopamine-derived toxins, such as aminochromes, the neurotoxicity of 6-OHDA has been well studied (68). Because 6-OHDA does not cross the blood–brain barrier, the compound must be administered directly into the CNS. Depending on the dosage, route and site of administration, and the animal species used, this agent produces reductions of catecholamine neurotransmitter levels that may be reversible or irreversible.

The primary targets of intraventricularly or intrastriatally administered 6-OHDA are nerve terminals (68). Introduction of 6-OHDA directly into the region of nigral cell bodies causes cell destruction (68). Because most studies of 6-OHDA involve only one or two injections, it could be argued that a model involving the slow, prolonged administration of 6-OHDA might more closely represent the pattern of exposure from an endogenously formed toxin and could produce pathological effects more similar to the disease. Unfortunately, no studies involving the slow or repeated administration of long-term, low-dose 6-OHDA have been reported.

Since 6-OHDA does not cross the blood–brain barrier, the major issue to be addressed in this chapter is whether or not 6-OHDA is produced endogenously. It is interesting to note that, in 1959, Senoh and colleagues (69) reported the formation of 6-OHDA in the brain of the rat after administration of tritiated dopamine; this compound accounted for about 0.5% of the administered radioactivity. Because the potent dopaminergic toxicity of this compound was recognized only later (68,70), this observation attracted little notice at the time. Given the potential importance of this finding, it is surprising that over 30 years have passed without a definitive resolution of the question of whether or not 6-OHDA is generated endogenously. If so, it could have profound implications for theories relating to the cause of Parkinson's disease.

There are several mechanisms by which the endogenous production of 6-OHDA could occur. For example, it could be produced as the result of the oxidation of dopamine to DOQ, and the subsequent reaction with water (Fig. 3, pathway I). Although dopamine can be electrochemically induced to undergo this reaction in 2 *M* acid (48,71) the rate of water addition is extremely slow.

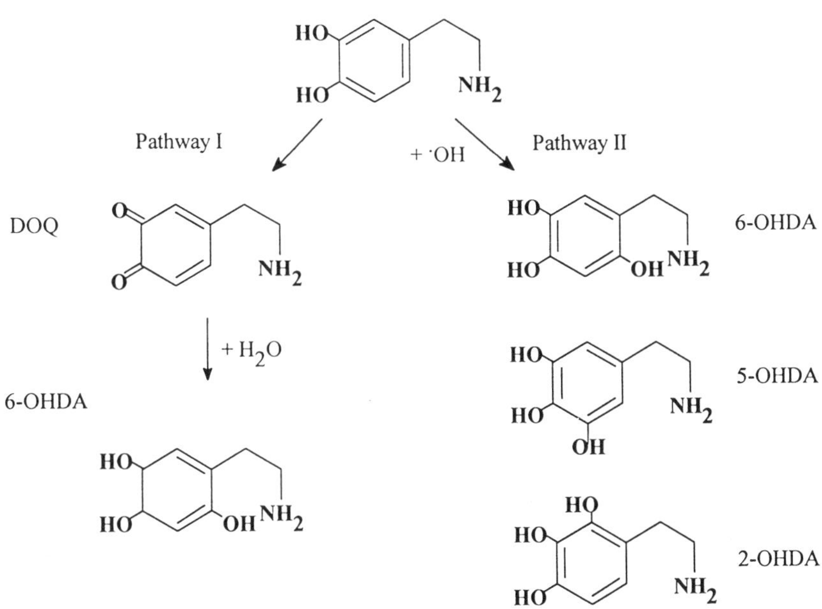

Figure 3 Possible pathways for the endogenous formation of 6-hydroxydopamine. Pathway I. Dopamine is oxidized to dopamine orthoquinone, which subsequently undergoes nucleophilic addition of water. Pathway II: Direct addition of hydroxyl radical to the benzene ring of dopamine. The radical addition is not specific for the 6 position and considerable amounts of 2- and 5-hydroxydopamine are also formed.

At physiological pH, the rate is probably three to four orders of magnitude slower than the internal cyclization reaction (aminochrome formation) and approximately six orders of magnitude less than the addition of sulfhydryl agents.

An alternative mechanism for the formation of 6-OHDA involves the direct addition of hydroxyl radical to dopamine (see Fig. 3, pathway II). The requisite hydroxyl radical could come from various sources, including superoxide or the interaction of Fe^{2+} with hydrogen peroxide (the Fenton reaction). The addition of hydroxyl radical to the phenyl ring of dopamine has been demonstrated to occur in vitro at approximately physiological pH (72). These studies demonstrated that, in the presence of a hydroxyl radical-generating system, dopamine is converted to a mixture of trihydroxylated derivatives, including 2-, 5-, and 6-OHDA. Interestingly, of the three possible isomers, 6-OHDA appeared to be formed in the least amounts. Given the known toxicity of 6-OHDA, the endogenous formation by any means of even minute amounts of this chemical could result in serious damage to dopamine neurons.

In spite of these considerations, however, whether or not 6-OHDA is formed endogenously remains somewhat controversial. The original observations of Senoh and colleagues (69), indicating that 6-OHDA is a product of the normal metabolism of dopamine, have not been replicated. Given the tremendous advances in analytical techniques that have been made in the past decades, it is surprising that a reinvestigation of this question in parkinsonian and normal brain has not been reported. Such a study, although difficult, would seem warranted, particularly if it included analysis for the 2- and 5-hydroxy derivatives as well. An analytical study to detect the presence of the glutathione adduct of 6-OHDA would also seem worthwhile, since this compound has been identified in brain following the stereotaxic injection of 6-OHDA in the rat (73).

An entirely different line of evidence supporting the argument that 6-OHDA can be formed endogenously comes from experimental work with the amphetamines. Amphetamine and methamphetamine are known to damage striatal dopamine terminals and produce persistent depletions of striatal dopamine (74–76). The toxic effects of methamphetamine are thought to involve the autoxidation of endogenous dopamine released from its storage sites in striatal terminals. This view is supported by studies showing that lowering endogenous dopamine concentrations by the administration of α-methyl-tyrosine before amphetamine treatment ameliorates toxicity in rats. Furthermore, inhibition of monoamine oxidase exacerbates amphetamine toxicity in rats (77). Thus, because amphetamine toxicity appears to involve endogenous dopamine, it represents one of the best possible experimental models in which to determine mechanisms of dopamine toxicity and to identify endogenous formation of neurotoxins.

In 1984, Seiden and Vosmer reported the formation of 6-OHDA in the caudate nucleus of the rat brain after a single large dose of methamphetamine (78). Seiden and colleagues have subsequently reported that methamphetamine-induced production of 6-OHDA is reduced by pretreatment with α-methyl-*p*-tyrosine (79) and increased by pretreatment of animals with MAO inhibitors (80,81). Together these results appear to support that endogenous formation of 6-OHDA can occur, at least as the result of amphetamine administration.

Controversy has emerged over these findings, however, as other investigators have not been able to replicate these results. For example, when using in vivo microdialysis, Rollema and colleagues (82) were unable to detect 6-OHDA in the striatum of methamphetamine-treated rats. Future clarification of this controversy will be important in understanding the relevance of 6-OHDA in Parkinson's disease. For the moment, however, it must be said that, although this hypothesis remains alive, it is far from being established.

E. Neuromelanin

Any discussion of possible dopamine-derived etiologic agents would be incomplete without mention of neuromelanin. Perhaps this section should have begun with neuromelanin, since this enigmatic substance has held the interest of neuropathologists for nearly a century. This black pigment represents one of the most obvious morphological features of nigral neurons. The presence of neuromelanin in the substantia nigra is apparent even on gross examination of the midbrain and forms the basis for the name of this nucleus (black substance).

Neuromelanin is present in cytoplasm of catecholaminergic neurons in the adult human brain. Indeed, the association of neuromelanin and catecholamine neurons is so close that the presence of neuromelanin is often used as a marker for these cells (83). It is widely accepted that the spontaneous oxidation of dopamine is involved in the deposition of neuromelanin in the substantia nigra (50,52,53). Thus, if nothing else, the presence of neuromelanin here furnishes a biological record of the autoxidation of dopamine in the perikarya of these neurons. The accumulation of neuromelanin in substantia nigra neurons is age-dependent (84–87).

Interestingly, despite that the terminals of nigrostriatal neurons contain dopamine concentrations equal to or greater than those found in the cell bodies, the deposition of neuromelanin occurs only in nigral perikarya. The accumulation of neuromelanin in the cell bodies, and not the striatal processes of these neurons, points to differing conditions or capacities in the two regions. Either the autoxidation of dopamine is greater in the cell bodies, or the mechanisms available to deal with "free" oxidized dopamine are frequently exceeded there.

Although there is general agreement that the genesis of neuromelanin involves the autoxidation of dopamine, there is considerable controversy over the role that the pigment itself plays in health and disease. Many investigators have suggested that the accumulation of neuromelanin could be associated with increasing compromise of cellular functions. In Parkinson's disease, this accumulation might reach a critical point, sufficient to interfere with cell function, ultimately causing cellular dysfunction, atrophy, and death. Barden (88) found that the Golgi network in nigral cells containing large amounts of neuromelanin was considerably reduced and argued that such reductions would produce functional damage to cells. Mann et al. (89) noted that the accumulation of neuromelanin in substantia nigra neurons was accompanied by a reduction in cytoplasmic RNA and a decrease in nucleolar volume, suggesting that this substance itself eventually so compromises cellular function that it might cause cell death. These investigators linked melanin accumulation to both nigral cell loss in aging (85) and in Parkinson's disease (89,90). The latter view has recently been reinforced by the findings of Hirsch and colleagues (91) who noted that, in Parkinson's disease, melanized neurons bear the brunt of the degeneration, although just the opposite has been reported by Gibb et al. (92).

Certain of the chemical properties of neuromelanin support the view that neuromelanin may be culpable in the degeneration of neurons within which it accumulates. For example, neuromelanin can bind redox-active metal ions in a way such as to increase their participation in oxygen radical-generating reactions, a process that could enhance the production of peroxide, superoxide, and hydroxyl radicals (93). Neuromelanin can also alter the oxidation state of metal ions to favor superoxide (94) and peroxide production (95), or it can interact directly with molecular oxygen to generate these (96,97). Finally neuromelanin might accumulate, then slowly release, a variety of potentially toxic agents within nigral neurons (98–104).

Although these results all suggest that neuromelanin may have deleterious effect on cells, other properties of melanin indicate that it might be protective, rather than destructive. Melanin (a) binds redox-active metal ions, thereby reducing their availability to participate in oxygen radical generation (93); (b) accumulates and retains potentially toxic compounds, thereby compartmentalizing them and protecting against their damaging effects; and (c) directly reacts with hydroxyl, superoxide, peroxide, and other damaging radical species, thereby functioning as a scavenger (105,106).

Given the list of "protective" properties, some investigators have suggested that neuromelanin could have a protective function within melanized cells and have speculated that the loss of pigmented cells with aging and in Parkinson's disease reflects a primary deficit in neuromelanin "function," with cell death as a consequence of pigment loss (52,107–109). In support of the latter view, at least one group has reported that the melanized cells in the substantia nigra are preferentially spared in Parkinson's disease (92).

This seemingly paradoxical nature of the physical and chemical properties of melanin may be accounted for by the fact that the exact structure of neuromelanin is unknown. Much of the experimental work has been done with eumelanin (derived from eye pigment), pheomelanin (derived from skin pigment), or with "test tube" polymers synthesized in various ways from catecholamine precursor amino acids or catecholamines. The composition of these polymers could vary considerably from that found in the brain. Thus, until the exact structure of human neuromelanin is known, any conclusions about its exact function must be considered tentative. Clearly, more also needs to be learned about the chemical microenvironment of melanin-containing cells in terms of the composition and content of metal ions present in melanin-containing cells, to better understand these interactions. Fortunately, progress is being made in both these areas (53,110).

F. Criticisms of the Dopamine Hypothesis

As should be obvious from the previous discussion, the hypothesis that oxidized dopamine or its derivatives are etiologically important in Parkinson's disease is a theoretically attractive one for several reasons. First, the precursor molecule is present in high concentrations in many of the affected cells. Second, the toxic products of dopamine oxidation discussed in this section are formed spontaneously. These dopamine-derived compounds could provide a mechanism for the pulsatile or continuous damage to nigrostriatal cells from successive fluxes and continual accumulation of potentially toxic products. Finally, the production of dopamine-derived endotoxins would be subject to a great number of secondary factors, such as the (a) availability and state (free versus chelated) of transition metal ions; (b) the rates of release, uptake, and metabolic degradation of dopamine; (c) modulation of dopamine transport, storage, release, or metabolism by exogenous agents, which could either increase or reduce the consequent risk or damage; (d) the presence of transient oxidative stress; or (e) genetically transmitted defects in one or more of these systems. In this scenario, Parkinson's disease, while caused by dopamine-derived endotoxins, could still arise out of one or more of these secondary factors.

In spite of these considerations the hypothesis that a dopamine-derived endotoxin, or dopamine oxidation, might be responsible for the development of Parkinson's disease suffers from several theoretical and practical problems. One problem is that these hypotheses focus exclusively on dopamine-containing neurons. Although the brunt of the damage in Parkinson's disease is delivered to the nigrostriatal dopaminergic system, the disease also includes the characteristic pathological involvement of various other catecholaminergic (locus coeruleus) and noncatecholaminergic nuclei. Marsden (86) pointed out that the characteristic pattern of cell degeneration found in Parkinson's disease correlates with the distribution of Lewy bodies in the brain. These characteristic intraneuronal inclusions are typically seen, not only in the substantia nigra, but also in the substantia inominata, the nucleus basalis, the hypothalamus, and in the dorsal motor nucleus of vagus (see Chapter 3). Yet there are no identified catecholaminergic neurotransmitters in many of these areas.

Additional doubts about the exclusive involvement of dopamine or dopamine-derived toxins also arise from experience with L-dopa, monoamine oxidase inhibitors, and other drugs used to manipulate dopamine concentrations (see previous discussion). Finally, in spite of the experimental models of cytotoxicity, there is no convincing animal model, using any of these agents, that produces a histopathological spectrum of cell damage that resembles Parkinson's disease. The lack of such a model compromises the attempts to move this theory beyond the realm of speculation.

III. SEROTONIN-RELATED NEUROTOXINS

In addition to the high concentrations of dopamine found in nigrostriatal dopamine neurons, the basal ganglia also contains substantial amounts of serotonin. There is considerable comingling of serotonergic with dopaminergic cell bodies in the basal ganglia of the primate (111) and rodent (112). There is also some coregionalization of serotonergic and dopaminergic terminals in the striatum.

Given the proximity of serotonergic and dopaminergic neuronal elements, it is not surprising that suspicion has been cast on serotonergic neurons as possible sources of endogenous toxins. Most of the proposed serotonin-related endogenous toxins have been suggested, based on their structural similarity to the parkinsonogenic neurotoxin MPTP or to its toxic metabolite the 1-methyl-4-phenylpyridinium ion (MPP^+).

It has been suggested that the catabolism of a methylated derivative of serotonin could lead directly to the production of an MPTP-like compound (113), or directly to an MPP^+-like compound (114) in the brain. Since MPTP represents one of the best models of Parkinson's disease to date, additional exploration of these specific neurotoxins would seem warranted. Studies with these compounds demonstrating their occurrence in vivo would be of great interest. Such work has not been forthcoming, however, and the hypothetical mechanism by which they might be formed has been questioned (115).

IV. ISOQUINOLINES

Although one subgroup of isoquinolines, the salsolinol series, is derived from dopamine, isoquinolines represent a departure from neurotransmitter-derived neurotoxins, since they are formed from a variety of other phenethylamines. Isoquinolines may have a number of different states of substitution or saturation (Fig. 4). In the fully oxidized isoquinoline, the nitrogen ring contains three double bonds. This ring may also contain two double bonds or a single double

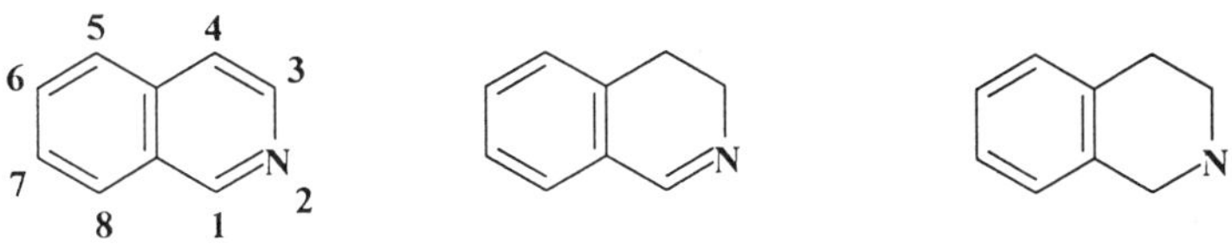

isoquinoline (IQ) 3,4-dihydroisoquinoline (DIQ) 1,2,3,4-tetrahydroisoquinoline (TIQ)

Figure 4 The simple isoquinolines, illustrating the numbering and naming conventions used for these compounds.

bond, giving rise to the dihydro- or tetrahydro- derivative. In addition there may be a variety of substituents on the ring. The positions of both saturation and substituents follows the numbering convention illustrated in Figure 4.

Fully oxidized isoquinolines substituted in the 2 position (Fig. 5) possess a quaternary nitrogen and bear a permanent positive charge (isoquinoliniums).

The primary formation of isoquinolines is thought to occur in vivo by spontaneous, or possibly enzymatic, cyclization reactions of phenethylamines. Additional isoquinolines arise by the metabolic transformation of these primary compounds. The primary source of biological isoquinolines is thought to be the Pictet–Spengler (Fig. 6a) condensation of β-phenethylamines with aldehydes, ketones, or keto acids, or the cyclization of β-phenethylamides (Bischler–Napieralski reaction; see Fig. 6b).

Once formed, isoquinolines undergo several enzymatic transformation reactions, including *O*-methylation of hydroxylated congeners by catechol-*O*-methyltransferase (COMT) (116), ring hydroxylation in the 4 position (117,118) *N*-methylation (118–120), or reduction and oxidation (118).

There is ample evidence that isoquinolines occur in the environment and endogenously. They have been isolated from many different sources, including both plants and animals. A number are present in foods rich in β-phenethylamine,

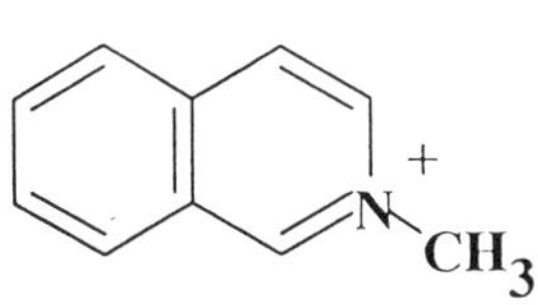

2-methylisoquinolinium

(MIQ+)

Figure 5 Quaternary isoquinolinium bearing a permanently charged nitrogen.

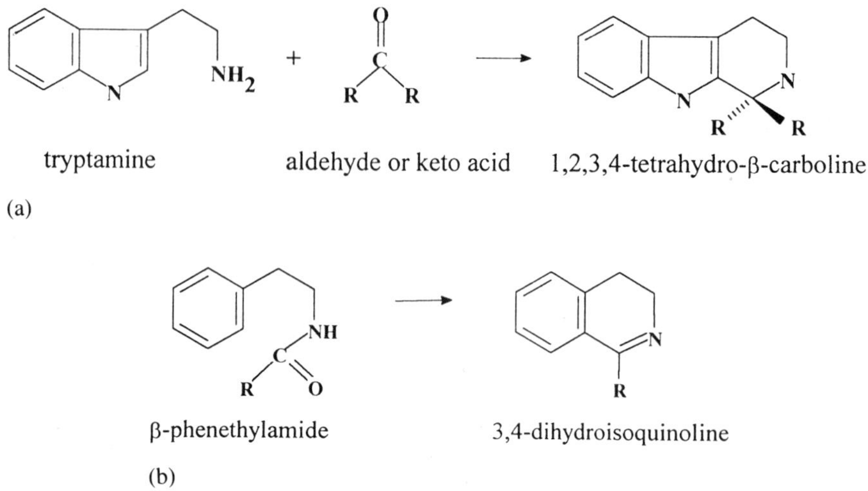

Figure 6 Possible routes for the endogenous formation of isoquinolines: (a) Pictet–Spengler condensation; (b) Bischer–Napieralski reaction.

such as cheese, wine, and cocoa (121–123). Several have been identified in various mammalian tissues, including brain (121,122,124–127).

Isoquinolines have already played a key historical role in Parkinson's research. Certain of the isoquinolines produced from the Pictet–Spengler condensation of catecholamines with aldehydes are intensely fluorescent. The exposure of tissue sections to reactive aldehydes (e.g., formaldehyde or glyoxylic acid) converts the catecholamines present in the tissue into these fluorophores. Examination of aldehyde-treated tissue using fluorescence microscopy reveals the location and distribution of the endogenous catecholamines. This phenomenon provides a chemical basis for fluorescence histochemical techniques that neuroscientists have exploited to delineate catecholaminergic pathways for the last 30 years (128–131).

Additional interest in the relation between Parkinson's disease and isoquinolines was generated by the observation of Sandler and colleagues (132) that two isoquinoline derivatives (salsolinol and tetrahydropapaverine) occur in patients taking L-dopa. This observation was subsequently expanded to include other isoquinoline metabolites as well (133). The suggestion has been made that one or more of these isoquinoline derivatives was important in either the therapeutic benefit (134) or the side effects of L-dopa therapy in the disease (135). Subsequent work has minimized the significance of these isoquinoline derivatives (136), and there is as yet no compelling evidence that isoquinoline formation during L-dopa therapy is either of benefit or detriment in the treatment of the disease.

Isoquinolines also received a great deal of attention during the late 1970s and early 1980s. Much of this interest was generated as a result of reports that exogenous alcohols, such as methanol or ethanol, enhanced the production of isoquinolines from endogenous amines (137–139). It has been speculated that because alcohols are metabolized to aldehydes, consumption of alcohol would be expected to greatly increase the precursor concentration for the Pictet–Spengler reaction. These observations heightened interest in the isoquinolines as possible factors in alcoholism and, as a result, there is a substantial literature on their chemistry, endogenous occurrence, biogenesis, and metabolism (125,140–142).

Perhaps the most intriguing suggestion that isoquinolines might represent endogenous toxins was reported by Osswald and colleagues (143). Working with condensation products of epinephrine and acetaldehyde, these investigators performed light and electron microscopic studies on adult and newborn rats injected with two of these products (143–145). Observed effects included marked alteration of nerve terminals, increased density of axoplasm, deposition of glycogen, absence of vesicles, disruption of neurotubules and mitochondrial abnormalities, and dense degeneration in the iris and heart, following two injections. These results are strikingly similar to the "chemical sympathectomy" seen after 6-hydroxydopamine administration. However, the doses used (10–50 mg/kg) were much larger than required for 6-hydroxydopamine. Furthermore, the products used in these studies were not chemically characterized or identified, and were referred to only as MA^3 and MA^4. Since that time, evidence has accumulated on several well-characterized isoquinolines; each of these are discussed in detail in the following section.

A. Salsolinol

Salsolinol represents one of the most extensively studied of the endogenously formed isoquinolines. It is thought to be formed from the condensation of pyruvate with dopamine and the successive decarboxylation and reduction of the carboxysalsolinol. The compound has been detected in tissues of rats, monkeys, and humans (146) and the simultaneous presence of salsolinol, carboxysalsolinol (147,148), as well as the 3,4-dihydroisoquinoline congener (148), all have been reported in human striata. The biosynthesis of salsolinol appears to be at least partly enzyme-mediated, since the product found in the urine of normal subjects is preponderantly a single stereoisomer (149,150).

The peripheral administration of 5–50 mg/kg of salsolinol has been reported to immediately lower brain dopamine concentrations by 15–25% in rats (151,152). Since this compound is not thought to cross the blood–brain barrier (153,154), the effects of peripherally administered salsolinol on central dopamine are puzzling. Because COMT inhibitors block this effect (152), it may be that salsolinol is converted to an *O*-methylated metabolite that crosses the blood–brain barrier and is the actual mediator of these neurochemical effects. Whether or not these effects are long-term remains to be determined. Long-term effects on striatal dopamine have not been noted, however, for the *N*-methylated analog of salsolinol in mice (155).

Prolonged administration of small amounts of salsolinol and other isoquinoline derivatives directly into the CNS by intracerebroventricular infusion does appear to produce long-lasting effects. Such infusions produce large increases in alcohol preference and consumption in models of alcohol preference. That these preference patterns are maintained in animals retested many months after discontinuation of infusion points to the possibility of long-term alterations in brain function induced by these compounds. Until there is better evidence on the effects of salsolinol, or one of its metabolites, on the dopaminergic nigrostriatal system, its role as a potential endogenous toxin will remain uncertain.

B. 2-Methyl-1,2,3,4-tetrahydroisoquinoline and 2-Methylisoquinolinium

In spite of the foregoing observations, the potential toxicity of isoquinolines did not attract much attention in the field of Parkinson's disease until the mid-1980s, when Nagatsu and colleagues (156,157), using an in situ preparation of rat striatal slices, examined the ability of MPP^+ and various quaternary analogs to inhibit tyrosine hydroxylase. Among the compounds tested in this screening system was the 2-methylisoquinolinium ion (2-MIQ^+), which exhibited activity similar to MPP^+, although it was only about one-tenth as potent. Although the ability of isoquinolines to inhibit tyrosine hydroxylase has been known for some time, the similarity of the effects of 2-MIQ^+ to MPP^+, a known parkinsongenic agent, when considered in light of the large number of known endogenous and naturally occurring isoquinolines, led this group to propose these compounds as candidate etiologic factors in Parkinson's disease. Several subsequent publications on isoquinolines have appeared, but only a handful of compounds have as yet been studied (see Fig. 7).

Rollema and colleagues (158,159) subsequently demonstrated that the 2-MIQ^+ is moderately toxic when infused through an in vivo microdialysis membrane into rat striata. Striatal infusion of 10 m*M* MIQ^+ for 150 min resulted in the characteristic massive release of dopamine and reductions of DOPAC seen after MPP^+ infusion. In addition, subsequent challenge of 2-MIQ^+-treated animals with MPP^+ 24 hr after the initial infusion failed to elicit increased dopamine release. The latter finding is interpreted as evidence of permanent damage to nigrostriatal terminals (160,161) induced by 2-MIQ^+. Although the effects of 2-MIQ^+ were similar to MPP^+ in this system, 2-MIQ^+ was again found to be less potent; the effects of MPP^+ are observed after a 15-min infusion of 10 m*M* whereas MIQ^+ required infusion for 2.5 hr. In addition, striatal terminals ap-

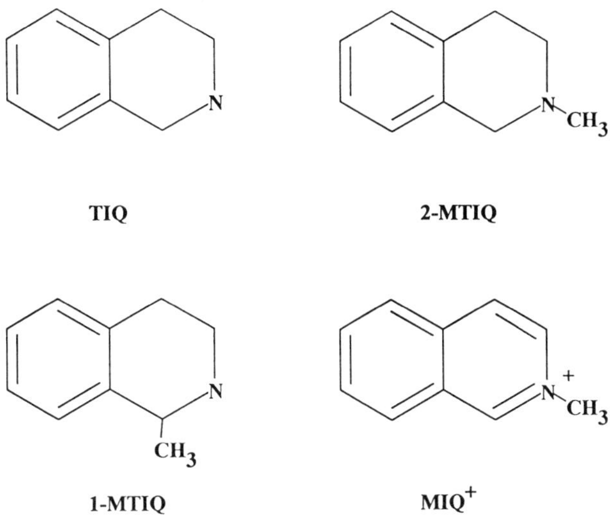

Figure 7 Isoquinolines that have been studied as possible endogenous neurotoxins involved in Parkinson's disease.

peared to be more preserved after 2-MIQ^+ than after MPP^+ infusion, since DA release on subsequent challenge was approximately ten times greater in 2-MIQ^+-lesioned animals than in MPP^+-lesioned rats.

Although these results suggest that 2-MIQ^+ is toxic to dopaminergic neurons, it is not likely to cross the blood–brain barrier and would have to be generated within the brain, possibly from a reduced precursor. In analogy with MPTP, which is biotransformed by MAO-B to MPP^+ (see chapter 13), 2-methyl-1,2,3,4-tetrahydroisoquinoline (2-MTIQ), the reduced form of 2-MIQ^+, is converted to 2-MIQ^+ in vitro, and this process is mediated by MAO (158,162). However, the rate of conversion is only about 3% of that seen with MPTP.

The next logical set of experiments would be to administer 2-MTIQ systemically to see if toxicity is observed. Indeed, such experiments have been carried out, but have yet to yield evidence that the systemic administration of this compound produces any adverse effects on the nigrostriatal system. In fact, the administration to mice of large doses of 2-MTIQ, over the course of 8 days, resulted in significant elevations of striatal dopamine (163). Perhaps even more importantly, similar studies in marmosets (164) failed to produce any behavioral, neurochemical, or neuropathological evidence of nigrostriatal damage. Although such results appear to argue against 2-MTIQ as a parkinsonogenic neurotoxin, these studies did not measure the levels of 2-MTIQ, or 2-MIQ^+, in the brain, so it is not possible to determine the extent to which it enters the brain or is converted to the isoquinolinium in vivo. Such experiments are clearly indicated before drawing a final conclusion about the potential importance of these compounds as compounds that might be important in Parkinson's disease. None of these experimental reports with MTIQ assessed the effects of long-term exposure. If small amounts of 2-MIQ$^+$ were formed in the brain over a long enough period, it still might be possible to induce degeneration of nigrostriatal neurons.

C. 1,2,3,4-Tetrahydroisoquinoline

Perhaps the most provocative studies on the isoquinolines as potential endogenous toxins come from a series of studies of 1,2,3,4-tetrahydroisoquinoline (TIQ) in primates. In 1988, Nagatsu and Yoshida reported that administration of TIQ (50 mg/kg) daily for 16 days produced parkinsonism in common marmosets (165); these behavioral changes were measured by scoring videotapes, based on 15 behavioral indices, including eating, climbing, facial expression, abnormal behaviors, and movements. The TIQ-treated animals had approximately 70% depletions of dopamine and biopterin in the substantia nigra relative to saline-injected animals. Nigral tyrosine hydroxylase activity was also reduced. In contrast with the nigral findings, only slight to moderate changes in these neurochemical parameters were observed in the striatum.

This same group later conducted a more extensive study on the effects of TIQ in squirrel monkeys (166). These studies employed lower doses (20 mg/kg) and longer drug administration times (up to 104 days). All TIQ-treated animals were reported to display significant disability and parkinsonian features. Behavioral deficits persisted up to 7 days after the last dose of TIQ and were reversed by levodopa. Neurochemical results were similar to those observed in marmosets, with marked differences between the nigra and the striatum. Dopamine, biopterin, and tyrosine hydroxylase were reduced 25–50% in the substantia nigra and normal or slightly increased in the striatum at all time points (1–7 days) after discontinuation of treatment.

The normal striatal dopamine observed in these experiments might be interpreted to suggest that TIQ treatment is not toxic and that the nigral effects were reversible, but a similar pattern of neurochemical changes (normal or increased striatal dopamine with depleted nigral dopamine) occurs during the first several days after MPTP treatment in monkeys (20), and these MPTP-treated animals go on to develop severe cell loss.

Yoshida and colleagues also reported measurements of striatal TIQ concentrations, after TIQ administration, in both marmosets (167) and squirrel monkeys (166). On the last day of a 16-day regimen, TIQ levels in marmosets were approximately 200 μg/g. Long-term TIQ treatment in squirrel monkeys resulted in levels of 3.9 ± 0.92 μg/g, 1 day after treatment. This represents nearly a 30-fold increase over the concentrations reported for control animals (0.150 μg/g). The TIQ appeared to be very persistent in monkey brain, and levels of the compound remained high (3.04 ± 1.04 μ/g), even 7 days after the last dose.

The persistence of TIQ in the brain of these TIQ-treated animals indicates the long-term retention of this agent in the CNS. Unfortunately, no TIQ measurements in other brain regions are reported. Comparative data on the levels of TIQ in the cortex or cerebellum would be useful to determine if TIQ is selectively or preferentially taken up or retained with the nigrostriatal regions. Although 2-MTIQ was identified as a metabolite in the brain of TIQ-treated marmosets (120), other potential metabolites of TIQ were not searched for. Such studies will be important if TIQ is acting as a protoxin. For example, it would be interesting to determine if TIQ or its 2-methylated metabolite (2-MTIQ) is converted to 2-MIQ$^+$ in the monkey CNS; although this conversion has been observed in vitro (119), Kikuchi and colleagues (118) were unable to detect evidence in rats of its formation in vivo. Likewise, it would be important to know if any of the other in vitro effects of TIQ, such as inhibition of mitochondrial respiration (168), are also at play in vivo.

Although these studies in primates are intriguing, definitive evidence that TIQ produces actual degeneration of nigral neurons has yet to be forthcoming. Furthermore, studies in humans have been limited and contradictory. Niwa and colleagues (124,169) reported that the concentration of TIQ in the brain of a 68-year-old woman who died of Parkinson's disease was approximately ten times higher than in an 81-year-old subject who did not have symptoms of the disease. However, Ohta and colleagues (127), in a study of four normal and four parkinsonian brains, were unable to replicate this observation. Although they found that the concentrations in the normal persons were comparable with those found in Niwa's case (about 1 ng/g), the average levels of TIQ in Parkinson's brains were approximately 50% less than in the control brain, although this difference did not reach statistical significance. No regional differences in TIQ concentrations between the frontal lobe and the caudate nucleus were noted.

One troubling issue in these studies is the apparent disparity between the levels of TIQ reported in patients compared with those in nonhuman primates. Niwa and colleagues (166,167) found concentrations of TIQ in control monkey brain in the range of 150 ng/g of tissue (see foregoing). This is more than two orders of magnitude higher than concentrations both groups found in control human brain (about 1 ng/g of tissue). It will be necessary to clarify if this tremendous discrepancy reflects rapid postmortem degradation of TIQ in autopsied human brain. Such an explanation is unlikely, however, since the levels in rodents (122,126) are more similar to the postmortem human concentrations. Thus, this disparity might reflect true differences in the normal levels of this compound in monkey and human brain, or problems in analytical methodology.

D. 1-Methyl-tetrahydroisoquinoline

In addition to TIQ, Ohta and colleagues (127) noted the appearance of another isoquinoline, 1-methyl-tetrahydroisoquinoline (1-MTIQ) in both control and Parkinson's brain. Large reductions (80–90%) of 1-MTIQ were noted in Parkinson's brain. This metabolite was lower in the caudate nucleus and frontal lobe, although these differences reached statistical significance only in the frontal lobe. These investigators also found a negative relation between age and 1-MTIQ concentrations in both the normal and parkinsonian brain. Given this decline of 1-MTIQ in aging and Parkinson's disease, these investigators proposed that this compound might serve as a marker for Parkinson's disease and aging. They further suggested that, rather than acting as an endogenous toxin, 1-MTIQ might play a protective role in the brain.

E. Implications for Parkinson's Disease

The isoquinolines are of particular interest as potential endogenous toxins, since they have been found in biological tissues of a variety of species, including rat (126), mouse (122), monkey (166,167), and postmortem human brain (124,127,169). However, as should be clear from the preceding discussion, the study of endogenous isoquinolines in normal and Parkinson-diseased brain is still in its infancy. Furthermore, there are a considerable number of experimental loose ends to be clarified. However, there is no doubt that many unexplored avenues of research relating to the study of these compounds exist. This is particularly true given that these studies have focused on such a small number of the many possible isoquinolines present in brain. Whether or not future measurements of the concentration of these compounds in postmortem tissue will provide evidence for a role of TIQ, or other isoquinolines, in Parkinson's disease, awaits additional investigation.

V. β-CARBOLINES

The next group of candidate agents, the β-carbolines, have much in common with the isoquinolines. The biogenesis of β-carbolines also involves the cyclization by the Pictet–Spenger or Bischler–Napieralski condensations. The precursor amines for the β-carbolines are indoleamines, instead of phenethylamines (Fig. 8).

Similar to the isoquinolines, β-carbolines also occur in a variety of different states of oxidation and different levels of substitution. The pyrido [*b*] ring may contain 1,2, or 3 double bonds, giving rise to tetrahydro, dihydro, or fully oxidized β-carboline. Depending on the nature of the starting tryptamine and aldehydes, various positions of the β-carboline ring may also bear substituents (e.g., methyl or other groups). The position of both saturation and substitution follows the numbering convention illustrated in Figure 9. Also, similar to the isoquinoliniums, fully oxidized β-carbolines substituted in the 2 position possess a quaternary nitrogen and bear a permanent positive charge (β-carboliniums; Fig. 10).

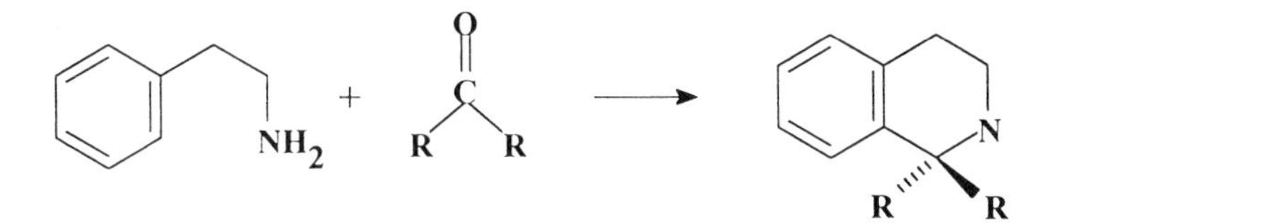

β-phenethylamine aldehyde or keto acid 1,2,3,4,-tetrahydroisoquinoline

(a)

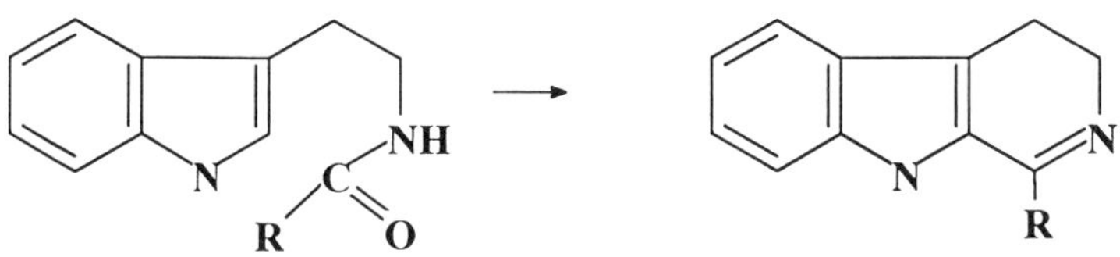

tryptamide 3,4-dihydro-β-carboline

(b)

Figure 8 Possible routes for the endogenous formation of β-carbolines: (a) Pictet–Spengler condensation; (b) Bischer–Napieralski reaction.

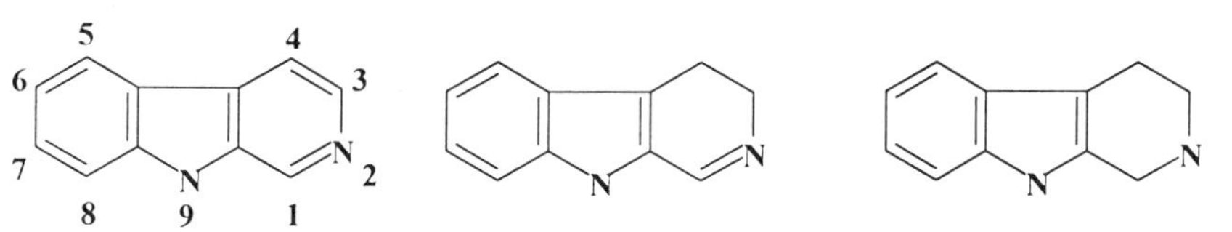

β-carboline (BC) 3,4-dihydro-β-carboline (DBC) 1,2,3,4-tetrahydro-β-carboline (TBC)

Figure 9 The simple β-carbolines, illustrating the numbering and naming conventions used for these compounds.

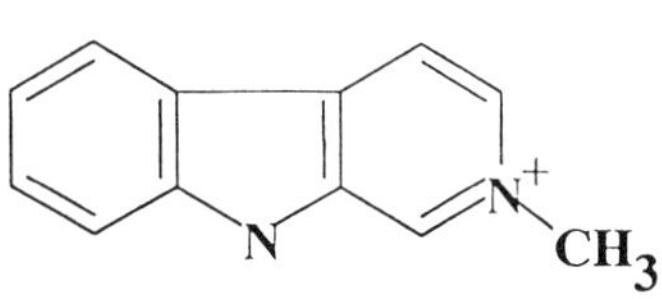

2-methyl-β-carbolinium ion

(MBC+)

Figure 10 Quaternary β-carbolinium bearing a permanently charged nitrogen.

β-Carbolines also have a historical relation to Parkinson's disease therapy. The drug harmine (1-methyl-7-methoxy-β-carboline), isolated from the seeds and stems of the plant *Peganum harmala*, was heralded in the 1920s as an especially useful drug in the treatment of the disease. Harmine was reported to improve "muscle rigor, chewing, speaking, eating and swallowing as well as movement of the arms, the capacity to walk and intellectualization of the facial expression" (170–173). For reasons that are not apparent, harmine disappeared from the clinical literature on Parkinson's disease in the mid-1930s. It is both interesting and ironic that some 60 years later, β-carbolines now attract interest as possible etiologic agents responsible for the disease.

The occurrence of many β-carbolines in animal and human tissue including brain is well documented (125,142,174–181). The concentration of these alkaloidal derivatives appears to be greater than that of isoquinolines. Although there has been some suggestion that β-carbolines might arise as a result of analytical procedures, careful deuterium-labeling experiments and gas chromatography–mass spectrometry have ruled out such artifactual formation during isolation.

The spontaneous formation of β-carbolines under "physiological conditions" has been studied by incubating various indoleamines and aldehydes or acids in buffer. A variety of β-carbolines have been shown to occur (182–186), and their spontaneous formation in these systems has been well demonstrated. Based on reports that brain homogenates appeared to enhance the formation of β-carbolines (187), an enzyme-mediated biogenesis has been suggested. Barker and colleagues (181) also argued in favor of the enzymatic synthesis of formaldehyde-derived TBCs, based on the observation that the ratios of TBC/indoleamine precursors present in the brain are orders of magnitude greater than similar ratios for TIQ/DA. Since spontaneous TIQ formation from dopamine and formaldehyde is about 100 times faster than the corresponding formation of TBC, such ratios are unlikely without some enzyme-catalyzed process. Various pathways have been postulated (177), but the definitive identity of enzymes or factors catalyzing the formation of β-carbolines in vivo remains unknown.

A. Implications for Parkinson's Disease

There is a considerable body of literature on β-carbolines, arising in part as a consequence of their potent benzodiazepine receptor activity and their possible role as anxiogenic and anxiolytic agents (125,142,177), their putative role in alcoholism (137), and their activity as MAO inhibitors (188). However, the suggestion that β-carbolines might play a possible role as endogenous toxins in Parkinson's disease arose as a consequence of the structural similarity of some of these compounds to MPTP and MPP^+ (115,159,189–192). Indeed, 2-methyl-1,2,3,4-tetrahydro-β-carboline (MTBC) and 2-methyl-β-carbolinium ion

(MBC^+) bear a striking resemblance to MPTP and MPP^+, modified only by the presence of a nitrogen bridge joining the pyridyl and benzene ring (Fig. 11).

This similarity led to the suggestion that, similarly to MPTP, tetrahydro-β-carbolines present in the brain might be converted to their fully oxidized quaternary form, and that the oxidized β-carbolinium species might exhibit properties similar to MPP^+, including uptake into dopaminergic neurons and inhibition of mitochondrial respiration. Some recent experimental studies lend support to this hypothesis.

MBC^+ has been shown to be an inhibitor of mitochondrial respiration in vitro (191,193). The ability of this compound to block mitochondrial respiration was about 1/20th that seen for MPP^+, but other β-carbolinium analogs were nearly as potent as MPP^+. Several β-carboliniums have also appeared to function as substrates for the catecholamine uptake carrier (194), although their activity is generally less than MPP^+.

Further evidence for the potential toxicity of MBC^+ comes from experiments demonstrating its ability to induce acute contralateral circling behavior, to deplete striatal dopamine, and to produce extensive nigral lesions when administered stereotactically into the SN of rats (195). These effects are similar to those seen when MPP^+ is administered by a similar route (196). The doses of MBC^+ used in these experiments were approximately 20 times as great as those required for MPP^+.

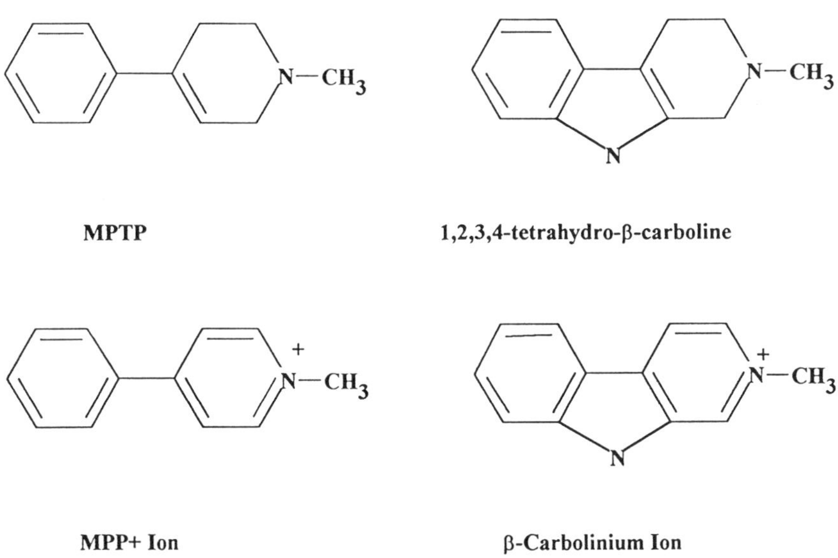

Figure 11 Chemical structures illustrating the similarity between the reduced and oxidized 2-methyl-β-carbolines and MPTP and MPP^+.

Rollema and colleagues (159,161) also demonstrated the toxicity of MBC^+ using in vivo microdialysis in rats. These investigators found that MBC^+ produced results similar to MPP^+, although longer infusion times were required for MBC^+ than for MPP^+ (10 versus 2.5 hr). Under these conditions, MBC^+ infusion into the striata produced the same immediate release of dopamine and reductions in DOPAC characteristic of MPP^+. In addition, MBC^+ and MPP^+ appeared to cause equivalent damage to nigrostriatal nerve terminals, assessed 24 hr after the infusion. Basal release of dopamine was not detectable, and basal DOPAC concentration were reduced by approximately 80%. Subsequent challenge with MPP^+ in both MBC^+-and MPP^+-perfused animals failed to produce the large dopamine release characteristic of undamaged neurons.

In contrast with the demonstrated toxic properties of MBC^+, studies with peripherally administered MTBC suggest that the tetrahydro-β-carboline is not likely to serve as a protoxin in a manner similar to MPTP. Peripheral administration of high (197) or moderate (163) doses of 2-methyl-1,2,3,4-tetrahydro-β-carboline have failed to produce depletions of striatal dopamine in mice. In owl monkeys, the administration of extremely large doses of MTBC over 20–23 days did not result in the characteristic parkinsonian features associated with MPTP (189). The only neurochemical effects observed in monkeys sacrificed after this prolonged high-dose MTBC treatment were depletions of DOPAC (-40%) and increases of serotonin (40%). No depletions in caudate dopamine were observed, nor was any evidence of cell loss present in the substantia nigra (189).

It is likely that the lack of toxicity of peripherally administered MTBC is due its poor MAO substrate properties (158). Indeed, MTBC itself may serve as an MAO inhibitor, thereby preventing its own metabolism. It is nonetheless possible that even the slow MAO-mediated oxidation of small amounts of MTBC, over a long period, could lead to the accumulation of sufficient amounts of MBC^+ to produce cell injury. Measurements of brain MBC^+ following the peripheral administration of MTBC would be helpful in evaluating the likelihood that MTBC is bioactivated in a manner similar to MPTP.

A wide variety of β-carbolines exist endogenously in the brain. No studies on their distribution in Parkinson's disease have been reported. Given the number of compounds in this family, it must be said that our current knowledge of their identity and distribution is limited. Although there is some evidence that, under certain conditions, β-carbolines can exert toxicity on the nigrostriatal system, our knowledge on the toxic properties of β-carbolines is even more limited. Whether or not the β-carboline hypothesis will flourish must await further investigation.

VI. EXCITATORY AMINO ACIDS

In spite of the great interest in excitatory amino acids (EAAs) as they relate to a variety of neurodegenerative diseases, there is as yet no experimental evidence that the administration of exogenous EAAs can produce a neuropathological picture similar to Parkinson's disease. The direct injection of kainate or *N*-methyl-D-aspartate (NMDA) agonists selectively destroys intrinsic striatal neurons with sparing of afferent (including dopaminergic) axons, thus producing a model that is more closely linked to Huntington's chorea than to Parkinson's disease.

Although there is as yet no experimental evidence that EAAs can induce direct damage to nigrostriatal dopamine neurons, they do appear to be involved in the mechanism of action of exogenous dopaminergic toxins. For example, recent reports indicate that treatment with noncompetitive NMDA receptor antagonists protect against amphetamine-induced dopamine depletions (198,199). A role for EAAs has also been proposed for the parkinsonogenic neurotoxin MPTP; however, there is still considerable controversy surrounding the experimental evidence for this (see Chapter 13).

A. Implications for Parkinson's Disease

Relative to Parkinson's disease itself, studies on various EAA markers in nigrostriatal neurons are incomplete. Although levels of excitatory amino acid transmitters have recently been reported to be reduced in the spinal fluid of parkinsonian patients, striatal glutamate levels appear to be unchanged (2,200,201).

Another approach involves the study of EAA receptors in the parkinsonian brain. Since the activation of EAA receptors is responsible for initiating EAA-mediated cell death, receptor binding studies would be expected to yield valuable information. On the one hand, if EAAs were endogenous toxins involved in Parkinson's disease, EAA receptor density in normal brain might be expected to be concentrated in areas considered the regional targets of the disease. As a corollary, one would anticipate reductions in receptor density in the disease, since target cells containing receptors would be expected to degenerate.

Studies of receptor binding of the selective NMDA noncompetitive agonist dizocilpine maleate (MK-801) in the caudate and putamen suggest that, although this region is rich in EAA receptors, there are no significant differences between Parkinson's disease and controls, despite the fact that all Parkinson's disease subjects were reported to have histopathologically confirmed Parkinson's disease and greater than 70% loss of dopamine and tyrosine hydroxylase. The failure to document a significant decline in binding in these studies indicates that the dopaminergic terminals that degenerate are not particularly rich in these receptors.

However, NMDA receptor binding in the striatum may not be the best maker for EAA toxicity, since it is possible that dopaminergic terminals may not possess these receptors. Currently, there is only a single paper in the literature on the density of EAA-binding sites in the substantia nigra. Difazio et al. (202) recently reported that, although the density of NMDA and α-ammo-3-hydroxy-5-methyl-

4-isoxazole propionic acid (AMPA) binding in the normal substantia nigra is extremely low, there is a marked reduction in receptor density in both the compacta and the reticulata in parkinsonian brain for both types of sites. Although these findings suggest the loss of EAA-positive cell bodies in Parkinson's disease, the reductions in receptor density might be explained by a variety of other causes, rather than cell death. Additional studies to confirm and clarify these results will be very important in pursuing this interesting observation.

VII. TRANSITION METALS

The final topic to be discussed in this chapter on potential endogenous toxins in Parkinson's disease is the transition metals, manganese, copper, and iron. These metal ions serve as cofactors for enzymes, are critical in many of the metabolic processes conducted by cells, and are essential for normal function. Although it might seem inappropriate to discuss such ubiquitous and obligatory cellular constituents as possible endogenous toxins, transition metals participate in redox reactions, enhancing the production of reduced oxygen species.

The capacity of transition metals to donate electrons and, thereby, promote the formation of reduced oxygen species has already been discussed in detail (see Chapter 4). Along with the emerging evidence for the involvement of oxygen-mediated damage in the degeneration seen in Parkinson's disease has come a proposed role for metals as endogenous agents responsible for the disease.

A. Manganese and Copper

There is some clinical basis to suspect copper or manganese in the disease. Environmental exposure to manganese among miners and brownstone millers has produced striatopallidal degeneration, reduction in striatal dopamine levels, and frank parkinsonism (203–206). The accumulation of high levels of copper in the basal ganglia in the genetic disorder of Wilson's disease has also been associated with parkinsonism (207).

However, these two clinical conditions each have features that are distinct from Parkinson's disease. Acute manganese poisoning presents with a marked psychiatric syndrome, which includes memory impairment, disorientation, anxiety, and hallucinations. Although chronic manganese poisoning does, indeed, induce a syndrome containing parkinsonian symptoms, dystonia is also a prominent feature. In addition, there is frequent involvement of the liver and other peripheral organs. Finally, the histopathological features of manganese intoxication, primarily involving the striatum and globus pallidus, are distinctly different from those seen in the idiopathic disease (208). Although manganese concentrations appear to be somewhat preferentially higher in the basal ganglia, there have been no demonstrated differences in the concentrations of manganese in Parkinson's disease patients versus controls (209).

In Wilson's disease, the liver bears the brunt of the copper-induced damage, and there is little evidence that Wilson's disease and Parkinson's disease share much in common. However, copper is a divalent cation, capable of participating in redox reactions, and little is known about its role in the brain. In normal brain, the substantia nigra contains the greatest amounts of this metal ion. Copper concentrations are reported to be significantly reduced (by about 30–45%) in this region in Parkinson's disease (210). In addition to these observations, however, there is little further evidence to implicate copper in Parkinson's disease. Given that little is known about the role of copper in the basal ganglia, this ion might perhaps deserve further consideration.

B. Iron

Unlike manganese or copper, the suggestion that iron might be involved in Parkinson's disease is not supported by any clinical observations in cases of iron exposure. Neither iron poisoning nor any of the known disorders of absorption, accumulation, or transport are commonly associated with neuropathological findings or symptomatology suggestive of this disease. Rather, advocates of iron generally cite the high concentrations of this metal in the basal ganglia and invoke its known participation in oxygen radical forming reactions.

1. Iron Concentrations in the Basal Ganglia

Recent data indicating increased concentrations of iron in the basal ganglia of Parkinson's disease patients have led to a focus on investigations of iron levels, and the emergence of several theories concerning its role in the disease (see Ref. 211). Most studies have focused on the levels of iron in tissue sections, whereas others have sought to identify and quantitate the subcellular localization and oxidation state of iron in Parkinson's and normal brain. There has been considerable disagreement among the various studies, however, over the results and the best techniques to assay this metal.

Earle (212), using X-ray fluorescence and studying formol-fixed brain from parkinsonian and control autopsies, noted a generalized increase in iron in parkinsonian brain. Iron was reported to be approximately twice as high in brains from Parkinson's disease patients than in controls, but no topographic differences in brain iron were reported. In addition, increased iron did not appear to be restricted to Parkinson's disease, since it was also found in Pick's disease and several other pathological conditions.

Dexter and colleagues (213) recently examined the concentration of iron and several other trace elements in tissue obtained from frozen autopsy brain, using inductively coupled plasma spectroscopy. Brains were studied from patients dying of Parkinson's disease and other neurodegenerative diseases, as well as nonneurological conditions. The normal basal ganglia was extremely rich in iron. The greatest levels were found in the substantia nigra, globus pallidus, and putamen. The levels in these areas were about two to three times as high as those found in the cerebellum or cortex. A marked and selective increase (approximately 35%) of iron in the substantia nigra and a decrease (29%) in the globus pallidus were found in Parkinson's brain. Neither the caudate nor the putamen showed differences in iron content between parkinsonian and normal brains.

Similar increases in iron in the substantia nigra were also noted in other degenerative disorders involving the basal ganglia, including progressive supranuclear palsy (PSP) and multisystem atrophy (MSA). However, in these other conditions, iron was also elevated in the caudate and putamen. Thus, increases in nigral iron appear to be generally associated with neurodegeneration involving the nigrostriatal systems. Although the case material included in this study presumably included a range of patients relative to severity and length of disease, no comment was made on the relation between these factors and iron content.

Riederer and colleagues (214), using X-ray fluorescence analysis of fresh tissue, also noted the preferential concentration of iron within the normal basal ganglia. These investigators found significant increases of iron concentration in the substantia nigra only in the most severe cases of Parkinson's disease, suggesting that changes in nigral iron might be a consequence, rather than a cause, of the disease process.

2. *Oxidation States of Iron*

The relative oxidation state of iron has also been examined and an increase in the proportion of Fe(III) has been reported (214,215) in PD. However, although the semiquantitative histological techniques employed can provide data on the oxidation states of iron, these techniques are among the least sensitive (216), and values on postmortem tissue may not reliably predict the situation in vivo. These observations have been extended, however, with the report of high-affinity binding of Fe(III) to synthetic dopamine melanin in vitro (217). Binding of $^{59}FeCl^{3}$ was not displaced by Fe(II), although Fe(III) chelators, such as desferroxamine, effectively inhibited binding, suggesting a specific binding site for this cation. Youdim and colleagues have provided an ambitious hypothesis relating all of these observations by proposing an interaction between iron, melanin, and the peroxide produced by MAO-mediated oxidation of dopamine as a possible scenario pointing to iron as an endogenous toxin in Parkinson's disease (218,219).

3. *Cellular Location of Iron*

Although increased iron concentration in the parkinsonian substantia nigra appears to be well documented by tissue analysis, the cellular and subcellular localization of iron is not established by this method. Given the known localization of iron, primarily within nonneuronal cells such as oligodendrocytes (220), increases in iron may simply reflect the increase of these nonneuronal cell types as a consequence of neurodegeneration. By using a variety of histochemical techniques, Jellinger and colleagues (221) found increased iron to be primarily localized to macrophages, astrocytes, and reactive microglia in the substantia nigra. Although iron was detected occasionally in the cytoplasm of nonpigmented neuronal cells, it was not detected in the cytoplasm of pigmented neurons (221). Nor was iron found to be associated with intraneuronal or extraneuronal melanin or with Lewy bodies, by this method. However, with the more sensitive methods of X-ray microanalysis to study the cellular distribution of iron, they found increased iron levels in neuromelanin of the substantia nigra of Parkinson's brain (222). No increases were noted in the cytoplasm of melanin-containing neurons in Parkinson's brain or in normal brain, nor was iron associated with Lewy bodies in the PD cases.

These results, however, are in contrast with those of Hirsch et al. (223), who also used X-ray microanalysis. These investigators reported that iron did not appear to vary between neuromelanin-and non–neuromelanin-containing regions of nigral cells in normal brain. In parkinsonian brain, iron was somewhat decreased (30–40%) in neuromelanin aggregates and dramatically increased (300%) in the cytoplasm of nigral neurons. No relation between these changes in iron and the severity of the disease was noted. The iron content of Lewy bodies was also even greater than the content of this metal in the nonpigmented areas. Recent data presented by Perl and Good (110), using laser microprobe mass analysis, tend to support the notion of increased iron content of neuromelanin in Parkinson's disease.

In summary, although there is considerable disagreement among the various studies on the topographic and cellular distribution of iron, the increased iron noted in the substantia nigra in Parkinson's disease calls for additional work to determine if these increases represent a causative factor, or whether they are simply the reaction and proliferation of cellular populations secondary to the degeneration in the disease.

4. *Iron-Binding Proteins: Ferritin*

Mechanisms for the binding and sequestration mechanisms for the storage, transport, and localization of metal ions have evolved to balance the requirement for metal ions against their potentially damaging effects to biological systems. Strictly speaking, any theory invoking transition metals as agents of damage must also involve a breakdown or alteration in the normal function of these mechanisms. One such mechanism is the iron-binding protein ferritin. Considerable attention has been paid to the concentration and distribution of this protein in the brain. However, there appears to be considerable disagreement here as well.

Dexter and colleagues (209,210,224), using a polyclonal antibody against human spleen ferritin, examined ferritin concentrations in parkinsonian and control brain obtained from autopsy, as well as in plasma and CSF of controls and parkinsonians. Patient levels of ferritin were significantly reduced (45–75%) in parkinsonian brain relative to controls. No significant differences were observed in the plasma or CSF. These reductions in brain ferritin were generalized and included the cerebellum, cortex, and all areas of the basal ganglia. In contrast with the levels of iron, which appear to be increased in many disorders involving the basal ganglia, such as PSP and MSA, the reductions in ferritin were specific for Parkinson's disease. They suggested that a disparity between iron binding (reduced) and iron concentrations (increased) favored elevations of "free" iron, which might enhance the formation of reduced oxygen species.

On the other hand, Jellinger and colleagues (214,221), using an immunohistochemical technique, based on an antibody raised against human liver ferritin, found a dramatic increase in the number of ferritin-positive microglia in the substantia nigra. Unfortunately, the results of these studies cannot be directly compared. The immunocytochemical studies do not yield a value for the regional ferritin concentration, and the radioimmunoassay (RIA) methodology gives no clue to the cellular location of the measured ferritin.

C. Summary

The emergence of more sensitive and accurate techniques for trace metal analysis can be expected to add greatly to our knowledge of iron content in the basal ganglia. It must also be said that our understanding of iron transport and distribution in the brain needs to be considerably expanded before the role of iron in the disease can be fully understood. Although the development of animal models of iron toxicity will accelerate this process, and have already provided some interesting preliminary results [utilizing the direct injection of iron into the brain (225,226) or the interaction of 6-OHDA and iron (227)], these too will need considerable additional study if they are to shed light on the role of iron in Parkinson's disease.

VIII. CONCLUSIONS

At the beginning of this chapter, the search for endogenous toxins that might be etiologic factors in Parkinson's disease was compared with a detective story, with the death of nigrostriatal dopaminergic neurons cast as the crime. In this review and the accompanying chapter on mechanisms of cell death in this volume (see chapter 4), an attempt has been made to survey the many suspects that might play a role in the death of dopaminergic neurons. As should be obvious by the number of compounds discussed, there is no shortage of potential offenders. Traces left behind at the site of nigral cell death, such as malondialdehyde or lipid peroxides, point to reduced oxygen species, such as superoxide and peroxide. Inhibition of mitochondrial enzymes involved in energy metabolism raise the specter of an agent that is still present, slowly robbing cells of their energy supplies. Neuromelanin continues to be an obvious place to look for clues. Perhaps this complex substance will be found to contain fragments left behind by reactive intermediates, such as dopamine quinones or aminochromes, that could be keys to solving the mystery of nigral cell death in Parkinson's disease.

Some of the chemical agents reviewed here, including neuromelanin and dopamine, have been under suspicion for decades. Although there are several problems with the hypotheses that invoke these compounds, our ignorance about even their most fundamental properties (e.g., the structure of neuromelanin, the occurrence of 6-hydroxydopamine in vivo), make it premature to rule them out as offenders. Similarly, the role of metal ions in the disease, although provocative, is poorly understood, and a great deal of additional work on their occurrence, transport, binding, reactions, and distribution is needed if we are to understand their participation in normal (let alone pathological) processes.

Although other endogenous chemicals, such as the isoquinolines and β-carbolines, have been studied for some time, they have only recently become suspect as possible etiologic agents in Parkinson's disease. Given the sophistication of our analytical techniques, it should now be possible to obtain reliable information on their status in Parkinson's disease. Such information will undoubtedly become available as research on these compounds continues.

Another important direction for future research will be to develop new and better animal models for neurodegenerative diseases. MPTP has already shown us how valuable an animal model can be, and has also provided insights into many aspects of the neurodegenerative process, including such variables as animal species, age, and route of administration, to neurotoxic outcome. Proposed endogenous agents should be subjected to the same rigorous study to determine their neurotoxic potential and relation to Parkinson's disease.

From a broader prospective, a common story among the compounds reviewed here has been for an agent (or hypotheses related to that agent) to ascend into prominence in the literature, only to disappear and reappear at later times. From a historical point of view, often the trail goes cold without an obvious reason. It is no doubt true that scientific frontiers often open and close with the availability of new instrumentation and technology. Such advances are likely to propel research forward in many of the areas discussed in this chapter. However, when it comes to the study of chronic neurodegenerative disease, it may be necessary for scientists studying these disorders to lengthen their attention span if definitive answers are to be obtained to many of these questions. If we bear in mind that the development of Parkinson's disease most likely occurs over the course of many years, it would do well to consider long-term animal studies with these agents before they are abandoned. Ultimately, new biomarkers for neuronal injury are likely to add support for one or more of the toxic mechanisms described in this chapter, or to provide evidence for other mechanisms, such as apoptosis or alterations in intracellular calcium. In our opinion, the field of neurotoxicology is likely to provide fertile ground for years to come in the search for endogenous or environmental agents that may lie at the heart of Parkinson's disease.

ACKNOWLEDGMENTS

The authors wish to thank Ms Wendy Bogart and Marina Fridlib for their assistance with the figures for this chapter, and David Rosner for his assistance in preparing the chapter. We would also like to thank Drs. Donato Di Monte, Martha Sandy, and Piu Chan for their reading and helpful comments.

REFERENCES

1. Bernheimer H, Birkmayer W, Hornykiewicz O, Jellinger K, Seitelberger F. Brain dopamine and the syndromes of Parkinson and Huntington. J Neurol Sci 1973; 20:415–455.
2. Agid Y, Cervera P, Hirsch E, et al. Biochemistry of Parkinson's disease 28 years later: a critical review. Mov Disord 1989; 4:S126–S144.
3. Cohen G. The pathophysiology of Parkinson's disease: biochemical aspects of dopamine neuron senescence. J Neural Transm 1983; 19:89–103.
4. Spina MB, Cohen G. Dopamine turnover and glutathione oxidation: implications for Parkinson disease. Proc Natl Acad Sci USA 1989; 86:1398–1400.
5. Werner P, Cohen G. Intramitochondrial formation of oxidized glutathione during the oxidation of benzylamine by monoamine oxidase. FEBS Lett 1991; 280:44–46.
6. Carlsson A, Winblad B. Influence of age and time interval between death and autopsy on dopamine and 3-methoxytryamine levels in human basal ganglia. J Neural Transm 1976; 38:271–276.
7. Hornykiewicz O. Dopamine changes in the aging human brain: functional considerations. In: Agnoli A, ed. Aging: aging brain and ergot alkaloids. New York: Raven Press, 1983:9–13.
8. McGeer PL, McGeer EG, Suzuki JS. Aging and extrapyramidal function. Neurology 1977; 34:33–35.
9. Robinson DS, Davis JM, Nies A, Ravaris CL, Sylwester D. Relation of sex and aging to monoamine oxidase activity of human brain, plasma, and platelets. Arch Gen Psychiatry 1971; 24:536–539.
10. Fowler CJ, Wilberg A, Oreland L, Marcusson J, Winblad B. The effect of age on the activity and molecular properties of human brain monoamine oxidase. J Neural Transm 1980; 49:1–20.
11. Hornykiewicz O. The mechanisms of action of L-dopa in Parkinson's disease. Life Sci 1974; 15:1249–1259.
12. Quinn NP, Parkes D, Janota I, Marsden CD. Preservation of the substantia nigra and locus ceruleus in a patient receiving levodopa (2 kg) plus decarboxylase inhibitor over a four-year period. Mov Disord 1986; 1:65–68.

13. Lesser RP, Fahn S, Snider SR, Cote LJ, Isgreen WP, Barrett RE. Analysis of the clinical problems in parkinsonism and the complications of long-term therapy. Neurology 1979; 29:1253–1260.
14. Langston JW, Ballard PA. Parkinsonism induced by 1-methyl-4-phenyl-1,2,5,6-tetrahydropyridine: implications for treatment and the pathophysiology of Parkinson's disease. Can J Neurol Sci 1984; 11:160–165.
15. Ballard PA, Tetrud JW, Langston JW. Permanent human parkinsonism due to 1-methyl-4-phenyl-1,2,3,6-tetrahydropyridine (MPTP): seven cases. Neurology 1985; 35:949–956.
16. Hoehn MM. Parkinsonism treated with levodopa: progression and mortality. J Neural Transm [Suppl] 1983; 19:253–264.
17. Markham CH, Diamond SG. Long-term follow-up of early dopa treatment in Parkinson's disease. Ann Neurol 1986; 19:365–372.
18. Blin J, Bonnet AM, Agid Y. Does levodopa aggravate Parkinson's disease. Neurology 1988; 38:1410–1416.
19. Blin J, Bonnet AM, Agid Y. Does levodopa aggravate Parkinson's disease. In: Fahn S, Marsden CD, Goldstein M, Calne DB, eds. Recent developments in Parkinson's disease, vol 2. Florham Park, NJ: Macmillan Healthcare Information, 1987:165–181.
20. Irwin I, DeLanney LE, Forno LS, Finnegan KT, Di Monte DA, Langston JW. The evolution of nigrostriatal neurochemical changes in the MPTP-treated squirrel monkey. Brain Res 1990; 531:242–252.
21. Zigmond MJ, Hastings TG. Neurochemical responses to 6-hydroxydopamine and L-dopa therapy: implications for Parkinson's disease. Ann NY Acad Sci 1992; 648:71–86.
22. Ricaurte GA, Langston JW, DeLanney LE, Irwin I, Peroutka SJ, Forno LS. Fate of nigrostriatal neurons in young mature mice given 1-methyl-4-phenyl-1,2,3,6,-tetrahydropyridine: a neurochemical and morphological reassessment. Brain Res 1986; 376:117–124.
23. Irwin I, DeLanney LE, Langston JW. MPTP and aging: studies in the C57BL/6 mouse. In: Narabayashi H, Nagatsu T, Yanagisawa N, Mizuno Y, eds. Parkinson's disease: from basic research to treatment. Proceedings of the 10th international symposium on Parkinson's disease. Adv Neurol 1992; 60:197–206.
24. Hefti F, Melamed E, Bhawan J, Wurtman RJ. Long-term administration of L-dopa does not damage dopaminergic neurons in the mouse. Neurology 1981; 31:1194–1195.
25. Perry TL, Yong VW, Ito M. Nigrostriatal dopaminergic neurons remain undamaged in rats given high doses of L-dopa and carbidopa chronically. J Neurochem 1984; 43:990–993.
26. Cotzias GC, Miller ST, Tang LC, Papavasiliou PS. Levodopa, fertility, and longevity. Science 1977; 200:549–551.
27. Papavasiliou PS, Miller ST, Thal LJ. Age-related motor and catecholamine alterations in mice on levodopa supplemented diet. Life Sci 1981; 28:2945–2952.
28. Blunt SB, Jenner P, Marsden CD. The effect of chronic L-DOPA treatment on the recovery of motor function in 6-hydroxydopamine-lesioned rats receiving ventral mesencephalic grafts. Neuroscience 1991; 40:453–464.

29. Steece-Collier K, Collier TJ, Sladek CD, Sladek JRJ. Chronic levodopa impairs morphological development of grafted embryonic dopamine neurons. Exp Neurol 1990; 110:201–208.
30. Tetrud JW, Langston JW. The effect of Deprenyl (selegiline) on the natural history of Parkinson's disease. Science 1989; 245:519–522.
31. The Parkinson Study Group. Effect of Deprenyl on the progression of disability in early Parkinson's disease. N Engl J Med 1989; 321:1364–1371.
32. Myllyla VV, Sotaniemi KA, Vuorinen JA, Heinonen EH. Selegiline as initial treatment in de novo parkinsonian patients. Neurology 1992; 42:339–343.
33. Elizan TS, Yahr MD, Moros DA, Mendoza MR, Pang S, Bodian CA. Selegiline use to prevent progression of Parkinson's disease: experience in 22 de novo patients. Arch Neurol 1989; 46:1275–1279.
34. Knoll J. Extension of life span of rats by long-term (-)Deprenyl treatment. Mt Sinai J Med 1988; 55:67–74.
35. Lichter D, Kurlan R, Miller C, Shoulson I. Does pergolide slow the progression of Parkinson's disease? A 7-year follow-up study [abstract]. Neurology 1988; 38:122.
36. Zimmerman T, Sage JI. Long-term pergolide treatment and progression of Parkinson's disease. Neurology 1989; 39:200.
37. Zimmerman T, Sage JI. Comparison of combination pergolide and levodopa to levodopa alone after 63 months of treatment. Clin Neuropharmacol 1991; 14:165–169.
38. Felten DL, Felten SY, Fuller RW. Chronic dietary pergolide preserves nigrostriatal neuronal integrity in aged-Fischer-344 rats. Neurobiol Aging 1992; 13:339–351.
39. Felten DL, Felten SY, Steece-Collier K, Date I, Clemens JA. Age-related decline in the dopaminergic nigrostriatal system: the oxidative hypothesis and protective strategies. Ann Neurol 1992; 32 (suppl): S133–S136.
40. Bird ED, Iversen LL. Huntington's chorea. Post-mortem measurement of glutamic acid decarboxylase, choline acetyltransferase and dopamine in basal ganglia. Brain 1974; 97:457–472.
41. Mackay AVP, Iversen LL, Rossor M. Increased brain dopamine and dopamine receptors in schizophrenia. Arch Gen Psychiatry 1982; 39:991–997.
42. Robinson DS, Sourkes TL, Nies A. Monoamine metabolism in human brain. Arch Gen Psychiatry 1977; 34:89–92.
43. Martin WRW, Palmer MR, Patlak CS, Calne DB. Nigrostriatal function in humans studied with positron emission tomography. Ann Neurol 1989; 26:535–542.
44. Sawle GV, Colebatch JG, Shah A, Brooks DJ, Marsden CD, Frackowiak RS. Striatal function in normal aging: implications for Parkinson's disease. Ann Neurol 1990; 28:799–804.
45. Calne DB, Calne JS. Normality and disease. Can J Neurol Sci 1988; 15:3–4.
46. Irwin I, Finnegan KT, DeLanney LE, Di Monte D, Langston JW. The relationships between aging, monoamine oxidase, striatal dopamine and the effects of MPTP in C57BL/6 mice: a critical reassessment. Brain Res 1992; 572:224–231.
47. McNeill TH, Koek LL. Differential effects of advancing age on neurotransmitter cell loss in the substantia nigra and striatum of C57BL/6N mice. Brain Res 1990; 521:107–117.

48. Tse DCS, McCreery R, Adams RN. Potential oxidative pathways of brain catecholamines. J Med Chem 1976; 19:37–40.
49. Fridovich I. Oxygen free radicals and tissue damage. Amsterdam: Excerpta Medica, 1979.
50. Graham DG. Oxidative pathways for catecholamines in the genesis of neuromelanin and cytotoxic quinones. Mol Pharmacol 1978; 14:633–643.
51. Graham DG, Tiffany SM, Bell WRJ, Gutknecht WF. Autoxidation versus covalent binding of quinones as the mechanism of toxicity of dopamine, 6-hydroxydopamine, and related compounds toward C1300 neuroblastoma cells in vitro. Mol Pharmacol 1978; 14:644–653.
52. Van Woert MH, Prasad KN, Borg DC. Spectroscopic studies of substantia nigra pigment in human subjects. J Neurochem 1967; 14:707–716.
53. Carstam R, Brinck C, Hindemith-Augustsson A, Rorsman H, Rosengren E. The neuromelanin of the human substantia nigra. Biochim Biophys Acta 1991; 1097:152–160.
54. Fornstedt B, Rosengren E, Carlsson A. Occurrence and distribution of 5-*S*-cysteinyl derivatives of dopamine, dopa and DOPAC in the brains of eight mammalian species. Neuropharmacology 1986; 25:451–454.
55. Rosengren E, Linder-Eliasson E, Carlsson A. Detection of 5-S-cysteinyl-DA in human brain. J Neural Transm 1985; 63:247–253.
56. Heacock RA, Powell BS. Adrenochrome and related compounds. In: Ellis GP, West GB, eds. Progress in medicinal chemistry 9. Amsterdam: North-Holland Publishing, 1973:275–339.
57. Bindoli A, Rigobello MP, Galzigna L. Toxicity of aminochromes. Toxicol Lett 1989; 48:3–20.
58. Pileblad E, Slivka A, Bratvold D, Cohen G. Studies on the autoxidation of dopamine: interaction with ascorbate. Arch Biochem Biophys 1988; 263:447–452.
59. Powell W, Heacock RA, Mattock GL, Wilson DL. Chemistry of the aminochromes. X. Some further observations on the reactions of aminochromes with thiols. Can J Chem 1969; 47:467–476.
60. Powell W, Heacock RA. Chemistry of the aminochromes. XVII. Formation of addition products with bisulphite and thiols. J Chem Soc 1973; 509–515.
61. Mattock GL. Reactions of adrenochrome with some thiols. Arch Biochem Biophys 1967; 120:170–174.
62. Mattock GL, Heacock RA. The chemistry of aminochromes. VI. The reaction of adrenochrome with glutathione. Can J Chem 1965; 43:119–125.
63. Heacock RA. The chemistry of adrenochrome and related compounds. Chem Rev 1959; 59:181–237.
64. Heacock RA, Mattock GL. The reaction of adrenochrome with glutathione. Arch Biochem Biophys 1964; 107:352–353.
65. Van der Wende C, Spoerlein MT. Oxidation of dopamine to melanin by an enzyme of rat brain. Life Sci 1963; 6:386–392.
66. Rodgers AD, Curzon G. Melanin formation by human brain in vitro. J Neurochem 1975; 24:1123–1129.
67. Sealy RC, Felix CC, Hyde JS, Swartz HM. Structure and reactivity of melanins:

influence of free radicals and metal ions. In: Pryor W, ed. Free radicals in biology, vol 4. New York: Academic Press, 1980:209–259.
68. Kostrzewa RM, Jacobowitz DM. Pharmacological actions of 6-hydroxydopamine. Pharmacol Rev 1974; 26:199–288.
69. Senoh S, Creveling CR, Udenfriend S, Witkop B. Chemical, enzymatic and metabolic studies on the mechanism of oxidation of dopamine. J Am Chem Soc 1959; 81:6236–6240.
70. Ungerstedt U. 6-Hydroxy-dopamine induced degeneration of central monoamine neurons. Eur J Pharmacol 1968; 5:107–110.
71. Sternson AW, McCreery R, Feinberg B, Adams RN. Electrochemical studies of adrenergic neurotransmitters and related compounds. Electroanal Chem Interfac Electrochem 1973; 46:313–321.
72. Slivka A, Cohen G. Hydroxyl attack on dopamine. J Biol Chem 1985; 260:15466–15472.
73. Liang YO, Plotsky PM, Adams RN. Isolation and identification of an in vivo reaction product of 6-hydroxydopamine. J Med Chem 1977; 20:581–583.
74. Seiden LS, Fischman MW, Schuster CR. Long-term methamphetamine-induced changes in brain catecholamines in tolerant rhesus monkeys. Drug Alcohol Depend 1975; 1:215–219.
75. Wagner GC, Ricaurte GA, Seiden LS, Schuster CR, Miller RJ, Westley J. Long-lasting depletion of striatal dopamine and loss of dopamine uptake sites following repeated administration of methamphetamine. Brain Res 1980; 181:151–160.
76. Ellison G, Eison MS, Huberman HS, Daniel F. Long-term changes in dopaminergic innervation of caudate nucleus after continuous amphetamine administration. Science 1978; 201:276–278.
77. Fuller RW, Hemrick-Luecke SK. Inability of monoamine oxidase inhibitors to prevent the persistent depletion of striatal dopamine by amphetamine in rats. Res Commun Subst Abuse 1984; 5:247–252.
78. Seiden LS, Vosmer G. Formation of 6-hydroxydopamine in caudate nucleus of the rat brain after a single large dose of methylamphetamine. Pharmacol Biochem Behav 1984; 21:29–31.
79. Axt KJ, Commins DL, Vosmer G, Seiden LS. α-Methyl-*p*-tyrosine pretreatment partially prevents methamphetamine-induced endogenous neurotoxin formation. Brain Res 1990; 515:269–276.
80. Marek GJ, Vosmer G, Seiden LS. The effects of monoamine uptake inhibitors and methamphetamine on neostriatal 6-hydroxydopamine (6-OHDA) formation, short-term monoamine depletions and locomotor activity in the rat. Brain Res 1990; 516:1–7.
81. Marek GJ, Vosmer G, Seiden LS. Pargyline increases 6-hydroxydopamine levels in the neostriatum of methamphetamine-treated rats. Pharmacol Biochem Behav 1990; 36:187–190.
82. Rollema H, De Vries JB, Westerink BHC, Van Putten FMS, Horn AS. Failure to detect 6-hydroxydopamine in rat striatum after the dopamine releasing drugs dexamphetamine, methylamphetamine and MPTP. Eur J Pharmacol 1986; 132:65–69.

83. Bogerts B. A brainstem atlas of catecholaminergic neurons in man, using melanin as a natural marker. J Comp Neurol 1981; 197:63–80.
84. Graham DG. On the origin and significance of neuromelanin. Arch Pathol Lab Med 1979; 103:359–362.
85. Mann DMA, Yates PO. Lipoprotein pigments—their relationship to ageing in the human nervous system—II. The melanin content of pigmented nerve cells. Brain 1974; 97:489–498.
86. Marsden CD. Neuromelanin and Parkinson's disease. J Neural Transm [Suppl] 1983; 19:121–141.
87. Shoffner JM, Watts RL, Juncos JL, Torroni A, Wallace DC. Mitochondrial oxidative phosphorylation defects in Parkinson's disease. Ann Neurol 1991; 30:332–339.
88. Barden H. Relationship of Golgi thiaminepyrophosphatase and lyososomal acid phosphatase to neuromelanin and lipofuscin in cerebral neurons of the aging rhesus monkey. J Neuropathol Exp Neurol 1970; 29:225–240.
89. Mann DMA, Yates PO, Barton CM. Neuromelanin and RNA in cells of substantia nigra. J Neuropathol Exp Neurol 1977; 36:379–383.
90. Mann DMA, Yates PO. Possible role of neuromelanin in the pathogenesis of Parkinson's disease. Mech Age Dev 1983; 21:193–203.
91. Hirsch EC, Graybiel AM, Agid Y. Selective vulnerability of pigmented dopaminergic neurons in Parkinson's disease. Acta Neurol Scand [Suppl] 1989; 126:19–22.
92. Gibb WRG, Fearnley JM, Lees AJ. The anatomy and pigmentation of the human substantia nigra in relation to selective neuronal vulnerability. In: Streifler MB, Korczyn AD, Melamed E, Youdim MBH, eds. Parkinson's disease: anatomy, pathology and therapy. Adv Neurol 1990; 53:31–34.
93. Miller DM, Buettner GR, Aust SD. Transition metals as catalysts of auto-oxidation reactions. Free Radical Biol Med 1990; 8:95–108.
94. Felix CC, Hyde JS, Sarna T, Sealy RC. Melanin photoreactions in aereated media: electron spin resonance evidence for production of superoxide and hydrogen peroxide. Biochem Biophys Res Commun 1978; 84:335–341.
95. Pilas B, Sarna T, Kalyanaraman B, Swartz HM. The effect of melanin on iron associated decomposition of hydrogen peroxide. Free Radical Biol Med 1988; 4:285–293.
96. Korytowski W, Hintz P, Sealy RC, Kalyanaraman B. Mechanism of dismutation of superoxide produced during auto-oxidation of melanin pigments. Biochem Biophys Res Commun 1985; 131:659–665.
97. Sarna T, Duleba A, Korytowksi W, Swartz HM. Interaction of melanin with oxygen. Arch Biochem Biophys 1980; 200:140–148.
98. Lyden A, Bondesson U, Larsson BS, Lindquist NG. Melanin affinity of 1-methyl-4-phenyl-1,2,3,6-tetrahydropyridine, and inducer of chronic parkinsonism in humans. Acta Pharmacol 1983; 53:429–432.
99. Irwin I, Langston JW. Selective accumulation of MPP^+ in the substantia nigra: a key to neurotoxicity? Life Sci 1985; 36:207–212.
100. Wu EY, Chiba K, Trevor AJ, Castagnoli N Jr. Interactions of the 1-methyl-4-phenyl-2,3-dihydrophyridinium species with synthetic dopamine–melanin. Life Sci 1986; 39:1695–1700.

101. Melamed E, Soffer D, Rosenthal J, Reches A, Pikarski E. Effect of intrastriatal and intranigral administration of synthetic neuromelanin on the dopaminergic neurotoxicity of MPTP in rodents. Neurosci Lett 1987; 83:41–46.
102. D'Amato RJ, Lipman ZP, Snyder SH. Selectivity of the parkinsonian neurotoxin MPTP: toxic metabolite MPP^+ binds to neuromelanin. Science 1986; 231:987–989.
103. D'Amato RJ, Benham DF, Snyder SH. Characterization of the binding of *N*-methyl-4-phenylpyridine, the toxic metabolite of the parkinsonian neurotoxin *N*-methyl-4-phenyl-1,2,3,6-tetrahydropyridine, to neuromelanin. J Neurochem 1987; 48:653–658.
104. D'Amato RJ, Alexander GM, Schwartzman RJ, Kitt CA, Price DL, Snyder SH. Evidence for neuromelanin involvement in MPTP-induced neurotoxicity. Nature 1987; 327:324–326.
105. Lindquist NG, Larsson BS, Lyden-Sokolowski A. Neuromelanin and its possible protective and destructive properties. Pigment Cell Res 1987; 1:133–136.
106. Swartz HM, Sarna T, Zecca L. Modulation by neuromelanin of the availability and reactivity of metal ions. Ann Neurol 1992; 32 (suppl):S69–S75.
107. Van Woert MH. DPNH oxidation by melanin: inhibition by phenothiazines. Proc Soc Exp Biol Med 1968; 129:165–171.
108. Gan EV, Haberman HF, Menon IA. Electron transfer properties of melanin. Arch Biochem Biophys 1976; 173:666–672.
109. Gan EV, Lam KM, Haberman HF, Menon IA. Oxidizing and reducing properties of melanins. Br J Dermatol 1977; 96:25–28.
110. Perl DP, Good PF. Comparative techniques for determining cellular iron distribution in brain tissues. Ann Neurol 1992; 32:S76–S81.
111. Lavoie B, Parent A. Immunohistochemical study of the serotoninergic innervation of the basal ganglia in the squirrel monkey. J Comp Neurol 1990; 299:1–16.
112. Steinbusch HWM. Serotonin-immunoreactive neurons and their projections in the CNS. In: Bjorklund A, Hokfelt T, Kuhar MJ, eds. Handbook of clinical neuroanatomy, vol 3: classical transmitters and transmitter receptors in the CNS, part II. Amsterdam: Elsevier Science Publishers, 1984:68–125.
113. Ramsden DB, Williams AC. Production in nature of compound resembling methylphenyltetrahydropyridine, a possible cause of Parkinson's disease. Lancet 1985; 1:215–216.
114. Fellman JH, Nutt JN. MPTP-like molecules and Parkinson's disease. Lancet 1985; 1:924.
115. Ohkubo S, Hiraro T, Oka K. Methyltetrahydro-beta-carbolines and Parkinson's disease. Lancet 1985; 1:1272–1273.
116. Creveling CR, Morris N, Shimizu H, Ong HH, Daly J. Catechol-*O*-methyltransferase. Mol Pharmacol 1972; 8:398-403.
117. Ohta S, Tachikawa O, Makino Y, Tasaki Y, Hirobe M. Metabolism and brain accumulation of tetrahydroisoquinoline (TIQ): a possible parkinsonism inducing substance, in an animal model of a poor debrisoquine metabolizer. Life Sci 1990; 46:599–605.
118. Kikuchi K, Nagatsu Y, Makino Y, Mashino T, Ohta S, Hirobe M. Metabolism

and penetration through blood–brain barrier of parkinsonism-related compounds: 1,2,3,4-tetrahydroisoquinoline and 1-methyl-1,2,3,4-tetrahydroisoquinoline. Drug Metab Dispos 1991; 19:257–262.

119. Naoi M, Matsuura S, Takahashi T, Nagatsu T. A *N*-methyltransferase in human brain catalyses *N*-methylation of 1,2,3,4-tetrahydroisoquinoline into *N*-methyl-1,2,3,4-tetrahydroisoquinoline, a precursor of a dopaminergic neeurotoxin, *N*-methylisoquinolinium ion. Biochem Biophys Res Commun 1989; 161:1213–1219.

120. Niwa T, Yoshizumi H, Tatematsu A. Endogenous synthesis of *N*-methyl-1,2,3,4-tetrahydroisoquinoline, a precursor of *N*-methylisoquinolinium ion, in the brains of primates with parkinsonism after systemic administration of 1,2,3,4-tetrahydroisoquinoline. J Chromatogr Biomed Appl 1990; 533:145–151.

121. Niwa T, Yoshizumi H, Takeda N, Tatematsu A, Matsuura S, Nagatsu T. Detection of tetrahydroisoquinoline, a parkinsonism-related compound, in parkinsonian brains and foods by gas chromatography–mass spectrometry. In: Nagatsu T, Fisher A, Yoshida M, eds. Basic, clinical, and therapeutic aspects of Alzheimer's and Parkinson's diseases, vol 1. New York: Plenum Press, 1990:313–316.

122. Makino Y, Tasaki Y, Ohta S, Hirobe M. Confirmation of the enantiomers of 1-methyl-1,2,3,4-tetrahydroisoquinoline in the mouse brain and foods applying gas chromatography/mass spectrometry with negative ion chemical ionization. Biomed Environ Mass Spectrom 1990; 19:415–419.

123. Makino Y, Ohta S, Tachikawa O, Hirobe M. Presence of tetrahydroisoquinoline and 1-methyl-tetrahydro-isoquinoline in foods: compounds related to Parkinson's disease. Life Sci 1988; 43:373–378.

124. Niwa T, Takeda N, Kaneda N, Hashizume Y, Nagatsu T. Presence of tetrahydroisoquinoline and 2-methyl-tetrahydroquinoline in parkinsonian and normal human brains. Biochem Biophys Res Commun 1987; 144:1084–1089.

125. Melchior C, Collins MA. The route and significance of endogenous synthesis of alkaloids in animals. Crit Rev Toxicol 1982; 9:313–354.

126. Kohno M, Ohta S, Hirobe M. Tetrahydroisoquinoline and 1-methyl-tetrahydroisoquinoline as novel endogenous amines in rat brain. Biochem Biophys Res Commun 1986; 140:448–454.

127. Ohta S, Kohno M, Makino Y, Tachikawa O, Hirobe M. Tetrahydroisoquinoline and 1-methyl-tetrahydroisoquinoline are present in the human brain: relation to Parkinson's disease. Biomed Res 1987; 8:453–456.

128. Falck G, Hillarp NA, Thieme G, Torp A. Fluorescence of catecholamines and related compounds condensed with formaldehyde. J Histochem Cytochem 1962; 10:348–354.

129. Corrodi H, Hillarp NA. Fluoreszenzmethoden zur histochemischen sichtbarmachung von Monoaminen. 2. Identifizierung des fluoreszierenden Produktes aus Dopamin und Formaldehyd. Helv Chim Acta 1964; 47:911–918.

130. Corrodi H, Hillarp NA. Fluoreszenzmethoden zur histochemischen sichtbarmachung von Monoaminen. I. Identifizierung fluoreszierenden Produkte aus modellversuchen mit 6,7-Dimethoxyisochinolinderivaten und Formaldehyd. Helv Chim Acta 1963; 46:2425–2430.

131. Bjorklund A. Fluorescence histochemistry of biogenic monoamines. In: Bjorklund

A, Hokfelt T, eds. Handbook of chemical neuroanatomy, vol 1: methods in chemical neuroanatomy. Amsterdam: Elsevier Science Publishers, 1983:50–121.

132. Sandler M, Carter SB, Hunter KR, Stern GM. Tetrahydroisoquinoline alkaloids: in vivo metabolites of L-dopa in man. Nature 1973; 241:439–443.
133. Coscia CJ, Burke W, Jamroz G. Occurrence of a new class of tetrahydroisoquinoline alkaloids in L-dopa-treated parkinsonian patients. Nature 1977; 269:617–619.
134. Sourkes TL. Possible new metabolites mediating actions of L-dopa. Nature 1971; 229:413–414.
135. Dougan D, Wade D, Mearrick P. Effects of L-dopa metabolites at a dopamine receptor suggest a basis for "on–off" effect in Parkinson's disease. Nature 1975; 254:70–72.
136. Hornykiewicz O. Parkinson's disease: from brain homogenate to treatment. Fed Proc 1973; 32:183–190.
137. Cohen G, Collins MA. Alkaloids from catecholamines in adrenal tissue: possible role in alcoholism. Science 1970; 167:1749–1751.
138. Davis VE, Walsh MJ. Alcohol, amines, and alkaloids: a possible biochemical basis for alcohol addiction. Science 1970; 167:1005–1007.
139. Hamilton MG, Blum K, Hirst M. Identification of an isoquinoline alkaloid after chronic exposure to ethanol. Alcohol Clin Exp Res 1978; 2:133–137.
140. Deitrich R, Erwin V. Biogenic amine–aldehyde condensation products: tetrahydroisoquinolines and tryptolines (beta-carbolines). Annu Rev Pharmacol Toxicol 1980; 20:55–80.
141. beta-Carbolines and tetrahydroisoquinolines—proceedings of a workshop held at the Salk Institute, La Jolla, California, Dec 12 and 13, 1981. Prog Clin Biol Res 1982; 90:1–490.
142. Rommelspacher H, Susilo R. Tetrahydroisoquinolines and beta-carbolines: putative natural substances in plants and animals. In: Jucker E, ed. Prog Drug Res 1985; 29:415–459.
143. Osswald W, Polonia J, Polonia MA. Preparation and pharmacological activity of the condensation product of adrenaline with acetaldehyde. Arch Pharmacol 1975; 275:290.
144. Osswald W, Azevedo I. Chemical sympathectomy due to tetrahydroisoquinolines derived from adrenaline. In: Begleiter H, ed. Biological effects of alcohol. New York: Plenum Press, 1980:131–146.
145. Azevedo I, Osswald W. Adrenergic nerve degeneration induced by condensation products of adrenaline and acetaldehyde. Arch Pharmacol 1977; 300:139–144.
146. Collins MA. Acetaldehyde and its condensation products as markers in alcoholism. In: Galanter M, ed. Recent developments in alcoholism, vol 6. New York: Plenum Press, 1988:387–403.
147. Sjoquist B, Magnusson E. Analysis of salsolinol and salsoline in biological samples using deuterium-labelled standards and gas chromatography/mass spectrometry. J Chromatogr 1980; 183:17–22.
148. Ung-Chhun N, Cheng BY, Pronger DA. Alkaloid adducts in human brain: coexistence of 1-carboxylated and noncarboxylated isoquinoline and beta carbolines in alcoholics and nonalcoholics. In: Collins MA, ed. Adducts in alcoholism. New York: Alan R. Liss, 1985:125–136.

149. Dostert P, Benedetti MS, Dedieu M. Ratio of enantiomers of salsolinol in human urine. Pharmacol Toxicol 1987; 60 (suppl 1):13.
150. Benedetti MS, Dostert P, Dedieu M. Ratio of enantiomers of salsolinol in human urine and effect of food [abstract]. 15th CINP congress, Puerto Rico, 12/14–17, book of abstracts 1986:56.
151. Collins MA, Weiner CD. Studies on the effects of tetrahydroisoquinoline derivatives of catecholamines and aldehydes on tyrosine hydroxylase. In: Thurman R, Williamson J, Drott H, eds. Alcohol and aldehyde metabolizing systems III. New York: Academic Press, 1977:511–526.
152. Collins MA, Hannigan JJ, Weiner C. Effects of catecholic tetrahydroisoquinolines on endogenous catecholamines. In: Galanter M, ed. Currents in alcholism, vol V. Biomedical issues and clinical effects of alcholism. New York: Grune & Stratton, 1979:53–59.
153. Reden J, Ripka WC, Rice KC, Brossi A. 4-Hydroxy-1,2,3,4-tetrahydroisoquinolines: potential reaction products of norepinephrine. In: Begleiter H, ed. Biological effects of ethanol. New York: Plenum Press, 1980:69–84.
154. Origitano T, Hannigan J, Collins MA. Rat brain salsolinol and blood–brain barrier. Brain Res 1981; 224:446–451.
155. Perry TL, Yong VW, Clavier RM, et al. Partial protection from the dopaminergic neurotoxin *N*-methyl-4-phenyl-1,2,3,6-tetrahydropyridine by four different antioxidants in the mouse. Neurosci Lett 1985; 60:109–114.
156. Hirata Y, Sugimura H, Takei H,Nagatsu T. The effects of pyridinium salts, structurally related compounds of 1-methyl-4-phenylpridinium ion (MPP^+), on tyrosine hydroxylation in rat striatal tissue slices. Brain Res 1986; 397:341–344.
157. Nagatsu T, Hirata Y. Inhibition of the tyrosine hydroxylase system by MPTP, 1-methyl-4-phenylpyridinium ion (MPP^+) and the structurally related compounds in vitro and in vivo. Eur Neurol 1987; 26(suppl 1):11–15.
158. Booth RG, Castagnoli NJ, Rollema H. Intracerebral microdialysis neurotoxicity studies of quinoline and isoquinoline derivatives related to MPTP/MPP^+. Neurosci Lett 1989; 100:306–312.
159. Rollema H, Johnson EA, Booth RG, et al. In vivo intracerebral microdialysis studies in rats of MPP^+ analogues and related charged species. J Med Chem 1990; 33:2221–2230.
160. Sayre LM, Singh MP, Arora PK, Wang F, McPeak RJ, Hoppel CL. Inhibition of mitochondrial respiration by analogues of the dopaminergic neurotoxin 1-methyl-4-phenylpyridinium: structural requirements for accumulation-dependent enhanced inhibitory potency on intact mitochondria. Arch Biochem Biophys 1990; 280:274–283.
161. Rollema H, De Vries JB, Damsma G, et al. The use of in vivo brain dialysis of dopamine, acetylcholine, aminoacids and lactic acid in studies on the neurotoxin 1-methyl-4-phenyl-1,2,3,6-tetrahydropyridine (MPTP). Toxicology 1988; 49:503–511.
162. Naoi M, Matsuura S, Parvez H, et al. Oxidation of *N*-methyl-1,2,3,4-tetrahydroisoquinoline into the *N*-methyl-isoquinolinium ion by monoamine oxidase. J Neurochem 1989; 52:653–655.
163. Perry TL, Yong VW, Wall RA, Jones K. Paraquat and two endogenous analogues

of the neurotoxic substance *N*-methyl-4-phenyl-1,2,3,6-tetrahydropyridine do not damage dopaminergic nigrostriatal neurons in the mouse. Neurosci Lett 1986; 69:285–289.

164. Perry TL, Jones K, Hansen S, Wall RA. 4-Phenylpyridine and three other analogues of 1-methyl-4-phenyl-1,2,3,6-tetrahydropyridine neurotoxicity in mice and marmosets. Neurosci Lett 1987; 75:65–70.
165. Nagatsu T, Yoshida M. An endogenous substance of the brain, tetrahydroisoquinoline, produces parkinsonism in primates with decreased dopamine, tyrosine hydroxylase and biopterin in the nigrostriatal regions. Neurosci Lett 1988; 87:178–182.
166. Yoshida M, Niwa T, Nagatsu T. Parkinsonism in monkeys produced by chronic administration of an endogenous substance of the brain, tetrahydroisoquinoline: the behavioral and biochemical changes. Neurosci Lett 1990; 119:109–113.
167. Niwa T, Takeda N, Tatematsu A, Matsuura S, Yoshida M, Nagatsu T. Migration of tetrahydroisoquinoline, a possible parkinsonian neurotoxin, into monkey brain from blood as proved by gas chromatography–mass spectrometry. J Chromatogr 1988; 452:85–91.
168. Suzuki K, Mizuno Y, Yoshida M. Inhibition of mitochondrial NADH–ubiquinone oxidoreductase and ATP synthesis by tetrahydroisoquinoline. Neurosci Lett 1988; 86:105–108.
169. Niwa T, Takeda N, Sasaoka T. Detection of tetrahydroisoquinoline in parkinsonian brain as an endogenous amine by use of gas chromatography–mass spectrometry. J Chromatogr 1989; 491:397–403.
170. Beringer K. Zur Banisterin und Harminfrage. Nervenarzt 1929; 2:548–549.
171. Beringer K. Uber ein neues, auf das extrapyramidal-motorische System wirkendes Alkaloid (Banisterin). Nervenarzt 1928; 1:265–275.
172. Gunn JA. Relations between chemical constitution, pharmacological actions, and therapeutic uses, in the harmine group of alkaloids. Arch Int Pharmacodynam 1935; 50:379–396.
173. Gunn JA. The pharmacological actions of tetrahydroharmine. Pharm Pharmacol 1930; 3:1–20.
174. Shoemaker DW, Cummins JT, Bidder TG, Boettger HG, Evans M. Identification of harman in the rat arcuate nucleus. Arch Pharmacol 1980; 310:227–230.
175. Schouten MJ, Bruinvels J. Endogenously formed nonharman (beta-carboline) in platelet rich plasma obtained from porphyric rats. Pharmacol Biochem Behav 1986; 24:1219–1223.
176. Peura P, Johnson JV, Yost RA, Faull KF. Concentrations of tryptoline and methtryptoline in rat brain. J Neurochem 1989; 52:847–852.
177. Airaksinen MM, Kari I. beta-Carbolines, psychoactive compounds in the mammalian body. Med Biol 1981; 59:190–211.
178. Bosin TR, Borg S, Faull KF. Harman in rat brain, lung and human CSF: effect of alcohol consumption. Alcohol 1989; 5:505–511.
179. Bosin TR, Faull KF. Indole derivatization procedures for electron capture negative chemical ionization mass spectrometry: identification of 1-methyl-1,2,3,4-tetrahydro-beta-carboline in rat brain and lung. Biomed Environ Mass Spectrom 1989; 18:247–252.

180. Beck O, Repke DB, Faull KF. 6-Hydroxymethtryptoline is naturally occurring in mammalian urine: identification by combined chiral capillary gas chromatography and high resolution mass spectrometry. Biomed Environ Mass Spectrom 1986; 13:469–472.
181. Barker SA, Harrison REW, Monti JA, Brown GB, Christian ST. Identification and quantification of 1,2,3,4-tetrahydro-beta-carboline, 2-methyl-1,2,3,4-tetrahydro-beta-carboline, and 6-methoxy-1,2,3,4-tetrahydro-beta-carboline as in vivo constituents of rat brain and adrenal gland. Biochem Pharmacol 1981; 30:9–17.
182. McIsaac WM. Formation of 1-methyl-6-methoxy-1,2,3,4-tetrahydro-2-carboline under physiological conditions. Biochim Biophys Acta 1961; 52:607–609.
183. Robbins JH. Possible alkaloid formation in alcoholism and other diseases. Clin Res 1968; 15:554.
184. Robbins JH. Alkaloid formation by condensation of biogenic amines with acetaldehyde. Clin Res 1968; 16:350.
185. Davis VE, Cashaw JL. Metabolism of tetrahydroisoquinolines and related alkaloids. Prog Clin Biol Res 1982; 90:99–111.
186. Kenyhercz TM, Kissinger PT. High-performance liquid chromatographic assay of isoquinoline alkaloid formation from reaction of biogenic amines and aldehydes. J Pharm Sci 1978; 67:112–113.
187. Saheb SE, Dajani RM. 1-Methyl-6-hydroxytetrahydrocarboline: a possible product of ethanol and tryptophan metabolism. Comp Gen Pharmacol 1973; 4:225–227.
188. Ho BT, McIsaac WM, Walker KE, Estevez V. Inhibitors of monoamine oxidase. Influence of methyl substitution on the inhibitory activity of beta-carbolines. J Pharm Sci 1968; 57:269–274.
189. Collins MA, Neafsey EJ. beta-Carboline analogues of *N*-methyl-4-phenyl-1,2,5,6-tetrahydropyridine (MPTP): endogenous factors underlying idiopathic parkinsonism. Neurosci Lett 1985; 55:179–184.
190. Testa B, Naylor R, Costall B, Jenner P, Marsden CD. Does an endogenous methylpyridinium analogue cause Parkinson's disease. J Pharm Pharmacol 1985; 37:679–680.
191. Hoppel CL, Greenblatt D, Kwok HK, Arora PK, Singh MP, Sayre LM. Inhibition of mitochondrial respiration by analogs of a 4-phenylpyridine and 1-methyl-4-phenylpyridinium cation (MPP^+), the neurotoxic metabolite of MPTP. Biochem Biophys Res Commun 1987; 148:684–693.
192. Rollema H, Johnson EA, Booth RG, et al. In vivo dopaminergic neurotoxicity of the 2-beta-methylcarbolinium ion, a potential endogenous MPP^+ analog. Eur J Pharmacol 1988; 153:131–134.
193. Albores R, Neafsey EJ, Drucker G, Fields JZ, Collins MA. Mitochondrial respiratory inhibition by *N*-methylated β-carboline derivatives structurally resembling *N*-methyl-4-phenylpyridine. Proc Natl Acad Sci USA 1990; 87:9368–9372.
194. Drucker G, Raikoff K, Neafsey EJ, Collins MA. Dopamine uptake inhibitory capacities of β-carboline and 3,4-dihydro-β-carboline analogs of *N*-methyl-4-phenyl-1,2,3,6-tetrahydropyridine (MPTP) oxidation products. Brain Res 1990; 509:125–133.
195. Neafsey EJ, Drucker G, Raikoff K, Collins MA. Striatal dopaminergic toxicity

following intranigral injection in rats of 2-methyl-norharman, a β-carbolinium analog of *N*-methyl-4-phenylpyridinium ion (MPP^+). Neurosci Lett 1989; 105:344–349.
196. Harik SI, Schmidley JW, Iacofano LA, Blue P, Arora PK, Sayre LM. On the mechanisms underlying 1-methyl-4-phenyl-1,2,3,6-tetrahydropyridine neurotoxicity: the effect of perinigral infusion of 1-methyl-4-phenyl-1,2,3,6-tetrahydropyridine, its metabolite and their analogs in the rat. J Pharmacol Exp Ther 1987; 241:669–676.
197. Collins MA, Neafsey EJ, Cheng BY. Endogenous analogs of *N*-methyl-4-phenyl-1,2,3,6-tetrahydropyridine: indoleamine derived tetrahydro-beta-carbolines as potential causative factors in Parkinson's disease. Adv Neurol, 1986; 45:179–182.
198. Sonsalla PK, Nicklas WJ, Heikkila RE. Role for excitatory amino acids in methamphetamine-induced nigrostriatal dopaminergic toxicity. Science 1989; 243:398–400.
199. Sonsalla PK, Riordan DE, Heikkila RE. Competitive and noncompetitive antagonists at *N*-methyl-D-aspartate receptors protect against methamphetamine-induced dopaminergic damage in mice. J Pharmacol Exp Ther 1991; 256:506–512.
200. Rinne JO, Halonen T, Riekkinen PJ, Rinne UK. Free amino acids in the brain of patients with Parkinson's disease. Neurosci Lett 1988; 94:182–186.
201. Perry TL, Agid FJ, Agid Y, Fibiger HC. Striatal GABAergic neuronal activity is not reduced in Parkinson's disease. J Neurochem 1983; 40:1120–1123.
202. Difazio MC, Hollingswoth Z, Young AB, Penney JBJ. Glutamate receptors in the substantia nigra of Parkinson's disease brains. Neurology 1992; 42:402–406.
203. Cotzias GC. Manganese in health and disease. Physiol Rev 1958; 38:503–529.
204. Cotzias GC, Papavasiliou PS, Ginos J, Steck A, Duby S. Metabolic modification of Parkinson's disease and of chronic manganese poisoning. Annu Rev Med 1971; 22:305–326.
205. Cotzias GC, Miller ST, Papavasiliou PS, Tang LC. Interactions between manganese and brain dopamine. Med Clin North Am 1976; 60:729–738.
206. Mena I. Manganese poisoning. In: Vinken PJ, Bruyn GW, Cohen MM, Klawans HL, eds. Handbook of clinical neurology, vol 36: intoxications of the nervous system, part 1. Amsterdam: North Holland Publishing, 1979:217–237.
207. Weiner WJ, Lang AE. Movement disorders: a comprehensive survey. Mount Kisco, NY: Futura Publishing, 1989:257–291.
208. Langston JW, Irwin I, Ricaurte GA. Neurotoxins, parkinsonism, and Parkinson's disease. Pharmacol Ther 1987; 32:19–46.
209. Dexter DT, Jenner P, Schapira AHV, Marsden CD. Alterations in levels of iron, ferritin, and other trace metals in neurodegenerative diseases affecting the basal ganglia. Ann Neurol 1992; 32(suppl):S94–S100.
210. Dexter DT, Carayon A, Javoy-Agid F. Alterations in the levels of iron, ferritin and other trace metals in Parkinson's disease and other neurodegenerative diseases affecting the basal ganglia. Brain 1991; 114:1953–1975.
211. Olanow CW, Cohen G, Perl DP, Marsden CD. Role of iron and oxidant stress in the normal and parkinsonian brain: proceedings of a symposium sponsored by the University of Florida, Nov 14–17, 1991. Ann Neurol 1992; 32(suppl):S2–S9.

212. Earle KM. Studies on Parkinson's disease including X-ray fluorescent spectroscopy of formalin fixed brain tissue. J Neuropathol Exp Neurol 1968; 27:1–14.
213. Dexter DT, Wells FR, Agid FJ. Increased nigral iron content in postmortem parkinsonian brain. Lancet 1987; 2:1219–1220.
214. Riederer P, Sofic E, Rausch WD, et al. Transition metals, ferritin, glutathione, and ascorbic acid in parkinsonian brains. J Neurochem 1989; 52:515–520.
215. Sofic E, Paulus W, Jellinger K, Riederer P, Youdim MB. Selective increase of iron in substantia nigra zona compacta of parkinsonian brains. J Neurochem 1991; 56:978–982.
216. Orrenius S, McConkey DJ, Jones DP, Nicotera P. CA^{2+}-activated mechanisms in toxicity and programmed cell death. ISI Atlas Sci Pharmacol 1988; 2:319–324.
217. Ben-Shachar D, Riederer P, Youdim MBH. Iron-melanin interaction and lipid peroxidation: implications for Parkinson's disease. J Neurochem 1991; 57:1609–1614.
218. Youdim MBH, Ben-Shachar D,Riederer P. Is Parkinson's disease a progressive siderosis of substantia nigra resulting in iron and melanin induced neurodegeneration? Acta Neurol Scand 1989; 126:47–54.
219. Youdim MB. Iron in the brain: implications for Parkinson's and Alzheimer's diseases [published erratu appears in Mt Sinai J Med (NY) 1988 Mar;55 (2): inside back cover]. Mt Sinai J Med 1988; 55:97–101.
220. Hill JM. Comments on ''putatitive biological mechanisms of the effect of iron deficiency on brain chemistry and behavior.'' Am J Clin Nutr 1989; 50:616–617.
221. Jellinger K, Paulus W, Grundke-Iqbal I, Riederer P, Youdim MB. Brain iron and ferritin in Parkinson's and Alzheimer's diseases. J Neural Transm Park Dis Dement Sect 1990; 2:327–340.
222. Jellinger K, Kienzl E, Rumpelmair G. Iron-melanin complex in substantia nigra of parkinsonian brains: an X-ray microanalysis. J Neurochem 1992; 59:1168–1171.
223. Hirsch EC, Brandel JP, Galle P, Javoy-Agid F, Agid Y. Iron and aluminum increase in the substantia nigra of patients with Parkinson's disease: an X-ray microanalysis. J Neurochem 1991; 56:446–451.
224. Dexter DT, Carayon A, Vidailhet M, et al. Decreased ferritin levels in Parkinson's disease. J Neurochem 1990; 55:16–20.
225. Sengstock GJ, Olanow CW, Dunn AJ, Menzies R, Arendash GW. Iron induces degeneration of substantia nigra neurons. Mov Disord 1991; 6:272.
226. Ben-Shachar D,Youdim MBH. Intranigral iron injection induces behavioural and biochemical ''parkinsonism'' in rats. J Neurochem 1991; 57:2133–2135.
227. Ben-Shachar D, Eshel G. Finberg JP,Youdim MB. The iron chelator desferrioxamine (Desferal) retards 6-hydroxydopamine-induced degeneration of nigrostriatal dopamine neurons. J Neurochem 1991; 56:1441–1444.

8

The Neuroepidemiology of Parkinson's Disease

Gustavo C. Román

National Institute of Neurological Disorders and Stroke, National Institutes of Health, Bethesda, Maryland

Zhen-Xin Zhang

National Institute of Neurological Disorders and Stroke, National Institutes of Health, Bethesda, Maryland, and Peking Medical College Hospital, Beijing, China

Jonas H. Ellenberg

National Institute of Neurological Disorders and Stroke, National Institutes of Health, Bethesda, Maryland

I. INTRODUCTION

Ayurveda, the ancient system of medicine practiced in India from 5000–3000 BC, described a category of disorders known as *vata*, characterized by tremors (*kampa*), stiffness (*stambha*), and depression (*vishada*) (1,2). Although these complaints as described could have been caused by essential tremor or arthritis, Ayurvedic recommendations for treatment of *kampavata* included ingestion of the seeds of *Mucuna pruriens* Bak (cowhage), a plant that has been recently confirmed to contain levodopa (L-dopa) (2). Some 2500 years ago, the first Chinese medical book *Nei Jing* described a disease characterized by "*Feng Yin Mo Ji*" (i.e., shaking "like the leaves of a tree") involving the extremities. Subsequently, on the basis of *Nei Jing*, medical writers of the dynasties Tang, Song, Ming, and Qing referred to this condition under the name "*Chan Zhen Zhen*," and distinguished three categories: (1) *Chan Zhen*, dominated by tremor; (2) *Jing Luan*, with stiffness; and (3) *Jin Ji*, with loss of movement, mutism, and staring into the distance (3). Writers since the Ming dynasty indicated that the disorder was rare in the young and occurred after middle age, particularly in the elderly.

However, it was not until 1817 that James Parkinson (4) described, in *An Essay on the Shaking Palsy*, the syndrome of akinesia, rigidity, tremor, and postural disturbances that bears his name. In 1895, Brissaud (5) first suggested that the substantia nigra could be the site of the lesion in Parkinson's disease, based on a case report by Blocq and Marinesco (6) of hemiparkinsonism, resulting from a contralateral tuberculoma of the midbrain. In 1919—more than 100 years after Parkinson's initial report—Trétiakoff (7) demonstrated the constant presence of lesions in the substantia nigra in postencephalitic parkinsonism and Parkinson's disease. Finally, in 1960, Ehringer and Hornykiewicz (8) identified a dopamine deficit in the striatum of patients with Parkinson's disease. This observation led to the introduction of an effective pharmacological treatment for Parkinson's disease and signaled the importance of the dopaminergic nigrostriatal pathway in the pathogenesis of the parkinsonian syndrome.

Parkinsonism may be the clinical manifestation of a variety of conditions. Idiopathic Parkinson's disease, sometimes called idiopathic parkinsonism or paralysis agitans, is the primary observable cause of this syndrome. The neuronal inclusion bodies described in 1912 by Lewy (9) appear to be the most important pathological marker to support the nosological identity of idiopathic Parkinson's disease. Cases with an identifiable cause of damage to the nigrostriatal system are termed *secondary parkinsonism*. Parkinsonism may also be part of widespread degenerative pathological abnormalities affecting other areas of the brain besides the substantia nigra, such as the multiple system degeneration. Gerstenbrand and Poewe (10) and Pahwa and Koller (see Chapter 1) discuss classification of the parkinsonian syndrome in detail.

Despite major research, the etiology of Parkinson's disease remains unknown. Epidemiological methods are useful in the etiological investigation of Parkinson's disease for two main reasons: First, descriptive epidemiology provides a definite profile of Parkinson's disease in terms of frequency, temporal occurrence, and distribution by age, sex, racial, and geographic characteristics. Not only must this profile of the disease be taken into account when etiologic hypotheses are proposed, but descriptive epidemiological observations by themselves may generate a first level of understanding of disease causation (e.g., based on geographic variation, environmental factors might be considered in the etiology of Parkinson's disease). Second, analytic epidemiology is used to disclose risk factors that may signal the existence of unexpected causal associations with the disease [e.g., investigation of a cluster of young-onset Parkinson's disease resulted in the discovery of MPTP-induced parkinsonism (11)]. Neuroepidemiology, therefore, provides useful research strategies to generate etiologic hypotheses for Parkinson's disease. There are, however, significant problems for the epidemiological study of Parkinson's disease.

II. PROBLEMS IN EPIDEMIOLOGICAL STUDIES OF PARKINSON'S DISEASE

There are many textbooks on epidemiological and statistical aspects in the design of studies for incidence, prevalence, etiology, and natural history of disease (12–14). Our ability to design appropriate research studies will depend, to a large degree, on our success in eliciting the answers to what appear to be very simple questions. These include: How do you define the disease? How do you identify cases? How do you identify risk factors? How do you quantify exposure to risk factors? How do you track natural history both before and after onset of clinical symptoms? In the short overview provided in this section we will attempt to highlight some of the complexities involved in responding to simple questions such as these. The design issues related to the study of Parkinson's disease will also be relevant to other neurodegenerative disorders, such as Alzheimer's disease.

A. Case Definition

Studies of Parkinson's disease are hampered by the lack of universal acceptance and by the inaccuracy of current clinical diagnostic criteria. Chapters 1 and 3 define Parkinson's disease both clinically and pathologically. The use of these definitions for epidemiological studies needs to be assessed in the context of each proposed study, with consideration of the level of neurological expertise available, the extent of contact with the subject, and the availability of autopsy material.

Clinical diagnosis of Parkinson's disease usually requires at least two of the following cardinal features: resting tremor, rigidity, bradykinesia, and impaired postural reflexes. A beneficial response to levodopa therapy is also considered to favor the diagnosis of Parkinson's disease. Essential tremor, secondary (symptomatic) parkinsonism, and parkinsonism in multiple system degeneration must be ruled out. These other disorders are usually unresponsive to levodopa therapy (10).

Pathological confirmation is currently the gold standard for the diagnosis of parkinson's disease, albeit not entirely without error (15,16). More often than not, autopsy material cannot be obtained for ethical reasons, lack of resources, logistical reasons, lack of family's cooperation, or time constraints. Therefore, we are usually confronted with the problem of objectively and uniformly applying a clinical definition of Parkinson's disease by potentially multiple investigators, often in different environments. Can we develop an accurate clinical definition, and can we expect to achieve reasonably uniform application of such an agreed on definition? The Parkinson's Epidemiology Research Committee (PERC; see

Neurology 1991; 41 (suppl 2):4) considers these as fundamental questions to be resolved. The PERC is developing a protocol to assess the accuracy of the clinical definition of Parkinson's disease and to measure and minimize inter- and intraobserver reliability in its application. The committee is in the process of obtaining videotapes of subjects with Parkinson's disease and other disorders that mimic the clinical signs and symptoms of this disease, for patients who also have autopsy data available. The study is designed to allow experts in movement disorders as well as nonneurologists to view the tapes and provide clinical diagnoses. The study will then assess how well the raters have fared in distinguishing idiopathic Parkinson's disease (as definitively diagnosed by autopsy) from other forms of parkinsonism. By examining which elements of the clinical features were associated with high levels of misclassification, it is hoped that a better working definition can be developed that researchers at various levels of expertise can use in future studies.

B. Case Identification

Unfortunately, Parkinson's disease is not a reportable disease in most countries, so identifying cases within a community, a state, or a country is a difficult aspect of any epidemiological research. Complete ascertainment of all cases of Parkinson's disease in a community may be extremely difficult to achieve for several reasons.

First, cases may remain undiagnosed because symptoms of Parkinson's disease may be considered part of the aging process, and patients may not seek medical care until late or when incapacitated by the disease. Therefore, case-finding based on hospital admissions or physicians' records may prove incomplete, since it is likely to exclude mild or early cases. In fact, such case-finding techniques resulted in underascertainment in 29 and 42% of Parkinson's disease series in community-based studies (17–18).

Second, correct diagnosis of Parkinson's disease depends on access to health services and neurological expertise, since it may be difficult to distinguish idiopathic Parkinson's disease in the best of circumstances (see Section II.A) from secondary parkinsonism, multiple system degeneration, or essential tremor, or even from other conditions frequently observed in the elderly, such as slowness of movement, or pain and stiffness from arthritis. Also, dementia and depression may be part of the clinical picture of Parkinson's disease (10,19–21), and bona fide Parkinson's disease patients may be misdiagnosed. For the foregoing reasons, false-positive diagnoses have been reported in 11–44% of subjects identified as Parkinson's disease cases after detailed clinical or pathological examination (22–26).

Third, variations in the diagnostic criteria and the classifications used in different studies also affect the measurement of disease frequency. For instance, studies of Parkinson's disease incidence and prevalence, such as those in Rochester, Minnesota (27–29), have included drug-induced parkinsonism, postencephalitic parkinsonism, and patients with cerebrovascular disease (see Tables 1–5).

Fourth, prevalence ratios are affected by the length of diagnostic delay, by the incidence of the disease, and by the survival rates (as a reflection of the quality of care for the elderly). Therefore, variations in the prevalence of Parkinson's disease in different countries may not reflect exactly true differences in incidence (30).

Fifth, death certificates appear to provide underestimates of Parkinson's disease death rates (31). For example, Kessler (32) found that Parkinson's disease was mentioned in only 38.7% of 186 death certificates from patients who died with Parkinson's disease during the period of study.

Finally, even when the foregoing problems can be overcome, because of the relatively low frequency of the disease large populations must be studied in epidemiological studies of Parkinson's disease, including a substantial segment of elderly subjects, to obtain accurate incidence, prevalence, and mortality rates.

C. Identification and Assessment of Risk Factors

It has been postulated that Parkinson's disease could result from excessive age-related attrition of neurons in the substantia nigra owing to environmental factors. The disease would be characterized by a long latency, lasting from several years to decades between a postulated exposure to a risk factor and appearance of symptoms, as the decrease in the neuronal population reaches a critical threshold (33). Epidemiological observations of parkinsonism–dementia complex on Guam (34,35), pugilistic encephalopathy (36), postencephalitic parkinsonism (37,38), chronic manganese poisoning (39,40), carbon monoxide toxicity (41), hemiatrophy–hemiparkinsonism (42,43), and familial parkinsonism (44,45) seem to support the concept of an environmentally induced acceleration of neuronal degeneration. Chapters 12–14 discuss putative exogenous risk factors for Parkinson's disease.

In the long latency period postulated for Parkinson's disease (46), there may be an environmental factor acting alone, or in conjunction with a genetic deficit (47), which exacerbates the chain of events leading to the appearance of clinical symptoms of Parkinson's disease. Although many risk factors have been nominated in observational clinical studies (see Chapter 12), the level of biochemical specificity necessary for detailed study of a particular mechanism of action has not been forthcoming, with one rare exception (see Chapter 13).

The long latency period makes it difficult to document specific exposures in analytical comparative studies. Relevant information must either be collected decades before the disease manifests itself, or elicited from elderly individuals with and without Parkinson's disease. At best, responses from these individuals are useful only in the broadest sense. Even if recall were accurate for a period of decades before disease onset, the specificity of the information might be limited. For example, in assessing pesticides as a risk factor for Parkinson's disease (see Chapter 12), a 75-year-old Parkinson's disease patient may be able to specify approximately the number of times per month pesticides were used to treat crops on his farm when he or she was 25 years old or younger. But the chemical being used for each crop being treated would likely not have been known to the subject, let alone its level of concentration. Another example is the hypothesis of well water (see Chapter 12) as a source of a toxicant. The 75-year-old patient may be quite specific that his or her house was or was not connected to the city water supply, but would not be likely to specify the particular chemicals or chemical by-products that occurred in the water table of his or her particular home site.

Another inherent difficulty in investigating the associations of risk factors with Parkinson's disease with its modal incidence later in life is that subjects may succumb to death of other causes before the onset of Parkinson's disease, causes that may or may not be related to the risk factor under study. In statistical parlance, this is termed the *competing risk* problem; that is, in a particular subject or group of elderly subjects, onset of Parkinson's disease is competing with death of other causes as to which occurs first.

This could cause problems, for example, in comparing prevalence in different geographic areas, each of which is racially homogeneous, but with race-specific and differing mortality rates for non-Parkinson's disease mortality. Certain races may have a lower life expectancy within a specific geographic region sufficient to reduce the prevalence of Parkinson's disease simply because a lower proportion of the population survives long enough to manifest the disorder. Attribution of any observed differences in prevalence of Parkinson's disease in the geographic areas to a racial risk factor might be incorrect (see Section III.A.1). This problem can even affect the direction of observed associations of putative risk factors with Parkinson's disease (see Chapter 11). Conclusions about race as a risk factor would depend on the ability to create a standardized age and ''other'' mortality-adjusted comparison between geographic groups. Statistical methodology is available to help ameliorate some aspects of this problem (48), but the methodological approaches require strong and sometimes untenable assumptions.

Conflicting reports of risk factors in the literature may partly be explained by differences in study design, insufficient sample size, or differences in study populations. For example, a case–control study among Chinese living in a nursing home in Hong Kong (49) found a fivefold increase in risk of Parkinson's disease among subjects who had lived in rural areas for over 40 years and in those who had farmed for 20 years. It was suggested that environmental factors associated with rural living and farming activities were responsible. However, another hospital-based case–control study among Chinese in Beijing and Guangzhou (50) found that subjects with rural residence and involved in wheat cultivation had a lower risk of Parkinson's disease. There were major differences in the size, sex distribution, and place of residence of the two populations. For instance, 69% of the 35 patients in the study by Ho et al. (49) were women in nursing homes, whereas 23% of the 100 patients in the study by Tanner et al. (50) were women being seen in an outpatient clinic. The small sample size in both of these studies resulted in low statistical power.

Most of the studies reporting putative risk factors for Parkinson's disease come from non–population-based studies; that is, the cohorts studied are not whole populations or at least a representative or random sample of the subjects from a specified geographic or otherwise defined population. Ellenberg and Nelson (51) have shown that associations in non–population-based studies not only tend to be nonreplicable, but often overstate the magnitude of associations.

D. Quantification of Exposure to Risk Factors

In addition to the difficulties in designing retrospective epidemiological studies that will yield specific risk factors, it has been difficult to obtain results relating the level of increased risk to the level of exposure of the putative risk factor. This situation may well remain unsolved without a long-term prospective clinical study. It would be extremely important to demonstrate a dose–response relation between a putative risk factor and either the likelihood of disease development or the severity of the outcome. Such a demonstration would add credibility to the potential agent for a cause-and-effect relationship, since a "one-hit, any level of exposure" toxicant is unlikely to be a primary cause of Parkinson's disease in the general population. An example of such lack of confirmation in a study is given by Golbe et al. (52) in a study during which the dose of the risk factor could be estimated in assessing the reported negative association between smoking and Parkinson's disease; they found "no correlation between any measure of smoking and any measure of Parkinson's disease severity."

In summary, the late onset of the disease militates against retrospective studies uncovering the level of exposure because of poor recall and the lack of available detailed knowledge of the putative agent(s) in the first place. If a factor is determined to be associated with Parkinson's disease, then secondary clinical and animal studies will need to be done to replicate the results and to attempt to demonstrate a dose–response relation to bolster the biological plausibility of the observational result.

E. Tracking Natural History of Parkinson's Disease Both Before and After Onset of Clinical Symptoms

A better understanding of the clinical, biochemical, and pathological course of Parkinson's disease, from its presymptomatic, through its symptomatic, and to its terminal stage, would undoubtedly lead to many insights about the etiology or etiologies of this disorder.

For this reason, and also to ameliorate many of the methodological difficulties encountered in the traditional cross-sectional, retrospective, and case–control clinical studies that are the hallmarks of epidemiological research, PERC is also examining the feasibility of undertaking a long-term prospective observational study of the presymptomatic and postsymptomatic course of Parkinson's disease (53) in an asymptomatic cohort. The study would be designed along the lines of the Framingham study (54,55) and would include several neurodegenerative disorders. It is understood that such an investigation would need to be a collaborative effort among researchers interested in the etiology and natural history of all disorders of aging.

Efforts are underway toward the presymptomatic diagnosis of the disease (46,53,56), using biomarkers related to disease progression and, one hopes, to disease etiology. The successful use of safe, noninvasive, and inexpensive biomarkers and other lines of evidence of subclinical degradation will be important elements in the design of studies of risk factors and of the natural history of Parkinson's disease. This is especially true in the context of the long-term follow-up study of a healthy cohort mentioned earlier. Some of the olfactory markers (57), the use of positron emission tomography with fluorodopa (58), or dopamine neuron antibody in the cerebrospinal fluid (CSF) (59) are promising. The ability to relate natural history chronologically to risk exposure and other clinical changes will undoubtedly help us in our understanding of the etiology of Parkinson's disease.

III. MAGNITUDE AND DISTRIBUTION

A. Prevalence

There are wide variations in the reported prevalence ratios of Parkinson's disease in different parts of the world. Even among Caucasians in Europe and North America, prevalence ratios for Parkinson's disease range from 60: 100,000–187: 100,000 population (27,60). It is unclear if these differences represent artifacts or true variations in the prevalence of Parkinson's disease. Some of the factors that could create artificial discrepancies in the reported figures have been discussed in the foregoing. We examined all the studies in Table 1, with the explicit assumption that no serious deficiencies in case ascertainment were present. We recognized that although this is a reasonable assumption for the studies that used door-to-door surveys for case ascertainment, assuming that all studies had reasonable case ascertainment is an unrealistic, albeit necessary assumption, to make some broad comparisons. It must also be recognized that there are limitations in the data obtained from the literature relative to uniformity of definition

Table 1 Prevalence Ratios of Parkinson's Disease per 100,000 Population From Selected Studies

Region	Study period	Population	Number of cases	Prevalence: Crude	Prevalence: Age-adjusted[a,b]
North America					
Rochester, Minn[e] (27)	1955	29,885	56	187	175 (132–228)
Rochester, Minn[e] (28)	1965	47,797	75	157	172 (135–215)
Copiah Co. MS[e,g,h] (18)	1978	23,597	31	131	98 (67–139)
Blacks		11,666	12	103	103 (53–181)
Whites		11,931	19	159	90 (54–140)
Baltimore, MD (141)	1967–69	2,070,000	1,630	79	
Canada (142)	1950–51			30	
British Columbia (26)	1988	80,000	55	69	
Northern Europe					
UK, Leeds[c] (60)	1952	485,903	288	60	
UK, Carlisle[c] (85)	1961	71,101	80	113	90 (71–112)
UK, Northampton (143)	1982	208,499	226	108	78 (69–89)
Scotland, Aberdeen (24)	1984		249	164	101 (89–145)
Sweden, Göteborg[c] (71)	1960	400,000	270	65	56 (49–63)
Iceland[f] (65)	1963	187,314	304	162	182 (163–204)
Finland, Turku[d] (23)	1971	402,988	484	120	95 (87–104)
Denmark, Arhus[d] (73)	1972	242,151	203	84	72 (62–83)
Northern Norway (144)	1986	48,091	59	133	
Western Europe					
France, Limousin[h] (145)	1985			350	
Northern Germany (146)	1987		1,018	183	
Spain[h] (147)	1987	7,417	21	283	
Eastern Europe					
USSR, Moscow (148)	1978			80–230	

Table 1 Continued

Region	Study period	Population	Number of cases	Prevalence	
				Crude	Age-adjusted[a,b]
Bulgaria, Sofia[c] (148)	1983	1,381,295	2,150	156	
Poland, Poznan (72)	1986	1,308,277	862	66	60 (56–64)
Southern Europe					
Sassari, Sardinia[d] (76)	1971	397,891	310	78	73 (65–82)
Nuoro, Sardinia[d] (77)	1972	273,421	193	71	67 (58–78)
Sardinia[d] (78)	1972	1,473,800	967	66	65 (61–69)
San Marino (17)	1986	22,322	34	152	113 (78–158)
Ferrara, Italy (66)	1987	38,360	73	190	127 (99–160)
Terrasini and Santa Teresa di Riva, Sicily[h] (149)	1987	14,376	38	246	
Southern Hemisphere					
New Zealand, Wellington[e] (22)	1962	124,000	131	106	
Australia, Victoria[e] (84)	1965	83,001	70	85	98 (77–124)
Asia					
Japan, Kyoto (150)	1978			46	
Japan, Sanin (151)	1980		191	48	
Japan, Yonago (74)	1982	125,291	101	81	73 (60–89)

Japan, Izumo (75)	1985	80,639	66	82	61 (47–78)
China, 6 cities[h] (70)	1983	63,195	28	44	57 (38–82)
China, 29 provinces[h] (69)	1986	3,869,162	566	15	18 (17–20)
India, Bombay, Parsis[h] (68)	1985	14,010	46	328	148 (108–197)
Saudi Arabia, Thugbah[h] (67)	1991	22,613	6	27	128 (47–279)
Africa					
Libya, Benghazi (79)	1985	518,745	163	31	57 (49–67)
Togo (152)	1989	20,000		15	
Nigeria, Igbo-Ora[h] (153)	1979	18,954	2	10	
S. Africa					
Johannesburg (154)	1977				
Whites				159	
Blacks				4	

[a]Prevalence age adjusted to 1970 U.S. total population and calculated from data given in the corresponding report for which age distribution was available (61).

[b]95% confidence interval given in parentheses was calculated from data given in the corresponding report.

[c]All parkinsonian cases included.

[d]Postencephalitic cases included.

[e]Arteriosclerotic and postencephalitic cases included.

[f]Arteriosclerotic cases included.

[g]Population screened older than age 39, prevalence based on entire population assuming no prevalent cases younger than aged 40.

[h]Population screening of defined geographic area.

of Parkinson's disease. Therefore, the comparisons and conclusions presented here should be considered only tentative.

The lack of international standards for epidemiological studies on Parkinson's disease reinforces the need to reach universal agreement on the definitions and methods to be used in future studies. In addition to the lack of consistent methodological approaches, discussed earlier, most investigators have reported crude prevalence rates. Crude rates cannot be used for comparison of populations from different geographic areas, nor of sex differences among populations from the same area, because of the uneven distribution of the age pyramids across regions. It is also impossible to compare worldwide figures using age-adjusted rates that were calculated based on different standard populations in the different studies. In the present review we have adjusted all studies (with published age distributions) to the 1970 U. S. population, computing directly standardized ratios (61), for which 95% confidence limits (CI) were obtained (62,63). Crude and age-adjusted prevalence ratios for Parkinson's disease in a worldwide review of the literature are presented in Table 1 and Figure 1. Age-specific prevalence ratios are summarized in Table 2 and Figure 2. These results have been previously reported in detail by Zhang and Román (64).

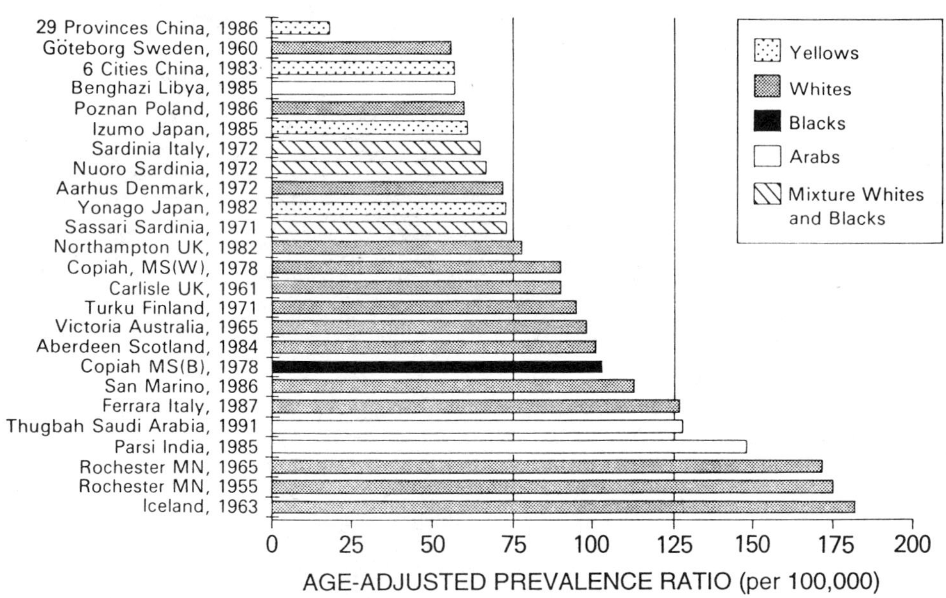

Figure 1 Worldwide comparison of age-adjusted prevalence ratios for Parkinson's disease by country for both sexes combined, adjusted to the 1970 U.S. population (see Table 1).

1. Geographic and Racial Variation

Despite the obvious limitations of these data—the only worldwide data available—we believe that this information should be used, with the caution and caveats mentioned in the previous section. Parkinson's disease has been reported throughout the world, in all ethnic groups. Given the limitations of the available data, we have grouped the worldwide age-adjusted prevalence ratios for Parkinson's disease into three broad categories: *low*, fewer than 75:100,000 population; *intermediate*, between 75:100,000 and 125:100,000; and *high*, more than 125:100,000 population.

High prevalences of Parkinson's disease ranging from 127:100,000 to 182:100,000 population were reported in Iceland (65); Rochester, Minnesota (27,28); Ferrara, Italy (66); Saudi Arabia (67), and among the Parsis in Bombay, India (68) (see Fig 1). In contrast, low ratios, ranging from 18:100,000 to 73:100,000 population were reported in China (69,70); Sweden (71); Poland (72); Denmark (73); Japan (74,75); Sardinia, Italy (76–78); and Benghazi, Libya (79). The differences between the highest and lowest reported prevalence ratios are statistically significant; the 95% confidence intervals (CI) for the highest ratios did not overlap with those of the lowest ratios (see Table 1), except for Saudi Arabia (67). However, of the six studies with the highest ratios, three included all types of parkinsonism. In the two Rochester surveys, crude prevalence ratios for postencephalitic parkinsonism and parkinsonism caused by arteriosclerotic brain disease were about 7–10 and 30% of the total ratios, respectively. Idiopathic Parkinson's disease represented about 60% of the total (i.e., 94:100,000 for the year 1965 and 112:100,000 for the year 1955; 27,28). In Iceland, the crude prevalence ratio for combined Parkinson's disease with parkinsonism caused by arteriosclerosis was 162:100,000, but for idiopathic Parkinson's disease the ratio would be reduced to 146:100,000 (65). The results reported for some of the lower prevalence areas [Sweden (71), and Sardinia (77,78)], would also need to be adjusted downward for an appropriate comparison of the idiopathic Parkinson's disease rates, although the two Sardinian studies included postencephalitics only and would be adjusted only moderately. Thus, some of the observed regional differences might be explained by differences in definition.

Observed geographic variations in Parkinson's disease frequency may be related to racial factors, with the lowest prevalence ratios found preponderantly in Asia (China and Japan), Africa (Nigeria and Libya), and in southern Europe (Sardinia). Yellow races (Orientals) appear to have the lowest prevalence rates for Parkinson's disease worldwide. The highest rates were observed in whites (Caucasians).

However, regional discrepancies in the prevalence of Parkinson's disease among similar races remain unexplained. These include low ratios among whites in Sweden and Denmark and high ratios in Iceland and Rochester, Minnesota;

Table 2 Age-Specific Prevalence of Parkinson's Disease per 100,000 for Both Sexes Combined From Selected Studies

	Age (yr)					
Region	≤39	40–49	50–59	60–69	70–79	80+
Northern and Eastern Europe						
Carlisle, UK 1961[d] (85)	0	145	162	315	614	444
Aberdeen, Scotland 1984 (24)	0	47	78	254	832	1925
Turku, Finland 1971[b] (23)	0.8	21	119	501	797	593
Sweden, Göteborg 1961[d] (71)	0	23	94	195	511	445
Arhus, Denmark 1972[b] (73)	0	12	126	362	582	374
Iceland, 1963[c] (65)	1.5	61	163	936	1584	1309[g]
Northampton, UK 1982 (143)		[≤49] 3	64	277	702	1136[g]
Noznan, Poland 1985–86 (72)		3.5	123	296	484	158
Southern Europe						
Nuoro, Sardinia 1972[b] (77)	0.6	74	216	347	245	65
Sardinia 1972[b] (78)	0.6	39	205	342	311	83
Ferrara, Italy 1987 (66)	0	57	38	327	1504[h]	
Sassari, Sardinia 1971[b] (76)	2	[30–39] 67	200	314	464	136[f]
San Marino 1986 (17)		[≤54] 0	[55–59] 80	468	1529	550

Australia						
Victoria 1965 [a] (84)	2	28	166	297	923[h]	
Africa						
Benghazi, Libya 1985 (79)	0.2	23	92	186	525[h]	
Asia						
Yonago 1980 (74)	1.3	40	86	245	698	753[f]
Izumo 1985 (75)	7.3	20	64	339	479	336[f]
Chinese 6 cities 1983[e] (70)	0	0	92	145	615[h]	
Saudi, Arabia 1991 (67)		[≤50] 5	[51–60] 520	[60+] 590		
North America						
Copiah Co. MS 1978 [a,e] (18)						
Whites	0	0	0	455	932	1013
Blacks	0	0	354	626	156	900
Rochester Minn 1955[a] (27)		[≤49] 5	[50–59] 239	[60–69] 758	[70–84] 1407	[85+] 2646
Rochester Minn 1965[a] (28)		8	25	661	1823	2162

[a]Arteriosclerotic and postencephalitic cases included.
[b]Postencephalitic cases included.
[c]Arteriosclerotic cases included.
[d]All parkinsonian cases included.
[e]Population screening of defined geographic area.
[f]Aged 80–89.
[g]Aged 80–99.
[h]Aged 70 and older.

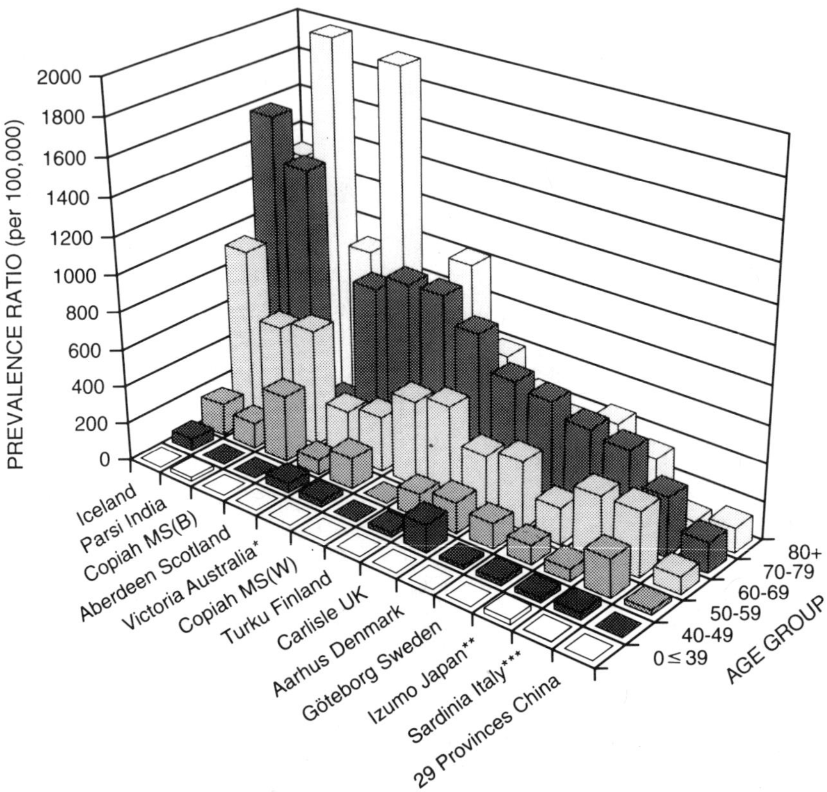

Figure 2 Age-specific prevalence ratios for Parkinson's disease for both sexes combined in selected countries in North America, Europe, Australia, and Asia (see Table 2). *Last bar indicates age group as older than 70 years; **first bar indicates age 30–39 years; ***last bar indicates age 80–89 years.

and high ratios among the Parsis in Bombay, India. This is an ethnic group that migrated from Iran (Persia) between the seventh and tenth centuries and are probably closer to Caucasians and Arabs than to Hindus. Low prevalence was reported among Arabs in Libya, in contrast with high ratios in Saudi Arabia.

Two studies among blacks, one in Igbo-Ora, Nigeria, Africa (80), and another in Copiah County, Mississippi, (18), used uniform diagnostic criteria and similar door-to-door screening procedures. In Nigeria, the age-adjusted prevalence ratio of Parkinson's disease for aged 40 years or older was 67:100,000 population (age adjusted using indirect method to the black population of Copiah County) i.e., one-fifth of the age-adjusted ratio for blacks 40 years and older in Copiah County (341:100,000). The confidence intervals (63) around the point prevalence ratios for Igbo-Ora (8:100,000–242:100,000) and Copiah County

(176:100,000–597:100,000) overlapped slightly. Schoenberg (80), using a different approach to compare the differences, showed a statistically significant difference ($p < 0.05$) in the proportionate increase in the prevalence ratios in the two populations. Despite the lack of a consistent significant difference, the point estimates would indicate a difference in the risk of Parkinson's disease among blacks in the United States, compared with blacks in Africa, which might relate to widely different environmental conditions.

Geographic variation, therefore, is unlikely to be exclusively due to racial factors. Further studies (e.g., on migrant populations) should help clarify variations of racial differences in susceptibility to Parkinson's disease and the factors accounting for the geographic distribution.

B. Incidence

Incidence may be a more suitable measure of disease frequency than prevalence when comparing the risk of Parkinson's disease in different populations and races. More likely, incident cases will be at an earlier stage of the disease than prevalent cases. In general, the cases also will likely be younger and have less comorbidity (such as dementia), making the diagnosis somewhat easier. Incident cases, with either a likelihood of early death related to the disease (81–83) or to the differences in populations being compared, will be included in an incidence cohort, since the period of observation is very short (usually 1 year). Incidence as a measure of disease frequency has been studied less often than prevalence because of the difficulties inherent in these types of studies. In addition to the problems described in Section II on classification and diagnosis of cases for prevalence studies, incidence studies require pinpointing of onset of Parkinson's disease to the time period within which incidence is being measured. This may be more difficult than the diagnosis itself, since often diagnosis is only "probable" until several clinical signs are present, so that the investigator must "predate" the time of diagnosis in many cases.

Crude incidence rates range worldwide from 2:100,000 to 24:100,000 per year in China and Rochester, respectively (27,69) (Table 3). The highest annual age-adjusted incidence rates, ranging from 18 to 22 new cases per 100,000 population, were observed in three studies in Rochester (27–29) and one in Iceland (65). Lower age-adjusted incidence rates were observed in Turku, Poznan, Carlisle, and Victoria, ranging from 8:100,000 to 12:100,000 per year (23,72,84,85). Although for Asia, Africa, and southern Europe, with the exception of China, data suitable for age adjustment are unavailable, the lowest crude incidence rates have been found in China, Japan, Libya, and Sardinia, ranging from 1.5:100,000 to 10.2:100,000 per year (69,74,76–79). The available figures show that the geographic distribution of incidence appears to be consistent with the information on prevalence.

Table 3 Average Annual Incidence Rates of Parkinson's Disease per 100,000 Population From Available Studies

Region	Study period	Number of cases	Incidence Crude	Incidence Age-adjusted[a,b]
North America				
Rochester (Minn)[e] (27)	1945–54	71	23.8	22.1 (17.2–27.8)
(28)	1935–66	191	17.9	18.1 (15.6–20.9)
(29)	1967–79	138	19.7	19.1 (16.1–22.6)
Males		64	20.2	24.9 (19.1–31.8)
Females		74	19.3	15.8 (12.4–19.9)
Northern and Eastern Europe				
Iceland[f] (65)	1954–63	272	16.0	18.2 (16.0–23.6)
Turku (Finland)[d] (23)	1968–70	179	14.8	11.7 (10.0–13.6)
Males		67	11.7	13.1 (10.1–16.6)
Females		112	17.6	11.9 (10.0–14.3)
Carlisle (U.K.)[c] (85)	1955–61	80	12.1	9.4 (7.2–12.1)
Göteborg (Swe)[c] (71)	1957–61	270	6	
Arhus (Denmark)[d] (73)	1967–71		8.7	
Bulgaria[c] (148)	1981		16.3	
Poznan (Poland) (72)	1986	163	12.6	11.5 (9.9–13.5)
Males		78	12.5	13.2 (10.4–16.5)
Females		81	12.1	10.0 (7.9–12.4)
Southern Europe				
Sardinia (Italy)[d] (78)	1961–71	796	4.9	
Males		437	5.4	
Females		359	4.5	

Sassari (Italy)[d] (76)	1961–71	257	5.9	
Males		134	6.2	
Females		123	5.7	
Nuoro (Italy)[d] (77)	1961–71	166	5.3	
Males		93	5.9	
Females		73	4.7	
Southern Hemisphere				
Victoria (Australia)[e] (84)	1959–64	35	7.0	7.9 (5.5–10.9)
Asia				
Yonago (Japan) (74)	1975–79	62	10.2	
Sanin (Japan) (151)	1980		5.4	
29 provinces (China) [g] (69)			1.5	1.9 (1.5–2.5)
Males	1986	58		
Females		30	1.5	2.1 (1.4–3.1)
Africa		28	1.4	1.7 (1.2–2.5)
Benghazi (Libya) (79)	1982–84	58	4.5	

[a]Average annual incidence rates age-adjusted to 1970 United States total population.
[b]95% confidence interval given in parentheses was calculated from data given in the corresponding report.
[c]All parkinsonian cases included.
[d]Postencephalitic cases included.
[e]Arteriosclerotic and postencephalitic cases included.
[f]Arteriosclerotic cases included.
[g]Population screening of defined geographic area.

C. Age-Related Morbidity

The prevalence and incidence rates of Parkinson's disease increase steadily with advancing age (Tables 4 and 5; Figs. 2 and 3). The age-specific incidence rates for Parkinson's disease in North American, European, and Australian whites are very low in those younger than 40 years of age and increase sharply to a peak in the age group 70–79 years, apparently decreasing afterward at ages 80–85 years.

Age-specific prevalence ratios also follow a parallel increase up to ages 70–79 years (see Fig 2). It is conceivable that the alleged rarity of Parkinson's disease in the general population before the beginning of the Industrial Revolution could be due to the characteristic age distribution of Parkinson's disease. In fact, at the turn of the 19th century, survival for a person older than 40 years was uncommon (86), which would have greatly reduced the population at risk for developing Parkinson's disease. With increasing life expectancy (87), there has been a considerable increase both in the proportion of elderly population as well as in the number of persons living to the age of higher risk for Parkinson's disease. The age–distribution curve is also consistent with the current concept that Parkinson's disease is a disorder of age-related neuronal vulnerability (34,37,56,88–90), as well as with the alternative explanation that Parkinson's disease would require a long preclinical phase (46).

The observed incidence and prevalence in the eighth decade of life, although generally higher than that observed in the fourth, fifth, or sixth decades of life, is lower then the peak rates observed in the seventh decade. This may reflect the natural history of Parkinson's disease, but alternatively, may reflect the difficulty of diagnosing Parkinson's disease in this age group. Subjects in this age group have a high frequency of extrapyramidal symptoms and a higher rate of dementia, making distinctions between Parkinson's disease and other disorders more difficult.

D. Gender Differences

On the basis of age-adjusted morbidity (to 1970 U.S. population) a slight male preponderance of Parkinson's disease is found in most studies (see Tables 4, 5, and Fig. 4). The male/female ratios for prevalence range from 4.25 to 0.86 (see Chapter 10 for further discussion).

E. Time Trends

Several population studies from Rochester, Minnesota reported the incidence of parkinsonism and idiopathic Parkinson's disease in incremental time periods, covering the years 1935–1988 (27–29,91). The most current one (91) reassessed all previously reported cases using "modern diagnostic criteria" for idiopathic Parkinson's disease. Age- and sex-adjusted incidence rates over the period show

Table 4 Age-Specific Incidence of Parkinson's Disease per 100,000 for Both Sexes from Available Studies

Region	Age (yr)					
	≤39	40–49	50–59	60–69	70–79	80+
Europe						
Carlisle, UK (1955–61)[a] (85)	0	7.1	20.0	43.1	65.0	37.3
Turku, Finland (1968–70)[b] (23)	0.1	2.6	19.8	62.3	92.6	49.4
Males	3	2.6	25.2	51.5	83.2	57.9
Females	0	2.5	15.6	70.0	97.7	46.1
Iceland (1954–63) [c] (71)	0.3	5.6	32.9	97.2	136.2	(80–99) 69.2
Poznan, Poland (1985–86) (72)		(≤49) 0.7	26.5	62.9	74.6	33.9
Males		0.6	28.9	61.6	108.1	44.1
Females		0.8	24.4	56.3	54.4	29.8
Asia						
Chinese 29 provinces (1986)[e] (69)	0	0.7	3.0	6.1	18.7	16.5
Males	0	0.5	3.3	6.6	20.9	21.2
Females	0	0.9	2.7	5.6	16.8	13.6

Table 4 Continued

Region	Age (yr) ≤39	40–49	50–59	60–69	70–79	80+
Southern Hemisphere						
Victoria Australia (1959–64)[d] (84)	0.3	6.1	15.8	24.7	58.8[f]	
North America						
Rochester Minn (1935–44)[d] (28)	2	3.0	27.0	24.0	121.0	90.0
(1945–54)	0	5.0	18.0	87.0	214.0	136.0
(1955–66)	0	7.0	13.0	70.0	181.0	211.0
(1935–66)	1	5.0	18.0	65.0	174.0	167.0
Rochester Minn (1945–54)[d] (27)	0	7.8	23.9	99.8	(70–84) 189.6	(85+) 211.6
Rochester Minn (1967–79)[d] (29)	(≤29) 0	(30–54) 5.3	(55–64) 32.2	(65–74) 113.5	(75–84) 254.4	(85+) 155.4
Males	(≤29) 0	(30–54) 6.5	(55–64) 41.0	(65–74) 147.1	(75–84) 345.6	(85+) 175.3
Females	(≤29) 0	(30–54) 4.1	(55–64) 26.0	(65–74) 94.7	(75–84) 209.5	(85+) 148.2

[a]All parkinsonian cases included.
[b]Postencephalitic cases included.
[c]Arteriosclerotic cases included.
[d]Arteriosclerotic and postencephalitic cases included.
[e]Population screening of a defined geographic area.
[f]Aged 70 and older.

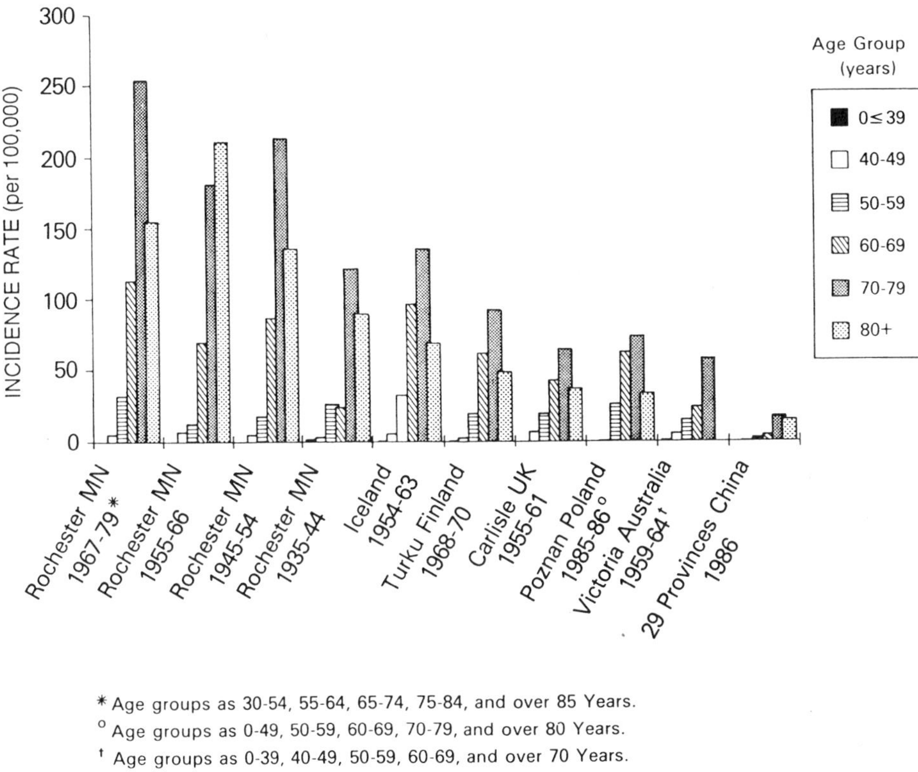

Figure 3 Average annual age-specific incidence rates for Parkinson's disease in seven countries (America, Europe, Australia, and Asia).

an upward, although not substantial, movement in the incidence rate. Tanner et al. (91) allow that even these modest changes over time may "reflect changing medical practice." Similarly, over a shorter time span (from 1961 to 1971) a slightly increasing rate has been observed in crude incidence rates in Italy. In contrast, in Iceland in the decade from 1954 to 1963 (65), the crude incidence rates appeared stable (Fig. 5). In a broad sense, these observations would suggest that, in these locations, Parkinson's disease has occurred at a relatively steady rate over the past 30 years.

F. Mortality Rate

Mortality data fails to adequately reflect the frequency of chronic neurological disorders, and this is particularly true for Parkinson's disease. In a Baltimore hospital survey (32), only 39% of deceased patients with Parkinson's disease

Table 5 Prevalence Ratios and Average Annual Incidence Rates of Parkinson's Disease per 100,000 Population by Sex From Available Studies

Region	Study period	Males		Females		Ratios M/F
		Crude	Age-adjusted[a,b]	Crude	Age-adjusted[a,b]	
Prevalence						
Northern America						
Baltimore MD						
Black (144)	1967–69	31	51 (40–65)	9	12 (7–21)	4.25[c]
White		128	14 (138–157)	121	103 (97–110)	1.43[c]
Copiah Co. MS[d,e] (18)	1978	116	96 (51–164)	145	96 (57–152)	1.00
Black		91	96 (31–223)	113	109 (43–224)	0.88
White		140	100 (43–196)	177	86 (43–154)	1.16
Europe						
Finland, Turku[f] (23)	1971	98	93 (81–108)	140	95 (85–107)	0.98
UK, Northampton (143)	1982	102	90 (74–109)	114	69 (58–83)	1.30
Scotland, Aberdeen (24)	1984		124 (103–151)		84 (71–100)	1.48[c]
Poland, Poznan (72)	1986	74	75 (68–83)	62	49 (45–55)	1.53[c]
Sassari, Sardinia[f] (76)	1971	83	81 (69–95)	73	66 (56–78)	1.23
Nuoro, Sardinia[f] (77)	1972	81	80 (66–97)	61	56 (45–69)	1.43

Sardinia[f] (78)	1972	74	76 (70–82)	58	55 (50–61)	1.38[c]
San Marino (17)	1986	154	129 (75–207)	150	104 (60–166)	1.24
Ferrara, Italy (66)	1987	160	133 (90–190)	219	123 (89–166)	1.08
Asia						
Japan, Yonago (74)	1982	63	67 (47–92)	97	78 (60–100)	0.86
Japan, Izumo (75)	1985	47	39 (23–61)	114	76 (56–102)	0.51
India, Parsis[d] (68)	1985	375	176	286	127	1.39
China, 29 provinces[d] (69)	1986	17	22 (20–25)	12	15 (13–17)	1.47[c]
Africa						
Libya, Benghazi (79)	1985	33	58 (47–72)	30	56 (44–70)	1.04
Incidence						
Rochester, MN[e] (29)	1967–79	20	25 (19–32)	19	16 (12–20)	1.58
Finland, Turku[f] (23)	1968–70	12	13 (10–17)	18	12 (10–14)	1.10
Poland, Poznan (72)	1985–86	13	13 (10–17)	12	10 (8–12)	1.32
China, 29 provinces[d] (69)	1986	1.5	2.1 (1–3)	1.4	1.7 (1–3)	1.24

[a]Age adjusted to 1970 United States total population and calculated from data given in the corresponding report.
[b]95% confidence interval given in parentheses was calculated from data given in the corresponding report.
[c]Indicates that the 95% confidence limits for the age-adjusted incidence rates for males and females did not overlap.
[d]Population screening of a defined geographic area.
[e]Arteriosclerotic and postencephalitic cases included.
[f]Postencephalitic cases included.

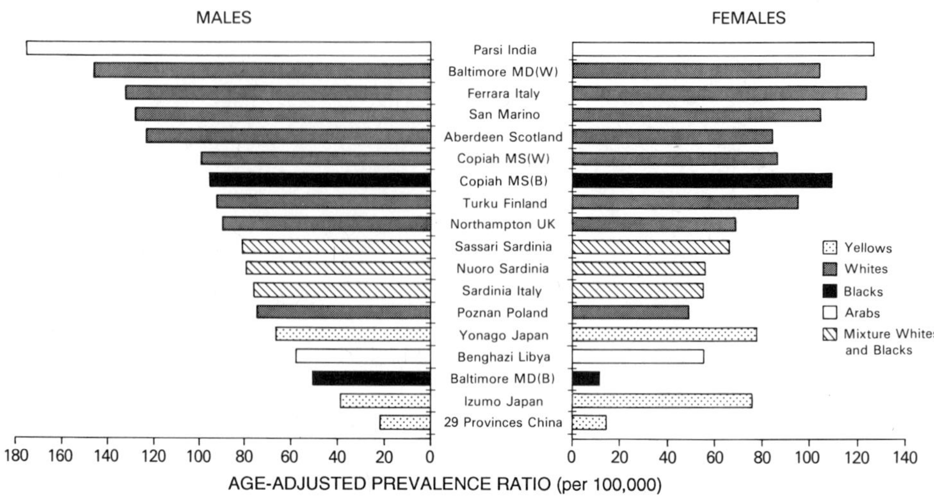

Figure 4 Worldwide comparison of sex distribution of age-adjusted prevalence ratios for Parkinson's disease by country, adjusted to the 1970 U.S. population (see Table 5).

had this diagnosis mentioned on their death certificates. Even when included on death certificates, the proportion of death certificates that indicated Parkinson's disease as the underlying cause of death was fairly low, with only a few studies observing rates above 35% (92,93). Moreover, death rates are a function of incidence, survival, comorbidity, prevalence at time of study, and other factors. Unfortunately, for large parts of the world, death records are the only source of information available on the frequency of Parkinson's disease.

A comparison of age-adjusted (direct method of standardization, using the 1950 U.S. population) mortality from Parkinson's disease for the years 1951–1958 in 33 countries ranged from a high of 3.8:100,000 for Australia to 0.5:100,000 for Mexico, Japan, Czechoslovakia, and nonwhites in the United States (94). The observed variation in death rates for Parkinson's disease in these countries must be considered only a rough measure of variation of disease frequency.

Keeping these limitations in mind, interesting geographic patterns for Parkinson's disease mortality have emerged from U.S. surveys. When the annual death rates of Parkinson's disease as an underlying cause of death in the United States from 1950 to 1984 were compared with Denmark from 1956 to 1985 (95,96), a clear excess is noted in Parkinson's disease mortality in both countries for men over women, and in the United States also for whites over blacks. An unexpected increase in the death rates was noted between 1976 and 1984 in both countries, for men and women, and was considered to be an indirect effect of available

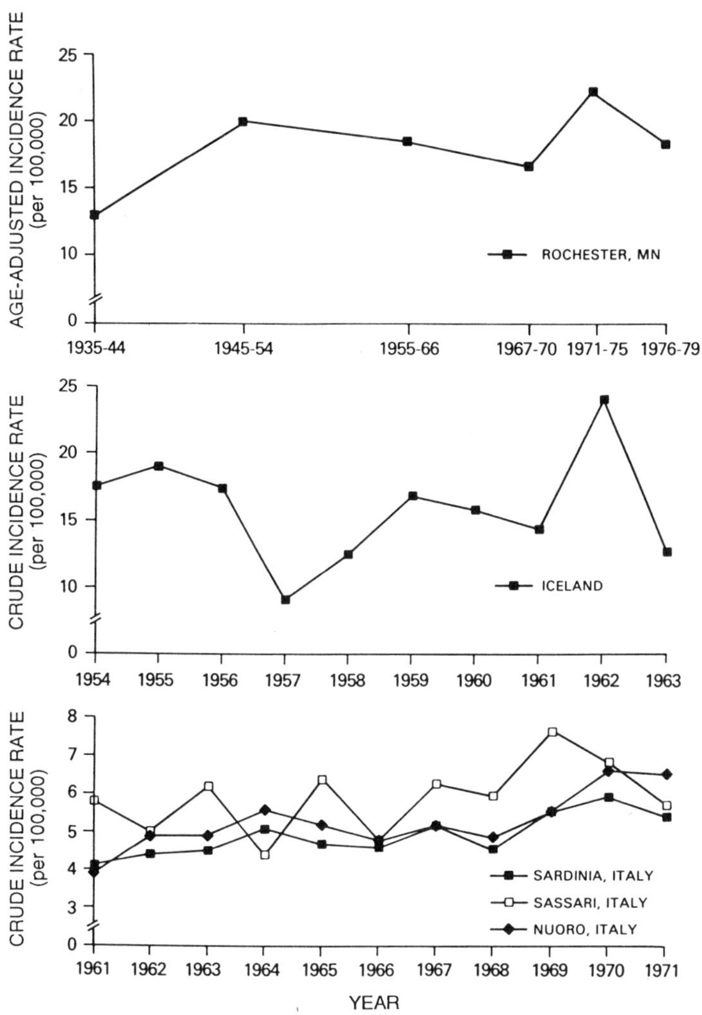

Figure 5 Average annual age-adjusted incidence rates over time for Parkinson's disease in Rochester, Minnesota (1935–1979), and crude incidence rates for Iceland (1954–1963) (65); and Sardinia (76), Sassari (77), and Nuoro (78), Italy (1961–1971).

treatment, which makes the condition more likely to be listed in the death certificate.

A north–south gradient of Parkinson's disease mortality has also been observed in the United States (Fig. 6) (97). The age-adjusted (to 1960 U.S. total white population) mortality rate from Parkinson's disease was 1.7:100,000 popu-

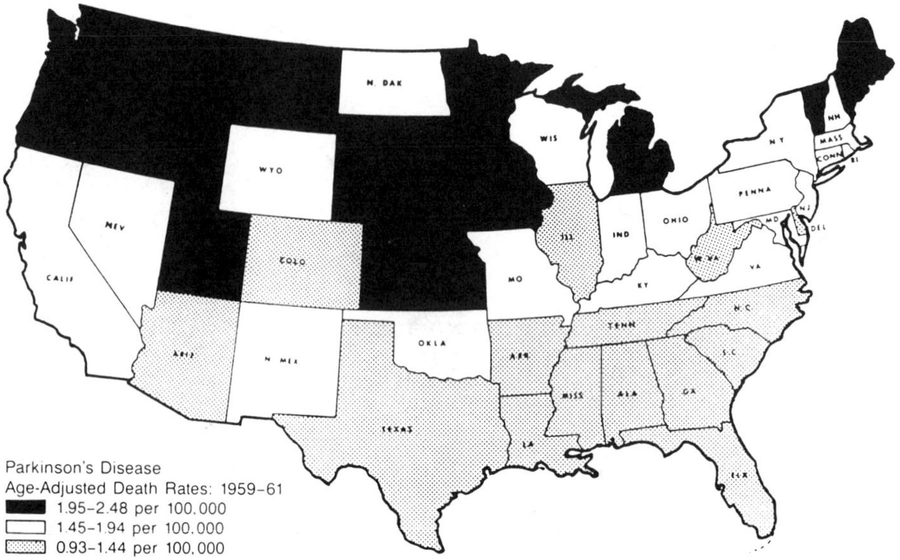

Figure 6 Age-adjusted (to 1960 U.S. total white population) average annual death rates per 100,000 population for Parkinson's disease by state of residence at death, whites only, coterminous United States, 1959–1961.

lation, among whites only, for the United States as a whole during the period 1959–1961. The lowest mortality rate (0.9) was found in Louisiana; in general, the states lying below the 37°–38° latitude north (i.e., the southern tier) showed a Parkinson's disease mortality rate at or below the national average. Conversely, the highest mortality rate (2.5:100,000) was found in Vermont. This north–south gradient of Parkinson's disease mortality within the United States is considered to be an argument in favor of an environmental cause for Parkinson's disease (97,98).

Geographic differences have also been reported among provinces in Canada, although the pattern is not as clear as the one observed in the United States (99). Rybicki and colleagues (100) examined geographic difference in Parkinson's disease death rates in Michigan counties and suggest "a geographic association in Parkinson's disease mortality and the industrial use of heavy metals."

Mortality rates for Parkinson's disease have remained relatively stable through the 1980s in the United States, England, and Wales (98,99,101–103). From 1959 to 1961, the age-adjusted mortality rate for Parkinson's disease in the United States was 1.7:100,000 population (range 0.9–2.5; 97); from 1962 to 1975, it ranged from 1.4 to 1.6 (101); and from 1979 to 1983, it reached 1.7 (95). This observation has been confirmed by incidence trends (see Fig.5).

However, from a mathematical model proposed by Gompertz in 1825, an increase in the annual crude Parkinson's disease mortality rate for men and women since 1980 has been demonstrated in the United States, in comparison with the stable mortality rates observed from 1955 to 1979 (104). Recent increased mortality for Parkinson's disease in the United States may reflect the "graying out" of the population, with progressively larger numbers of elderly subjects surviving into advanced age as well as improved diagnosis or improved reporting as potential reasons.

The overall stability in Parkinson's disease mortality rates up to the 1980s masks differential age-specific mortality rates for Parkinson's disease in the United States that showed substantial decline for the middle-aged, but notable increases for the elderly among whites and nonwhites of both sexes (103). The rates have increased steadily with advancing age, reaching a peak at ages 77–80 years, in the 1960s, and at ages 82–85 in the 1980s (96).

IV. WESTERN PACIFIC PARKINSONISM–DEMENTIA AND AMYOTROPHIC LATERAL SCLEROSIS: AN EPIDEMIOLOGICAL CASE STUDY

A prototypic example of the usefulness of epidemiological research is the study of the neurodegenerative disorders found in the western Pacific islands. Parkinsonism–dementia complex (PDC) and amyotrophic lateral sclerosis (ALS) (105–109) are observed with extremely high prevalence among inhabitants of Guam, New Guinea (Irian Jaya, Indonesia), and Japan (Kii Peninsula, Honshu). Amyotrophic lateral sclerosis was called *lytico* or *paralítico* by the native Chamorros in the island of Guam. In 1931, the diagnosis of ALS appeared on death certificates. In 1945, the occurrence of these cases among Chamorros was first confirmed at autopsy by Zimmerman (110). Subsequent reports on the extremely high incidence of ALS among native Chamorros attracted the attention of investigators and prompted the first epidemiological surveys in 1953. During the 1950s, surveys for ALS disclosed patients presenting with a combination of parkinsonism and dementia; this was recognized as a new entity, designated the parkinsonism–dementia complex (PDC) (111). A possible case of PDC was reported as early as 1936 (112), and the disease was known locally as *Lytico-Bodig* or *rayput*. From the pathological viewpoint, PDC is clearly different from Parkinson's disease, with presence of characteristic neurofibrillary tangles, rather than Lewy bodies (113). Both ALS and PDC occurred with high incidence, often in the same family and, occasionally, in the same individual. Years of investigation of western Pacific ALS–PDC have provided important clues about the etiology and pathogenesis of Parkinson's disease and other age-related neurodegenerative diseases.

During the past 30 years downward trends in age-adjusted incidence rates for

ALS–PDC were documented, ranging from over 60:100,000 in 1959–1961 to 11:100,000 per year in 1983–1985 for men, and from over 20:100,000 in 1956–1958 to fewer than 5:100,000 per year in 1983–1985 for women (34). Concurrently, an upward trend in age at onset was seen for Chamorros of both sexes (34,109,114). Since 1980, new cases have occurred only among persons older than 50 years of age, whereas a younger age at onset had been noted in the past (34). Changes in the epidemiological pattern may also be reflected in the increasing prevalence of dementia in recent years, associated with a decline in the frequency of the PDC type among older Chamorros (115). During 1956 through 1985, the highest rates of PDC for both sexes combined were found in the southern and central districts (Umatac, Inarajan, Sinajana, Yona, and Barrigada); the lowest rates in northern and western districts (Dededo, Piti, Santa Rita, Asan, and Tamuning; Fig. 7) (116). On Guam, during 1956–1985, there was a high level of familial aggregation for PDC, with approximately 42% of cases being familial; also the risk of PDC in susceptible sibships was 12 times higher than that in the general population for districts with the highest incidence rates, and 92 times higher for districts with the lowest incidence rates (116). The high familial aggregation of PDC was inconsistent with monogenic inheritance (116–120). It suggests a common exposure within the family unit, or common exposures in the presence of hereditary susceptibilities.

In the past few years there have been changes not only in the epidemiological patterns observed, but also in the clinical and pathological profiles of the disease. These include increased development of supranuclear disturbances of gaze in Chamorros with PDC, impairment of olfactory function in the aging population on Guam, and presence of a pigmentary retinopathy resembling posterior ophthalmomyiasis interna in Chamorros with ALS–PDC. These findings might indicate that the clinical characteristics of the disease are changing (121–123). In neuropathological features, senile plaques have been found in some Chamorro patients in addition to Alzheimer's neurofibrillary tangles, suggesting that the pattern of lesions is moving toward that of Alzheimer's disease (123,124). The involvement of pontine regions in a PDC case was similar to that seen in patients with progressive supranuclear palsy (124), and many neurons containing Pick bodies were found in a patient with clinical diagnosis of PDC (125).

These observations, combined with birth cohort analysis and migration surveys (from and to Guam), strongly suggest that PDC is an acquired condition. Environmental factors associated with socioeconomic status appear to play an important role in the occurrence of PDC (126). Moreover, evidence suggests that the length of the preclinical period may range from several years to decades, and it seems to have increased with time; the risk of acquiring PDC has declined since the late 1950s. The critical age of exposure to an unknown factor in the environment on Guam appears to have been during adolescence or adulthood (34).

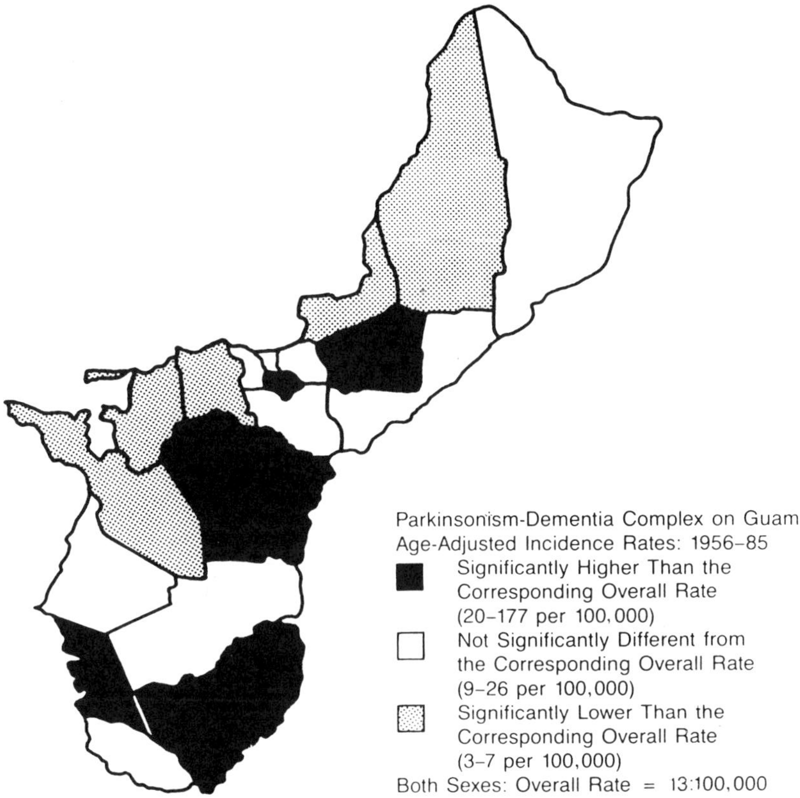

Figure 7 Distribution of average annual age-adjusted incidence rates of parkinsonism–dementia complex by district for all residents of Guam and both sexes combined. The patterns are based on comparisons of the district-specific rates with the corresponding overall rates for Guam.

Over the past 30 years, several etiological hypotheses of ALS–PDC have been developed; those linked to cycad use and to metal exposure remain actively studied. In 1987, Spencer and colleagues (127) reported that the excitotoxin β-*N*-methylamino-L-alanine (BMAA), found in *Cycas circinalis*, induced spasticity and bradykinesia in primates associated with pathological changes of motoneurons. The major new observation is the detection of two neurotoxins (cycasin and BMAA) in Chamorro cycad flour obtained from 17 Chamorro residents of nine districts of Guam (128). Cycasin is the major component of cycad seed (2–4 %), conversely BMAA is present in low concentrations in Chamorro flour. They noted that the content of cycasin in Chamorro flour from several districts was significantly correlated with incidence rates of PDC in the various districts

(Pearson correlation coefficient $= 0.99$, $p < 0.000001$). However, there was no statistically significant association for BMAA (Table 6). The relation between cycad and neurodegeneration as well as the presence of long latency has received epidemiological support (129–131). Although the human equivalent to the very large doses of BMAA used in animal experiments seem unlikely to have been used by local people (132,133), this hypothesis is currently under active research.

Recently, contamination with zinc of cycad flour prepared in the traditional Guamanian way has been demonstrated (134). Neurotoxicity to cultured neurons from mesencephalon and cerebellum was not dependent on the BMAA content, but on the concentration of zinc in the flour (134). This observation would give further support to the potential role of metals in neurodegenerative diseases (135). Deficient nutritional intakes of calcium, associated with absorption and neuronal deposition of aluminum, iron, and other ions, have also been advanced as potential causes (136–139). Some difficulties exist to conform the epidemiological patterns of PDC on Guam to these two hypotheses (116,132,140). Further epidemiological and laboratory investigations are needed to better understand the cause of PDC on Guam (see also Chapter 12).

Table 6 Pearson's Correlation Coefficients Between Average Annual Age-Adjusted Incidence Rates of PDC, 1956–1985, and Content of Cycad Toxins in Flour Samples Obtained From Nine Districts on Guam

		Average concentration[b]	
	Incidence rates[a] (per 100,000)	BMAA (μg/g)	Cycasin (μg/g)
Umatac	177	2.20	63.67
Inarajana	41	13.31	11.39
Sinajana	32	2.50	7.01
Merizo	26	18.39	7.89
Talofofo	24		0.63
Mongmong	13	1.18	7.23
Yigo	11	4.90	6.33
Agat	10	1.02	0.004
Tumon	7		0.43
Correlation coefficient		−0.14	0.99
p value		0.8	0.000001

Source:
[a]Derived from Ref. 116.
[b]Derived from Ref. 128. Values are the mean (μ/g flour) for each district.

V. CONCLUSIONS

Epidemiological studies of Parkinson's disease are fraught with difficulties, but provide both a framework for future etiologic studies and a number of useful research tools. However, there is the need to establish universally accepted diagnostic criteria and methods for the design of epidemiological studies of Parkinson's disease to undertake the task of accurately studying the frequency, natural history, and etiology of this disorder.

The possible etiology of Parkinson's disease should be considered within the framework of the following tentative findings derived from descriptive studies: (1) There are significant *geographic differences* reported in the frequency of Parkinson's disease occurrence throughout the world, ranging from a low age-adjusted prevalence ratio of 18:100,000 in China, to a high of 182:100,000 in Iceland. Whether this observed ten fold difference is artifactual or due to racial or environmental differences remains to be clarified. (2) In favor of a smaller role for genetic factors is the observation that blacks in the United States have higher age-adjusted Parkinson's disease prevalence ratios than blacks in Africa. (3) Common to all ethnic groups is the slight preponderance of Parkinson's disease in men and the substantial increase in disease risk with age, reaching a peak of incidence at age 70–79 years and falling thereafter.

In the final analysis, the etiology of Parkinson's disease will probably be found to result from the interplay of factors in the classic triad of epidemiological causation: host (genetic susceptibility), agent, and environment. Analytic epidemiological approaches should help in the task of defining which ones, among the multitude of naturally occurring potential neurotoxic and infectious agents that have surrounded human environments for centuries, are important determinants in the pathogenesis of Parkinson's disease.

REFERENCES

1. Gourie-Devi M, Ramu MG, Venkataram BS. Treatment of Parkinson's disease in 'Ayurveda' (ancient India system of medicine): discussion paper. J R Soc Med 1991; 84:491–492.
2. Vaidya AB, Rajagopalan TG, Mankodi NA, et al. Treatment of Parkinson's disease with the cowhage plant—*Mucuna pruriens* Bak. Neurology (India) 1978; 26:171–176.
3. Huang Di. Huang Di Nei Jing plain question. Beijing: People's Health Press, 1963:538–539.
4. Parkinson J. An essay on the shaking palsy. London: Whittingham and Rowland for Sherwood, Neely, Jones 1817.
5. Brissaud E. Leçons sur les maladies nerveuses. Paris: Masson et Cie, 1895.
6. Blocq P, Marinesco G. Sur un cas de tremblement parkinsonien hémiplégique

symptomatique d'une tumeur du peduncule cérébral. Mem Soc Biol 1893; 45:105–111.
7. Trétiakoff C. Contribution à l'étude de l'anatomie pathologique du locus niger de Soemmering avec quelques deductions relatives a la pathogenie des troubles du tonus musculaire et de la maladie de Parkinson. 1919.
8. Ehringer H, Hornykiewicz O. Verteilung von Noradrenalin und Dopamin (3-Hydroxytyramin) in Gehirn des Menschen und ihr Verhalten bei Erkrankungen des extrapyramidalen Systems. Klin Wochenschr 1960:1236–1239.
9. Lewy FH. Paralysis agitans. I Pathologische Anatomie. In: Lewandowsky M, ed. Handbuch der Neurologie. Berlin: Springer, 1912:920–933.
10. Gerstenbrand F, Poewe WH. The classification of Parkinson's disease. In: Stern G, ed. Parkinson's disease. London: Chapman & Hall, 1990:315–331.
11. Langston JW, Ballard PA, Tetrud JW, Irwin I. Chronic Parkinsonism in humans due to a product of meperidine-analog synthesis. Science 1983; 219:979–980.
12. Rothman K. Modern epidemiology. Boston: Little Brown & Co, 1986.
13. Kelsey JL, Thompson WD, Evans AS. Methods in observational epidemiology. New York: Oxford University Press, 1986.
14. MacMahon B, Pugh TF. Epidemiology—principles and methods. Boston: Little, Brown & Company, 1970.
15. Forno LS. Pathology of Parkinson's disease, the importance of the substantia nigra and the Lewy bodies. In: Stern G, ed. Parkinson's disease. London: Chapman & Hall, 1990:185–238.
16. Gibb WRG, Lees AJ. The relevance of the Lewy body to the pathogenesis of idiopathic Parkinson's disease. J Neurol Neurosurg Psychiatry 1988; 51: 745–752.
17. D'Alessandro R, Gamberini G, Granieri E, Benassi G, Naccarato S, Manzaroli D. Prevalence of Parkinson's disease in the Republic of San Marino. Neurology 1987; 37:1679–1682.
18. Schoenberg BS, Anderson DW, Haerer AF. Prevalence of Parkinson's disease in the biracial population of Copiah County, Mississippi. Neurology 1985; 35:841–845.
19. Marder K, Mayeux R. The epidemiology of dementia in patients with Parkinson's disease. Adv Exp Med Biol 1991; 295:439–445.
20. Cooper B. The epidemiology of primary degenerative dementia and related neurological disorders. Eur Arch Psychiatry Clin Neurosci 1991:240:223–233.
21. Cummings JL. Depression and Parkinson's disease: a review. Am J Psychiatry 1992; 149:443–454.
22. Pollock M, Hornabrook RW. The prevalence, natural history and dementia of Parkinson's disease. Brain 1966; 89:429–448.
23. Marttila RJ, Rinne U. Epidemiology of Parkinson's disease in Finland. Acta Neurol Scand 1976; 53:81–102.
24. Mutch WJ, Dingwall-Fordyce I, Downie AW, Paterson JG, Roy SK. Parkinson's disease in a Scottish city. Br Med J 1986; 292:534–536.
25. Hughes AJ, Daniel SE, Kilford L, Lees AJ. Accuracy of clinical diagnosis of idiopathic Parkinson's disease: a clinico-pathological study of 100 cases. Neurol Neurosurg Psychiatry 1992; 55:181–184.

26. Snow B, Wiens M, Hertzman C, Calne DB. A community survey of Parkinson's disease. Can Med Assoc J 1989; 141:418–422.
27. Kurland LT. Epidemiology: incidence, geographic distribution and genetic considerations. In: Field WS, ed. Pathogenesis and treatment of parkinsonism. Springfield, IL: Charles C Thomas, 1958:5–49.
28. Nobrega FT, Glattre E, Kurland LT, Okazaki H. Comments on the epidemiology of parkinsonism including prevalence and incidence statistics for Rochester, Minnesota, 1935–1966. In: Barbeau A, Brunette JR, eds. Progress in neuro-genetics. Proceedings of the international congress of neuro-genetics and neuro-opthalmology. Amsterdam: Exerpta Medica, 1969:474–485.
29. Rajput AH, Offord KP, Beard CM, Kurland LT. Epidemiology of parkinsonism: incidence, classification, and mortality. Ann Neurol 1984; 16:278–282.
30. Hoehn MM, Yahr MD. Parkinsonism: onset, progression and mortality. Neurology 1967; 17:427–442.
31. Chandra V, Bharucha E, Schoenberg BS. Mortality data for the US for deaths due to and related to twenty neurologic diseases. Neuroepidemiology 1984; 3:149–168.
32. Kessler II. Epidemiologic studies of Parkinson's disease. II. A hospital-based survey. Am J Epidemiol 1972; 95:308–318.
33. Langston JW. Predicting Parkinson's disease. Neurology 1990; 40(suppl):70–74.
34. Zhang ZX, Anderson DW, Lavine L, Mantel N. Patterns of acquiring parkinsonism–dementia complex on Guam: 1944 through 1985. Arch Neurol 1990; 47:1019–1024.
35. Garruto RM, Gajdusek DC, Chen KM. Amyotrophic lateral sclerosis among Chamorro migrants from Guam. Ann Neurol 1980; 8:612–619.
36. Mawdsley C, Manc MB, Ferguson FR. Neurological disease in boxers. Lancet 1963; 2:795–801.
37. Calne DB. Options for the etiology of Parkinson's disease: the association with dementia. Mt Sinai J Med 1988; 55:58–61.
38. Duvoisin RC, Yahr MD. Encephalitis and parkinsonism. Arch Neurol 1965; 12:227–239.
39. Abel EN, Nassanein M. Neuropsychiatric manifestations of chronic manganese poisoning. J Neurol Neurosurg Psychiatry 1965; 28:282–285.
40. Mena I, Marin O, Fuenzalida S, Cotzias G. Chronic manganese poisoning. Clinical picture and manganese turnover. Neurology 1967; 17:128–136.
41. Ringel S, Klawans H. Carbon monoxide induced parkinsonism. J Neurol Sci 1972; 16:245–251.
42. Klawans HL Jr. Hemiparkinsonism as a late complication of hemiatrophy. A new syndrome. Neurology 1981; 31:625–628.
43. Buchman AS, Goetz C, Klawans H. Hemiparkinsonism with hemiatrophy. Neurology 1988; 38:527–530.
44. Calne S, Schoenberg BS, Martin W, Uitti RJ, Spencer P, Calne DB. Familial Parkinson's disease: possible role of environmental factors. Can J Neurol Sci 1987; 14:303–305.
45. Ward CD, Duvoisin RC, Ince SE, Nutt JD, Eldridge R, Calne DB. Parkinson's disease in 65 pairs of twins and in a set of quadruplets. Neurology 1983; 33:815–824.

46. Koller WC, Langston JW, Hubble JP, et al. Does a long pre-clinical period occur in Parkinson's disease? Neurology 1991; 41(suppl 2):8–13.
47. Factor SA. Letter to the Editor. Mov Disord 1989; 4:284–285.
48. Cox DR, Oakes D. Analysis of survival data. New York: Chapman & Hall, 1993.
49. Ho SC, Woo J, Lee CM. Epidemiologic study of Parkinson's disease in Hong Kong. Neurology 1989; 39:1314–1318.
50. Tanner CM, Chen B, Wang WZ, et al. Environmental factors and Parkinson's disease: a case–control study in China. Neurology 1989; 39:660–664.
51. Ellenberg JH, Nelson KB. Sample selection and the natural history of disease. JAMA 1992; 1980:1337–1340.
52. Golbe LI, Cody RA, Duvoisin RC. Smoking and Parkinson's disease. Search for a dose–response relationship. Arch Neurol 1986; 43:774–778.
53. Langston JW, Koller W. The next frontier in Parkinson's disease: presymptomatic detection. Neurology 1991; 41(suppl 2):5–7.
54. Ellenberg JH. Preclinical detection in studies of the etiology, natural history, and treatment of Parkinson's disease. Neurology 1991; 41(suppl 2):14–22.
55. Dawber TR. The Framingham study—the epidemiology of atherosclerotic disease. Cambridge: Harvard University Press, 1980.
56. Koller WC. When does Parkinson's disease begin? Neurology 1992; 42(suppl 4):27–31.
57. Doty RL, Perl DP, Steele JC, et al. Odor identification deficit of the parkinsonism–dementia complex of Guam: equivalence to that of Alzheimer's and idiopathic Parkinson's disease. Neurology 1991; 41(suppl 2):77–80.
58. Brooks DJ. Detection of preclinical Parkinson's disease with PET. Neurology 1991; 41(suppl 2):24–28.
59. Carvey PM, McRae A, Flint TF, et al. The potential use of a dopamine neuron antibody and a striatal-derived neurotrophic factor as diagnostic markers in Parkinson's disease. Neurology 1991; 41(suppl 2):53–60.
60. Garland HG. Refresher course for general practitioners: parkinsonism. Br Med J 1952; 1:153–155.
61. Pickle LW, Mason TJ, Howard N, Hoover R, Fraumeni JF. Atlas of U.S. cancer mortality among whites: 1950–1980. NIH (87–2900), 1987:6.
62. Kahn HA. An introduction to epidemiologic methods. Oxford: Oxford University Press, 1983:25–37.
63. Schoenberg BD. Calculation of confidence intervals for rates and ratios: simplified method utilizing tabular values based on the Poisson distribution. Neuroepidemiology 1983; 2:257–265.
64. Zhang ZX, Román GC. Worldwide occurrence of Parkinson's disease: an updated review. Neuroepidemiology 1993; 12:195–208.
65. Gudmundsson KR. A clinical survey of parkinsonism in Iceland. Acta Neurol Scand [Suppl] 1967; 33:1–61.
66. Casetta I, Granieri E, Govoni V, et al. Epidemiology of Parkinson's disease in Italy. A descriptive survey in the U.S.L. of Cento, province of Ferrara, Emilia-Romagna. Acta Neurol (Naples) 1990; 12:284–291.
67. Bademosi O, Al-Rajeh IH, Awada A, et al. Prevalence of Parkinson's disease

(PD) in an Arab community: the Thugbah study. In: Congrés de neurologie tropicale. Sept 26–28, 1991. Limoges: Recherche en Neurologie Tropicale Press, 1991:27.
68. Bharucha NE, Bharucha EP, Bharucha AE, Bhise AV, Schoenberg BS. Prevalence of Parkinson's disease in the Parsi community in Bombay, India. Arch Neurol 1988; 45:1321–1323.
69. Wang Y, Shi Y, Wu S He Y, Zhang B. Parkinson's disease in China. Chin Med J 1991; 960–964.
70. Li SC, Schoenberg BS, Wang CC, et al. A prevalence survey of Parkinson's disease and other movement disorders in the People's Republic of China. Arch Neurol 1985; 42:655–657.
71. Broman T. Parkinson's syndrome, prevalence and incidence in Goteborg. Acta Neurol Scand [Suppl] 1963; 4:95–101.
72. Wender M, Pruchnik D, Kowal P, Florczak J, Zalejski M. [Epidemiology of Parkinson disease in the Pozna'n province]. Przegl Epidemiol 1989; 43:150–155.
73. Dupont E. Epidemiology of parkinsonism. The Parkinson investigation, Arhus, Denmark (preliminary results). In: Worm-Peterson J, Bottcher J, eds. Symposium on parkinsonism. Denmark: Merck, Sharp & Dohme, 1977:65–75.
74. Harada H, Nishikawa S, Takahashi K. Epidemiology of Parkinson's disease in a Japanese city. Arch Neurol 1983:40:151–154.
75. Okada K, Kobayashi S, Tsunematsu T. Prevalence of Parkinson's disease in Izumo City, Japan. Gerontology 1990; 36:340–344.
76. Rosati G, Granieri E, Pinna L, et al. Parkinson's disease. Prevalence and incidence in the Province of Sassari, North Sardinia. Acta Neurol (Naples) 1978; 33:201–207.
77. Rosati G, Granieri E, Pinna L, Devoto MC. The frequency of Parkinson's disease in the province of Nuoro (Sardinia). Acta Neurol Scand 1979; 1:303–308.
78. Rosati G, Granieri E, Pinna L, et al. The risk of Parkinson's disease in Mediterranean people. Neurology 1980; 30:250–255.
79. Ashok PP, Radhakrishnan K, Sridharan R, Mousa ME. Epidemiology of Parkinson's disease in Benghazi, north-east Libya. Clin Neurol Neurosurg 1986; 88:109–113.
80. Schoenberg BS, Osuntokun BO, Adeuja AO, et al. Comparison of the prevalence of Parkinson's disease in black populations in the rural United States and rural Nigeria: door-to-door community studies. Neurology 1988; 38:645–646.
81. Diamond SG, Markham CH, Hoehn MM, McDowell FH, Muenter MD. Effect of age at onset on progression and mortality in Parkinson's disease. Neurology 1989; 39:1187–1190.
82. Diamond SG, Markham CH, Hoehn MM, McDowell FH, Muenter MD. An examination of male–female differences in progression and mortality of Parkinson's disease. Neurology 1990; 40:763–766.
83. Ebmeier KP, Calder SA, Crawford JR, Stewart L, Besson JOA, Mutch WJ. Mortality and causes of death in idiopathic Parkinson's disease: results from the Aberdeen whole population study. Scott Med J 1990; 35:173–175.

84. Jenkins AC. Epidemiology of parkinsonism in Victoria. Med J Aust 1966; 2:496–502.
85. Brewis M, Poskanzer DC, Rolland C, Miller H. Neurological disease in an English city. Acta Neurol Scand [Suppl] 1966; 24:1–89.
86. U. S. Bureau of the Census. Historical statistics of the United States, colonial times to 1957—Card A 60–9150. Washington: Library of Congress, 1960.
87. U. S. Bureau of the Census. Statistical abstract of the United States. Washington: Bureau of the Census, 1991.
88. Brizzee KR. Risk factors for senility. In: Rothschild H, ed. Pathophysiology of aging. New York: Oxford University Press, 1984:44–62.
89. Forno LS, Alford EC Jr. The pathology of parkinsonism. Some observations and new correlations. Contemp Neurol 1971; 8:120–130.
90. Hornykiewicz O. Parkinson's disease and its chemotherapy. Biochem Pharmacol 1975; 24:1061–1065.
91. Tanner CM, Thelen JA, Offord KP, Rademacher D, Goetz CG, Kurland LT. Parkinson's disease (PD) incidence in Olmsted County, MN: 1935–1988. Neurology 1992; 42: (suppl 3):194.
92. Kessler II. Parkinson's disease: perspectives on epidemiology and pathogenesis. Prev Med 1973; 2:88–105.
93. Marmot M. Mortality and Parkinson's disease. In: Rose FC, Capildeo R, eds. Research progress in Parkinson's disease. Kent: Tunbridge Wells, 1981:9–16.
94. Goldberg ID, Kurland LT. Mortality in 33 countries from diseases of the nervous system. World Neurol 1972; 3:444–463.
95. Sethi KD, Meador KJ, Loring D, Meador MP. Neuroepidemiology of Parkinson's disease: analysis of mortality data for the U. S. A. and Georgia. Int J Neurosci 1989; 46:87–92.
96. Kurtzke JF, Murphy FM. The changing patterns of death rates in parkinsonism. Neurology 1990; 40:42–49.
97. Lux WE, Kurtzke JF. Is Parkinson's disease acquired? Evidence from a geographic comparison with multiple sclerosis. Neurology 1987; 37:467–471.
98. Kurland LT, Kurtzke JF, Goldberg ID, Choi NW, Williams G. Parkinsonism. In: Epidemiology of neurologic and sense organ disorders. Cambridge: Harvard University Press, 1973:41–63.
99. Svenson LW. Geographic distribution of deaths due to Parkinson's disease in Canada: 1979–1986. Mov Disord 1990; 5:322–324.
100. Rybicki BA, Johnson CC, Uman J, Gorell JM. Parkinson's disease mortality and the industrial use of heavy metals in Michigan. Mov Disord 1993; 8:87–92.
101. Kurtzke JF, Kurland LT. The epidemiology of neurologic disease. In: Baker AB, Baker LH, eds. Clinical neurology. Philadelphia: Harper & Row, 1985: 455–460.
102. Duvoisin RC, Schweitzer MD. Paralysis agitans mortality in England and Wales 1855–1962. Br J Prev Soc Med 1966; 20:27–33.
103. Lilienfeld DE, Chan E, Ehland J, et al. Two decades of increasing mortality from Parkinson's disease among the US elderly. Arch Neurol 1990; 47: 731–734.
104. Riggs JE. Longitudinal gompertzian analysis of Parkinson's disease mortality in the U. S., 1955–1986: the dramatic increase in overall mortality since 1980 is the

natural consequence of deterministic mortality dynamics. Mech Age Dev 1990; 55:221–233.

105. Kurland LT, Mulder DW. Epidemiologic investigations of amyotrophic lateral sclerosis. I. Preliminary report on geographic distribution, with special reference to the Mariana Island, including clinical and pathologic observations. Neurology 1954; 4:355–378.
106. Gajdusek DC. Motor-neuron disease in natives in New Guinea. N Engl J Med 1963; 268:474–476.
107. Shiraki H, Yase Y. Amyotrophic lateral sclerosis. In: Vinken P, Bruyn G, eds. Handbook of clinical neurology, vol. 22. System disorders and atrophies, part II. Amsterdam: Elsevier, 1975:353–419.
108. Garruto RM, Yase Y. Neurodegenerative disorders of the western Pacific: the search for mechanisms of pathogenesis. Trends Neurosci 1986; 9:368–374.
109. Reed D, Labarthe D, Chen KM, Stallones R. A cohort study of amyotrophic lateral sclerosis and parkinsonism–dementia on Guam and Rota. Am J Epidemiol 1987; 125:92–100.
110. Zimmerman HM. Monthly report to medical officer in command. U S Naval Medical Research 1945; 2.
111. Reed D, Plato C, Elizan T, Kurland LT. The amyotrophic lateral sclerosis/parkinsonism–dementia complex: a ten years follow-up on Guam. I. Epidemiology studies. Am J Epidemiol 1966; 83:54–73.
112. Okaya N. A case of paralysis agitans in the Chamorro people (Micronesian) of the U. S. Territory of Guam. Tokyo Med J 1936; 2997:2517–1518.
113. Hirano A, Malamud N, Kurland LT. Parkinsonism–dementia complex, an endemic disease on the island of Guam. II. Pathological features. Brain 1961; 84:662–679,
114. Garruto RM, Yanagihara R, Gajdusek DC. Disappearance of high-incidence amyotrophic lateral sclerosis and parkinsonism–dementia on Guam. Neurology 1985; 35:193–198.
115. Chen KM. Dementias other than ALS/PDC occuring on Gaum. Presented at international symposium on neurodegenerative disorders in the western Pacific region, on Guam, Feb 17–18, 1992.
116. Zhang ZX, Anderson DW, Mantel N. Geographic patterns of parkinsonism–dementia complex on Guam: 1956 through 1985. Arch Neurol 1990; 47:1069–1074.
117. Plato CC, Garruto RM, Fox KM, Gajdusek DC. Amyotrophic lateral sclerosis and parkinsonism–dementia on Guam: a 25-year prospective case–control study. Am J Epidemiol 1986; 124:643–656.
118. Plato CC, Cruz MT, Kurland LT. Amyotrophic lateral sclerosis–parkinsonism dementia complex of Guam: further genetic investigations. Am J Hum Genet 1969; 21:133–141.
119. Plato CC, Reed DM, Elizan TS, Kurland LT. Amyotrophic lateral sclerosis–parkinsonism–dementia complex of Guam. IV. Familial and genetic investigations. Am J Hum Genet 1967; 19:617–632.
120. Reed DM, Torres JM, Brody JA. Amyotrophic lateral sclerosis and parkinsonism–dementia on Guam, 1945–1972. II. Familial and genetic studies. Am J Epidemiol 1975; 101:302–310.

121. Lepore FE, Steele JC, Cox TA, et al. Supranuclear disturbances of ocular motility in Lytico–Bodig. Neurology 1988; 38:1849–53.
122. Hirano A. Cytopathology of amyotrophic lateral sclerosis. Adv Neurol 1991; 56:91–101.
123. Cox TA, McDarby JV, Lavine L, Steele JC, Calne DB. A retinopathy on Guam with high prevalence in Lytico–Bodig. Ophthalmology 1989; 96:1731–5.
124. Perl D. An appraisal of recent cases of ALS/PDC in Guam. Int ALS–MND Update 1989; 2Q:14.
125. Bergeron C, Steele JC. Guam Parkinson–dementia complex and amyotrophic lateral sclerosis: clinic-pathological correlation of seven cases. Int ALS–MND Update 1989; 2Q:13–14.
126. Reed DM, Brody JA. Amyotrophic lateral sclerosis and parkinsonism–dementia on Guam, 1945–1972. I. Descriptive epidemiology. Am J Epidemiol 1975; 101:287–301.
127. Spencer PS. Guam ALS/parkinsonism–dementia: a long-latency neurotoxic disorder caused by "slow toxin(s)" in food. Can J Neurol Sci 1987; 14:347–357.
128. Kisby GE, Ellison M, Spencer PS. Content of the neurotoxins cycasin (methylazoxymethanol β-D-glucoside) and BMAA (β-N-methylamino-L-alanine) in cycad flour prepared by Guam Chamorros. Neurology 1992; 42:1336–1340.
129. Whiting MG. Food practices in ALS foci in Japan, the Marianas and New Guinea. Fed Proc 1964; 23:1343–1345.
130. Kurland LT. An appraisal of the neurotoxicity of cycad and the etiology of amyotrophic lateral sclerosis on Guam. Fed Proc 1972; 31:1540–1542.
131. Dastur DK. Cycad toxicity in monkeys: clinical, pathological, and biochemical aspects. Fed Proc 1964; 23:1368–1369.
132. Garruto RM, Yanagihara R, Gajdusek DC. Cycads and amyotrophic lateral sclerosis/parkinsonism–dementia. Lancet 1988; 2:1079.
133. Duncan MW, Steele JC, Kopin IJ, Markey SP. 2-Amino-3-(methylamino)-propionic acid (BMAA) in cycad flour: an unlikely cause of amyotrophic lateral sclerosis and parkinsonism–dementia of Guam. Neurology 1990; 40:767–772.
134. Duncan MW, Marini AM, Watters R, Kopin IJ, Markey SP. Zinc, a neurotoxin to cultured neurons, contaminates cycad flour prepared by traditional Guamanian methods. J Neurosci 1992; 12:1523–1537.
135. Garruto RM. Pacific paradigms of environmentally-induced neurological disorders: clinical, epidemiological and molecular perspectives. Neurotoxicology 1991; 12:347–378.
136. Yase Y. The pathogenesis of amyotrophic lateral sclerosis. Lancet 1972; 2:292–296.
137. Perl DP, Gajdusek DC, Garruto RM, Yanagihara RT, Gibbs CT, Jr. Intraneuronal aluminum accumulation in amyotrophic lateral sclerosis and parkinsonism–dementia of Guam. Science 1982; 217:1053–1055.
138. Garruto RM, Yanagihara R, Gajdusek DC, Arion DM. Concentrations of heavy metals and essential minerals in garden soil and drinking water in the western Pacific. In: Chen KM, Yase Y, eds. Amyotrophic lateral sclerosis in Asia snd Oceania. Taiwan, Republic of China: National Taiwan University, 1984:265–329.

139. Chen KM, Yase Y. Parkinsonism–dementia, neurofibrillary tangles and trace elements in the western Pacific. In: Hutton JT, Kenny AD, eds. Senile dementia of the Alzheimer type. New York: AR, Liss, 1985:153–173.
140. Spencer PS, Kisby G, Ludolph A. Slow toxins, biologic markers, and long-latency neurodegenerative disease in the western Pacific region. Neurology 1991; 41(suppl 2):62–66.
141. Kessler II. Epidemiologic studies of Parkinson's disease. III. A community-based survey. Am J Epidemiol 1972; 96:242–254.
142. DeJong D. Parkinson's disease—V.A.–D.V.A. study group Part I. Biostatistics and case reporting. Med Ser J Can 1960; 3–12.
143. Sutcliffe RL, Prior R, Mawby B, McQuillan WJ. Parkinson's disease in the district of the Northampton Health Authority, United Kingdom. A study of prevalence and disability. Acta Neurol Scand 1985; 72:363–379.
144. Bekkelund SI, Selseth B, Mellgren SI. [Parkinson's disease in a population group in northern Norway]. Tidsskr Nor Laegeforen 1989; 109:561–563.
145. Dumas M, Munoz M, Boutros-Toni F, et al. Neuroepidemiological study in Limousin (France). J Neurol 1985; 232(suppl):76.
146. Vieregge P, Kleinhenz J, Fassl H, Jorg J, Kompy D. Epidemiology and outpatient care in Parkinson's disease: results from a pilot-study in northern Germany (Schleswig-Holstein). J Neural Transm 1991; 33 (suppl):115–118.
147. Acosta J. Epidemiology of Parkinson's disease: record of patients in our rural medium: Verjel de la Frontera. Ninth international symposium on Parkinson's disease. 1988:57.
148. Chalmanov VN. Epidemiological studies of parkinsonism in Sofia. Neuroepidemiology 1986; 5:171–177.
149. Rocca WA, Morgante L, Grigoletto F, et al. Prevalence of Parkinson's disease (PD) and other parkinsonisms: a door-to-door survey in two Sicilian communities. Neurology 1990; 40(suppl 1):422.
150. Kondo K, Shibasaki H. Epidemiology of Parkinson's disease: clues for etiology. Excerpta Medica 1981; 548:233.
151. Harada H, Nishikawa S, Takahashi K. An epidemiological study of Parkinson's disease in the Sanin district, Sanin, Japan. 12th world congress of neurology. 1981; series 548:30.
152. Grunitzky KE, Dumas M, Tatagan-agbi K, et al. Prevalence et distribution des principles affections neurologiques au Togo. In: Congrés de neurologie tropicale. Sept 26–28,1991. Limoges: Groupe Francophone d'étude et de Recherche en Neurologie Tropicale Press, 1991:16.
153. Osuntokum BO, Adeuja AOG, Schoenberg BS, et al. Prevalence of neurological disorders in a community in Nigeria. J Neurol 1985; 232(suppl):196.
154. Reef HE. Prevalence of Parkinson's disease in a multiracial community. In: Jage HWA, Bruyn GW, Heihstee APJ, eds. Eleventh world congress of neurology. Int Congr Ser 427, Amsterdam: Excepta Medica, 1977:125.

9

Comorbidity as It Relates to the Etiology of Parkinson's Disease

Caroline M. Tanner

The Parkinson's Institute, Sunnyvale, California

Matthew M. Zack

Centers for Disease Control and Prevention, Atlanta, Georgia

I. INTRODUCTION

Comorbidity, or the simultaneous presence of more than one disease state, may influence nearly every aspect of the natural history of Parkinson's disease. For example, survival, response to medication, or functional capacity, all may differ in persons with both Parkinson's disease and a second disorder, compared with those with Parkinson's disease alone. Although these topics are important, their consideration is beyond the scope of this volume. Rather, this chapter will consider only those comorbid conditions that have been proposed to relate to the cause of Parkinson's disease.

Theoretically, comorbid conditions could affect the etiology of Parkinson's disease in a variety of ways, including (1) a comorbid illness could be the direct cause of Parkinson's disease, as diabetes mellitus directly causes both neuropathy and retinopathy; (2) a comorbid condition and Parkinson's disease could have the same etiology, just as the etiologic agent, tobacco smoke, can cause pulmonary emphysema and squamous cell carcinoma of the lungs, bladder, or oropharynx; (3) a comorbid condition could alter vulnerability to risk factors for Parkinson's disease, as human immunodeficiency virus (HIV) increases the likelihood of infection following exposure to *Toxoplasma gondii*. In addition to these direct etiologic relations, a comorbid condition could be associated with Parkinson's disease if its presence changes the natural history of Parkinson's disease, such as "unmasking" Parkinson's disease by causing symptoms at an earlier point in the preclinical period. Identification of associations between Parkinson's disease and other disorders therefore, might provide important clues to the cause of Parkinson's disease. However, no other condition is yet known to be etiologically related to Parkinson's disease.

Since the cause of Parkinson's disease is unknown, consideration of the etiologic contribution of any comorbid condition must be somewhat conjectural. In judging whether an association may be etiologically related to Parkinson's disease, the general criteria for causality as originally proposed by Bradford Hill (1) can be useful. Of these, perhaps the most inviolate is temporality; that is, if a comorbid condition causes Parkinson's disease, its occurrence should precede the onset of this disorder. This timing may be very difficult to determine for two reasons. First, persons with Parkinson's disease may find it hard to pinpoint the date of onset of their disease. Second, there is an asymptomatic preclinical or latent period, of unknown length, but lasting months or years, during which neural degeneration occurs, but no signs or symptoms of disease occur(2–4). Since there is now no way to identify persons during this latent period, it is not possible to be certain that a comorbid condition preceded Parkinson's disease.

Mathematical approaches are commonly used to test the strength of an association. However, the separate cumulative risks of Parkinson's disease and of many other diseases, conditions, disabilities, and injuries, all increase with increasing age. The longer one lives, therefore, the more likely one is to have experienced both Parkinson's disease and some other disorder, coincidentally. Comparisons of the prevalence of the comorbid disorder among persons with Parkinson's disease and controls should account for this age dependency in the design. Multivariate statistical techniques may also be helpful, but they are not cure-alls for poor designs. Additional factors come into play when analyzing reports of familial associations. Age of living relatives and age at death are important in determining the meaningfulness of an association. The size of the family and the degree of relatedness among family members studied are also important. As an example, comparison of a family with 20 first-degree relatives, living to age 80 or older, with a second family, with four first-degree relatives, each of whom dies before age 30, would be biased against finding an adult-onset disorder in the second family, both because of the smaller size of the family and because of the early age at death of family members.

A further problem is posed by difficulties in defining the clinical syndrome of Parkinson's disease. In addition to motor abnormalities, Parkinson's disease includes many nonmotor signs, such as altered gastrointestinal motility, orthostatic hypotension, seborrheic dermatitis, and decreased olfaction. Moreover, subtle motor changes may predispose to accidental injury, even before the diagnosis of Parkinson's disease is made. With these and similar problems, the comorbid disorder is a manifestation of the underlying disease process, and not a truly distinct comorbid disorder. Failure to make such distinctions could lead to erroneous etiologic postulates.

Finally, any proposed cause for Parkinson's disease should have both specific and biologically plausible effects. If the only known effects of a proposed comorbid condition are on structures remote from the substantia nigra, the biological rationale for an etiologic association is more tenuous. If the clinical findings or pathological changes accompanying a proposed casual comorbid condition are very general, causing parkinsonism along with other signs, the proposed association is less likely to be a cause of Parkinson's disease. For example, parkinsonian signs may follow carbon monoxide exposure, but cognitive impairment and other motor changes are also usually present, and pallidal injury is most prominent pathologically. These differences make carbon monoxide an unlikely cause of Parkinson's disease, despite that parkinsonism can result from carbon monoxide poisoning.

This chapter will review the evidence for and against specific comorbid conditions proposed as causes for Parkinson's disease. These conditions include endocrine and metabolic disorders, other neurological and psychological conditions, arteriosclerosis, physiological stress, and trauma. Disorders associated with symptomatic parkinsonism (rather than Parkinson's disease) will not be considered. The interested reader is referred to Chapter 1, as well as to several excellent texts (5,6). Risk factors for Parkinson's disease are addressed in Chapters 6 and 10–12.

II. ENDOCRINE AND METABOLIC DISORDERS

Over the years, investigators have proposed a relation between disorders outside the central nervous system and Parkinson's disease. Although no association has been proved to be causative, the possibility that a systemic abnormality may cause Parkinson's disease continues to tantalize investigators.

A. Thyroid Disease

Thyroid disease is the endocrine dysfunction most frequently proposed to be associated with Parkinson's disease. Barbeau and his colleagues (7,8) proposed a cause-and-effect relation between thyroid disease and Parkinson's disease, based on their surveys in Quebec, Canada. Thyroid disease was identified more commonly in persons with Parkinson's disease onset younger than age 40. Similar differences were observed in their family members (1.3%) when compared with control families of persons without neurological disease (0.9%). The reports were not sufficiently detailed to allow determination of the statistical significance of these observations. Hyperthyroidism was associated with a dominantly inherited, essential tremor-associated subgroup, and hypothyroidism with a recessively inherited akinetic–rigid subgroup. Thyroid biochemistry in ten young-onset Parkinson's disease subjects, although normal, showed more low-normal results in the akinetic–rigid patients, and high-normal in the tremor–associated patients. Two subsequent studies supported this proposed association. One case–control study (9), conducted in Israel, found thyroid disease (type not specified) to be associated with an increased risk of Parkinson's disease. A medical records review of 406 Parkinson's disease patients found some thyroid disorder requiring thyroidectomy in 21 persons (10). Thyroid disease preceded parkinsonism in 70%.

Several possible etiologic mechanisms for a cause-and-effect relation between thyroid disease and Parkinson's disease were proposed (7,8,11). First, a direct effect of thyroid hormone on dopamine neurotransmission was postulated, following from the observation that thyroid dysfunction causes reversible symptomatic worsening in established Parkinson's disease. Second, postthyroidectomy hypoparathyroidism was proposed as an etiologic mechanism, following from the few secondary cases of hypoparathyroid-induced parkinsonism with associated basal ganglia calcification.

Despite these intriguing metabolic hypotheses, the association between thyroid disease and Parkinson's disease failed to be reproduced in numerous studies in other populations (12–15). Fewer studies investigated familial associations (12,14), so that the rare occurrence of a familial association between young age at onset of Parkinson's disease and thyroid disease cannot be eliminated, given current information. In conclusion, available information does not support a primary etiologic relation between Parkinson's disease and thyroid disease. Nonetheless, since hyperthyroidism can worsen existing parkinsonism, it is conceivable that hyperthyroidism might also cause an earlier expression of symptoms in preclinical Parkinson's disease.

B. Diabetes Mellitus

Diabetes mellitus has been proposed to have both an etiologic association with Parkinson's disease and the converse: protection against the development of Parkinson's disease. Familial diabetes mellitus was associated with the akinetic–rigid form of young-onset Parkinson's disease proposed by Barbeau and Pourcher (7), based on a study of 32 personal cases and 135 identified by mail survey. A later, larger investigation failed to find such an association (8). Investigations of other populations also did not find an increased association of diabetes and Parkinson's disease (12,14–17).

An opposite hypothesis was put forth by Di Monte and his colleagues (18), who found that fructose blocks 1-methyl-4-phenyl-1,2,3,6-tetrahydropyridine (MPTP) toxicity in isolated hepatocytes. If this observation can be extended to the brain, increased glucose levels would be expected to block MPTP-induced neurotoxicity. If one assumes a parallel between MPTP-induced injury and the pathogenesis of Parkinson's disease, diabetics would be predicted to be less likely to develop Parkinson's disease. Israeli investigators (19) recently explored this issue, comparing Parkinson's disease patients with demented controls, matched for age, sex, and country of origin, and found diabetes mellitus to be more common (20%) in the controls than the parkinsonian (12%) patients. A similar trend that was not statistically significant was seen in two other studies (16,17). Since these investigations counted prevalent cases of each disorder, the observed associations could result if persons with both Parkinson's disease and diabetes mellitus have shortened survival. Clarification of this awaits studies in which information is collected prospectively.

C. Other Metabolic Abnormalities

Various metabolic abnormalities have been associated with Parkinson's disease, including dysfunction of several specific hepatic enzymes. In this instance, comorbidity does not refer to a symptomatic abnormal health state, since affected individuals are unaware of the abnormality unless challenged with a substrate to the enzyme (most typically a drug). Similar conditions include phenylketonuria, malignant hyperthermia, and Refsum's disease, in which disease occurs only after exposure to a precipitating agent. In Parkinson's disease, a clinically asymptomatic enzyme dysfunction may increase susceptibility to nerve cell death. A more detailed discussion is given in Chapter 6.

1. Cytochrome P450 2D6

In 1969, Barbeau (20) proposed that hepatic enzyme abnormalities might cause Parkinson's disease. Impaired function of a specific hepatic cytochrome P450 enzyme (CYP 2D6 in current nomenclature) was later reported by Barbeau and colleagues (7,21) to be increased in persons with Parkinson's disease, particularly those with young age at Parkinson's disease onset, based on the ability of subjects to metabolize a fixed dose of the drug debrisoquin. However, only a few studies were reported to support these observations, whereas others concluded that there were no differences between persons with Parkinson's disease and those without (22–26,187). These conclusions may have been, in part, artifacts of study design, such as small sample sizes, differing definitions of "poor metabolizer phenotype" among reported studies, or differences in the clinical protocols. For example, the combined results of the three studies shown in Table 1 (22,26,187) are consistent with a modest increase in risk of Parkinson's disease associated with the defective phenotype, although the confidence intervals for the odds ratios cross 1, lowering certainty that this is a real effect.

Interest in the association between this polymorphism and Parkinson's disease was revived when the identification of the human gene for CYP 2D6 was located on chromosome 22q11.2-qter (27). Several groups have now used molecular genetic techniques to observe an association between Parkinson's disease and

Table 1 Some Studies Investigating the Risk of Parkinson's Disease Associated With Cytochrome P450 2D6

Study	Cases +	Cases −	Controls +	Controls −	Study odds ratios (95% CI)	Summary odds ratio (95% CI)
Studies of phenotype						
Risk of PD for nonextensive metabolizers						
Kallio et al. (187)	24	73	33	143	1.43 (0.79,2.58)	
Tanner et al. (22)	15	20	5	13	1.95 (0.58,6.61)	1.51 (0.91,2.48)
Meillard et al. (26)	11	9	6	7	1.43 (0.35,5.78)	
Studies of genotype						
Risk of Parkinson's disease if one or more CYP 2D6 *B* alleles present						
Armstrong et al. (28)	22	84	15	129	2.25 (1.19,4.53)	
Smith et al. (29)	205	639	572	2308	1.29 (1.08,1.55)	1.39 (1.18,1.65)
Kurth et al. (186)	33	67	44	176	1.97 (1.16,3.34)	
Risk of Parkinson's disease if two CYP 2D6 *B* alleles present						
Armstrong et al. (28)	1	52	0	72	2.76 (0.27,28.38)	
Smith et al. (29)	46	376	69	1371	2.43 (1.66,3.55)	2.39 (1.65,3.45)
Kurth et al. (186)	5	45	6	104	1.93 (0.57,6.52)	

The first section of Table 1 categorizes subjects using the system in Barbeau's original report, as *extensive metabolizers* (EM), defined as those subjects with a ratio of debrisoquin to debrisoquin hydroxylase ≤ 1 or *not extensive metabolizers* (nonEM), defined as those subjects with a debrisoquin to debrisoquin hydroxylase ratio > 1. The three studies listed are the only studies for which the actual metabolic ratios are available. Using the Mantel–Haenszel method of stratified analysis (177), the estimated summary odds ratio for these three studies is 1.51, but confidence limits span 1. The second and third section examine the pooled results of genotyping studies reporting the most frequent allelic variant of CYP 2D6 in whites. The *B* allele results from a point mutation (G to A) and produces impaired metabolic activity. For these genotype studies, the pooled analyses show a consistently increased risk, and 95% confidence intervals, for the combined odds ratios do not span 1. Key: +, Presence of the risk factor (nonEM phenotype, *B* allele or homozygous CYP 2D6 B genotype); −, absence of the risk factor, in accordance with preceding.

an abnormal *CYP 2D6* allele, corresponding to the phenotypic abnormalities previously described.

Numerous allelic variants have been described, and these vary across racial groups, both in character and frequency (28–33,186). In whites, a mutation producing an allelic variant called the *B* allele is the most common of these. The second and third sections of Table 1 examine the pooled results of genotyping studies reporting the most frequent allelic variant of CYP 2D6 in whites. The combined results of the three studies of the *B* allele show a modest increase in risk of Parkinson's disease associated with the defective genotype. In each instance the confidence interval for the odds ratio is greater than 1, and the risk for the homozygous *B* allele genotype is greater than for heterozygous. If the distribution of defective alleles across all populations is assumed to be 10%, then the attributable risk (34) for an odds ratio of 2.5 is about 0.13 (that is, about 13% of all cases of Parkinson's disease are likely attributable to this single factor).

Interest in this association is increased because there is some preliminary evidence of scientific plausibility to support a possible relation between this abnormal enzyme function and the development of Parkinson's disease. First, the nigral toxicant MPTP is itself a substrate of the specific P450 enzyme metabolizing human debrisoquin, although this is not the primary route of metabolism (35,36). Moreover, CYP 2D6 is present in the nigrostriatal system, and appears to function as a low-affinity dopamine reuptake system (37). Since the 1-methyl-4- phenylpyridinium ion (MPP^+) exerts its selective toxic effect on substantia nigra neurons only after uptake into the neuron (38), a central abnormality of this enzyme might somehow increase transport of a toxicant into nigral dopaminergic neurons. Alternatively, impaired hepatic CYP 2D6 function might produce inadequate detoxification of nigral toxicants outside of the nervous system, permitting an increased dose to cross the blood–brain barrier and cause nigral injury. In either event, the likely mechanism would be an interaction between a genetic predisposition and an exposure. Whether these or other hypotheses will clarify this intriguing association awaits further investigation. A quarter century later, the hypothesis posed in Barbeau's 1969 paper (20) still merits investigation: "Therefore we would like to propose, as a working hypothesis warranting *much* further investigation, that Parkinson's disease results from a generalized disorder in specialized transport systems across cell membranes or in tissue binding mechanisms and that the defective mechanisms responsible should be looked for in the *liver*." [Italics are Barbeau's.]

2. *Other Hepatic Enzyme Abnormalities*

Other P450 enzymes suggested to increase the risk of Parkinson's disease have not shown consistent associations in phenotypic investigations (39–41). A defect in sulfoxation has been associated with an increased vulnerability for Parkinson's disease in one study of phenotype (24). Theoretically, it is plausible that several enzyme abnormalities may, either separately or in combination, participate in the sequence of events leading to Parkinson's disease. However, evaluation of each proposed association is impractical, if not impossible, with clinical metabolic methods. Evaluation of the importance of these proposed associations awaits more precise methods, such as molecular genetic assays for specific genetic markers.

Application of these simpler techniques will enable a more accurate assessment of many individuals, avoiding the lengthy and less reliable metabolic measures used to determine phenotype.

3. *Mitochondrial Dysfunction*

The activity of complex I of the mitochondrial respiratory chain has been reported to be decreased in postmortem substantia nigra (42) and in platelets and muscle of living persons with Parkinson's disease, compared with control subjects (43–45). Further investigations have so far yielded contradictory results (46–48). Molecular genetic analyses have not clarified this controversy, failing to identify a specific abnormality of mitochondrial DNA in Parkinson's disease (49–52). Moreover, similar abnormalities of mitochondrial respiration have been identified in other neurological diseases (53,54), without associated parkinsonian signs. An underlying defect of energy metabolism is scientifically plausible in view of current theories of neurodegeneration (see Ref. 55 for review). Yet despite appealing theoretical arguments, a compelling clinical association between Parkinson's disease and mitochondrial dysfunction has not yet been provided.

III. OTHER NEURODEGENERATIVE DISORDERS: IS THERE A COMMON ETIOLOGY?

Several neurodegenerative disorders have been proposed to share etiologic factors with Parkinson's disease. In the following sections, the evidence for and against an etiologic relation between each disorder and Parkinson's disease will be considered separately. In the final section, several global hypotheses, proposing a shared pathogenesis for multiple neurodegenerative syndromes, will be presented.

A. Essential Tremor

Essential tremor is the term most commonly applied to a tremor that is predominant with use of the affected part, although, in severe cases, tremor may persist at rest (56). This is in distinction to the tremor of Parkinson's disease, which is most prominent at rest, and absent or minimized with activity (56). The term "essential" emphasizes the lack of other signs of neurological dysfunction. Terms used synonymously include *benign tremor* (emphasizing the typical clinical outcome), *senile tremor* (reflecting the increased frequency of this tremor with increasing age), and *familial tremor* (reflecting the dominant pattern of inheritance observed in some families). The proposal that there is an association between essential tremor and Parkinson's disease has fueled controversy for decades. Since the diagnostic differentiation of the two disorders is made by clinical observation, confusion stems partly from the practice of some physicians of including all cases of tremor as Parkinson's disease (57–59). Others have taken an opposite approach—diagnosing those persons with Parkinson's disease who have both postural and resting tremor as having two disorders, both Parkinson's disease and essential tremor (60). This broad variation in diagnostic criteria for essential tremor (ET) makes interpretation of proposed etiologic relations between Parkinson's disease and ET particularly challenging.

Barbeau, from studies of clinic patients with Parkinson's disease beginning younger than age 40, suggested an association between familial essential tremor and risk for young-onset Parkinson's disease (7,61,62). His several publications on this topic did not provide sufficient information to allow an independent assessment of the data relative to the observed associations. For example, the sizes of the families studied, the vital status of family members, and their current ages, or ages at death, were not provided. Since essential tremor is a common disorder, especially in the aging population (59,63), critical analysis of a proposed association must take into account the ages of the population studied. Similarly, larger family size would increase the probability of a chance association between the two disorders.

Several subsequent studies contradicted Barbeau et al.'s results. Marttila found no statistically significant differences in the prevalence of Parkinson's disease or essential tremor in the families of 52 persons with young-onset Parkinson's disease (64). Essential tremor occurred in 1.2% of first-degree relatives of Parkinson's disease cases and in 0.9% of first-degree relatives of matched controls. Taddei and Ludin found only 2 distant relatives of 41 essential tremor patients to be reported to have Parkinson's disease (65). Lazzarini et al. (66) found essential tremor in only 1.9% of first-degree relatives of Parkinson's disease patients with one or more relatives who had Parkinson's disease. In contrast, Lang and colleagues (67) found a family history of essential tremor in 3.8% of Parkinson's disease patients and 4.4% of dystonia patients, but in no controls. In a study of familial Parkinson's disease (defined as families with more than one case of Parkinson's disease), Maraganore et al. (68) found ET in 5.3% of first-degree relatives. Lou and Jankovic (69) reported parkinsonism in a family member of 4.6% of a 350-member, clinic-based group of persons with ET. In a second study by Jankovic et al. (70), a history of tremor in a first-degree relative was reported by 5.1% of Parkinson's disease patients, 23.4% of essential tremor patients, 20.7% of patients with both postural tremor and parkinsonism, but in only 2.6% of patients with progressive supranuclear palsy and 2.2% of normal controls. Some of the variation in these results may be explained by differences in age and in kindred size, as discussed earlier. All of these observations were based on patients attending specialty clinics. Different referral practices could contribute to differing results. Importantly, unusual cases, such as those with family histories of tremor, might be overrepresented in such clinics, when compared with the whole population. Nonetheless, investigation of the possibility that some families are at increased risk for both Parkinson's disease and essential tremor deserves further exploration.

Other authors suggested that persons with essential tremor might be at increased risk of later developing Parkinson's disease. Geraghty et al. (60) studied 130 consecutive patients with essential tremor identified from a referral practice. Twenty-five also had Parkinson's disease. They concluded that the prevalence of Parkinson's disease in persons with essential tremor is 24 times greater than expected. Because their cases were referred to a specialty practice in movement disorders, it is likely that this figure greatly overestimates the true association, as is seen in the population-based studies cited earlier. In several other clinical series, the association was not detectable despite a 2- to 5-year follow-up of 200 persons with essential tremor in Italy (71), or 1-year follow-up of 237 cases from Chicago and London (72).

Also compelling are the results of several well-designed, population-based studies. These studies, which are not subject to the bias introduced into a clinic-derived series, for which unusual cases are more likely to be referred, found no association between Parkinson's disease and essential tremor (59,63,73). In their study of a population-based and clinic-based sample of more than 300 persons with essential tremor, Marttila et al. (74) also did not find evidence supporting an increased frequency of concurrent essential tremor and Parkinson's disease. Because essential tremor and Parkinson's disease are both increasingly common with increasing age, a chance association of these two disorders would not be unusual. From Finnish population-based prevalence rates, they estimated that the coincidental association of Parkinson's disease in a person older than 40 with essential tremor would be about 0.3%, and of essential tremor in a person with Parkinson's disease about 5%. These rates were similar to those observed in their patients.

However, in a recent retrospective review of 350 persons with essential tremor, referred to a single, movement disorders center, Lou and Jankovic (69) found 20% who developed Parkinson's disease 5 or more years after the onset of essential tremor. Koller and his colleagues (75), reporting on 307 ET cases from one movement disorders center and 371 collected by mail questionnaires completed by 80 other neurologists, found that 6.1% of those with essential tremor had concurrent parkinsonism. Differences in these results may reflect methodological differences between the studies, including differing diagnostic criteria and different sources of referral in different practices. Both groups concluded that the observed association between ET and Parkinson's disease was higher than would be expected. However, although direct comparisons are not possible, the finding of 6.1% of essential tremor patients with parkinsonism (75) is similar to the 5% estimated by Marttila for Finland (74).

In summary, clinic-based and population-based surveys, when taken as a whole, do not provide conclusive evidence that essential tremor is a risk factor for Parkinson's disease. The failure to find any pathological abnormality (and, in particular, any pathological changes of Parkinson's disease) at postmortem in eight well-characterized essential tremor cases (76) further detracts from the theory that persons with essential tremor are at greater risk of Parkinson's disease. Similar indirect support is provided by the observation of cerebellar, rather than nigrostriatal, dysfunction in positron emission tomography (PET) studies of persons with familial and sporadic postural tremor (77,78), in contrast with the demonstration of decreased nigrostriatal function in persons with Parkinson's disease and in those with sporadic resting tremor (78). Also, olfactory dysfunction is common in Parkinson's disease, but was not observed in 16 essential tremor patients matched for age and gender (79). For all of these reasons, it seems likely that, on the whole, persons with essential tremor, or their relatives, are not at increased risk of developing Parkinson's disease.

Nonetheless, it is possible that a familial subgroup may exist in whom both Parkinson's disease and essential tremor share genetic determinants. Alternatively, a "benign progressive" form of parkinsonism, characterized by a long monosymptomatic (tremor only) stage, may sometimes occur. The continuing association of parkinsonism and tremor in large series do not allow this possibility to be eliminated completely. Clarification will require careful family studies, ideally coupled with genetic markers. Even if such a familial subgroup were very rare, elucidation of the pathogenesis of essential tremor and parkinsonism in these families could provide important clues to the cause of each disorder.

B. Motor Neuron Disease

The clinical syndromes of motor neuron dysfunction and parkinsonism (either alone or with an associated dementia) have been described to occur together in numerous situations. First, both syndromes sometimes followed encephalitis lethargica infection (80). Moreover, persons who have the high-prevalence neurodegenerative disorder found in the western Pacific, amyotrophic lateral sclerosis (ALS)–parkinsonism–dementia complex (ALS–PDC), commonly have signs of motor neuron disease along with parkinsonism or dementia (81). Both sporadic and familial cases have also been reported in whom both motor neuron dysfunction and parkinsonism occur in a single individual (80,82–87). In addition, other families show an increase in both disorders, presenting as separate syndromes (84,85,87,88). In one survey of persons with sporadic motor neuron disease,

Parkinson's disease was reported more frequently in first-degree relatives of patients than in those of controls, although descriptions of family composition were not provided, limiting interpretation of this finding (89). In a recent case–control study of persons with sporadic ALS, the frequency of relatives with another neurodegenerative disorder was similar between cases and controls (90).

These observations do not argue strongly for a direct etiologic association between Parkinson's disease and motor neuron disease As was true for essential tremor, however, the association in some families raises the possibility that subgroups may have shared pathogenetic mechanisms, and that these, at least partly, may be genetically determined. The recent observation that abnormalities of the gene coding for the enzyme superoxide dismutase (91), which protects against oxidative injury, provides an intriguing hypothetical example of how such a shared mechanism could occur. Although abnormalities of this gene have not been shown in Parkinson's disease, a deficit in superoxide dismutase function could theoretically contribute to the oxidative injury proposed to underlie Parkinson's disease (see later discussion, and other chapters in this volume).

C. Alzheimer's Disease

Alzheimer's disease is a specific, dementing illness of adults. Like Parkinson's disease, definitive diagnosis can be made only at autopsy by the presence of characteristic changes, such as neurofibrillary tangles and neuritic plaques (92). An etiologic association between Alzheimer's disease and Parkinson's disease has been proposed for several reasons. First, the clinical syndromes overlap. Parkinsonian motor dysfunction, particularly rigidity and bradykinesia, occur commonly in those meeting clinical criteria for senile dementia of the Alzheimer's type (SDAT; 93–95), although these signs are rarely responsive to antiparkinsonian therapy. Dementia also occurs more frequently in persons with Parkinson's disease than in others of the same age and gender. Recent estimates of the prevalence of dementia in Parkinson's disease range from 8 to 20% (96–98). The association of dementia and Parkinson's disease is even stronger when the incidence of dementia in Parkinson's disease is considered (99). For example, Stern and his associates (100) diagnosed new dementia in 29.6% of 250 medical records of persons with Parkinson's disease within a 2.5-year period. The strong relation between parkinsonism and dementia is more apparent when incidence, rather than prevalence, is measured, because survival is shortened when Parkinson's disease and dementia are comorbid.

Family studies also lend some support to an etiologic association between Parkinson's disease and Alzheimer's disease. In a comparison of demented and nondemented persons with Parkinson's disease, Marder and her colleagues (99) found dementia to be more than six times more likely in first-degree relatives of persons with comorbid dementia and parkinsonism. In a case–control study comparing persons with Alzheimer's disease with age-and gender-matched controls, Parkinson's disease occurred nearly three times more commonly in relatives of those with Alzheimer's disease (101).

Even though dementia clearly occurs more often than expected in Parkinson's disease, whether or not the dementia is caused by Alzheimer's disease is less certain. The syndrome of dementia, like parkinsonism, may have many causes, and differentiation on clinical grounds can be difficult. Parkinsonism and dementia commonly coexist in disorders such as striatonigral degeneration (102) or progressive supranuclear palsy (103). Severe dementia and parkinsonism may be associated with diffusely distributed Lewy bodies, but no Alzheimer's-like changes, at postmortem (104,188). The cognitive deficits most commonly found in Parkinson's disease are clinically distinct from those typical of Alzheimer's disease (106–109). Although careful clinical evaluation may be helpful, the correct diagnosis of coexisting parkinsonism and dementia may not be possible without an autopsy (102,110,111). The true prevalence of comorbid Alzheimer's disease and Parkinson's disease cannot be determined accurately by current clinical diagnostic techniques.

The comorbid presence of Parkinson's disease and Alzheimer's disease has been sought in several autopsy studies. Typical changes of Alzheimer's disease [neuritic plaques (NP) and neurofibrillary tangles (NFT)] are often found in the brains of those with pathologically typical Parkinson's disease (112–118; Table 2). The presence and, to some extent, the severity of the Alzheimer's pathology also correlate with the presence of dementia before death. The converse association also occurs—pathological changes typical of Parkinson's disease may be found in the brains of persons dying of Alzheimer's disease (119–121), sometimes in association with clinical signs of parkinsonism. However, interpretation of the meaning of these associations must be judged against age-matched control populations. The frequencies of both Parkinson's disease and Alzheimer's disease increase markedly with increasing age (122,126). Both disorders are believed to have latent periods of months to years, during which pathological changes would be present, but clinical signs not yet diagnosed (4,126). A small number of Lewy bodies (102,124,125) or neuritic plaques and neurofibrillary tangles (123) may be found at postmortem in clinically normal persons. It is possible that the association between Alzheimer's pathology and Parkinson's pathology reflect, at least in part, the coexistence of two common diseases of aging, rather than a shared etiology. For example, Gibb and Lees (102) found the prevalence of Lewy bodies in Alzheimer's disease brains to be similar to that in age-matched controls (10.7 vs. 9.3%).

In summary, the clinical and pathological literature do not provide strong support for a shared etiology between Parkinson's disease and Alzheimer's disease. As is true for the other neurodegenerations considered here, exceptions

Table 2 Prevalence of Alzheimer's Pathology in Parkinson's Disease

Study	Comments	Parkinson's disease cases with Alzheimer's pathology: No dementia	Dementia
Hakim and Mathieson (112)	Minor AD changes acceptable	15/15	18/19
Boller et al. (113)		3/13	Severe dementia: 9/9 Mild dementia: 3/7
Heston (178)	Occasional NP or NFT in 8/12		0/12
Gaspar and Gray (114)		7/14	17/18
Perry et al. (115)		0/4	3/10
Paulus and Jellinger (116)	Quantitative study	10/19	23/26
Xuereb et al. (117)	Occasional NP or NFT in 4 non-demented and 9 demented	0/17	2/15
Ince et al. (118)	Quantitative study	5/12 cases, not differentiated by dementia	

NP, neuritic plaque; NFT, neurofibrillary tangle.

may be individual families in whom both disorders coexist. Pursuit of these exceptional cases may provide insight into the pathogenesis of neurodegeneration as a whole.

D. Hypotheses Proposing Shared Causes of Neurodegeneration

The argument that all neurodegenerations share a common pathogenesis, and that the expression of this process differs as the result of the specific characteristics of the neurons affected, has been proposed, in various forms, for nearly a century. Gowers (105) proposed most simply that ". . . many degenerative diseases of the nervous system [were the] result of a defect in vitality . . ." of those nerve cells sharing a common function. This loss of vitality was the factor underlying the selective degeneration of specific nerve cell groups observed in abiotrophies. He included motor neuron disease, "simple mental failure" and paralysis agitans in his list of senile abiotrophies. Although the pathogenetic defects proposed have changed a little over the intervening decades, the idea that these disorders might share a common pathogenesis continues to capture the imaginations of scientists. A full examination of the many hypotheses proposed is beyond the scope of this chapter, although many of these hypotheses are considered in other chapters in this volume. A summary of some of these hypotheses is provided in Table 3. Many of the scientific arguments underlying these unifying theories of

Table 3 Some Examples of Unified Hypotheses of Neurodegeneration

Study	Diseases	Hypothesis
Gowers (105)	PD MND Dementia	Neurons with shared function may have a common defect in vitality, causing a common tendency to decay, given an appropriate stimulus.
Gajdusek and Gibbs Jr. (179)	PD MND AD	A transmissible infectious agent, such as those causing the spongiform encephalopathies. Later considered unlikely based on experimental evidence (180).
Appel (181); Stewart and Appel (182)	PD MND AD	A deficiency of a disorder-specific trophic hormone, elaborated in the normal state by the target of the degenerating neurons, results in a retrograde degeneration.
Calne et al. (2)	PD MND AD	Localized neuronal damage resulting from environmentally induced injury does not produce symptoms until after several decades of age-related neuronal compromise and attrition.
Cadet (183)	PD AD Schizophrenia	Oxyradical formation, and possibly formation of other reactive chemical species, cause neurodegeneration.
Barker (184)	PD AD MND	An early-life viral infection caused chronic autoimmune destruction of trophic peptidergic neurotransmission. This insult, coupled with natural aging, causes neurodegeneration.
Eisen and Calne (185)	PD MND AD	Phylogenetic disturbances of neocortical cells result in deranged glutamate metabolism and consequent secondary degeneration of postsynaptic neurons.
Beal et al. (55)	PD AD HD CD	Defects in mitochondrial energy metabolism or oxidative defects cause deteriorations in membrane potentials. NMDA receptors are persistently activated by endogenous glutamate, and excitotoxic nerve cell death ensues.

PD, Parkinson's disease; AD, Alzheimer's disease; MND, motor neuron disease; CD, cerebellar degenerations; HD, Huntington's disease; NMDA, *N*-methyl-D-aspartate.

neurodegeneration are compelling. Nonetheless, clinical evidence in support of any specific hypothesis still remains patchy.

IV. PERSONALITY AND MOOD DISORDERS

Both "normal" and diseased states have been associated with the subsequent development of Parkinson's disease. Measurement of these proposed associations is particularly difficult, since assessments are generally performed retrospectively, and exclusion of bias based on disease-produced changes in personality is impossible. Moreover, in each case it is debatable whether the personality profile or mood disorder reflects a separate, comorbid condition, or a manifestation of the nerve cell injury and consequent neurochemical changes of Parkinson's disease. Resolution of this puzzle is presently impossible, and awaits carefully designed longitudinal studies.

A. "Preparkinsonian" Personality

A lifelong characteristic personality type has often been associated with Parkinson's disease. Compared with nondisease controls or those with other illnesses, those with Parkinson's disease have been found to be rigid, conservative, introverted, law-abiding, non–risk-taking, hard working, and conforming individuals (127–134). Similar personality differences were described as early as age 8 in retrospective interviews of monozygotic twins discordant for Parkinson's disease (135). Another characteristic of persons with Parkinson's disease is a tendency to be nonsmokers (136–139) and, possibly, nondrinkers of alcohol (129). If these observations are correct, the more conservative personality could be an early manifestation of Parkinson's disease. Alternatively, the preparkinsonian personality could predispose an individual to behaviors that increase the risk of developing Parkinson's disease (see also other chapters this volume).

B. Other Disorders of Personality or Mood

Depression (140) and anxiety (134) occur commonly in Parkinson's disease. Each disorder may precede the development of parkinsonian motor abnormalities (140–142). Persons developing familial parkinsonism may be especially likely to have antecedent anxiety disorders (143). A diagnosis of psychoneurosis or psychosomatic illness was also associated with an increased risk for Parkinson's disease in one case–control study (15). The association between Parkinson's disease and antecedent mood disorder has been suggested to represent a clinical subgroup (141). Whether such subgroups might share common etiologies, perhaps leading to nerve cell loss in nondopaminergic regions relatively early in the course of illness, will require more investigation.

V. OTHER DISORDERS

A. Stroke and Atherosclerosis

Arteriosclerotic parkinsonism was proposed by Critchley (144) in 1929. He described a syndrome distinct from Parkinson's disease, occurring in association with arterial hypertension, believed to be the result of multiple vascular lesions in the basal ganglia. In subsequent decades, clinical distinctions blurred, and arteriosclerosis was commonly proposed to be an important pathogenetic mechanism in Parkinson's disease, until the advent of levodopa therapy provided an additional means of differentiation. In 1974, therapeutic response to the dopamine precursor levodopa was proposed to distinguish Parkinson's disease (presynaptic lesions) from arteriosclerotic parkinsonism (both pre- and postsynaptic lesions) (145). This was based on the pharmacological requirement of an intact postsynaptic receptor to allow therapeutic benefit. Since then, arteriosclerotic parkinsonism has generally been thought to be an unusual cause of parkinsonism. Although parkinsonism can occasionally occur as the result of cerebrovascular disease, these patients can typically be distinguished from Parkinson's disease by an abrupt onset of disability, other signs of vascular disease or stroke, and appropriate lesions on computed tomograph (CT) or magnetic resanance (MR) imaging (146). Arteriosclerosis is no longer considered a possible cause of Parkinson's disease.

Struck et al. (16) proposed an opposite association: persons with Parkinson's disease have less risk of stroke. This is contradicted by other reports (17,147), however, and may be an artifact of the control population used in the former study. Recently, Gottlieb and Melamed (148) proposed that, in some cases, a cerebrovascular injury might ". . . contribute to the development of Parkinson's disease, perhaps by acceleration and decompensation of a pre-existing subclinical illness." In their study, only 45 of 1655 Parkinson's disease patients also had stroke. Although comorbid stroke might occasionally unmask an existing lesion, such an association would not be a direct etiologic relationship.

B. Cancer

Surveys of persons attending Parkinson's disease clinics have suggested an inverse association between Parkinson's disease and cancers (10,149,150). The lower smoking rate in persons with Parkinson's disease or a third, shared pathogenetic factor have been proposed to explain this association. Barbeau et al. (150), for example, proposed that the poor metabolizer phenotype for CYP 2D6 might account not only for the increased risk for Parkinson's disease, but the decreased risk for cancer, since the extensive metabolizer phenotype has been associated with increased risk for some cancers. Although these explanations are plausible, the association of lower cancer rates and Parkinson's disease has been questioned, based on a failure to demonstrate such a relation in postmortem (151), death certificate (152), and population-based (15) studies. An association between Parkinson's disease and thyroid disease has been proposed (see Section II. A) and, in one study, thyroid tumors were more common than expected (10). Because levodopa is a precursor to melanin, an increased risk for melanoma in Parkinson's disease has been proposed (153). In the same clinic-based study, melanoma occurred more often than expected in patients with Parkinson's disease (10). Neither of these associations have been replicated in other studies (15,151,152), and both may reflect the selected nature of the referral population studied. Alternatively, comorbidity of cancer and Parkinson's disease may alter the clinical course of Parkinson's disease. For example, persons with both Parkinson's disease and cancer might die before the Parkinson's disease is diagnosed. Prospective studies of the incidence of each disorder, and their comorbidity, would help to clarify these questions.

VI. PHYSIOLOGIC STRESS

The extreme emotional and physical hardship of concentration camp imprisonment has been proposed to increase the risk of developing Parkinson's disease, based on observations of holocaust survivors living in Israel and on English survivors of prisoner of war camps in Southeast Asia (9,154). Eatough et al. (127) found persons with Parkinson's disease to have suffered more adverse life events, such as bereavement, serious illness or injury, or geographic dislocation during childhood, but not adulthood, when compared with a control group with rheumatoid arthritis. Stress has been proposed to increase dopamine turnover which, in turn, could cause oxidative injury to nigral dopamine neurons (155–157). Whether these or other physiological consequences of extreme stress, particularly in predisposed individuals, could be related to the development of Parkinson's disease awaits further investigation. In persons with Parkinson's disease, stress is known to cause transient worsening, but does not appear to cause permanent increases in disease severity (158). Unfortunately, the retrospective investigation of severe emotional or physical stress poses significant methodological challenges.

VII. HEAD TRAUMA

Repeated trauma, such as occurs in professional boxers, can cause a syndrome of dementia and parkinsonism, with associated neuropathological changes of neurofibrillary tangles, gliosis, and nerve cell loss (159). Despite the clinical and pathological distinctions between this disorder and Parkinson's disease, head injury has remained a commonly proposed cause of Parkinson's disease. Many case–control studies, using retrospective interviews, found an association between head trauma and Parkinson's disease (139,160,161). Often the trauma was mild, and preceded the onset of disease by decades. In the only case–control study using prospectively collected information (15), head trauma was not associated with the subsequent development of Parkinson's disease. Similarly, a population-based follow-up study of persons with head trauma did not identify an increased number of cases with Parkinson's disease (162). Although the stress associated with head trauma might have triggered a process resulting decades later in Parkinson's disease, this is not supported by the current literature. Rather, because the two studies with no possibility of recall bias are both negative, such a bias may have contributed to the associations reported in the other studies. Given current evidence, head trauma does not seem likely to be etiologically associated with Parkinson's disease.

VIII. DRUG USE

Transient reversible parkinsonism has occasionally been associated with many different drug treatments (142,163). Only a few of these drug exposures have been proposed to have an etiologic relation with Parkinson's disease. These are considered in the following sections.

A. Dopamine Receptor-Blocking Agents and Dopamine-Depleting Agents

Drugs that decrease central dopaminergic function can cause reversible parkinsonism. These include drugs, such as reserpine and tetrabenazine, that deplete presynaptic stores of biogenic amine neurotransmitters, including dopamine (164). The more commonly used are neuroleptic drugs, such as the phenothiazines, butyrophenones, and substituted benzamides, all of which block dopamine receptors and, consequently, can cause parkinsonism (164,165). Individual susceptibility to the development of drug-induced parkinsonism varies, and may be partly determined by genetic susceptibility (166–168). Elderly persons are more prone to develop drug-induced parkinsonism (164). If acute neuroleptic therapy can cause reversible parkinsonism, can chronic neuroleptic exposure cause permanent parkinsonism?

Anecdotal associations between neuroleptic treatment and Parkinson's disease are provided in several case reports, each describing persons with acute neuroleptic-induced parkinsonism. The parkinsonism resolved with drug withdrawal, only to be followed by Parkinson's disease years later (169,170). A similar association was reported by Rajput (171), who described two persons with neuroleptic-induced parkinsonism. In each, symptoms resolved when neuroleptic treatment was stopped. At postmortem, each showed the typical pathological changes of Parkinson's disease. These few case reports suggest a cause-and-effect relation between neuroleptic exposure and Parkinson's disease. However, another interpretation is more likely. The persons described in these observations could have been in the latent or preclinical phase of Parkinson's disease at the time they were exposed to neuroleptics. In the absence of the drugs, they showed no signs of parkinsonism, although they already had some degree of substantia nigra injury. Following neuroleptic therapy, the pharmacologically induced reduction in dopaminergic neurotransmission caused severe parkinsonism, an unmasking of the asymptomatic nigral lesion. When drugs were withdrawn, parkinsonism resolved. In the first instances, progression of the preclinical nigral lesion eventually resulted in clinical parkinsonism. In the latter cases, death preceded the development of clinical parkinsonism, but typical changes were identified at autopsy.

Several other facts argue against an etiologic relation between neuroleptic treatment and Parkinson's disease. Neuroleptics were not available until the middle of this century, but Parkinson's disease was clearly described more than 150 years ago. At present, neuroleptics are commonly prescribed in several settings, including persons with psychosis, elderly persons with behavioral disturbances associated with cognitive decline, and persons with certain gastrointestinal disorders. Yet case–control studies have not yet identified prior exposure to neuroleptics or dopamine-depleting agents as risk factors for Parkinson's disease. Therefore, it seems more likely that neuroleptic treatment may at times unmask preclinical Parkinson's disease than that neuroleptic treatment actually causes the nigral injury. Nonetheless, the analysis of existing information can neither prove nor disprove a relation. Determination of the actual relation between treatment with neuroleptic drugs and Parkinson's disease awaits evaluation in a prospective study.

B. Illicit Drug Use

Parkinsonism resulting from intravenous injection of the meperidine analogue MPTP is very similar to, but distinct from, Parkinson's disease (172) (see Chapter 13). Ross has described parkinsonism after exposure to multiple licit and illicit drugs (173) with broadly similar chemical structures. Reversible parkinsonism has been associated with meperidine in one case (174). Chronic exposure to amphetamine causes dopamine depletion in experimental animals (175), but an association with human parkinsonism has yet to be demonstrated. The similarities between the permanent parkinsonism caused by MPTP and Parkinson's disease make the search for a related drug exposure intriguing. However, evidence in support of such an etiologic association has not yet been presented.

IX. CONCLUSION

Several of the associations reviewed here may account for small fractions of Parkinson's disease, but, from current information, none likely contribute to more than a few of all cases of Parkinson's disease. Particularly intriguing are the proposed associations in families. Although families with multiple cases of neurodegenerative disease are unusual, identification of a genetic mechanism in even one family may provide important insights into disease pathogenesis. Many of the associations proposed are based on clinically derived studies. Because persons attending referral practices may not represent all persons with Parkinson's disease, the strength of the association may be over- or underestimated. Similarly, proposed associations based on observations of prevalent cases will miss or underestimate the association of diseases that shorten Parkinson's disease survival. The significance of these biases, and the true strength of associations between Parkinson's disease and other illnesses, require prospective observation, with identification of incident cases. Carefully designed investigations of this type may provide important pieces to the etiologic puzzle.

REFERENCES

1. Rothman KJ. Modern epidemiology. Boston Little, Brown & Co., 1986.
2. Calne DB, Eisen A, McGeer E, Spencer P. Alzheimer's disease, Parkinson's disease, and motoneurone disease: abiotrophic interaction between ageing and environment. Lancet 1986; 2:1067–1070.
3. Langston JW. Predicting Parkinson's disease. Neurology 1990; 40(suppl 3):70–74.
4. Koller WC, Langston JW, Hubble JP, et al. Does a long pre-clinical period occur in Parkinson's disease? Neurology 1991; 41(suppl 2):8–13.
5. Stern M, Koller WC. Parkinsonian syndromes. New York: Marcel Dekker, 1993.
6. Weiner WJ, Lang AE. Movement disorders: a comprehensive survey. Mount Kisco, NY: Futura Publishing, 1989. 257–291.
7. Barbeau A, Pourcher E. Genetics of early onset Parkinson's disease. Amsterdam: Excerpta Medica 1983:1–16.
8. Roy M, Boyer L, Barbeau A. A prospective study of 50 cases of familial Parkinson's disease. Can J Neurol Sci 1983; 10:37–42.
9. Treves TA, Rabey JM, Korczyn AD. Case–control study, with use of temporal approach, for evaluation of risk factors for Parkinson's disease (PD) [abstract]. Mov Disord 1990; 5:11.
10. Jansson B, Jankovic J. Low cancer rates among patients with Parkinson's disease. Ann Neurol 1985; 17:505–509.
11. Foster HD. Disease family trees: the possible roles of iodine in goitre, cretinism, multiple sclerosis, amyotrophic lateral sclerosis, Alzheimer's and Parkinson's diseases and cancers of the thyroid, nervous system and skin. Med Hypotheses 1987; 24:249–263.
12. Quinn N, Critchley P, Marsden C. Young onset Parkinson's disease. Mov Disord 1987; 2:73–91.
13. Kondo K. Epidemiological clues for the etiology of Parkinson's disease. Adv Neurol 1984; 40:345–351.
14. Lima B, Neves G, Nora M. Juvenile parkinsonism: clinical and methobolic characteristics. J Neurol Neurosurg Psychiatry 1987; 50:345–348.

15. Rajput AH, Offord KP, Beard CM, Kurland LT. A case–control study of smoking habits, dementia, and other illnesses in idiopathic Parkinson's disease. Neurology 1987; 37:226–232.
16. Struck LK, Rodnitzky RL, Dobson JK. Stroke and its modification in Parkinson's disease. Stroke 1990; 21:1395–1399.
17. Levine RL, Jones JC, Bee N. Stroke and Parkinson's disease. Stroke 1992; 23:839–842.
18. Di Monte DA, Sandy MS, Blank L, Smith MT. Fructose prevents 1-methyl-4-phenyl-1,2,3,6-tetrahydropyridine (MPTP)-induced ATP depletion and toxicity in isolated hepatocytes. Biochem Biophys Res Commun 1988; 153:734–740.
19. Dikman M, Leibowitz Y. Association of diabetes, hypertension and arteriosclerotic heart disease with Parkinson's disease: a pilot study. Book of abstracts, 9th international symposium on Parkinson's disease, 1988.
20. Barbeau A. Parkinson's disease as a systemic disorder. In: Gillingham FJ, Donaldson IML, eds. Third symposium on Parkinson's disease. Edinburgh: Livingstone, 1969:66–73.
21. Barbeau A, Cloutier T, Roy M, Plasse L, Paris S, Poirier J. Ecogenetics of Parkinson's disease: 4-hydroxylation of debrisoquine. Lancet 1985; 2:1213–1216.
22. Tanner CM, Chen B, Wang WZ, et al. Environmental factors in the etiology of Parkinson's disease. Can J Neurol Sci 1987; 14:419–423.
23. Benitez J, Ladero JM, Jiminez-Jiminez FJ, et al. Oxidative polymorphism of debrisoquine in Parkinson's disease. J Neurol Neurosurg Psychiatry 1990; 53:289–292.
24. Steventon GB, Heafield MTE, Waring RH, Williams AC. Xenobiotic metabolism in Parkinson's disease. Neurology 1989; 39:883–887.
25. Gudjonsson O, Sanz E, Alvan G, Aquilonius SM, Reviriego J. Poor hydroxylator phenotypes of debrisoquine and *S*-mephenytoin are not over-represented in a group of patients with Parkinson's disease [letter]. Br J Clin Pharmacol 1990; 30:301–302.
26. Meillard MN, Bentué-Ferrer D, Brunet-Bourgin F, Morel G, Allain H. Étude de l'hydroxylation de la débrisoquine dans la maladie de Parkinson. Presse Méd. 1990; 19:947–949.
27. Gonzalez FJ, Skoda RC, Kimura S, et al. Characterisation of the common genetic defect in humans deficient in debrisoquine metabolism. Nature 1988; 331:442–446.
28. Armstrong M, Daly AK, Cholerton S, Bateman DN, Idle JR. Mutant debrisoquine hydroxylation genes in Parkinson's disease. Lancet 1992; 339:1017–1018.
29. Smith CAD, Gough AC, Leigh PN, et al. Debrisoquine hydroxylase gene polymorphism and susceptibility to Parkinson's disease. Lancet 1992; 339:1375–1377.
30. Kondo I, Kanazawa I. Debrisoquine hydroxylase and Parkinson's disease. In: Narabayashi H, Nagatsu T, Yanakisawa N, Mizuno Y, eds. Parkinson's disease: from basic research to treatment. Adv Neurol 1993; 60:338–342.
31. Tsuneoka Y, Matsuo Y, Iwahashi K, Takeuchi H, Ichikawa Y. A novel cytochrome P-450IID6 mutant gene associated with Parkinson's disease. J Biochem 1993; 114:263–266.
32. Evans WE, Relling MV, Rahman A, McLeod HL, Scott EP, Lin J-S. Genetic

basis for a lower prevalence of deficient CYP2D6 oxidative drug metabolism phenotypes in black Americans. J Clin Invest 1993; 91:2150–2154.
33. Wang SL, Huang JD, Lai MD, Liu BH, Lai ML. Molecular basis of genetic variation in debrisoquin hydroxylation in Chinese subjects: polymorphism in RFLP and DNA sequence of CYP2D6. Clin Pharmacol Ther 1993; 53:410–418.
34. Armitage P, Berry G. Statistical methods in medical research. Oxford: Blackwell Scientific Publications, 1987.
35. Fonne-Pfister R, Bargetzi MJ, Meyer UA. MPTP, the neurotoxin inducing Parkinson's disease, is a potent competitive inhibitor of human and rat cytochrome P450 isozymes (P450bufI, P450db1) catalyzing debrisoquine 4-hydroxylation. Biochem Biophys Res Commun 1987; 148:1144–1150.
36. Smith MT, Ekström G, Sandy MS, Di Monte D. Studies on the mechanism of 1-methyl-4-phenyl-1,2,3,6-tetrahydropyridine cytotoxicity in isolated hepatocytes. Life Sci 1987; 40:741–748.
37. Niznik HB, Tyndale RF, Sallee FR, et al. The dopamine transporter and cytochrome P450IID1 (debrisoquine 4-hydroxylase) in brain: resolution and identification of two distinct [^{3}H] GBR-12935 binding proteins. Arch Biochem Biophys 1990; 276:424–432.
38. Langston JW, Irwin I. MPTP: current concepts and controversies. Clin Neuropharmacol 1986; 9:485–507.
39. Ferrari MD, Peeters EA, Haan J, et al. Cytochrome P450 and Parkinson's disease. Poor parahydroxylation of phenytoin. J Neurol Sci 1990; 96:153–157.
40. Factor SA, Weiner WJ, Hefti F. Acetaminophen metabolism by cytochrome P450 monooxygenases in Parkinson's disease. Ann Neurol 1989; 26:286–288.
41. Koller WC, Rope SD, Huber SJ, Blumenthal DC, Blumenthal HJ. Metabolism of glucurolactone to glucarate in Parkinson's disease. Neurology 1992; 42:1807–1808.
42. Schapira AHV, Cooper JM, Dexter D, Jenner P, Clark JB, Marsden CD. Mitochondrial complex I deficiency in Parkinson's disease. Lancet 1989; 1:1269.
43. Parker WD, Boyson SJ, Parks JK. Abnormalities of the electron transport chain in idiopathic Parkinson's disease. Ann Neurol 1989; 26:719–723.
44. Bindoff LA, Birch-Machin MA, Cartlidge NEF, Parker WD Jr, Turnbull DM. Mitochondrial function in Parkinson's disease. Lancet 1989; 2:49.
45. Shoffner JM, Watts RL, Juncos JL, Torroni A, Wallace DC. Mitochondrial oxidative phosphorylation defects in Parkinson's disease. Ann Neurol 1991; 30:332–339.
46. Mann VM, Cooper JM, Krige D, Schapira AHV, Marsden CD. Brain skeletal muscle and platelet homogenate mitochondrial function in Parkinson's disease. Brain 1992; 115:333–342.
47. DiMonte DA, Sandy MS, Jewell SA, Adornato B, Tanner CM, Langston JW. Oxidative phosphorylation by intact muscle mitochondria in Parkinson's disease. Neurodegeneration 1993; 2:275–281.
48. Mann VM, Cooper JM, Krige D, Daniel SE, Schapira AHV, Marsden CD. Brain, skeletal muscle and platelet homogenate mitochondrial function in Parkinson's disease. Brain 1992; 115:333–342.

49. Ikebe S, Tanaka M, Ohno K, et al. Increase of deleted mitochondrial DNA in the striatum in Parkinson's disease and senescence. Biochem Biophys Res Commun 1990; 170:1044–1048.
50. Schapira AH, Holt IJ, Sweeney M, Harding AE, Jenner P, Marsden CD. Mitochondrial DNA analysis in Parkinson's disease. Mov Disord 1990; 5:294–297.
51. Lestienne P, Nelson J, Riederer P, Jellinger K, Reichmann H. Normal mitochondrial genome in brain from patients with Parkinson's disease and complex I defect. J Neurochem 1990; 55:1810–1812.
52. Sandy MS, Langston JW, Smith MT, Di Monte DA. PCR analysis of platelet mtDNA: lack of specific changes in Parkinson's disease. Mov Disord 1993; 8:74–82.
53. Rosing HS, Hopkins LC, Wallace DC, Epstein CM, Weidenheim K. Maternally inherited mitochondrial myopathy and myoclonic epilepsy. Ann Neurol 1985; 17:228–237.
54. Wallace DC, Singh G, Lott MT, et al. Mitochondrial DNA mutation associated with Leber's hereditary optic neuropathy. Science 1988; 242:1427–1430.
55. Beal MF, Hyman BT, Koroshetz W. Do defects in mitochondrial energy metabolism underlie the pathology of neurodegenerative diseases? Trends Neurosci 1993; 16:125–131.
56. Salisachs P, Findley LJ. Problems in the differential diagnosis of essential tremor. In: Findley LJ, Capildeo R, eds. Movement disorders: tremor. London: Macmillan, 1984:219–224.
57. Allan W. Inheritance of the shaking palsy. Arch Intern Med 1937; 60:424–436.
58. Mjönes H. Paralysis agitans. Acta Psychiatr Neurol Scand [Suppl] 1949; 54:1–195.
59. Rautakorpi I, Takala J, Marttila RJ, Sievers K, Rinne UK. Essential tremor in a Finnish population. Acta Neurol Scand 1982; 66:58–67.
60. Geraghty JJ, Jankovic J, Zetusky WJ. Association between essential tremor and Parkinson's disease. Ann Neurol 1985; 17:329–333.
61. Barbeau A, Roy M. Familial subsets in idiopathic Parkinson's disease. Can J Neurol Sci 1984; 11:144–150.
62. Barbeau A, Pourcher E. New data on the genetics of Parkinson's disease. Can J Neurol Sci 1982; 9:53–60.
63. Haerer AF, Anderson DW, Schoenberg BS. Prevalence of essential tremor. Results from the Copiah County study. Arch Neurol 1982; 39:750–751.
64. Marttila RJ, Rinne UK. Parkinson's disease and essential tremor in families of patients with early-onset Parkinson's disease. J Neurol Neurosurg Psychiatry 1988; 51:429–431.
65 Taddei IM, Ludin HP. Essential tremor: a follow-up study. Schweiz Arch Neurol Psychiatr 1988; 139:33–46.
66. Lazzarini AM, Myers RH, Zimmerman TR Jr, et al. A clinical genetic study of Parkinson's disease: evidence for dominant transmission. Neurology 1994; 44:499–506.
67. Lang AE, Kierans C, Blair RD. Family history of tremor in Parkinson's disease compared with those of controls and patients. In: Parkinson's disease. Adv Neurol 1985; 45:313–316.
68. Maraganore D, Harding A, Marsden C. A clinical and genetic study of familial Parkinson's disease. Mov Disord 1991; 6:205–211.

69. Lou J-S, Jankovic J. Essential tremor: clinical correlates in 350 patients. Neurology 1991; 41:234–238.
70. Jankovic J, Beach J, Schwartz K. Tremor and longevity in relatives of patients with Parkinson's disease, essential tremor and control subjects [abstract]. Neurology 1994; 44(suppl 2):A368.
71. Martinelli P, Gabellini AS, Gulli MR, Lugaresi E. Different clinical features of essential tremor: a 200 patient study. Acta Neurol Scand 1987; 75:106–111.
72. Cleeves L, Findley LJ, Koller W. Lack of association between essential tremor and Parkinson's disease. Ann Neurol 1988; 24:23–26.
73. Rajput AH, Offord K, Beard CM, Kurland L. Essential tremor in Rochester, Minnesota: a 45 year study. J Neurol Neurosurg Psychiatry 1984; 47:466–470.
74. Marttila RJ, Rautakorpi I, Rinne UK. The relation of essential tremor to Parkinson's disease. J Neurol Neurosurg Psychiatry 1984; 47:734–735.
75. Koller WC, Busenbark K, Miner K, essential tremor study group. The relationship of essential tremor to other movement disorders: Report on 678 patients. Ann Neurol 1994; 35:717–723.
76. Rajput AH, Rozdilsky B, Ang L, Rajput A. Clinicopathologic observations in essential tremor: report of six cases. Neurology 1991; 41:1422–1424.
77. Colebatch JG, Findley LJ, Frackowiak RS, Marsden CD, Brooks DJ. Preliminary report: activation of the cerebellum in essential tremor. Lancet 1990; 336:1028–1030.
78. Brooks DJ, Playford ED, Ibanez V, et al. Isolated tremor and disruption of the nigrostriatal dopaminergic system: an ^{18}F-dopa PET study. Neurology 1992; 42:1554–1560.
79. Busenbark KL, Huber SJ, Greer G, Pahwa R, Koller WC. Olfactory function in essential tremor. Neurology 1992; 42:1631–1632.
80. Brait K, Fahn S, Schwarz G. Sporadic and familial parkinsonism and motor neuron disease. Neurology 1973; 23:990–1002.
81. Kurland LT, Hirano A, Malamud N, Lessell S. Parkinsonism–dementia complex, an endemic disease on the island of Guam. Clinical, pathological, genetic and epidemiological features. Trans Am Neurol Assoc 1961; pp 115–120.
82. Bonduelle M, Bouygues P, Escourolle R, Lormeau G. Simultaneous development of amyotrophic lateral sclerosis, Parkinson's syndrome and progressive dementia. Apropos of 2 anatomoclinical cases. Attempted interpretation. J Neurol Sci 1968; 6:315–332.
83. Amato L, Cuffaro F, Lupo I, Nava L, Rizzo M. Discussion of a clinical case of associated amyotrophic lateral sclerosis–parkinsonism–dementia. Acta Neurol Scand 1986; 8:310–313.
84. Schmitt HP, Emser W, Heimes C. Familial occurrence of amyotrophic lateral sclerosis, parkinsonism, and dementia. Ann Neurol 1984; 16:642–648.
85. Hudson AJ. Amyotrophic lateral sclerosis and its association with dementia, parkinsonism and other neurological disorders: a review. Brain 1981; 104: 217–247.
86. Perticoni GF, Pezzella F, Ferroni A. The problem of parkinsonism associated with motor neuron disease. Clinical report on 11 sporadic cases. Riv Patol Nerv Ment 1977; 98:159–170.
87. Kondo K. Motor neuron disease: changing population patterns and clues for etiol-

ogy. In: Neurological epidemiology: principles and clinical applications. Adv Neurol 1978; 19:509–543.
88. Alter M, Schaumann B. A family with amyotrophic lateral sclerosis and parkinsonism. J Neurol 1976; 212:281–284.
89. Deapen DM, Henderson BE. A case–control study of amyotrophic lateral scherosis. Am J Epidemiol 1986; 123:790–797.
90. Armon C, Kurland LT, Daube JR, O'Brien PC. Epidemiologic correlates of sporadic amyothrophic lateral sclerosis. Neurology 1991; 41:1077–1084.
91. Siddique T, Figlewicz DA, Pericak-Vance MA, et al. Linkage of a gene causing familial amyotrophic lateral sclerosis to chromosome 21 and evidence of genetic-locus heterogeneity. N Engl J Med 1991; 324:1381–1384.
92. Terry R, Katzman R. Alzheimer disease and cognitive loss. In: Katzman R, Rowe JW, eds. Principles of geriatric neurology. Philadelphia: FA Davis, 1992:207–265.
93. Chui HC, Teng EL, Henderson VW, Moy AC. Clinical subtypes of dementia of the Alzheimer type. Neurology 1985; 35:1544–1550.
94. Mayeux R, Stern Y, Spanton S. Heterogeneity in dementia of the Alzheimer type: evidence of subgroups. Neurology 1985; 35:453–461.
95. Mölsä PK, Marttila RJ, Rinne UK. Extrapyramidal signs in Alzheimer's disease. Neurology 1984; 34:1114–1116.
96. Brown RG, Marsden CD. How common is dementia in Parkinson's disease? Lancet 1984; 2:1262–1265.
97. Mayeux R, Stern Y, Rosenstein R, et al. An estimate of the prevalence of dementia in idiopathic Parkinson's disease. Arch Neurol 1988; 45:260–262.
98. Girotti F, Soliveri P, Carella F, et al. Dementia and cognitive impairment in Parkinson's disease. J Neurol Neurosurg Psychiatry 1988; 51:1498–1502.
99. Marder K, Flood P, Cote L, Mayeux R. A pilot study of risk factors for dementia in Parkinson's disease. Mov Disord 1990; 5:156–161.
100. Stern Y, Marder K, Tang MX, Mayeux R. Antecedent clinical features associated with dementia in Parkinson's disease. Neurology 1993; 43:1690–1692.
101. Hofman A, Schulte W, Tanja RA, et al. History of dementia and Parkinson's disease in 1st-degree relatives of patients with Alzheimer's disease. Neurology 1989; 39:1589–1592.
102. Gibb WRG, Lees AJ. The significance of the Lewy body in the diagnosis of idiopathic Parkinson's disease. Neuropathol Appl Neurobiol 1989; 15:27–44.
103. Golbe L. Parkinsonian syndromes. In: Stern MB, Koller WC, eds. Progressive supranuclear palsy. New York: Marcel Dekker, 1993:227–247.
104. Yoshimura N, Yoshimura I, Asada M, et al. Juvenile Parkinson's disease with widespread Lewy bodies in the brain. J Neuropathol 1988; 77:213–218.
105. Gowers WR. A lecture on abiotrophy. Lancet 1902; 2:1003–1007.
106. Sagar HJ. Clinical similarities and differences between Alzheimer's disease and Parkinson's disease. J Neural Transm 1987; 24:(suppl):87–99.
107. Huber S, Shuttleworth E, Freidenberg D. Neuropsychological differences in the dementia of Alzheimer's and Parkinson's disease. Arch Neurol 1989; 46:1287–1291.
108. Cummings JL. The dementias of Parkinson's disease: prevalence, characteristics,

neurobiology, and comparison with dementia of the Alzheimer type. Eur Neurol 1988; 28(suppl 1):15–23.
109. Pillion B, Dubois B, Ploska A, Agid Y. Severity and specificity of cognitive impairment in Alzheimer's, Huntington's and Parkinson's diseases and progressive supranuclear palsy. Neurology 1991; 41:634–643.
110. Rajput AH, Rozdilsky B, Rajput A. Accuracy of clinical diagnosis in parkinsonism—a prospective study. Can J Neurol Sci 1991; 18:275–278.
111. Hughes AJ, Daniel SE, Kilford L, Lees AJ. Accuracy of the clinical diagnosis of Parkinson's disease: a clinicopathological study of 100 cases. J Neurol Neurosurg Psychiatry 1992; 55:181–184.
112. Hakim AM, Mathieson G. Dementia in Parkinson disease: a neuropathologic study. Neurology 1979; 29 (9 pt 1):1209–1214.
113. Boller F, Mizutani T, Roessmann U, Gambetti P. Parkinson disease, dementia, and Alzheimer disease: clinicopathological correlations. Ann Neurol 1980; 7:329–335.
114. Gaspar P, Gray F. Dementia in idiopathic Parkinson's disease. A neuropathological study of 32 cases. Acta Neuropathol 1984; 64:43–52.
115. Perry EK, Curtis M, Dick DJ, et al. Cholinergic correlates of cognitive impairment in Parkinson's disease: comparisons with Alzheimer's disease. J Neurol Neurosurg Psychiatry 1985; 48:413–421.
116. Paulus W, Jellinger K. The neuropathologic basis of different clinical subgroups of Parkinson's disease. J Neuropathol Exp Neurol 1991; 50:743–755.
117. Xuereb JH, Tomlinson BE, Irving D, Perry RH, Blessed G, Perry EK. Cortical and subcortical pathology in Parkinson's disease: relationship to parkinsonian dementia. In: Streifler MB, Korczyn AD, Melamed E, Youdim MBH, eds. Parkinson's disease: anatomy, pathology and therapy. Adv Neurol 1990; 53:35–40.
118. Ince P, Irving D, MacArthur F, Perry RH. Quantitative neuropathological study of Alzheimer-type pathology in the hippocampus: comparison of senile dementia of Alzheimer type, senile dementia of Lewy body type, Parkinson's disease and non-demented elderly control patients. J Neurol Sci 1991; 106:142–152.
119. Bergeron C, Pollanen M. Lewy bodies in Alzheimer disease—one or two diseases. Alzheimer Dis Assoc Disord 1989; 3:197–204.
120. Leverenz J, Sumi SM. Parkinson's disease in patients with Alzheimer's disease. Arch Neurol 1986; 43:662–664.
121. Ditter SM, Mirra SS. Neuropathologic and clinical features of Parkinson's disease in Alzheimer's disease patients. Neurology 1987; 37:754–760.
122. Tanner CM. Epidemiology of Parkinson's disease. Neurol Clin 1992; 10:317–329.
123. Katzman R, Terry R, DeTeresa R, et al. Clinical, pathological, and neurochemical changes in dementia: a subgroup with preserved mental status and numerous neocortical plaques. Ann Neurol 1988; 23:138–144.
124. Forno LS. Concentric hyalin intraneuronal inclusions of Lewy type in the brains of elderly persons (50 incidental cases): relationship to parkinsonism. J Am Geriatr Soc 1969; 17:557–575.
125. Gibb WRG. The epidemiology of Lewy bodies. In: Fahn S, Marsden CD, Calne DB, Goldstein M, eds. Recent developments in Parkinson's disease, vol 2. New Jersey: Macmillan Healthcare Information, 1987:1–13.

126. Katzman R, Terry R. Normal aging of the nervous system. In: Katzman R, Rowe JW, eds. Principles of geriatric neurology. Philadelphia: FA Davis, 1992:18–58.
127. Eatough VM, Kempster PA, Stern GM, Lees AJ. Premorbid personality and idiopathic Parkinson's disease. In: Parkinson's disease: anatomy, pathology and therapy. Adv Neurol 1990; 53:335–337.
128. Kondo K. Epidemiological clues for the etiology of Parkinson's disease. In: Hassler RG, Christ F, eds. Parkinson-specific motor and mental disorders, role of the pallidum: pathophysiological, biochemical, and therapeutic aspects. Adv Neurol 1984; 40:345–351.
129. Pollock M, Hornabrook RW. The prevalence, natural history and dementia of Parkinson's disease. Brain 1966; 89:429–448.
130. Poewe W, Karamat E, Kemmler GW, Gerstenbrand F. The premorbid personality of patients with Parkinson's disease: a comparative study with healthy controls and patients with essential tremor. In: Parkinson's disease: anatomy, pathology and therapy. Adv Neurol 1990; 53:339–342.
131. Poewe W, Gerstenbrand F, Ransmayr G, Plörer S. Premorbid personality of Parkinson patients. J Neural Transm 1983; 19(suppl):215–224.
132. Uono M, Segawa M, Aoyama M. [Symposium: metabolism in neurological disorders. 1. Parkinsonism four pedigrees of familial parkinsonism—mainly on DOPA metabolism]. Nippon Naika Gakkai Zasshi 1972; pp 1136–1138.
133. Paulson G, Dadmehr N. Is there a premorbid personality typical for Parkinson's disease? Neurology 1991; 41(suppl 2):73–76.
134. Menza M, Forman NE, Goldstein HE, Golbe LI. Parkinson's disease, personality and dopamine. J Neuropsychiatry Clin Neurosci 1990; 2:282–287.
135. Ward CD, Duvoisin RC, Ince SE, et al. Parkinson's disease in twins. In: Parkinson-specific motor and mental disorders, role of the pallidum: pathophysological, biochemical, and therapeutic aspects. Adv Neurol 1984; 40:341–344.
136. Kahn HA. The Dorn study of smoking and mortality among U. S. veterans: report on eight and one-half years of observation. In: Haenszel W, ed. Epidemiological approaches to the study of cancer and other chronic diseases. Bethesda, MD: US Health, Education and Welfare, National Cancer Institute, Monogr 19, 1966:1–27.
137. Kessler II, Diamond EL. Epidemiologic studies of Parkinson's disease. I. Smoking and Parkinson's disease: a survey and explanatory hypothesis. Am J Epidemiol 1971; 94:16–25.
138. Nefzger MD, Quadfasel FA, Karl VC. A retrospective study of smoking in Parkinson's disease. Am J Epidemiol 1968; 88:149–158.
139. Godwin-Austen RB, Lee PN, Marmot MG, Stern GM. Smoking and Parkinson's disease. J Neurol Neurosurg Psychiatry 1982; 45:577–581.
140. Mayeux R, Stern Y, Rosen J, Leventhal J. Depression, intellectual impairment, and Parkinson disease. Neurology 1981; 31:645–650.
141. Santamaria J, Tolosa E, Valles A. Parkinson's disease with depression: a possible subgroup of idiopathic parkinsonism. Neurology 1986; 36:1130–1133.
142. Ross RT. Drug-induced parkinsonism and other movement disorders. Can J Neurol Sci 1990; 17:155–162.

143. Lauterbach EC, Duvoisin RC. Anxiety disorders in familial parkinsonism [letter]. Am J Psychiatry 1991; 148:274.
144. Critchley M. Arteriosclerotic parkinsonism. Brain 1929; 52:23–83.
145. Parkes J, Marsden C, Rees J, Carjon M. Parkinson's disease, cerebral arteriosclerosis, and senile dementia. Q J Med 1974; 43:49–61.
146. Hurtig H. Vascular parkinsonism. In: Stern MB, Koller WC, eds. Parkinsonian syndromes. New York: Marcel Dekker, 1993:81–92.
147. Marttila RJ, Rinne UK. Arteriosclerosis, heredity, and some previous infections in the etiology of Parkinson's disease. A case–control study. Clin Neurol Neurosurg 1976; 79:46–56.
148. Gottlieb D, Melamed E. Is there a relationship between Parkinson's disease and stroke [abstract]. Nineth international symposium on Parkinson's disease, 1988:117–110.
149. Doshay LJ. Problem situations in the treatment of paralysis agitans. JAMA 1954; 156:680–684.
150. Barbeau A, Roy M, Cloutier T. Smoking, cancer, and Parkinson's disease. Ann Neurol 1986; 20:105–106.
151. Pritchard PB 3d, Netsky MG. Prevalence of neoplasms and causes of death in paralysis agitans. A necropsy study. Neurology 1973; 23:215–222.
152. Hoehn MM, Yahr MD. Parkinsonism: onset, progression and mortality. Neurology 1967; 17:427–442.
153. Fermaglich J, Delaney P. Parkinson's disease, melanoma and levodopa. J Neurol 1977; 215:221–224.
154. Gibberd FB, Simmonds JP. Neurological disease in ex-Far-East prisoners of war. Lancet 1980; 2:135–137.
155. Spina MB, Cohen G. Dopamine turnover and glutathione oxidation: implications for Parkinson disease. Proc Natl Acad Sci USA 1989; 86:1398–1400.
156. Snyder AM, Stricker EM, Zigmond MJ. Stress-induced neurological impairments in an animal model of parkinsonism. Ann Neurol 1985; 18:544–551.
157. Urakami K, Masaki N, Shimoda K, Nishikawa S, Takahashi K. Increase of striatal dopamine turnover by stress in MPTP-treated mice. Clin Neuropharmacol 1988; 11:360–368.
158. Goetz CG, Stebbins GT. Effects of head trauma from motor vehicle accidents on parkinson's disease. Ann Neurol 1991; 29:191–193.
159. Lampert PW, Hardman JM. Morphological changes in brains of boxers. JAMA 1984; 251:2676–2679.
160. Stern MB. Head trauma as a risk factor for Parkinson's disease. Mov Disord 1991; 6:95–97.
161. Factor SA, Weiner WJ. Prior history of head trauma in Parkinson's disease. Mov Disord 1991; 6:225–229.
162. Williams DB, Annegers JP, Kokeman E, O'Brien PC, Kurland LT. Brain injury and neurologic sequelae: a cohort study of dementia, parkinsonism, and amyotrophic lateral sclerosis. Neurology 1991; 41:1554–1557.
163. Crane GE, Smeets RA. Tardive dyskinesia and drug therapy in geriatric patients. Arch Gen Psychiatry 1974; 30:341–343.
164. Hubble JP. Drug-induced parkinsonism. In: Stern MB, Koller WC, eds. Parkinsonian syndromes. New York: Marcel Dekker, 1993:111–122.

165. Hall R, Jackson R, Swan J. Neurotoxic reactions resulting from chlorpromazine administration. JAMA 1956; 161:214–218.
166. Metzer WS, Newton JEO, Steele RW, et al. HLA antigens in drug-induced parkinsonism. Mov Disord 1989; 4:121–128.
167. Myrianthopoulos N, Kurland A, Kurland L. Hereditary predisposition in drug-induced parkinsonism. Arch Neurol 1962; 6:5.
168. Myrianthopoulos NC, Waldrop IN, Vincent BL. A repeat study of hereditary predisposition in drug-induced parkinsonism. In: Barbeau A, Brunette JB, eds. Progress in neurogenetics. Amsterdam: Excerpta Medica, 1969:486–491.
169. Goetz CG. Drug-induced parkinsonism and idiopathic Parkinson's disease [letter]. Arch Neurol 1983; 40:325–326.
170. Hardie RJ, Lees AJ. Neuroleptic-induced Parkinson's syndrome: clinical features and results of treatment with levodopa. J Neurol Neurosurg Psychiatry 1988; 51:850–854.
171. Rajput AH, Rozdilsky B, Hornykiewicz O. Reversible drug-induced parkinsonism. Arch Neurol 1982; 39:644–646.
172. Ballard PA, Tetrud JW, Langston JW. Permanent human parkinsonism due to 1-methyl-4-phenyl-1,2,3,6-tetrahydropyridine (MPTP): seven cases. Neurology 1985; 35:949–956.
173. Ross RT. Young age parkinsonism and common drugs [letter]. Can J Neurol Sci 1989; 16:366–367.
174. Lieberman A, Goldstein M. Reversible parkinsonism related to meperidine. N Engl J Med 1985; 8:509.
175. Seiden LS, Fischman MW, Schuster CR. Long-term methamphetamine-induced changes in brain catecholamines in tolerant rhesus monkeys. Drug Alcohol Depend 1975; 1:215–219.
176. Osuntokun BO, Bademosi O, Ogunremi K, Wright SG. Neuropsychiatric manifestations of typhoid fever in 959 patients. Arch Neurol 1972; 27:7–13.
177. Schlesselman J. Case–control studies: design, conduct, analysis. New York: Oxford University Press, 1982.
178. Heston LL. Dementia associated with Parkinson's disease: a genetic study. J Neurol Neurosurg Psychiatry 1980; 43:846–848.
179. Gajdusek DC, Gibbs CJ. Attempts to demonstrate a transmissible agent in kuru, amyotrophic lateral sclerosis, and other sub-acute and chronic nervous system degenerations of man. Nature 1964; 204:257–259.
180. Gibbs CJ Jr, Gajdusek DC. An update on long-term in vivo and in vitro studies designed to identify a virus as the cause of amyotrophic lateral sclerosis, parkinsonism dementia and Parkinson's disease. In: Rowland L, ed. Human motor neuron diseases. Adv Neurol 1982; 36:343–353.
181. Appel SH. A unifying hypothesis for the cause of amyotrophic lateral sclerosis, parkinsonism, and Alzheimer disease. Ann Neurol 1981; 10:499–505.
182. Stewart SS, Appel SH. Trophic factors in neurologic disease. Ann Rev Med 1988; 39:193–201.
183. Cadet JL. A unifying theory of movement and madness: involvement of free radicals in disorders of the isodendritic core of the brainstem. Med Hypotheses 1988; 27:59–63.

184. Barker R. Substance P and Parkinson's disease: a causal relationship. J Theor Biol 1986; 120:353–362.
185. Eisen A, Calne D. Amyotrophic lateral sclerosis, Parkinson's disease and Alzheimer's disease: phylogenetic disorders of the human neocortex sharing many characteristics. Can J Neurol Sci 1992; 19(suppl 1):117–123.
186. Kurth MC, Kurth, JH. Variant cytochrome P450 CYP2D6 allelic frequencies in Parkinson's disease. Am J Med Genet 1993; 48:166–168.
187. Kallio J, Marttila RM, Rinne UK, Sonninen V, Syvalahti E. Debrisoquine oxidation in Parkinson's disease. Acta Neurol Scand 1991; 83:194–197.
188. Byrne EJ, Lennox G, Lowe J, Godwin-Austen RB. Diffuse Lewy body disease: clinical features in 15 cases. J Neurol Neurosurg Psychiatry 1989; 52:709–717.

10

Early Life and Demographic Factors Predisposing to Parkinson's Disease

Jonas H. Ellenberg

National Institute of Neurological Disorders and Stroke, National Institutes of Health, Bethesda, Maryland

I. INTRODUCTION

Are there groups of subjects who are more vulnerable than others for *onset* of Parkinson's disease? The word onset is used with some feeling of unease. Manifestation of Parkinson's disease may be evident only at the time of observable clinical symptomatology, but the subclinical *process* that causes clinical signs to become evident may precede, by decades, the first presentation of clinical signs (1). With the promising research in the area of presymptomatic markers (2), and the potential for recognition of early clinical signs not directly related to the movement malfunction of Parkinson's disease, the distinction between process and outcome is becoming somewhat blurred. For purposes of the current discussion, we will use onset to mean clinical symptomatology of Parkinson's disease, since that is the outcome measure used in the research reports we will be examining.

There are a host of fundamental questions related to the issues of predisposition that include the following: Is there a group or are there groups of subjects who are more susceptible than others? Does the susceptibility operate in the form of a simple increase in the likelihood of onset of symptoms, or does it manifest itself by lowering the threshold of tolerance against environmental or endogenous attacks on the system that protects against onset? Does heritability play any role in these questions? Data are not yet available to address most of these questions relating to the etiology of this disorder. However, several factors potentially defining susceptible groups have been studied, including sex, race, premorbid personality, and blood type. The examples of demographic markers determined before birth and early-life factors considered in this chapter are distinguished from endogenous biochemical deficiencies examined in Chapters 4 and 6. This short review will focus on the methodological approaches used in the reports on these factors and the effect of the methodology on the validity of the stated conclusions.

II. SEX DIFFERENTIALS

Diamond et al. (3) have indicated recently that "most studies find Parkinson's disease to be more common in men than in women, with male:female ratios reported as 1.36(4), 1.45(5), 1.51(6), 1.53(7), 2.13(8), 2.32(9), 2.64(10), 3.3(11), and 3.7(12)." They go on to state that "A few studies have found more Parkinson's disease in women than men, presenting male: female ratios of 0.75(13) and 0.81(14), although the latter (14) concludes that age-adjusted prevalence ratios for men and women are essentially the same."

The characteristics of the studies that Diamond et al. use in support of the male preponderance hypothesis are presented in Table 1. Of the 11 studies referenced, only 3 (7,12,13) were designed to measure prevalence and demographic characteristics of subjects with Parkinson's disease. The other eight studies, were "selected" samples of subjects, with study objectives relating to either etiology, or survival and morbidity under different treatment regimens. None of the authors of these eight studies presented their data on the male/female distribution as a result, but rather as a description of their sample. Diamond et al.'s, inappropriate interpretation (3) of most of these reports is unfortunate. It is also interesting that the one population-based prevalence study showing no differential (14) is highlighted almost disparagingly by Diamond et al., for its very appropriate use of age adjustment.

In general, comparisons of frequency of disease among different groups would best be done using incidence, rather than prevalence. *Prevalence* is a measure of frequency of disease in a population at a point in time and a function of, among other things, both incidence and mortality. *Incidence*, on the other hand, is the frequency of new cases in a defined time period. Thus, group differences in prevalent morbidity could represent underlying differences of frequency of disease, or differences in mortality. Unfortunately, studies of incidence are inherently more difficult to undertake. Both in this section and in the section on race that follows, assessment of the available prevalence data is undertaken, although the principles involved in evaluating studies of incidence would be similar.

The several studies in the literature that were designed to allow examination of differentials between male and female prevalence of Parkinson's disease, and that also provided absolute prevalence levels for each sex, will be reviewed.

Table 1 Reports Selected by Diamond et al. (3) in Support of the Hypothesis of Differences in Prevalence of Parkinson's Disease Between Men and Women

First author	Study design
Bauer (4)	Observational follow-up study of patients with significant impairment, presenting for care at a large city hospital
Golbe (5)	Case–control study of patients referred to university hospital
Hoehn (6)	Observational follow-up study of patients with mild to severe impairment presenting for care at a large city hospital
Bharucha (7)	Door-to-door survey of neurological disorders in an entire community
Sweet (8)	Observational follow-up study of patients with moderate to severe impairment, presenting for care at a university hospital
Diamond (9)	Observational follow-up study of patients with mild to severe impairment, presenting for care at a university hospital
Barbeau (10)	Observational follow-up study of patients primarily with severe impairment and receiving experimental therapy at a teaching hospital
Tanner (11)	Case–control study of patients presenting for care at neurology outpatient clinics
Li (12)	Door-to-door survey of neurological disorders in defined geographic areas
Marttila (13)	Observational follow-up study of patients with mild to severe impairment, presenting for care at a university hospital
Schoenberg (14)	Door-to-door survey of neurological disorders in an entire community

The prevalence reports given in Table 2 include many, but not all, studies that provide information on the prevalence of Parkinson's disease for men and women separately. The many reports based on death certificate data were not included, for example, since such data have been shown to markedly underestimate prevalence. In the past, Parkinson's disease as an underlying cause of death, or as a contributory cause of death, has not been reported on death certificates in a large proportion of subjects known to have died with Parkinson's disease (see Chapter 8 and Ref. 6). There is no recent evidence to indicate substantial changes in reporting practice.

Most of the studies reported relied on providers of medical care for case ascertainment. Schoenberg (14) noted that approximately 40% of subjects classified as having Parkinson's disease identified through a door-to-door household survey, had "not previously received medical attention," leading one to be cautious about reliance on medical care providers for comprehensive detection of all cases in a given geographic area. This would be especially important where there may be impediments to access to medical care, societal reasons for not

Table 2 Reports of Prevalence of Parkinson's Disease: Sex Differentials and Methodology

				Prevalence/100,000			Notes[a]		
Study	First author	Country	Year	Male	Female	p^*	Case ascertainment	Diagnosis	Age standardization
A.	Kurland (41)	USA	1955	115	113	—	a–c, g, j	a, b, d	c
B.	Gudmundsson (42)	Iceland	1963	157	133	—	a–d, j, g	a, b, d	c
C.	Kessler (17)	USA: White	1965–7	28	23	n.s.	a, j	a, b, f, g	b
D.		Black		31	5	4	n.s.		
E.	Kessler (19)	USA: White	1967–9	128	121	n.s.	b, c, g, j	a, b, e	b
F.		Black		31	9	<0.05			
G.	Dupont (43)	Denmark	1971	80	87	—	a–c, f, g, j	a, c, e	c
H.	Marttila (16)	Finland	1971	114	116	—	a–e, g, j	a, c, e	a
I.	Rosati (44)	So. Europe	1971	56	77	<0.001	a–c, e, g, j	a, c, e	a
J.	Schoenberg (14)	USA	1978	350	345	—	g, h, k	a, c, e	b
K.	Harada (45)	Japan	1980	63	97	—	a, e, g, j	a, c, d	c
L.	Sutcliffe (46)	UK	1982	102	114	n.s.	a, b, g, j	a, b, d	c
M.	Ashok (23)	Libya	1985	58	62	—	a, e, f, g, j	a, c, d	b
N.	Bharucha (47)	India	1985	235	154	—	g, h	a, d, c	b
O.	Wang (48)	China	1986	18	12	<0.0001	g, i	a, c, d n	a
P.	Casetta (49)	Italy	1987	161	212	n.s.	a–d, g, j	a, c, d	b

*p value for statistical test of difference reported by author: —indicates test not performed; n.s. indicates test not significant, usually at 0.05 level.

[a]*Notes*:

Case ascertainment
a. Hospital records
b. General practitioners
c. Specialists
d. Pharmacies
e. Health insurance or national medical care records
f. Long-term care institutions
g. Defined geographic area
h. Comprehensive survey
i. Stratified random sampling
j. Prevalence based on estimated population from which cases were identified
k. Evaluated population aged 40 or older only

Diagnosis
a. Neurologist or other physician confirmation
b. Medical record review
c. In-person examination
d. IPD only
e. Postencephalitic Parkinson's disease included
f. Drug-induced Parkinson's disease included
g. Arteriosclerotic Parkinson's disease included

Age standardization
a. Direct age standardization to total surveyed population using available published data (15)
b. Age standardized by original authors
c. Unadjusted

seeking medical care, or differential inclinations to seek medical care in the groups under study (e.g., men vs. women). There are other problems with reliance on medical care providers for identification of cases: Parkinson's disease patients are not generally treated as inpatients for long-term care, and comorbid conditions may be included only on discharge diagnoses as outpatients; busy private practitioners are likely to have to rely on their memory for case identification, absent a sophisticated computer data base; and patients with Parkinson's disease may see many physicians and double-counting might occur. These types of problems and their severity vary within and between countries, and although we should not exclude all but complete door-to-door surveys, results of prevalence (and incidence) studies must be evaluated while taking into account the completeness of case identification.

Diagnostic confirmation is another evaluative criterion for judging the generalizability or usefulness of results. Generally accepted definitions of Parkinson's disease should be employed, with neurologist or at least physician confirmation. In-person examination is optimal, but examination of complete histories, including results of neurological examinations may be acceptable. Exclusions should be clearly defined at the beginning of an investigation. Drug-induced Parkinson's disease (e.g., phenothiazines), or postencephalitic cases, should be identified separately or excluded.

Since men and women have different age distributions, it is important to provide age-adjusted prevalence estimates. These adjustments may vary in approach, but in general, take account of the different age distributions between men and women, especially in the older-aged brackets in whom Parkinson's disease is more prevalent. If the authors did not provide age-adjusted estimates, when possible we used their published data to provide "direct" standardization (15), using the distribution of the combined male plus female age distribution as the standard.

We have chosen those studies for presentation that demonstrated an awareness of the foregoing issues. Few of the studies were without substantial methodological flaws, but the investigators made attempts to ameliorate problems expected because of them. For example, most studies were not door-to-door comprehensive surveys of a defined geographic area. However, multiple resources were frequently used for case finding, such as hospitals, private practitioners, long-term care facilities, insurance and disability rolls, or others, to assure the highest possible level of case ascertainment. The methods of case ascertainment for each study are given in Table 2.

Marttila (16) concisely states the problems of selected samples and the use of age adjustments for obtaining reliable estimates of frequency of Parkinson's disease as follows:

> Clinical series have suggested that the sexes are affected differently by Parkinson's disease; a male predominance has most often been observed.

However, several sources of bias may distort sex distribution in such series. More reliable data can be obtained in epidemiologic studies, and even then the crude prevalence or incidence rates are not free from bias, since female and male age structures are seldom identical. Therefore, age- and sex-specific prevalence, or preferably incidence, is the most reliable indicator in estimating the risk of Parkinson's disease in the sexes.

The studies reviewed here have made reasonable attempts to achieve these goals. In any event, readers can use the design descriptions given to help decide for themselves the adequacy of the different studies.

If we can accept the prevalence values presented in Table 2 at face value, several observations can be made. First, for both sexes the studies report dramatic differences in absolute levels of Parkinson's disease point prevalence. The highest levels, reported by Schoenberg et al. (14), can probably be attributed to their use of only the older than 40-year-old population. The low levels reported by Kessler(17) in 1965–1967 can likely be attributed to the use of only hospital-based ascertainment in that particular study. Only three of the eight studies in which tests of significance were performed in the comparison of male versus female prevalence ratios indicated statistical significance, with conflicting results.

Within each study, when possible, the 95% confidence intervals about the age-adjusted point prevalence were derived for men and women separately from the data available in the published reports (Fig. 1). Given the low prevalence of Parkinson's disease, the large sample approximation for the estimation of the mean of the Poisson distribution was used to construct the confidence limits (18). These limits are not symmetrical about the point prevalence for the studies with smaller sample sizes. Since the study designs were relatively heterogeneous, a combined estimate of prevalence for each sex was not undertaken. However, from Figure 1, the large width of the confidence bands provided by most of the studies, and the overlap of the confidence bands in all but three of the studies do not present convincing existing evidence for an important difference in prevalence between the sexes, if any exists. Ignoring the differences in the absolute prevalence levels among the studies, the ratios of prevalence for men to women within each study (given below horizontal axis in Fig. 1) also do not support a consistent dominance for either sex. The observed sex ratios were unity in three studies and were suggestive of female (less than unity) and male (greater than unity) dominance in six and seven of the remaining studies, respectively.

The differences in prevalence levels between countries and within the United States may be ascribed to the differences in methodologies of case ascertainment, diagnosis, and age standardization already discussed and described in Table 2. The differences may also represent true geographic disparities in prevalence. The variation in absolute levels of prevalence, although different between studies, are similar within studies, even when either sex dominates.

It is probably reasonable to assume that the differences in study design that

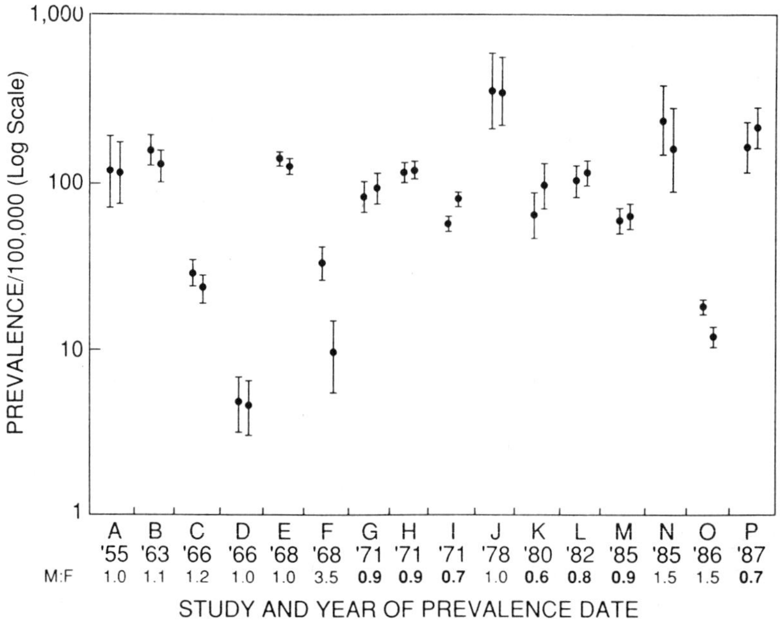

Figure 1 Prevalence of Parkinson's disease by sex (logarithmic scale): 95% confidence intervals and point prevalence estimates indicated by lower and upper bar and dot, respectively, for men and women, respectively, for each study. Letters on *x* axis refer to study in Table 2. The ratio of the absolute prevalence for men/women is given for each study, below the *x* axis.

may be the cause of between-study differences would not have differentially affected the results between the sexes within studies in a major way. If this is so, then the current studies best able to detect a susceptibility to Parkinson's disease, based on gender, do not provide convincing evidence that it exists.

III. RACIAL DIFFERENTIALS

Dramatic racial differences were seen in the two Kessler studies (17,19), the Paddison and Griffith study (20), and the Lombard study(21), all of which relied solely on medical care records for identification of cases (Table 3). The Paddison and Griffith and the Lombard studies should be considered the least definitive of these reports, since no appropriate attempts at determining prevalence in a defined geographic area were made. These studies report only the number of hospitalized patients (black and white), and provide prevalence of black and white patients with Parkinson's disease among all hospitalized patients.

Table 3 Prevalence of Parkinson's Disease: Race Differentials and Methodology

				Prevalence/100,000			Notes[b]		
Study	First author	Country	Yr	White	Black	p^*	Case ascertainment	Diagnosis	Age standardization
A.	Paddison (20)	USA	1959–69	146	22	<0.001	a	b	b
B.	Kessler (17)	USA: Male	1965–67	28	5	<0.05	a, j	a, b, e, f, g	a
C.		Female		23	4	<0.05			
D.	Kessler (19)	USA: Male	1967–69	128	31	<0.05	b, c, g, j	b, e	a
E.		Female		121	9	<0.05			
F.	Lombard (21)	Africa	1973–76	79	4	—	a	b, f, g	b
G.	Haerer (22)	USA[a]	1978	353	338	—	g, h, k	a, c, e	a
H.	Ashok (23)	Libya	1985		60	—	a, e, f, g, j	a, c, d	a
I.	Schoenberg (24)	Nigeria	1986		67	—	g, h, k	a, c, e	a

[a]Possible and definite Parkinson's disease cases are combined by authors.
$^*p$ values for statistical tests of significance reported by author: —indicates statistical test not performed.
[b]*Notes*:

Case ascertainment
a. Hospital records
b. General practitioners
c. Specialists
d. Pharmacies
e. Health insurance or national medical care records
f. Long-term care institutions
g. Defined geographic area
h. Comprehensive survey
i. Stratified random sampling
j. Prevalence based on estimated population from which cases were identified
k. Evaluated population aged 40 or older only

Diagnosis
a. Neurologist or other physician confirmation
b. Medical record review
c. In person examination
d. IPD only
e. Postencephalitic Parkinson's disease included
f. Drug-induced Parkinson's disease included
g. Arteriosclerotic Parkinson's disease included

Age standardization
a. Age standardized by original authors
b. Unadjusted

In the only population-based comprehensive survey of an entire community in the United States, with both white and black residents (50.1% white, 49.1% black) (22), there were no differences seen in the age-adjusted rates of Parkinson's disease (possible and definite combined) between blacks and whites. When the authors considered definite Parkinson's disease cases only, the age-adjusted prevalence for whites was higher than for blacks in this study. However, there was only a 40% differential, as contrasted with the fivefold increases in prevalence among blacks seen in the other studies (17,19–21).

Within each study, the 95% confidence intervals were derived for whites and blacks separately, based on the information available from the published reports. [Both Ashok (23) and Schoenberg et al.(24) report only on prevalence in blacks]. The method for deriving the confidence bands has been described previously. The results along with the ratio of prevalence rates for whites to blacks are given in Figure 2. The nonoverlapping confidence bands for most of the studies are indicative of a statistical indication of a racial disparity in Parkinson's disease prevalence, with rate ratios ranging from 4 to 19 in favor of whites. However, these observations (if not their direction, at least their magnitude) may be influenced by biases introduced by the study designs used.

In the Copiah County study (22), some 40% of the Parkinson's disease subjects had not been seen for medical attention before their detection in the survey. Although the absolute number of cases was small, the number not previously seen for medical care was approximately equally divided between whites and blacks. With the latter observation in mind, it may be difficult to impute the large racial disparities seen in the non–community-based studies to differential access to medical care. However, Copiah County is a small rural community, with all of its physicians as "family practitioners," and it is perhaps not a sound assumption that the observed *equal* lack of receipt of medical attention between the races for Parkinson's disease in Copiah County be translated to equal access to medical care in different types of communities, such as Baltimore, a large urban community (17,19).

The community-based survey in Nigeria (24) used the same techniques for case ascertainment as in Copiah County and indicated a considerably lower prevalence in blacks in Nigeria from that seen in both whites and blacks in Copiah County. In commenting on this disparity, Schoenberg et al., remind us that observed prevalence is related to both the occurrence of new cases and the survival of both old and new cases. However, he states that the results of two community-based surveys in these two different countries, which demonstrated a "five-fold increase in age-adjusted prevalence ratios between Igbo-Ora and Copiah County is unlikely to reflect variations in survival and probably is a result of a difference in incidence rates . . . and that these findings are consistent with the hypothesis that an environmental agent (or agents) may be responsible for the observed differences."

Paddison and Griffith (20), on the basis of their non–community-based results

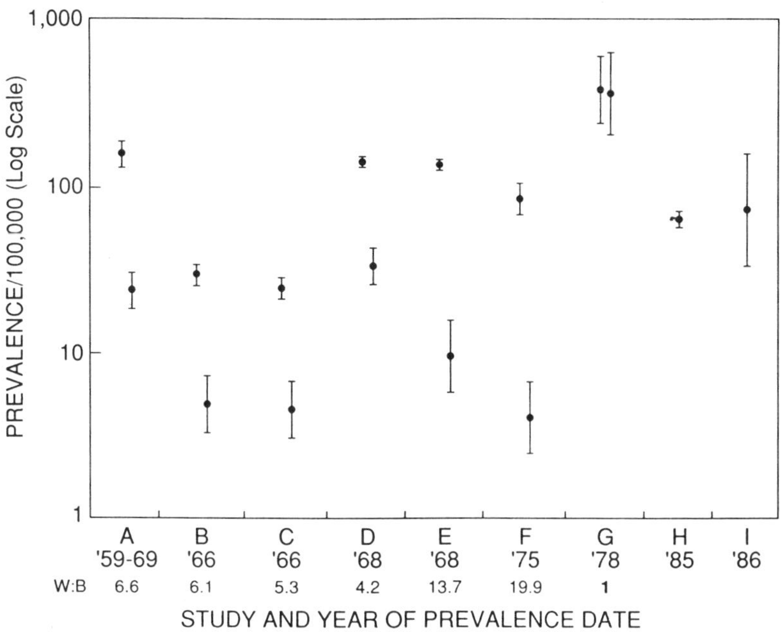

Figure 2 Prevalence of Parkinson's disease by race (logarithmic scale): 95% confidence intervals and point prevalence estimates indicated by lower and upper bar and dot, respectively, for whites and blacks, respectively, for each study. Letters on *x* axis refer to study in Table 3. The Ashok (23) and Schoenberg (24) studies did not provide data for whites. The ratio of the absolute prevalence for whites/blacks is given for each study, below the *x* axis.

reporting racial differences, suggest further studies of the melanin metabolic pathways and catecholamine metabolism in black people, and Kessler (17) would extend such investigations to the "possible pathway between these (biogenic) amines and nicotine."

The Copiah County study (22), with its appropriate study design (door-to-door survey) and direct comparison of whites and blacks in the same community, stands as the most methodologically appropriate study yet available to address the question of racial differences. This study does not support the other evidence for an important black–white differential for racial susceptibility to Parkinson's disease. Schoenberg et al. caution the reader that these results may not apply to other populations. However, having seen the enormous distortion in results that can result from selected, rather than community-based sampling schemes (25), it can be argued that a racial susceptibility has not been consistently nor convincingly seen, and that only another community-based survey will clarify this issue.

IV. PREMORBID PERSONALITY TRAIT

In their twin study, Ward et al. (26) did retrospective premorbid personality assessments of monozygous (MZ) twin pairs discordant for Parkinson's disease. The original cohort of twins was developed using advertisements in newsletters of lay Parkinson's disease organizations (27), which were the most successful, through "adult twin registries in the United States and through notices in medical journals . . . announcements at neurology meetings, and informal inquiries among professional colleagues" (28). Of the 121 twin pairs so identified 77 (64%) were available for confirmation of diagnosis. Seventeen of these pairs were eliminated because of failure to confirm a Parkinson's disease diagnosis, leaving 60 twins, of which two-thirds were MZ. From this MZ group, 20 were selected, in an unspecified fashion, for premorbid personality testing. The detail of the sample selection is outlined here so that the reader can be aware of the potential for selection bias, from the initial nonrandom contact of 121 twin pairs down to the 20 pairs used for the study, that could influence the results.

Nineteen traits were assessed with self-reporting of each twin as well as cross-reporting by their twin counterpart. After accounting for multiple comparisons in the statistical analyses, several of the traits discriminated between the twin with and without Parkinson's disease. Well before onset, in the first decades of life, the affected twin was found to be more "self-controlled," less likely to be the leader, and more nervous. In later life, but still a decade before manifestation of Parkinson's disease, the affected twin was "less aggressive," "more quiet," "less confident," and "less light-hearted." Kondo (29) reported on a matched case–control study of preclinical personality among 166 parkinsonism patients in Japan, using language that implies the results relate to premorbid status only. His results indicate similarities to those of Ward et al., with Parkinson's disease patients being "introversive, excessively responsible, urged toward perfect fulfillment of tasks, keeping an exact schedule for daily activities." No time frame for the presence of these features before onset of symptoms is given. Ward et al. (28) conclude "An implication of chronic, possibly life long personality differences between discordant twins is that a long-term neurochemical difference may precede the onset of Parkinson's disease." These changes or differences may be manifested in a predisposition for Parkinson's disease among persons with certain personality traits.

Lees (30) states "A high frequency of depressive illness occurring many years before the onset of Parkinson's disease has been reported in some studies (Celesia and Wanamaker)"; (31). The cited report (31) on 170 Parkinson's disease patients indicates that 57 of these patients (37%) had depressive symptoms at the time of or within 1 year of initial evaluation. However, only 5 of these Parkinson's disease patients "also had a history of one or more episodes of severe depression preceding the onset of Parkinson's symptoms."

Poewe et al. (32), in a case–control study of 38 patients with Parkinson's disease and 17 controls also reported premorbid personality traits among Parkinson's disease patients of "introversion, rigidity, and inflexibility." The interviews used were repeated with a significant other, for confirmation.

Eatough et al. (33), in a study of 30 young-onset Parkinson's disease patients (average age 46.1 years), matched to normal subjects and patients with rheumatoid arthritis for age, sex, and occupational status, presented data indicating that "the Parkinsonians were less flexible and more cautious" and "scored considerably higher for bereavement and personal injury in childhood." The methods section did not clearly describe how efforts were made to attribute these traits to the premorbid state.

In a case–control study of 118 incident Parkinson's disease cases, each matched to two controls, Rajput et al. (34) observed an increased risk of Parkinson's disease for those with combined diagnoses of preclinical personality disorder or mental retardation. However, the number of cases ($n = 3$) among those with Parkinson's disease was small, and the reported results do not indicate how many of the three are personality disorders.

Smythies (35) compared the responses of Parkinson's disease patients, admitted for stereotactic surgery, on an instrument to measure "psychological disturbance", with sex- and age-matched chronic respiratory hospitalized patients. He concluded that "there is no correlation between a disturbed childhood, a previous tendency to neurotic symptomatology, or a difficult adjustment to life and the onset of parkinsonism." Significant others were not used to corroborate interview responses. Mjönes (36), in an early investigation, also did not demonstrate any "pre-morbid personality of note" among Parkinson's disease patients.

Menza et al. (37), in a study of 20 Parkinson's disease patients, administered the Tridimensional Personality Questionnaire (TPQ) to subjects, asking them to respond currently and as they saw themselves two decades before onset of Parkinson's disease. In addition, spouses were asked to complete the TPQ for the subjects as they felt the patient would have responded 20 years before onset. Premorbid novelty seeking was significantly different between Parkinson's disease patients and a group of matched controls. The spouse and subject's premorbid ratings were not significantly different. The authors linked the novelty-seeking trait to dopamine depletion in animal models.

Todes and Lees (38) conclude appropriately, I believe,

> The inherent problem however, remains the difficulty in distinguishing between pre-morbid personality characteristics and those which develop following the appearance of the classical symptoms of the illness. However, this should not prevent further attempts at assessing pre-morbid personality by means of the newer hostility and personality rating scales and by structured interviews with spouses and other family members. Attempts to

correlate life-events with depression and subsequent Parkinsonism, particularly in the young onset cases would also be of interest.

There will be extreme difficulties faced by investigators obtaining demonstrably reliable preclinical data on early personality traits in further study of this hypothesis. Definitive conclusions cannot be made based on the scope and validity of the data presented to date. But the usefulness of an early premorbid personality trait for the understanding of the pathogenesis and natural history of Parkinson's disease, and for its early clinical detection, argues strongly for its further study.

V. ABO BLOOD GROUP DISTRIBUTION

Only two major reports on blood type have been published (39,40) Strang (39) indicated an excess of blood group O in 450 Swedish Parkinson's patients (approximately half men), compared with controls. Kak et al. (40), in a study of 187 Parkinson's disease patients from Northern Ireland (approximately half men), reported an excess of group B and fewer than expected numbers of patients with group A when compared with controls, but no disparity in expected group O in Parkinson's disease patients. The controls for the Strang study were 10,457 subjects obtained from "paternity material," whereas those from Kak et al. were derived from a series of 27,650 blood donors, presumably of both sexes. The distribution of subjects in the four ABO blood groups was considerably different in the two control series (Table 4).

Kak concluded, 20 years ago after comparing the results from both studies, that "further studies are needed in different geographical areas on similar lines before any deductions can be put forward." Whether there is increased susceptibility among specific ABO blood groups remains an open question, since no further studies appear to have been done, and we cannot extricate the observed differences in results between these two studies from ethnic or other confounding factors.

VI. CONCLUSIONS

It is difficult to strictly distinguish between a factor, such as premorbid personality, that may be indicative of a susceptibility for onset of clinical Parkinson's disease and one that is an early clinical sign of the disease. Furthermore, the etiology of Parkinson's disease remains elusive, and could be multifactorial, with involvement of genetics, environment, and acquired or inborn endogenous deficits. Nonetheless, ability to distinguish groups at high risk for Parkinson's disease could greatly contribute to an understanding of the natural history of the

Table 4 ABO Blood groups and Parkinson's Disease Percentage Distribution

	Strang (50)		Kak and Gordon (40)	
Blood group[a]	Subjects *N*-245	Controls *N*-10,457	Subjects *N*-187	Controls *N*-27,650
	44.4			
O	38.0	53.5	54.0	
A	41.8	47.2	25.7	33.1
B	9.3	9.9	16.0	10.0
AB	4.4	4.8	4.8	2.9
Total	99.9	99.9	100.0	100.0

[a]Computed $X^2(3)$ for comparison of distribution of blood types in the two control groups less than tabled value at the $p = 0.001$ level.

disease and, in particular, to the process of neuronal degeneration leading to Parkinson's disease.

From the literature currently available, there does not appear to be compelling evidence to indicate that race, sex, or blood type are important cofactors in the search for etiology. Conversely, some of the work on premorbid personality is enticing and seems worthy of further pursuit. A future study, with appropriate case-finding techniques, an acceptible diagnostic approach, and unbiased sample selection, may provide definitive results for the race and sex questions. If differentials exist, such a study should have sufficient sample size not only to demonstrate a difference, but also to quantify the magnitude of the differential with reasonable precision.

REFERENCES

1. Koller WC, Langston JW, Hubble JP, et al. Does a long pre-clinical period occur in Parkinson's disease? Neurology 1991; 41(suppl 2):8–13.
2. Langston JW, Koller W. The next frontier in Parkinson's disease: presymptomatic detection. Neurology 1991; 41(suppl 2):5–7.
3. Diamond SG, Markham CH, Hoehn MM, McDowell FH, Muenter MD. An examination of male–female differences in progression and mortality of Parkinson's disease. Neurology 1990; 40:763–766.
4. Bauer RB, Stevens C, Reveno WS, Rosenbaum H. L-Dopa treatment of Parkinson's disease: a ten-year follow-up study. J Am Geriatr Soc 1982; 30:322–325.
5. Golbe LI, Farrell TM, Davis PH. Case–control study of early life dietary factors in Parkinson's disease. Arch Neurol 1988; 45:1350–1353.
6. Hoehn MM, Yahr MD. Parkinsonism: onset, progression and mortality. Neurology 1967; 17:427–442.
7. Bharucha NE, Bharucha EP, Bharucha AE, Bhise AV, Schoenberg BS. Parkinson's

disease in the Parsi community of Bombay, India. Arch Neurol 1988; 45:1321–1323.
8. Sweet RD, McDowell F. Five years' treatment of Parkinson's disease with levodopa. Ann Intern Med 1975; 83:456–463.
9. Diamond SG, Markham CH, Treciokas LJ. Long-term experience with L-dopa: efficacy, progression and mortality. In: Birkmayer W, Hornykiewicz O, eds. Advances in Parkinsonism. Basel: Roche, 1976:444–455.
10. Barbeau A. Six years of high-level levodopa therapy in severely akinetic parkinsonian patients. Arch Neurol 1976; 33:333–338.
11. Tanner CM, Chen B, Wang WZ, et al. Environmental factors and Parkinson's disease: a case–control study in China. Neurology 1989; 39:660–664.
12. Li SC, Schoenberg BS, Wang CC, et al. A prevalence survey of Parkinson's disease and other movement disorders in the People's Republic of China. Arch Neurol 1985; 42:655–657.
13. Marttila RJ, Rinne U, Siirtola T, Sonninen V. Mortality of patients with Parkinson's disease treated with levodopa. J Neurol 1977; 216:147–153.
14. Schoenberg BS, Anderson DW, Haerer AF. Prevalence of Parkinson's disease in the biracial population of Copiah County, Mississippi. Neurology 1985; 35:841–845.
15. Rothman KJ. Modern epidemiology. Boston: Little, Brown, & Co, 1986.
16. Marttila RJ. Epidemiology. In: Koller WC, ed. Handbook of Parkinson's disease. New York: Marcell Dekker, 1992:35–57.
17. Kessler II. Epidemiologic studies of Parkinson's disease. II. A hospital-based survey. Am J Epidemiol 1972; 95:308–318.
18. Haight Frank A. Handbook of the Poisson distribution. New York: John Wiley & Sons, 1967:85.
19. Kessler II. Epidemiologic studies of Parkinson's disease. III. A community-based survey. Am J Epidemiol 1972; 96:242–254.
20. Paddison RM, Griffith RP. Occurrence of Parkinson's disease in black patients at Charity Hospital in New Orleans. Neurology 1974; 24:688–690.
21. Lombard A, Gelfand M. Parkinson's disease in the African. Cent Afr J Med 1978; 24:5–8.
22. Haerer AF, Anderson DW, Schoenberg BS. Survey of major neurologic disorders in a biracial United States population: the Copiah County study. South Med J 1987; 80:339–343.
23. Ashok PP, Radhakrishnan K, Sridharan R, Mousa ME. Epidemiology of Parkinson's disease in Benghazi, north-east Libya. Clin Neurol Neurosurg 1986; 88:109–113.
24. Schoenberg BS, Osuntokun BO, Adeuja AO, et al. Comparison of the prevalence of Parkinson's disease in black populations in the rural United States and rural Nigeria: door-to-door community studies. Neurology 1988; 38:645–646.
25. Ellenberg JH, Nelson KB. Sample selection and the natural history of disease. JAMA 1992; 1980:1337–1340.
26. Ward CD, Duvoisin RC, Ince SE, et al. Parkinson's disease in twins. In: Parkinson-specific motor and mental disorders, role of the pallidum: pathophysological, biochemical, and therapeutic aspects. Adv Neurol 1984; 40:341–344.
27. Eldridge R, Rocca WA. Parkinson disease: In: King R, Rotter J, Motulsky A, eds. The genetic basis of common disease. New York: McGraw-Hill, 1990; 38:775–791.

28. Ward CD, Duvoisin RC, Ince SE, Nutt JD, Eldridge R, Calne DB. Parkinson's disease in 65 pairs of twins and in a set of quadruplets. Neurology 1983; 33:815–824.
29. Kondo K. Epidemiological clues for the etiology of Parkinson's disease. In: Hassler RG, Christ F, eds. Parkinson-specific motor and mental disorders, role of the pallidum: pathophysiological, biochemical, and therapeutic aspects. Adv Neurol 1984; 40:345–351.
30. Lees AJ. Early diagnosis of Parkinson's disease. Br J Hosp Med 1981; 26:511–512, 517–518.
31. Celesia G, Wanamaker W. Psychiatric disturbances in Parkinson's disease. Dis Nerv Syst 1972; 33:577–583.
32. Poewe W, Karamat E, Kemmler GW, Gerstenbrand F. The premorbid personality of patients with Parkinson's disease: a comparative study with healthy controls and patients with essential tremor. In: Parkinson's disease: anatomy, pathology and therapy. New York: Raven Press, 1990:339–342.
33. Eatough VM, Kempster PA, Stern GM, Lees AJ. Premorbid personality and idiopathic Parkinson's disease. In: Parkinson's disease: anatomy, pathology and therapy. Adv Neurol 1990; 53:335–337.
34. Rajput AH, Offord KP, Beard CM, Kurland LT. A case–control study of smoking habits, dementia, and other illnesses in idiopathic Parkinson's disease. Neurology 1987; 37:226–232.
35. Smythies JR. The previous personality in parkinsonism. J Psychosom Res 1967; 11:169–171.
36. Mjönes H. Paralysis agitans: a clinical and genetic study. Acta Psychiatr Neurol 1949; 54:1–195.
37. Menza M, Forman NE, Goldstein HE, Golbe LI. Parkinson's disease, dopamine, and personality [abstract]. J Neuropsychiatry Clin Neurosci 1990; 2:282–287.
38. Todes CJ, Lees AJ. The pre-morbid personality of patients with Parkinson's disease. J Neurol Neurosurg Psychiatry 1985; 48:97–100.
39. Strang RR. The ABO blood-group distribution of 450 Swedish patients with Parkinson's disease. Neurology 1966; 16:1051–1052.
40. Kak VK, Gordon DS. ABO blood groups and Parkinson's disease. Ulster Med J 1970; 39:132–134.
41. Kurland LT. Epidemiology: incidence, geographic distribution and genetic considerations. In: Field WS, ed. Pathogenesis and treatment of parkinsonism. Springfield, IL: Charles C Thomas, 1958:5–49.
42. Gudmundsson KR. A clinical survey of parkinsonism in Iceland. Acta Neurol Scand [Suppl] 1967; 33:1–61.
43. Dupont E. Epidemiology of parkinsonism. The Parkinson investigation, Arhus, Denmark (preliminary results). In: Worm-Peterson J, Bottcher J, eds. Symposium on parkinsonism. Denmark: Merck, Sharp & Dohme, 1977:65–75.
44. Rosati G, Granieri E, Pinna L, et al. The risk of Parkinson's disease in Mediterranean people. Neurology 1980; 30:250–255.
45. Harada H, Nishikawa S, Takahashi K. Epidemiology of Parkinson's disease in a Japanese city. Arch Neurol 1983; 40:151–154.
46. Sutcliffe RL, Prior R, Mawby B, McQuillan WJ. Parkinson's disease in the district

of the Northampton Health Authority, United Kingdom. A study of prevalence and disability. Acta Neurol Scand 1985; 72:363–379.
47. Bharucha NE, Bharucha EP, Bharucha AE, Bhise AV, Schoenberg BS. Prevalence of Parkinson's disease in the Parsi community in Bombay, India. Arch Neurol 1988; 45:1321–1323.
48. Wang YS, Shi YM, Wu ZY, He Y, Zhang BZ. Epidemiologic survey—Parkinson's disease in China. Chin Med J 1991; 104:960–964.
49. Casetta I, Granieri E, Govoni V, et al. Epidemiology of Parkinson's disease in Italy. A descriptive survey in the U.S.L. of Cento, province of Ferrara, Emilia-Romagna. Acta Neurol (Naples) 1990; 12:284–291.
50. Strang RR. ABO blood-groups in Parkinson's disease. Acta Pathol Microbiol Scand 1965; 65:653.

11

Prediction of Parkinson's Disease

Jonas H. Ellenberg

National Institute of Neurological Disorders and Stroke, National Institute of Health, Bethesda, Maryland

I. INTRODUCTION

The usefulness for predicting the onset of Parkinson's disease can be viewed from at least two perspectives. The first, a macro public health point of view, might encompass predictive methods for the assessment of the effect of change for a given risk factor on the development of a disease in a population. Risk factor modifications might include, for example, planned or unplanned intervention (e.g., treatment or communicable infection), environmental changes (e.g., introduction or elimination of known toxins), or changes in the characteristics of the population (e.g., increase in life expectancy). The second, a microlevel perspective, might involve predictive methods for the assessment of the risk of an individual patient contracting a disease. Decisions on prophylactic medical management could benefit from information derived from appropriate predictive models. Although the objectives of these different perspectives may require differences in the nature and performance of predictors and predictive models and the methodology used to find and evaluate them, their distinction in terms of actions taken may not be very different. Whichever perspective is being considered, it will be important in understanding the natural history of the disease to attempt to distinguish, where possible, between predictors of outcome, causative agents, and clinical signs or laboratory measures that are early manifestations of the disease process. Langston in a recent review (1) laments our current inability to "identify high-risk" subjects in view of the recent results concerning the potential prophylactic effects of selegiline (2). There exists an enormous literature on putative risk factors associated with Parkinson's disease. However, none of these factors can be considered dependably predictive, let alone demonstrably causal. Putative risk factors may themselves be causal, be part of a causal chain of events, or be part of a multifactorial etiology, involving heritability, environment, and endogenous defects. Conversely, an observed association may not be the result of a causal relationship, or may not be the basis for reliable prediction. It may merely reflect the association of unknown factors related to both the risk factor and the outcome, or it may appear as an artifact of a particular study design. Even if some factors reported to be associated with onset of Parkinson's disease are casual, there is no reason to believe any major proportion of cases can be accounted for by any individual factor or group of factors.

It is the intent of this review to examine approaches for evaluation of reports on risk factors that might be predictors, and to highlight the necessity for their use in critical assessment of studies in the literature. As a pedagogical approach, reports were reviewed on one well-studied predictor, smoking. The analysis presented here suggests that the widely reported observation of a negative association of smoking with Parkinson's disease may possibly be a result of an artifact of the study designs used.

II. ASSESSMENT OF PREDICTORS

There are many ways of measuring the association between potential predictors and disease outcome. The weaknesses and limitations of such measures, as well as approaches for evaluation of their predictive ability will be reviewed. Although the measures discussed are but a sample of those available, approaches to judgment of their quality and cautions in their use will be readily transferable to the myriad of other measures (see Refs. 3–5). The approaches to evaluation outlined should be useful to both writers and readers of research reports. Unfortunately, authors often do not uniformly report evaluative measures of putative predictors and, furthermore, may not present enough information for interested readers to make their own assessments.

To begin, consider the results of a hypothetical cross-sectional study relating a single dichotomous risk factor (possibly a predictor) to the outcome of Parkinson's disease. In such a cross-sectional study, all members of a defined cohort would be assigned into one of the four cells in Table 1.

By using the notation in Table 1, the risk of disease in those exposed and those not exposed can be defined

$$I_e = \frac{a_1}{(a_1 + a_2)} = \text{risk of disease in subjects exposed to the putative risk factor}$$

$$I_u = \frac{a_3}{(a_3 + a_4)} = \text{risk of disease in subjects not exposed to the putative risk factor}$$

Table 1 Schematic Representation of Results of a Cross-sectional Study of the Association of a Risk Factor With Parkinson's Disease

		Parkinson's disease		
		Yes	No	Total
Risk Factor	Yes	a_1	a_2	$a_1 + a_2$
	No	a_3	a_4	$a_3 + a_4$
	Total	$a_1 + a_3$	$a_2 + a_4$	$a_1 + a_2 + a_3 + a_4$

and then the ratio of these two measures is the relative risk

$$R = \frac{I_e}{I_u}$$

taking on possible values from 0 to ∞. Values close to unity would indicate little association of the risk factor with the outcome, and values higher than 1 would indicate increased risk of the disease, with the magnitude of R higher than 1 a measure of the heightened risk. Conversely, values lower than 1 would indicate a factor that might be protective.

For case–control studies, a fixed number of subjects with a disease (cases) is selected, a fixed number of subjects without the disease (controls) is selected, and then an assessment is made in cases and controls as to whether the risk factor is present or absent. This design is fundamentally different from a cross-sectional study, during which a group of subjects is examined unselected relative to their disease or their risk factor status. One result of this difference between a cross-sectional and case–control study design is that, in the former, one can directly estimate the absolute levels of risks of disease in both the exposed (I_e) and unexposed (I_u) and, hence, their ratio, R. In the case–control study, this is not possible (4). Instead, the odds ratio (OR) is used as a measure of association. When the population prevalence of the disease is low, the odds ratio closely approximates the relative risk. The use of either study design and a measure such as relative risk is a reasonable first step in developing the components of a predictive model for a disease. The simple paradigm in Table 1 will be maintained without considering other issues, such as statistical significance, or predictor variables that either have multiple levels or are continuous.

If you assume that the odds ratio or relative risk for a risk factor is not close to 1, what further evidence would identify a factor as a useful predictor? Other measures, such as sensitivity and specificity, can help. *Sensitivity* is the proportion of subjects with the disease who also have the risk factor. It measures the expected degree to which the risk factor can be used to identify all cases with the disease. *Specificity* is the proportion of subjects without the disease who do not have the risk factor.

With the notation of Table 1 we have:

$$\text{Sensitivity} = \frac{a_1}{(a_1 + a_3)}$$

$$\text{Specificity} = \frac{a_4}{(a_2 + a_4)}$$

One minus specificity, a measure of the degree to which noncases are identified as cases (i.e., an error) is termed the *false-positive rate*. One minus sensitivity, an analogous measure of the degree to which cases are identified as noncases, is termed the *false-negative rate*. High specificity and high sensitivity would produce low error rates of either kind. For a given risk factor to be a useful predictor, it would need to have reasonably high sensitivity and specificity. High values would indicate few observations in the nonconcordant cells of the schematic in Table 1 (i.e., a_2, a_3) or few errors in using the presence or absence of a risk factor to classify a subject as developing or not developing a disease.

It is not always important for sensitivity and specificity to be simultaneously high. For example, if the goal of prediction was early detection of a disease that could be prevented or delayed with intervention, then one would want sensitivity to be extremely high so that one does not miss many potential cases. However, if the intervention being considered was benign, and inexpensive, say diet modification for the prevention of colon cancer, there may be little concern if subjects were identified at high likelihood of having the disease when such was not preordained. Low specificity here (high false-positive rate) would probably be acceptable. Since the existence of a harmless and inexpensive intervention is likely the exception, rather than the rule, most situations require a predictor that makes few errors of either kind. This type of assessment would be similar from the perspectives of both public health policy and treatment of an individual patient.

Another measure of predictive ability, population attributable risk (PAR), takes account of both the heightened risk in those with a putative risk factor and the prevalence of the risk factor in the population under consideration. The measure, with appropriate caveats (3) of assumptions on causation and interactions of the risk factor with other factors in the causal link, can quantify within a population the amount of disease that is attributable to a risk factor. Elimination or reduction in prevalence of an identified risk factor would theoretically reduce the prevalence of the disease by the percentage (or some fraction thereof for incomplete elimination of the risk factor) indicated by the PAR. This measure has a macro or public health orientation. By assessing the effect of reduction of disease prevalence owing to reduction in risk factor prevalence in a total population, the PAR is an indirect measure of predictive ability. The concept has been put forward by numerous authors with perhaps the most well-known formula given as follows:

$$\text{PAR} = \frac{(I_t - I_u)}{I_t}$$

where I_u has already been defined, and

$$I_t = \frac{(a_1 + a_3)}{(a_1 + a_2 + a_3 + a_4)} = \text{the prevalence of the disease in the total population.}$$

The measure is defined for cross-sectional studies, but can be approximated from case–control studies (4–6). Miettinen defined an equivalent measure called the prevented fraction (PF) for factors that might be preventive and "can be interpreted as the proportion of the potential cases (in the absence of exposure) that was prevented by exposure" (7) where:

$$\text{PF} = \frac{(I_u - I_e)}{I_u}$$

A usual next step in evaluation of a predictor would be the development of a prediction model. In the context of Parkinson's disease, a likely choice would be the logistic regression model. This model has gained widespread popularity in the prediction of two-state outcomes (disease present, disease absent) because of its similarity to linear regression models in terms of interpretation; its ability to examine one or several risk factors while taking account of covariates (factors that may affect the relationship between the prognostic factor of interest and the outcome); and its ready accessibility through "packaged" computer software.

The model is

$$I_t = \frac{1}{[1 + \exp - (\alpha_0 + \alpha_1 x_1 + \ldots + \alpha_k x_k)]}$$

where x_1 is a proposed predictor variable, and $x_2, \ldots, x_k$, are $k - 1$ covariates which may be related to x_1 and also influence the risk of disease. More complicated models might involve synergistic relations among the predictor variable x_1 and the covariates $x_2, \ldots, x_k$ relative to risk of outcome. The model is readily generalizable to the simultaneous examination of multiple predictors.

The degree of success of a predictor in the context of a logistic model can be measured, by correlating for each of the subjects in a cohort, the estimated risk of Parkinson's disease (I_t) with the presence or absence of the disease. This multivariate modeling approach is very powerful and very sophisticated (and can be employed in the context both of public health policy and of the individual patient).

With this necessarily brief coverage of the statistical measures used to identify and quantify the quality of predictors, we can now look at one example of studies of a risk factor for Parkinson's disease in the literature.

III. SMOKING: AN EXAMPLE

Several matched case–control studies have reported on a negative association of smoking with clinical manifestation of Parkinson's disease (8–23). A summary of ten of the these reports that provided data from reasonably comparable study designs is given in Table 2. Six of the ten studies matched Parkinson's disease cases with one control; four used multiple controls. All studies matched on age, most on sex, and four on race.

In a case–control study the levels of risk for those with and without the risk factor is not available and, therefore, the relative risk is not directly estimable. The odds ratio, however, can be used as an estimate of the relative risk of a disease for a given risk factor when the disease itself is rare (4,24), as for Parkinson's disease. The interpretation of the computed odds ratio, the likelihood of obtaining the disease in individuals with the risk factor relative to those without the risk factor, is the same as the relative risk.

The results from the studies presented in Table 2 have, in some cases, been consolidated or restructured from more comprehensive published analyses to allow cross-study comparisons of similar measures. As indicated by the table notes, the studies are not strictly comparable. An odds ratio close to 1 would indicate no relation between smoking and Parkinson's disease, odds ratios greater than unity would imply a positive association, possibly causal. All of the observed odds ratios are less than 1 (i.e., smoking may be protective), with those studies showing smaller odds ratios indicating more profound preventive or possibly "therapeutic" value.

The odds ratios presented for many of the case–control studies are deemed statistically significant by the authors. Since the absolute levels of risk for those who smoke, and those who do not, cannot be estimated, the increase in risk of Parkinson's disease among nonsmokers implied by the odds ratios less than unity may not be clinically meaningful. For example, an odds ratio of 0.67 could be an estimate of an underlying population relative risk of $R = I_e/I_u = 0.004/0.006$, or $0.0004/0.0006$, or $0.00004/0.00006$.

Before interpreting the results of these data as indicative of a protective effect of smoking, it is useful to examine these study results using other measures, in addition to the odds ratios. A first look at the measure of sensitivity from each study is illuminating. Recall that sensitivity is the likelihood that if a subject has a disease, he or she will also have the risk factor. In the example of smoking, since the odds ratios are less than 1 for all the studies, we define *not* smoking as the putative risk factor for Parkinson's disease. With not smoking as a risk factor, the computed values of sensitivity are given in Table 3. With some exceptions these sensitivity measures had moderate values relative to the maximum possible value of unity.

Nine of the ten matched case–control studies provided data in only an unmatched format. In general, it is inappropriate to perform an unmatched analysis

Table 2 Matched Case–Control Studies of the Association of Smoking with Parkinson's Disease

Authors	Approximate time frame	Number of cases[b]	Odds ratios			Notes[a]	Country
			Males	Females	Total		
Nefzger et al. (9)	1965–66	198 +	0.44	–	–	1, 4	United States
Kessler et al. (10)	1965–67	468*	0.65	0.68	0.66	2	United States
Marttila et al. (11)	1971	443*	–	–	0.74	4	Finland
Bauman et al. (12)	1975–78	237†	0.68	0.19	0.46	1, 2, 3	United States
Godwin-Austin et al. (13)	1981	350†	–	–	0.52	2	England
Bharucha et al. (14)	1980	31*	–	–	0.60	1, 2	United States/ Canada
Rajput et al. (15)	1967–79	104	–	–	0.70	1, 2, 3	United States
Stern et al. (26)	1980s	149*	–	–	0.60	1, 2	United States
Tanner et al. (16, 17)	1980s	100	–	–	0.67	1, 2, 3	China
Sasco et al. (23)	1970s	79	–	–	0.70	2, 3, 5	United States

[a]*Notes*:
1. Ever smoked cigarettes if note is present, otherwise ever smoked any tobacco product.
2. Odds ratio computed, accounting for matching.
3. $>$1:1 matching.
4. Odds ratio computed from data available in published report in unmatched formats.
5. Study protocol provided for neurologist or physician confirmation of diagnosis.

[b](*, †) Reported p value for test of significance of difference between cases and controls at (<0.05 and <0.01) levels, respectively, for combined results of both sexes.

Table 3 Sensitivity[a] Derived From Matched Case–Control Studies of the Association of Not Smoking With Parkinson's Disease

Authors	Sensitivity
Nefzger et al. (9)	0.30
Kessler et al. (10)	0.57
Marttila et al. (11)	0.74
Baumann et al. (12)	0.63
Godwin–Austin et al. (13)	0.45
Bharucha et al. (14)	0.58
Rajput et al. (15)	0.63
Stern et al. (26)	0.55
Tanner et al. (17)	0.59
Sasco et al. (23)	0.18

[a]Note that since smoking has an observed negative association with Parkinson's disease, sensitivity is defined relative to absence of this factor. Sensitivity computed from data available in unmatched form from published reports.

on data from matched case–control studies (4). Since the data are not available in matched format, a summary of the results of all the studies is based on an analysis without considering the matching. The effect of treating the studies as unmatched will tend to "underestimate the deparature of the relative risk from unity (25)," which will not be critical for the purposes of this exposition. The unmatched data from all of the studies were combined to produce a Mantel–Haenszel estimate of the odds ratio (4) of 0.65 (95% confidence limits: 0.57, 0.73).

The sensitivity for the combined data from all studies was 0.56, with a specificity of 0.56. Even if we believed the association to be biologically plausible, use of "not smoking" as a predictor for onset of Parkinson's disease would be incorrect in a large proportion of cases, both in classifying cases as noncases and noncases as cases. The errors that would be made make the use of smoking as a predictor not much better than flipping a coin.

Is smoking history a good candidate for a predictor of Parkinson's disease? Although the odds ratios are quite consistent in direction, other evaluative measures, such as sensitivity and specificity, do not support the potential of not smoking as a good predictor from either of the perspectives of individual or public health risk assessment.

We also need to recognize the potential pitfalls in assessing an association of any disease with smoking histories. These problems sometimes, but not always, may be reflected in study design features, such as the definitions used for smoking exposure; the mechanisms in place for amelioration of recall bias of smoking history; the differential degrees of confirmation of disease diagnoses; or the potential for bias produced by the selection process for the cohorts (e.g., hospital-based or referral-based).

Concerning the last point on selection bias, several of the studies reviewed are reports from cohorts that were highly selected (e.g., hospital-based, twins). Many of the studies, however, were based on reasonably complete enumerations of Parkinson's disease cases from defined geographic areas.

The form of the published data allows neither ready computation of population attributable risk nor logistic analysis with covariates. Therefore, it is important to note that the population-based study from the Mayo Clinic (15), which used both univariate analysis and also multivariate logistic regression with covariates, did not demonstrate a statistically significant protective effect of smoking.

Some clinical observations raised by several of the cited authors concerning protective or etiologic linkage of smoking and Parkinson's disease follow:

1. "Smoking might have a protective effect on the development of PD, but there is as yet no direct evidence (pathophysiologic model) to support this hypothesis" (14).
2. "Another possibility is that the pathophysiologic phenomena of Parkinson's disease are active long before clinical manifestations appear. Perhaps they are manifest as personality traits" (12).
3. "Because Parkinson's disease may stem from an environmental insult (for example, an infection), smoking might alter the attack rate or sequelae from this insult" (12).
4. "The mortality and morbidity associated with smoking far outweighs any benefit from a possible lowering of risk of Parkinson's disease" (13)

Golbe et al.(19), Rajput et al.(15), and Stern et al.(26), in some of the more recent reports on this topic, have concluded respectively that ". . . smoking is probably not a benefit in preventing, delaying, or ameliorating PD.", ". . . smoking had no effect on the development of IPD [idiopathic Parkinson's disease]," and "studying the effect of cigarette smoke on animal models of PD and understanding the pathophysiology of human disease will ultimately determine whether or not components of cigarette smoke have a significant physiologic effect that can explain the inconsistent epidemiologic observations." In addition, there may be other unknown or unmeasured factors in the "casual chain" relating to smoking and Parkinson's disease that may account for the appearance of the observed negative association in these studies. Nonetheless, we have a number of reports indicating a negative association of smoking with Parkinson's disease.

A. A Possible "Nonetiologic" Explanation for the Observed Negative Association of Smoking History With Parkinson's Disease

Rajput(15) and others suggest that the observed negative associations result because smoking "differentially and negatively affects the mortality of those persons destined to get Parkinson's disease, thereby leaving fewer smokers who were destined to get Parkinson's disease alive at older ages, when the incidence of Parkinson's disease is higher." Godwin-Austin et al.(13) argue that this is unlikely since ". . . the negative association was seen as clearly in younger and early onset patients, where selective mortality is of little significance, as it was in older and late onset patients."

A critical look at these opposing arguments suggest that it is possible that both are incorrect. Consider a representation of a complete population, for which, for the sake of simplicity, it is assumed that life events can include only the following: alive with Parkinson's disease; alive without Parkinson's disease; death following onset of Parkinson's disease; and death without onset of Parkinson's disease. The schematic of the status of our hypothetical population at year end 1995 can be seen in Table 4.

If one were to undertake a cross-sectional or case–control study at year end, then attempts would be made to obtain information on

1. The $A_1 + A_2$ subjects with Parkinson's disease alive at year-end 1995.
2. The $B_1 + B_2$ living unaffected subjects at year-end 1995.
3. The $C_1 + C_2$ subjects who had died with Parkinson's disease, anytime before year-end 1995.
4. The $D_1 + D_2$ subjects who died without Parkinson's disease, anytime before year-end 1995.

Absent the prospective follow-up of this population beginning several decades before 1995, success in obtaining reliable information on subjects in either of groups 3 or 4 would depend on retrospective data. The presence or absence of disease would be based on sources such as death certificates and medical records, and the ability to obtain accurate smoking history posthumously would depend on sources such as interviews with "significant others."

Table 4 Status of a Population at Year-End 1995

	Morbidity / Mortality			
Smoking history	Alive with PD	Alive without PD	Death with PD	Death without PD
Ever smoked	A_1	B_1	C_1	D_1
Never smoked	A_2	B_2	C_2	D_2

In all of the reports listed in Table 2, the theoretical cohorts of patients $C_1 + C_2$ and $D_1 + D_2$ in Table 4 were not evaluated. Why is the absence of representation from these groups important? Simply because we cannot assess the potential effect of selective mortality on the results of the reported studies if data on these groups are not available. Godwin-Austin et al.(13) argue that if the reported case–control smoking differential is maintained at time of onset and 20–30 years before onset, then differential early mortality in smokers would not have had a chance to affect the findings. However, these backward looks at comparative smoking rates decades before time of onset are made *only on surviving Parkinson's disease cases and controls* (i.e., A_1, A_2, B_1, B_2).

Empirical evidence does suggest the possibility of some process of selective mortality. Stern et al.(26) and Rajput et al. (15) both looked at their cohorts stratified by age of onset of Parkinson's disease. In both studies, whereas the odds ratios for smoking history and Parkinson's disease did not differ significantly between young- and old-onset patients, the odds ratios were lower in the older than in the younger age of onset groups. In the Rajput et al. study, the odds ratios were monitonicaly increasing to 2.5 (positive association) inversely with age of onset.

The feasibility of obtaining reliable information about the groups C_1, C_2, D_1, D_2 to empirically demonstrate a selection bias is certainly questionable. Nonetheless, it can still be demonstrated that the observations suggesting a protective effect of smoking against Parkinson's disease may indeed be a function of selective mortality of smokers. It will be seen that the possible selection bias in the case–control studies that have shown this negative association may not, however, be due to the differential life expectancy of smokers and nonsmokers before onset of Parkinson's disease (27), as has been suggested(13,15), but may be due to a differential life expectancy after onset. To explore this possibility, first consider the actual versus the ideal sampling scenarios represented in Table 5.

Assume that information was obtainable on all living subjects in the population, then one could construct the 2 × 2 contingency table given in Table 6.

Ideally, one should be examining data from the complete cohort of subjects in Table 7.

Table 5 Actual Versus Ideal Sample Selection From Population in Table 4

Smoking history	Morbidity	Sampling frames: Actual	Ideal	Selection fraction
Ever smoked	PD	A_1	A_1+C_1	$\emptyset_1=A_1/(A_1+C_1)$
	No PD	B_1	B_1+D_1	$\emptyset_2=B_1/(B_1+D_1)$
Never smoked	PD	A_2	A_2+C_2	$\emptyset_3=A_2/(A_2+C_2)$
	No PD	B_2	B_2+D_2	$\emptyset_4=B_2/(B_2+D_2)$

Table 6 Observed Contingency Table for Study of Smoking History and Parkinson's Disease

Smoking history	Disease status PD	No PD
Ever smoked	A_1	B_1
Never smoked	A_2	B_2

The odds ratio computed from Table 6 is A_1B_2/B_1A_2, whereas the correct odds ratio should be from Table 7,

$$\text{OR} = \frac{(A_1 + C_1)(B_2 + D_2)}{(B_1 + D_1)(A_2 + C_2)} = \tag{1}$$

$$\left(\frac{\phi_2\ \phi_3}{\phi_1\ \phi_4}\right)\left(\frac{A_1B_2}{B_1A_2}\right) = \phi(A_1B_2/B_1A_2) \tag{2}$$

using the notation from Table 5, and $\phi = \left(\frac{\phi_2\ \phi_3}{\phi_1\ \phi_4}\right)$

If none of the population died in the decades before 1995 then C_1, C_2, D_1, and D_2 would all be equal to zero, the actual and ideal sampling frames would be the same, and the potential for selective mortality bias would be nonexistent (i.e., $\phi = 1$). However, there obviously will be deaths in the different groups before the observation of the cohort in 1995, so the ϕ_is in Table 5 will never be equal to unity. The sampling fractions ϕ_i can be thought of as the survival rates in each of the four smoking-by-morbidity groups. The nature of the differences among the group selection fractions will determine the extent of and nature of the selective mortality bias.

To examine the potential for bias, consider in Figure 1 a cohort of healthy 40-year-old subjects in 1965 and postulate 30-year survival probabilities to the year 1995. The three panels depict 30-year survival conditioned on smoking

Table 7 Ideal Contingency Table for Study of Smoking History and Parkinson's Disease

Smoking history	Disease status PD	No PD
Ever smoked	$A_1 + C_1$	$B_1 + D_1$
Never smoked	$A_2 + C_2$	$B_2 + D_2$

history at aged 40, and on onset of Parkinson's disease. The first panel shows a decrease in likelihood of survival among those who ever smoked, but the decrease in survival is the same, regardless of whether the subjects developed Parkinson's disease. A decrease in survival is seen in the middle panel related to smoking and a decrease related to development of Parkinson's disease, for which the effect of Parkinson's disease on survival is the same in both smoking groups. The final panel demonstrates a synergistic effect on survival of both smoking and development of Parkinson's disease. The decrease in survival among Parkinson's disease patients is disproportionately greater among those who smoked before onset than among those who did not.

In the first instance, where the negative impact of smoking on survival is the same, regardless of onset of Parkinson's disease, the sampling fractions would be $\phi_1 = \phi_2$ and $\phi_3 = \phi_4$ [i.e., $\phi = 1$ in Eq. (2)]. Although smoking would

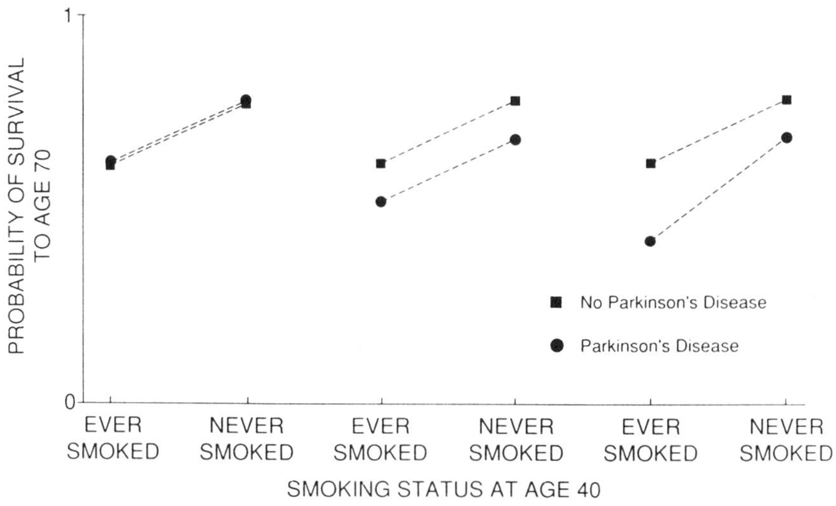

Figure 1 Probability of survival past age 70 by smoking status at age 40 and by development of Parkinson's disease. The circles with connecting dashed lines represent subjects who developed Parkinson's disease and the lines connecting the solid squares represent subjects who did not. The three panels of the graph represent, from left to right, respectively: a decrease in survival related to smoking, but no effect of development of Parkinson's disease on survival ($\phi = 1$); a decrease in survival related to smoking and also to development of Parkinson's disease, but the effects of development of Parkinson's disease on survival are the same in the smoking and nonsmoking groups ($\phi = 1$); and the final panel represents a decrease in survival related to both smoking and development of Parkinson's disease. The decrease in survival among Parkinson's disease patients is disproportionately greater among those who smoked before onset than among those who did not ($\phi > 1$).

produce selective mortality (i.e., $ø_1 < ø_3, ø_2 < ø_4$), it would affect the selective survival in the same way among the Parkinson's disease and no Parkinson's disease groups, providing a correct estimate of OR in Eq. (2).

In the second instance, the negative effect of smoking on survival is constant between the two disease groups, and the hypothetical effect of Parkinson's disease on survival is negative, but equal, in the two smoking groups. This would be equivalent to an equal proportionate reduction in survival, for example, a reduction of α (where $\alpha < 1$), between the Parkinson's disease and no Parkinson's disease groups, so that $ø_1 = \alpha ø_3$ and $ø_2 = \alpha ø_4$. Substituting in Eq. (2), it is seen that the factor ø is again equal to 1, and the estimate of OR is correct.

Finally, consider the example for which there is a negative synergistic effect on survival of smoking and developing Parkinson's disease. That is, survival is decreased dramatically among those Parkinson's disease patients who smoked before onset of Parkinson's disease. Here, the estimate of the actual OR will not be correct, but will be multiplied by some factor, dependent on the magnitude of this synergism [i.e., $ø_1 = \alpha ø_3$, $ø_2 = \alpha' ø_4$, where $\alpha, \alpha' < 1, \alpha < \alpha'$ and $ø > 1$ in Eq. (2)] (28). Thus, the observed odds ratio ø (A_1B_2/B_1A_2) will be an underestimate of the true odds ratio ø (A_1B_2/B_1A_2), where $ø > 1$. If the mortality among Parkinson's disease patients is disproportionately greater for those who smoked before onset than those who did not (i.e., $ø > 1$), then the observed negative association between smoking and Parkinson's disease may be an artifact.

B. A Hypothetical Numerical Example of Differential Postmorbidity Mortality

To examine the previously hypothesized selective mortality bias in a derived numerical example, the hypothetical cohort of 40-year olds in panel 3 of Figure 1 is equated to a cohort of the U.S. population 25 years ago. There were approximately 12.5 million persons in the age range 40–44 alive in 1965 (29). The rates of smoking by sex for this narrow age range are not readily accessible. However, in 1965 by the fourth decade of life, close to 80% of males had *ever smoked* and 40% of women had *ever smoked* (30).

If we use the 80% ever smoked rate for males and the 40% ever smoked rate for females, the first numeric column in Table 8, column A, "Cohort alive in 1965," gives a rough approximation of the sex by smoking status distribution of the 40- to 44-year-old cohort in 1965.

Next, the morbidity and mortality status of the 40- to 44-year-old cohort over the next 25–30 years is simulated. First, it is assumed that there is no mortality between ages 45 and 69. Then estimates of expected incidence of Parkinson's disease for the aging cohort are introduced, using cumulative incidence for ages 45–69 of 905:100,000 and 760:100,000 for men and women, respectively. These estimates were derived from unpublished data for this specific age range from the Rajput et al., study (31). These rates were applied *equally to the smoker*

Table 8 Expected Number of Survivors of a Cohort of 40- to 44-year olds and Their Disease Status

		A	B		C	D
		Cohort alive in 1965[a] ages 40–44 (1,000s)	Cohort by Parkinson's disease status 1966–1995[b] ages 45–69		Expected survival through age 69[c]	Alive in 1996[d] ages 70+ (1,000s)
Sex	Smoking status		N (1,000s)	PD Status		
Men	Ever	4,972	45	Yes	0.3710	17
			4,927	No	0.6184	3,047
	Never	1,243	11	Yes	0.6267	7
			1,232	No	0.7834	965
Women	Ever	2,499	19	Yes	0.4295	8
			2,480	No	0.7159	1,775
	Never	3,749	28	Yes	0.7030	20
			3,721	No	0.8788	3,270
Total	Ever	7,471	64	Yes		25
			7,407	No		4,822
	Never	4,992	40	Yes		27
			4,952	No		4,235
Total		12,463	12,463			9,109

[a]Approximation based on data from the Statistical Abstract of the United States, 1990 (29); Tables 11–12.

[b]Estimates based on Rajput et al (31) with unpublished data on the age range 50–69 for incident cases of 760:100,000 for women and 905:100,000 for men. Assumes no mortality in this period.

[c]Expected sex × smoking status survival rates for subjects without Parkinson's disease given by Rogers and Powell-Griner (27). Survival rates for subjects with Parkinson's disease are modifications of the rates given by Rogers and Powell-Griner, accounting for the increased force of mortality accompanying onset of Parkinson's disease.

[d]Estimates based on Rogers and Powell-Griner (27): conditional likelihood of reaching age 70 given a subject has reached age 40–44, by smoking and disease status. (column B multiplied by column C).

and nonsmoker groups, which provided the results in Table 8 column B labeled "Cohort by Parkinson's disease status 1966–1995."

Relaxing the "no mortality" assumption, the expected survival of the 40- to 44-year-old cohort after aged 70 can be approximated. Rogers and Powell-Griner (27) give smoking by sex-specific survival estimates conditioned on attained age. Their results relate to the general population, without consideration of the presence or absence of specific morbidity. These rates can be used as rough approximations to expected survival after aged 70 for patients without Parkinson's disease. The survival estimates are given in column A of Table 9.

Next the potential for differential mortality after onset of Parkinson's disease between those subjects who smoked and those who did not before onset of disease, as indicated by panel 3 of Figure 1, needs to be taken into account. Several recent reports have demonstrated a dramatic age-adjusted decrease in life expectancy among patients with Parkinson's disease as contrasted with subjects without Parkinson's disease (32–34). This decrease occurs in both men and women, and has been estimated to decrease the expected age-specific survival rates from two to four times that in the general population. The survival rates to age 70 of the cohort of 40- to 44-year-old nonsmokers for subjects without Parkinson's disease are, therefore, modified by superimposing an additional force of mortality of 20% caused by the onset of Parkinson's disease. For example, for women who developed Parkinson's disease, but never smoked, the expected survival up to age 70 dropped by 20% from 0.8788 (column A, Table 9) to 0.7030 (column B, Table 9).

Finally it is assumed that survival among smokers after onset of Parkinson's

Table 9 Expected Survival After Age 70 of a Cohort of 40- to 44-Year Olds by Sex, Smoking Status, and Disease Status

Sex	Smoking status	Expected survival after age 70[a] A No PD	Expected survival after age 70[a] B PD
Men	Ever smoked	0.6184	0.3710
	Never smoked	0.7834	0.6267
Women	Ever smoked	0.7159	0.4295
	Never smoked	0.8788	0.7030

[a]Expected sex × smoking status survival rates for subjects without Parkinson's disease given by Rogers and Powell-Griner (27). Survival rates for subjects with Parkinson's disease modify the rates given by Rogers and Powell-Griner accounting for the increased force of mortality accompanied by onset of Parkinson's disease.

disease would have a more dramatic reduction in survival to aged 70 of 40%. For example, for men who ever smoked the expected survival up to age 70 dropped from 0.6184 (column A, Table 9) to 0.371 (column B, Table 9). The expected survival rates thus derived are given for sex by smoking status, by disease status in Table 8 column C. For each sex, the hypothetical survival rate differences between the cases with and without Parkinson's disease by smoking group (column C) now reflect the paradigm demonstrated by the third panel in Figure 1. The tableau of survival rates given in Table 9 would produce a value of $\phi = 1.33$ from Eq. (2) in Section III.A.

To our knowledge, there is no empirical evidence that the constructed survival rates *following* onset of Parkinson's disease represent an accurate differential of mortality risk between smokers and nonsmokers. We are not aware of published mortality studies of cohorts involving subjects with and without Parkinson's disease classified by prior smoking status. Thus, for our example, increased mortality owing to onset of Parkinson's disease is postulated in support of a possible explanation of the observed negative relation between smoking and Parkinson's disease. If a disorder such as myocardial infarction (MI) is considered, however, an empirical example exists of a negative synergistic effect of a risk factor on postmorbidity survival: having an MI and having been a smoker before the MI. Kannel et al. (35) showed a 30% increase in all-cause mortality for both women and men surviving an MI for 30 days when prior (to MI) smokers are compared to prior nonsmokers.

Next, the expected sex by smoking by disease status mortality rates in column C were applied to the 12,463,000 45- to 69-year-old subjects in column B of Table 8 to produce column D. Column D then, gives the expected survival and disease status of a cohort of 12.4 million 40- to 44-year-olds followed 25–30 years in which two principal assumptions were operating: (1) the development of Parkinson's disease was assumed *not* to be affected by smoking status; but (2) *postmorbidity* mortality was assumed to be higher in smokers with Parkinson's disease than in nonsmokers. It represents the observation of a cohort, as depicted in Table 6, without benefit of knowledge of the mortality pattern over time. This observation can now be contrasted with the observation had we the ideal situation represented by Table 7.

The simple 2×2 table for testing the hypothesis of association between smoking and Parkinson's disease for both sexes combined is given in Table 10 based on column D of Table 8 with an estimated OR of 0.75 using the Mantel–Haenzel method (4) for combining the results for men and women. Thus, in spite of the fact that the cumulative incidence rates for Parkinson's disease were assumed equal in the groups who smoked and those who did not (i.e., assumption (1): smoking and Parkinson's disease are unrelated or OR $= 1$), the force of selective mortality from both smoking *and* Parkinson's disease produced a cohort demonstrating a protective effect of smoking. From Eq. (2) we see

Table 10 Expected Morbidity of 40- to 44-Year-Old Cohort at Age 70+ When Smoking is Not Related to Risk of Parkinson's Disease

(1000s)					
		PD status 70+			
		Yes	No	Total	Risk of PD
Smoking status age 40–44	Ever	25	4,822	4,847	0.0052
	Never	27	4,235	4,262	0.0063
	Total	52	9,057	9,109	

immediately that the observed odds ratio of 0.75 is biased downward from the true OR of 1 by a factor of ($1/\o = 1/1.33 = 0.75$).

A similar effect was not seen when only the putative risk factor (smoking) had a differential mortality (i.e., $\o = 1$; panels 1 and 2 in Fig. 1). It is the synergism of differential mortality in both the risk factor and the outcome itself that has created this anomaly (i.e., $\o > 1$; see third panel in Fig. 1).

In the foregoing example, we assumed that the cumulative incidence rates for Parkinson's disease among smokers and nonsmokers was equal, with selective mortality producing an observed odds ratio less than 1. This same approach was used applying theoretical *unequal* cumulative incidence rates to smokers and nonsmokers, with a *10% increase* in risk for Parkinson's disease among smokers. With the same differential mortality in Table 9, the Mantel–Haenszel odds ratio was 0.83, again below 1. Even in the face of a *positive* association of smoking with onset of Parkinson's disease, the selective mortality resulted in the observation of a negative association.

It is important to note that an example has been constructed using available population data, assuming differential mortality owing to smoking and presence of Parkinson's disease to demonstrate how selective mortality might have produced the observed negative association of Parkinson's disease with smoking. An attempt was made to provide prevalence, incidence, and survival expectations, based as far as possible on empirical results, rather than a purely theoretical set of figures. Different assumptions could provide even more extreme results.

Given the foregoing demonstration, the observed statistical evidence from the multiple studies that purport to show a negative association between smoking and the risk of Parkinson's disease may be explained as an artifact of sampling. In addition, the pursuit of clinical, pathophysiological, or other related explanations for the observed results has not provided a convincing explanation of a causal link. The contrived example was put forth to question the face validity of the observations from studies reporting a negative association between Parkinson's disease and smoking. It should remind investigators that the axiom that assessment of risk factors in only a single dimension (i.e., with measures of statistical association) is dangerous, and other aspects such as sampling techniques, biological rationale, and so forth must be incorporated into the evaluation process. Recent work by Grandinetti et al. (35a) examining 8006 men enrolled in the Honolulu Heart Program, in contrast to the cross-sectional studies presented here, is a prospective follow-up of a fixed cohort and also reports a negative association between Parkinson's disease and smoking. The initial published report does not give detailed information on the success of their follow-up over the 26-year period of observation of the cohort. Whether subjects lost to follow-up, lack of ascertainment of information on healthy and diseased cases not seeking medical care, and so forth may have had an impact on the data available on C_1, C_2, D_1, D_2 needs to be evaluated. Nonetheless, it is encouraging that the issue of this particular association has been examined in the context of a prospective study, in principle not subject to the bias postulated.

The reader is referred to other material on bias in the use of hospital-based subjects for case–control studies when the likelihood of subjects appearing for care at hospitals differs for the putative risk factor and the outcome being studied (4,5,36,37).

IV. CONCLUDING REMARKS

The types of measures that can be used in evaluation of putative risk factors for Parkinson's disease have been described, as well as the way these measures might be evaluated, depending on the circumstances for which prediction is intended. An example of the reported negative association of smoking with Parkinson's disease was presented and examined relative to how statistical measures of association might not correctly reflect the underlying process because of a type of selection bias. The contrived example was presented to demonstrate the potential for bias that would not necessarily be readily apparent by even the most acute observer. Furthermore, the presence of such bias cannot be proved, given the available data in the literature. However, since many decisions on use of scarce resources for future research and clinical decision making are predicated on the published literature, caution and skepticism are recommended in reviewing research results. Even those studies that are confirmed with replication may simply be replication of an artifact.

There are relatively few papers that deal specifically with the prediction of Parkinson's disease, although there are hundreds of reports on the association of risk factors with Parkinson's disease. In general, the available reports on association have not examined the usefulness of risk factors in predicting Parkinson's disease by using the types of measures outlined herein.

An area ripe for exploration with prediction models is preclinical detection of Parkinson's disease through the use of biomarkers and other measures before onset of clinical symptoms. A recent conference on this topic demonstrated the intense interest in this area (38). The statistical issues in the assessment of markers for preclinical detection of Parkinson's disease and the assessment of risk factors for Parkinson's disease are essentially equivalent. For example, studies to evaluate potential presymptomatic markers should be designed such that they do not introduce artifacts that create a spurious or inflated association; and factors related to both markers and Parkinson's disease need to be appropriately employed in adjusting observed associations to account for potential confounding. Langston and Koller (38) observe that "The implications of diagnosing the disease before symptoms develop could be profound . . . the closer (patients) can be identified to the time of exposure to precipitating factors, the more likely that an association between the disease and the causative factor(s) will be made." Thus, discovery of reliable preclinical markers is not yet necessarily an end in itself, although with the potential for prophylaxis, it could be. Rather, it may be seen as an opportunity to explore the clinical–pathological relevance of the marker to the neurodegenerative process.

Langston (1) gives early cognitive dysfunction, seborrhea, and electrophysiological abnormalities as promising biomarkers. If such markers are reasonable predictors as assessed by measures in this chapter, then they may be very useful in the design of studies of early environmental or other early-life risk factors for Parkinson's disease. Given the late onset of Parkinson's disease, there is great difficulty in obtaining retrospective information concerning life events decades before onset. It would be extraordinarily useful in case–control studies of early-life risk factors for Parkinson's disease to be able to use a cohort of subjects who have been identified by the presence or absence of a preclinical marker—a marker indicating eventual Parkinson's disease, but at a much younger age than the actual clinical onset. The problems of long-term recall and other retrospective evaluations would be considerably ameliorated.

The major emphasis of this chapter has been on the use of observed associations and prediction models in evaluating risk factors for Parkinson's disease. Studies of risk factors for this disorder often require the identification of existent cases and noncases of Parkinson's disease in a defined population as the first step in establishing a cohort for whom a protocol can be designed for a case–control study. The potential selection biases that attend the use of clinic- or hospital-based cases, as contrasted with selection of cases and controls from a defined population, can produce misleading results (see Refs. 4 and 39). Generally, it is relatively inexpensive to obtain cases from subjects seeking health care at medical institutions, and very expensive to examine an entire population from a geographically defined area to identify cases.

The screening of an entire population using medical examinations to determine case status will likely require a prohibitively large use of resources. Simple screening questionnaires, with second-stage confirmatory medical examinations of those subjects considered likely to have Parkinson's disease is an approach to identification of the prevalent Parkinson's disease cases in a cohort. This is not prediction in the sense of determining whether a particular risk factor or preclinical marker can identify a subject who will eventually develop the symptoms of Parkinson's disease. Instead, factors are used to identify (or predict) the current disease status of subjects. The factors will primarily be clinical symptoms specific to Parkinson's disease, in a screening program, as contrasted with risk factors, which may not be clinical, in a prediction model.

As with preclinical markers, the concepts of evaluation of the screening procedure are analogous with that for prediction—an attempt to minimize errors of classification. Those types of errors to be minimized have been defined previously as the false-positive rate (1 minus specificity) and the false-negative rate (1 minus sensitivity). The first error arises when the screen results in the nomination of a noncase as a possible case and the second is the screen resulting in the nomination of a case as a noncase. The former error has implications for tremendous costs of in-person medical examinations, and the latter type of error has implications for not deriving enough cases for sufficient power of a study to detect existing associations or differences.

In our search for the etiology of Parkinson's disease, reliable predictors will undoubtedly be very useful. Increased emphasis should be placed on appropriate research design for the evaluation of candidate predictors. The pros and cons of various study approaches, such as prospective versus retrospective designs, case–control versus cross-sectional studies, and so forth, are discussed in detail in standard texts (7). Appropriate study design in studies of Parkinson's disease is especially critical, since this disorder appears to have a large share of potential problem areas, including difficulty of diagnosis, difficulty of assessing risk factors predating onset by many years, and death from other causes before onset of disease. The future looks promising, with the potential for using biomarkers and neuroimaging techniques that may help in both diagnosis and early detection.

REFERENCES

1. Langston JW. Predicting Parkinson's disease. Neurology 1990; 40 (suppl):70–74.
2. The Parkinson Study Group. Effect of Deprenyl on the progression of disability in early Parkinson's disease. N Engl J Med 1989; 321:1364–1371.
3. Ellenberg JH. The extrapolation of attributable risk to new populations. Stat Med 1988; 7:717–725.
4. Schlesselman J. Case–control studies: design, conduct, analysis. New York: Oxford University Press, 1982.
5. Fleiss J. Statistical methods for rates and proportions. New York: John Wiley & Sons, 1981.

6. Taylor J. Simple estimation of population attributable risk from case–control studies. Am J Epidemiol 1977; 106:260.
7. Rothman K. Modern epidemiology. Boston: Little, Brown & Co, 1986.
8. Hammond E. Smoking in relation to the death rates of one million men and women. Natl Cancer Inst Monogr 19 166:127–204.
9. Nefzger MD, Quadfasel FA, Karl VC. A retrospective study of smoking in Parkinson's disease. Am J Epidemiol 1968; 88:149–158.
10. Kessler II, Diamond EL. Epidemiologic studies of Parkinson's disease. I. Smoking and Parkinson's disease: a survey and explanatory hypothesis. Am J Epidemiol 1971; 94:16–25.
11. Marttila RJ, Rinne UK. Smoking and Parkinson's Disease. Acta Neurol Scand 1980; 62:322–325.
12. Baumann RJ, Jameson HD, McKean HE, Haack DG, Weisberg LM. Cigarette smoking and Parkinson disease: I. A comparison of cases with matched neighbors. Neurology 1980; 30:839–843.
13. Godwin-Austen RB, Lee PN, Marmot MG, Stern GM. Smoking and Parkinson's disease. J Neurol Neurosurg Psychiatry 1982; 45:577–581.
14. Bharucha NE, Stokes L, Schoenberg BS, et al. A case–control study of twin pairs discordant for Parkinson's disease: a search for environmental risk factors. Neurology 1986; 36:284–288.
15. Rajput AH, Offord KP, Beard CM, Kurland LT. A case–control study of smoking habits, dementia, and other illnesses in idiopathic Parkinson's disease. Neurology 1987 37:226–232.
16. Tanner CM, Chen B, Wang WZ, et al. Environmental factors and Parkinson's disease: a case–control study in China. Neurology 1989; 39:660–664.
17. Tanner CM, Chen B, Wang WZ, et al. Environmental factors in the etiology of Parkinson's disease. Can J Neurol Sci 1987; 14:419–423.
18. Yong VW, Perry TL. Monoamine oxidase B, smoking, and Parkinson's disease. J Neurol Sci 1986; 72:265–272.
19. Golbe LI, Cody RA, Duvoisin RC. Smoking and Parkinson's disease. Search for a dose–response relationship. Arch Neurol 1986; 43:774–778.
20. Siemers E, Robbins B, Hui S. Environmental agents associated with Parkinson's disease. Meeting of the American Neurological Association, 1989; 13.
21. Burch PR. Cigarette smoking and Parkinson disease [letter]. Neurology 1981; 31:500–501.
22. Kirch DG, Alho A, Wyatt JW. Hypothesis: a nicotine–dopamine interaction linking smoking with Parkinson's disease and tardive dyskinesia. Cell Mol Neurobiol 1988; 8:285–291.
23. Sasco A, Paffenbarger R. Smoking and Parkinson's disease. Epidemiology 1990; 6:460–465.
24. Walter S. Calculation of attributable risks from epidemiological data. J Epidemiol 1978; 7:175–182.
25. Armitage P. Statistical methods in medical research. New York: John Wiley & Sons, 1971.
26. Stern M, Dulaney E, Gruber S. Risk factors for Parkinson's disease: a case–control study in young and old onset PD patients [abstract]. Ann Neurol 1990; 28:294.

27. Rogers R, Powell-Griner E. Life expectancies of cigarette smokers and nonsmokers in the United States. Soc Sci Med 1991; 32:1151–1159.
28. Kleinbaum DG, Kupper LL, Morgenstern H. Epidemiologic research: principles and quantitative methods. Belmont: Wadsworth, 1982.
29. U. S. Bureau of the Census. Statistical abstract of the United States. Washington, DC: Bureau of Census, 1990.
30. U. S. Bureau of the Census. Statistical abstract of the United States. Washington, DC: Bureau of Census, 1969.
31. Rajput AH, Offord KP, Beard CM, Kurland LT. Epidemiology of parkinsonism: incidence, classification, and mortality. Ann Neurol 1984; 16:278–282.
32. Diamond SG, Markham CH, Hoehn MM, McDowell FH, Muenter MD. Effect of age at onset on progression and mortality in Parkinson's disease. Neurology 1989; 39:1187–1190.
33. Diamond SG, Markham CH, Hoehn MM, McDowell FH, Muenter MD. An examination of male–female differences in progression and mortality of Parkinson's disease. Neurology 1990; 40:763–766.
34. Ebmeier KP, Calder SA, Crawford JR, Stewart L, Besson JOA, Mutch WJ. Mortality and causes of death in idiopathic Parkinson's disease: results from the Aberdeen whole population study. Scott Med J 1990; 35:173–175.
35. Kannel WB, Wolf PA, Garrison RJ. The Framingham study. NIH Publ 88–2969 1988.
35a. Grandinetti A, Morens DM, Reed D, MacEachern D. Prospective study of cigarette smoking and the risk of developing idiopathic Parkinson's disease. Am J Epidemiol 1994; 139:1129–1138.
36. Roberts R, Spitzer W, Delmore T, Sackett D. An empirical demonstration of Berkson's bias. J Chronic Dis 1978; 31:119–128.
37. Sackett D. Bias in analytic research. J Chronic Dis 1979; 32:51–63.
38. Langston JW, Koller W. The next frontier in Parkinson's disease: presymptomatic detection. Neurology 1991; 41(suppl 2):5–7.
39. Ellenberg JH, Nelson KB. Sample selection and the natural history of disease. JAMA 1992; 1980:1337–1340.

12

Environmental Agents and Parkinson's Disease

Peter S. Spencer and Patricia G. Butterfield

Oregon Health Sciences University, Portland, Oregon

I. INTRODUCTION

Although use of Sir James Parkinson's surname to characterize the disease of interest may lead one to imagine the operation of a single causal agent, it seems equally possible that idiopathic Parkinson's disease is not a single disease entity, but a uniform clinical syndrome, a reflection of the brain's limited repertoire for the expression of nigrostriatal damage, irrespective of cause. Just as current knowledge on the multifarious etiologies of stocking-and-glove neuropathy would make a mockery of a suggestion of a unitary causation for this syndrome, so may numerous factors—heritable, infectious, traumatic, toxic—be at the seat of Parkinson's disease. If this is true, attempts to elucidate Parkinson's disease etiology will be greatly complicated, and clever detective work in linking cause and effect in individual cases may play an important role in the discovery of causation.

It may seem surprising that environmental chemicals should be considered in the etiology of Parkinson's disease. Chemicals certainly have the potential to elicit a large number of disparate neurological disorders (1), but neurotoxic conditions usually have the cardinal property of stabilizing or regressing—not progressing—once exposure has terminated. Parkinson's disease, by contrast, is a disease that progresses whether or *not* the individual remains in the environment in which it first appeared. Ergo, idiopathic Parkinson's disease is not caused by environmental chemicals.

This type of conventional wisdom has been challenged by two observations suggesting that environmental chemicals are linked to diseases with features comparable with Parkinson's disease. One is the unequivocal demonstration that exposure to 1-methyl-4-phenyl-1,2,3,6-tetrahydropyridine (MPTP) damages the substantia nigra and induces irreversible parkinsonism in humans and primates (see Chapter 13). Whether the human disease is progressive or stationary following cessation of exposure has yet to be established. Second, the western Pacific amyotrophic lateral sclerosis (ALS) and parkinsonism–dementia (P–D) complex, a nontransmissible disorder lacking an obvious hereditable pattern, has declined in young subjects as affected regions have undergone environmental advancement. This suggests the operation of a disappearing environmental factor that is peculiar to the lifestyle of the affected populations. Use for food and medicine of the poisonous seed of the neurotoxic cycad plant is a possible causal factor (2,3), and the etiology of this disease has also been linked to the accumulation of aluminum in affected nerve cells of Guam cases (4). Etiology notwithstanding, the important observation for the present purpose is that western Pacific P–D is likely to be an environmentally triggered, long-latency, *progressive* neurological disorder with parkinsonian and other clinical features. Nonchemical environmental factors (i.e., transmissible agents) linked to parkinsonian disorders (i.e., postencephalitic parkinsonism) have been largely excluded in western Pacific P–D (5). Although the specific causal agent(s) has yet to be identified, it seems likely that an environmental chemical will prove to have a central etiologic role.

Although formal epidemiological studies are of great potential importance in associating environmental factors with disease, it is noteworthy they were *not* required to link MPTP with parkinsonism (6,7), or cycad with western Pacific ALS–P–D (8). Just as John Snow in 19th century London required none of the armamentarium and data-crunching capability of the modern epidemiologist to link cholera with consumption of contaminated drinking water from the Broad Street pump (9), the role of specific environmental factors in sporadic Parkinson's disease may well be solved by a modern-day sleuth with Snow's zeal, logical thinking, and observational powers.

II. THE CHEMICAL UNIVERSE

A sleuth in search of the etiology of Parkinson's disease must be prepared to explore the universe of chemical substances to seek environmental factors linked to Parkinson's disease. The association between cycad–aluminum and ALS–P–D serves as a reminder that naturally occurring as well as synthetic (e.g., MPTP) chemicals may be the root cause of certain types of neurodegenerative disease. Gajdusek (10) emphasized this point when he linked unknown environmental factors to the high prevalence of ALS–P–D in a pre-Industrial Age Papua New

Guinean population, which was subsequently linked by one of us (PSS) to the employment of cycad seed as a medicine (11,12).

There is direct evidence from both human and veterinary neurology that some plant and fungal agents target basal ganglia. Ingestion of mildewed sugar cane is a recognized cause of basal ganglia degeneration among Chinese children (13). Those who recover from the gastrointestinal and encephalopathic signs of acute poisoning may subsequently develop a severe dystonia associated with bilateral putaminal necrosis. Although an hypoxic element during coma cannot be ruled out in these cases, the primary trigger is the fungal toxin 3-nitropropionic acid (NPA), which arrests energy transformation by inhibiting succinic dehydrogenase activity. While cases of human disease outside China are undescribed, NPA is a widely distributed plant mycotoxin, with manifold possibilities for human contact (14).

Veterinary neurology contributes equine nigropallidal encephalomalacia, a disease featured by bilateral necrosis of the anterior globus pallidus and zona reticulata of the substantia nigra found in horses (but not in cattle or sheep) that graze on the Yellow Star thistle *(Centaurea solstitialis),* a weed of the western United States (15). Although the culpable agent has yet to be identified, two chemicals (cynaropicrin and 3-*O*-acetylsolstitialin) with cytotoxic potential in rat fetal brain cultures (derived from substantia nigra, striatum, cerebral cortex, and raphe nuclei) have been identified (16). Once the responsible neurotoxin has been found, it will be important to determine whether it is able to enter animal products (e.g., cow's milk) used by humans for food.

III. CRITERIA FOR CHEMICAL NEUROTOXICITY

Establishment of criteria by which to assess the strength of association between chemicals and disease processes is an essential point of departure in the search for environmental agents associated with Parkinson's disease. The story of Minamata disease, a widespread neurotoxic disorder of humans and animals caused by consumption of fish contaminated with methylmercury (17), illustrates the hurdles to be overcome before a suspect environmental contaminant is accepted as the culpable agent. In brief, the neurological illness seen in humans and cats was reproduced in the latter both by feeding methylmercury-contaminated fish and by administering authentic samples of the suspect chemical agent. Because pure methylmercury was able experimentally to induce in cats a neurological picture indistinguishable from that seen in the affected feline population of Minamata Bay, and the nature of the feline disorder clearly paralleled the attendant human disease, it was possible to draw strong conclusions about the etiological relation between methylmercury and Minamata disease. Thus, in the absence of human experimentation or controlled exposures (as with therapeutic agents), the strongest foundation for establishing chemical culpability is the experimental induction in animals, under controlled conditions, of a disorder equivalent to that seen in human subjects exposed to the compound under scrutiny.

At least six "confidence classes" may be proposed to define the relation between environmental factors and human neurological disorders, the strength of the association between agent and disease diminishing as one descends through the list:

Class 0. Effects in controlled human studies (applicable to drugs only)
Class 1. Effects in controlled mammalian studies, with similar effects following uncontrolled exposures of humans
Class 2. Effects in humans following uncontrolled exposures, but evidence from controlled animal studies unavailable
Class 3. Effects in controlled exposure studies in an appropriate animal species, with unknown effects in humans
Class 4. Possible effects in humans (e.g., case reports), but supporting experimental evidence weak or absent
Class 5. Epidemiological associations with effects unknown in humans and untested in animals

In relation to extrapyramidal disorders, the literature demonstrates that several agents have the potential to cause extrapyramidal damage with the clinical expression of parkinsonism or dystonia (Table 1), but only MPTP is known to induce discrete nigrostriatal damage resembling Parkinson's disease in humans and mammals. Chemically induced disorders of the basal ganglia are largely self-limiting although, with the attrition of nerve cells in basal ganglia with age (18), they likely advance slowly with the passage of time. However, no chemical agent has been shown to induce a neurodegenerative disorder of progressively increasing severity comparable with Parkinson's disease, although a putative factor of this type ("slow toxin") is sought in western Pacific ALS–P–D (19). The epidemiological association between Parkinson's disease and chemical groups (e.g., insecticides, herbicides), mixtures (well water), or practices (farming) represent clues for further research and provide no evidence of cause–effect relationships.

Another important qualification relates to the internal consistency of the proposed association between a chemical and a neurological disorder. Although idiosyncratic reactions may occur rarely, individual chemicals usually produce a stereotyped pattern of disease within a given dose range and duration of exposure. For example, in all tested animals, brief exposures to large concentrations of the compound *n*-hexane induce narcosis, whereas extended exposures to smaller concentrations elicit peripheral neuropathy (20). Furthermore, within the dose range required to induce peripheral neuropathy, the extent of axonal degeneration (and severity of neuropathy) is a function of dosage and time. Since

Table 1 Distribution of Chemicals and Mixtures by Confidence Class and Disease Entity

Class	Parkinson's disease	Nigrostriatal	Extrapyramidal	Neurotoxic
1		MPTP	Carbon disulfide/disulfiram	Aluminum
				Thallium salts
			Carbon monoxide	*N*-Hexane
			Manganese compounds	Pesticides[a]
			Mercurials	
			3-Nitropropionic acid	
2	(Cigarette smoking)		Hexachlorobenzene	
			Methyl bromide	
			Methyl iodine	
			Thallium salts	
3			β-*N*-Methylamino-L-alanine	Cycasin
4			Hexachlorobenzene	
			N-Hexane	
5	Pesticides (insecticides and herbicides)		Cycad	
	Rural living		Aluminum	
	Well water			
	Farming			
	Wood-related work			

Class 1–5. Strength of association between environmental chemical/mixture and disease entity (described in text): 1, very strong positive association vs. 5, very weak. *Parkinson's disease*: Agents positively or negatively associated with idiopathic Parkinson disease in epidemiological studies. *Nigrostriatal*: Agents linked to selective damage of substantia nigra pars compacta and nigrostriatal pathway. *Extrapyramidal:* Agents linked to selective damage to one or more of the following: putamen, globus pallidus, substantia nigra pars reticulata, subthalamic nucleus, and caudate. *Neurotoxic*: Agents that, at elevated levels, produce diverse neurological responses.
Note that (1) disorders induced by certain agents (e.g., mercurials and manganese compounds) are responsive to L-dopa, and (2) cigarette smoking shows an inverse association with Parkinson's disease risk, (3) cycad and aluminum are linked to western Pacific ALS–P–D, and (d) MPTP, 1-methyl-4-phenyl-1,2,3,6-tetrahydropyridine.
[a]Certain pesticides have neurotoxic potential (see section VI.A.6.)

neuropathy is also seen in humans comparably exposed to *n*-hexane (20), it follows that (1) the expected neurotoxic effect of *n*-hexane in humans is peripheral neuropathy, and (2) heavily exposed subjects will have severe clinical deficits. Thus, the recent suggestion (21,22) of a causal relation between *n*-hexane and severe parkinsonism in a single patient heavily exposed to mixed solvents, including the alkane, with only electromyographic evidence of peripheral neuropathy, must remain sub judice until concrete experimental evidence is brought forth.

A relation between dosage and degree of effect must be demonstrated to provide solid evidence to incriminate the chemical as the causal factor.

IV. CHEMICAL INTERACTIONS AND TOXIC POTENCY

Caution is also merited in specifying the chemical causation of a neurotoxic disorder when the patient has been significantly exposed to more than one agent. Health professionals sometimes step beyond their limited training in toxicology to assign causation to the wrong agents. Compounds such as methyl *n*-butyl ketone (MBK) and methyl isobutyl ketone (MIBK) may sound sufficiently similar to be treated as one and the same, but MBK is a class 1 human neurotoxicant for peripheral neuropathy, whereas MIBK has been experimentally proven to lack comparable neurotoxic potential (20).

Other sources of confusion may arise from the interactive toxic properties of chemical substances. For example, if four chemicals (a–d) are arbitrarily assigned the following numerical values: $a = 0$ (no effect); $b = 1$; $c = 2$; and $d = 3$, then the toxicity of two in combination acting . . .

additively, i.e., $b + c = 1 + 2 = 3$
(e.g., certain pesticides);

synergistically, i.e., $b + d = 1 + 3 = >> 4$
(e.g., ethanol + carbon tetrachloride);

antagonistically, i.e., $c + d = 2 + 3 = 1$
(e.g., certain nerve-membrane toxins);

and

by potentiation, i.e., $a + d = 0 + 3 = >> 3$
(e.g., methyl ethyl ketone + *n*-hexane)

The final example serves to illustrate the potential for mistaken indictment. In the 1970s, 18 cases of severe peripheral neuropathy developed in a group of glue-sniffers several months after the addition of 11% methyl ethyl ketone (MEK) to the abused glue formulation and a corresponding reduction of the *n*-hexane concentration from 31% to 16%. No cases were recognized among solvent abusers who had used the original formulation (containing 31% *n*-hexane) for 7 years. Additionally, after removal of MEK from the new glue formulation, no new cases of neuropathy occurred, except for one individual who continued to inhale the MEK-containing solvent (23). Although it seems reasonable to deduce from this incident that MEK causes peripheral neuropathy, that conclusion is wrong. The correct interpretation, as shown by the results of experimental animal studies, is that MEK alone is unable to induce neuropathy, but greatly increases the neurotoxic potential of *n*-hexane (24), a class 1 agent for peripheral neuropathy. This episode teaches the need for caution before specific substances are indicted as causes of neurological disease.

V. SPECIFIC CHEMICALS AND SELF-LIMITING EXTRAPYRAMIDAL DISEASE

Although the strongest possible evidence has been marshalled to demonstrate that MPTP is a class 1 parkinsonian agent (see Chapter 13), evidence to support the proposal that either the agent or a derivative has a role in Parkinson's disease has not been forthcoming (see Section V.A.1). MPTP was not the first agent recognized to induce an extrapyramidal disorder with clinical features resembling Parkinson's disease in humans and animals. Three other compounds lay claim to this dubious distinction: manganese dioxide, carbon disulfide, and carbon monoxide; these agents were first linked with parkinsonism in 1837, 1856, and 1926 (25–27), respectively, the former only 20 years after Parkinson published his *Essay on the Shaking Palsy*. These three compounds and a number of additional substances linked to related extrapyramidal disorders are examined in the following sections. The neurological conditions associated with these materials differ from Parkinson's disease; they are more akin to extrapyramidal disorders triggered by global brain energy compromise. MPTP, by contrast, may act by energy compromise *regionally restricted* to nigrostriatal neurons (discussed in the following).

Energy transformation is the sequential biochemical process by which glucose is converted to adenosine triphosphate (ATP). The acetyl group of acetyl-coenzyme-A, which is derived from glucose oxidation by glycolysis, is enzymatically degraded by the tricarboxylic acid cycle in the mitochondrion to form two molecules of carbon dioxide and four pairs of hydrogen atoms. Electrons from these atoms are fed into a series of electron carriers, the four complexes (I–IV) of the respiratory chain. The ensuing process of electron transport to molecular oxygen proceeds with a very large decline in free energy, much of which is conserved by the phosphorylation of adenosine diphosphate (ADP) to yield ATP, in the process of oxidative phosphorylation (28). An uninterrupted supply of ATP is an absolute requirement for many neuronal functions.

Agents that disrupt the electron transport chain have a propensity to compromise brain function and induce extrapyramidal dysfunction. This appears to result from energy compromise that is either global (common) or regionally selective (rare).

Global energy compromise often results in tardive extrapyramidal dysfunction; the attendant clinical manifestations may be labeled parkinsonism because of their similarity to Parkinson's disease, but the brunt of neuronal degeneration occurs in regions other than the nigrostriatal pathway. Parts of the basal ganglia vulnerable to global energy deficits include bilaterally the putamen, globus pallidus, substantia nigra pars reticulata, and subthalamic nuclei. These areas receive major neuroexcitatory inputs in which glutamate is the proven or likely neurotransmitter. Given the increased sensitivity of energy-compromised neurons to glutamate excitotoxicity (29), it is reasonable to postulate that selective neuronal damage in these regions of the basal ganglia, to some extent, involves the neurotoxic potential of glutamate acting through excitatory amino acid (EAA) receptors on target neurons. Additionally, acute intoxication, leading to convulsions, may trigger the release of glial stores of glutamate, resulting in massive neuronal damage.

Although the substantia nigra pars compacta receives no major glutamatergic input, systemic intoxication (with MPTP) conceivably may lead to regionally selective energy compromise sufficient to render dopaminergic nerve cells susceptible to the neurotoxic potential of normal transmitter levels of glutamate. A priori, the existence of multiple sites of mitochondrial vulnerability (complexes I–IV) suggests a role for a range of disparate substances able to gain selective entry to nigrostriatal neurons. An alternative postulate recognizes the selective increase in iron content in the substantia nigra pars compacta of Parkinson's disease patients and the possibility that free ferric ion participates in autoxidation of dopamine, resulting in the generation of hydrogen peroxide and toxic free oxygen radicals (30). Both hypotheses predict a state of oxidation stress selective to the substantia nigra.

Whether tissue energy deficits are regional or global in the brain, the net result is likely to be supraphysiological excitation of neurons equipped with glutamate receptors of the *N*-methyl-D-aspartate (NMDA)-preferring subclass, failure of their homeostatic mechanisms, and nerve cell (excitotoxic) degeneration (29,31). Fast cell death (within minutes) would ensue from continuous activation of ion channels coupled to EAA receptors, intracellular influx of Na^+ and Cl^-, and entry of water down the resulting osmotic gradient. Slow cell death (hours to days) would be caused by calcium entry, inappropriate activation of proteases, or the intracellular formation of toxic superoxide free radicals.

A. Regional Brain Mitochondrial Dysfunction?

1. 1-Methyl-4-phenyl-1,2,3,6-tetrahydropyridine

Regional oxidative stress may be linked to nigrostriatal degeneration and parkinsonism (30). This is suggested by the induction of human parkinsonism by the 1-methyl-4-phenylpyridinium ion (MPP^+, a metabolite of MPTP), which is selectively taken up by the dopamine transport system of nigrostriatal neurons and concentrated in mitochondria, where it inhibits complex I of the respiratory chain (32), possibly by a free-radical mechanism (33). Consistent with this idea are reports of complex I deficiency in Parkinson's disease (34), its apparent anatomical selectivity to the substantia nigra, and the absence of this mitochondrial defect in multiple system atrophy (35). Viewed from this perspective, therefore, Parkinson's disease may be causally linked to a mitochondrial gene abnormality, to a mitochondrial toxin that selectively gains access to nigrostriatal neurons, or to a combination of both. These concepts are discussed in greater detail in Chapter 13.

2. 1-Methyl-4-phenyl-1,2,3,6-tetrahydropyridine Analogues

Two groups of chemicals, the isoquinolines and the β-carbolines, have received attention in the search for chemicals with structure and properties comparable with those of MPP^+. Although isoquinolines and β-carbolines occur naturally in certain plants, research interest has focused on the possibility that neurotoxic derivatives are formed in the brain as endogenous metabolites, mostly by *N*-methylation, which reportedly is increased in Parkinson's disease (7).

Another structural relative of MPP^+ that has attracted attention is the herbicide paraquat; however, the primary target tissue of paraquat is the lung, and a movement disorder associated with selective nigrostriatal damage is not recognized. Two of these compounds, isoquinolines and β-carbolines, are discussed in much greater detail in Chapter 7.

Tetrahydroisoquinolines. The MPTP structural relatives 1-methyl-1-2,3,4,-tetrahydroisoquinoline (TIQ), 1-methyl-TIQ, and 2-methyl-TIQ are mammalian endogenous metabolites present in normal human and Parkinson's disease brains (37,38). TIQ is a specific inhibitor of complex I (39). TIQ and 2-methyl-TIQ induce experimental parkinsonism, whereas 1-methyl-TIQ is claimed to lack neurotoxicity and to prevent parkinsonism-like effects (38,40). *N*-Methylation of TIQ produces *N*-methyl-TIQ which, through the action of monoamine oxidase, forms the *N*-methyl-isoquinolinium ion ($NMIQ^+$), a possible direct neurotoxin comparable with MPP^+ (41).

β-Carbolines. β-Carbolines are heterocyclic, dehydrogenated derivatives of tryptophan, formed in plants and possibly in animals (42,43). The structural overlap between MPP^+ and the indole-derived β-carboline compounds that are methylated on the 2-nitrogen has stimulated interest in a possible role for 2-methylated-β-carbolines in Parkinson's disease (44). β-Carbolines that are close structural analogues of MPP^+, such as 2-*N*-methyl- and 2,9-*N*,*N'*-dimethylharminium and -harmolium derivatives, inhibit mitochondrial respiration (complexes I–III) and are toxic to dopaminergic and other cells (45). Mammalian brain appears to possess *S*-adenosylmethionine-dependent *N*-methyltransferases, which have the potential sequentially to *N*-methylate the β- and indole-nitrogens of norharman and harman (present in brain) to the corresponding 2,9-*N*,*N'*-dimethyl-β-carbolines, agents that mimic MPP^+ in their mode of mitochondrial uptake, extent of mitochondrial respiratory inhibition, and neurotoxic potency (46).

1,1'-Dimethyl-4,4-bipyridinium Ion (Paraquat). The structural relationship between MPP^+ and paraquat has been the object of scientific interest since the association between MPTP and parkinsonism was made in 1983. Paraquat, known commercially as Weedol and a host of other commercial labels, is a widely used herbicide. A compound of high acute toxicity, paraquat accumulates in lungs where it interacts with oxygen to cause spectacular free radical-induced lung injury in several species, including humans. Diquat, a related bipyridal herbicide, does not accumulate in lung or cause significant pulmonary damage (47).

Hundreds of cases of accidental and suicidal poisonings with paraquat show that effects in humans are similar to those in animals. Regardless of the route of exposure, fatally poisoned humans exhibit gastrointestinal irritation; hepatic, renal, and cardiac dysfunction; followed by a gradual onset and progression of respiratory difficulties, culminating in death (47). Convulsions, ataxia, and impaired consciousness may occur, and hemorrhagic leukoencephalopathy may be found at autopsy (48). Occupational exposures are associated with dermatitis and nail deformities, conjunctivitis, ocular damage, and respiratory compromise.

There is no evidence that paraquat induces parkinsonism, although extrapyramidal compromise may occur. Rajput and Uitti (49) found no increase in Parkinson's disease prevalence with the heavy use of paraquat in Saskatchewan, Canada. Neurological sequelae following ingestion of paraquat are contained in two reports. One describes eight family members in Naples with subacute paraquat poisoning: two died of "cardiobreathing attacks," and the remaining six were monitored prospectively. Six months following exposure, one developed rigidity in the right arm, whereas the others remained asymptomatic (50). In a second report, Grcevic and colleagues (51) described clinical and neuropathological findings of two patients following ingestion of paraquat. Both patients developed psychomotor disturbances and hand tremor within several days; death occurred 9 and 11 days following exposure. Neuropathological examination revealed accumulation of lipofuscin-like material that was most pronounced in the pallidum, thalamus, corpus geniculatum lateralis, substantia nigra, dentate and fastigial nuclei of the cerebellum, Purkinje cells, nuclei of motor cranial nerves, and inferior olivary nucleus. Chromatolytic changes and swelling of nerve cell bodies were noted in the dentate nucleus, substantia nigra, locus coeruleus, oculomotor nuclei, motor trigeminal nucleus, and facial and hypoglossal nuclei.

These reports show the toxic properties of paraquat are distinct from those of MPP^+. It is unclear whether the neurological effects attributed to paraquat are associated with a neurotoxic property of the compound or, more likely, reported changes are secondary to respiratory compromise, causing global brain hypoxia. The following section explores the relation between this phenomenon and extrapyramidal disorders that are distinct from Parkinson's disease.

B. Global Brain Energy Dysfunction and Related Disorders

Extrapyramidal signs are encountered in adults who are subjected to acute intoxication with chemical agents or hypoxic episodes that temporarily, but severely, interrupt the generation of chemical energy required for the maintenance of neuronal integrity. Combinations of hypoxia and ischemia, such as occurs after cardiorespiratory arrest, give rise to widespread neuropathological changes that depend on the survival time following the insult and the differential vulnerability of neuronal groups (52–54). Among the most vulnerable are neurons in the hippocampal subfields H1 and H3–5 (Sommer's sector and end folium); the Purkinje and basket cells of the cerebellum, layers 3,5, and 6 of the neocortex, especially of the parietal and occipital lobes where laminar necrosis is most prominent; the outer halves of the head and body of the caudate nucleus and the outer half of the putamen; the inferior colliculi, inferior olives, and the reticular zone of the substantia nigra (55). Note the pars compacta is absent from this list.

Several environmental chemicals directly or indirectly induce global brain energy deficiency and, thereby, cause extrapyramidal dysfunction, with a distribution of basal ganglia damage distinct from that seen in Parkinson's disease. Chemicals in this class include carbon monoxide (indirect) and NPA (direct); single exposures to these compounds may lead to seizures and coma, followed by the appearance of severe extrapyramidal disease resembling parkinsonism and dystonia, respectively. Acute intoxication with other agents, such as cyanide, hydrogen sulfide, and formate (a metabolite of methanol; 56), each of which terminates energy production by inhibiting cytochrome oxidase, may cause striatal damage culminating in a movement disorder, such as dystonia (57–60). Other substances associated with extrapyramidal dysfunction, including carbon disulfide, manganese compounds, and mercurials, interfere with various biochemical pathways, including energy transformation.

1. Carbon Monoxide

Emissions of this ubiquitous air pollutant result primarily from fuel combustion in motor vehicles, aircraft, vessels, and stationary sources (coal, fuel oil, natural gas, wood), various industrial processes, solid-waste combustion, forest fires, miscellaneous technological sources, and cigarette smoke (61). The solvent methylene chloride is metabolized to carbon monoxide.

Fuel combustion in settings with limited ventilation is a common cause of acute carbon monoxide intoxication. Inhaled carbon monoxide rapidly enters the pulmonary blood, where it binds with the ferrous ion complex of protoporphyrin IX in hemoglobin and blocks its physiological role of binding oxygen. Carbon monoxide also blocks ATP production by binding to the terminal oxidase (cytochrome a_3) of the mitochondrial chain. When blood contains greater than 50% carboxyhemoglobin, coma, convulsions, cardiorespiratory failure, and death may result. If resuscitation of comatose subjects is achieved, a small proportion may first recover and, between 2 days and 6 weeks (usually 2–3 weeks) later, develop global neurological deterioration. Parkinsonian rigidity, akinesia, and tremor may feature in this pathological process (27,62).

> Grinker (27) first described this remarkable condition in a 58-year-old woman with inoperable gastric carcinoma who attempted suicide with

> illuminating gas (12–20% carbon monoxide, 10–20% methane, 40–50% hydrogen). She was initially comatose but rapidly regained consciousness and appeared at first neurologically unremarkable. Some 26 days later, however, she became poorly oriented and apathetic, exhibited a masked facies, greatly accentuated muscle tone, and absence of spontaneous limb movements, and walked with a small-stepped gait. She had slow monotonous speech and impaired remote memory. Later, she became completely akinetic and mute. She died 2 months after the initial illness. At autopsy, she was found to have bilateral, symmetrical necrotic lesions of the globus pallidus . . . and . . . a diffuse demyelinating process involved the entire subcortical hemispheral white matter. . . . (Ginsberg; 63).

Klawans and colleagues (64) described the onset of parkinsonism in a 50-year-old woman 2 months following carbon monoxide poisoning. Signs of micrographia, simian posture, difficulty rising from a chair, and propulsion were resistant to treatment with levodopa, but responded to anticholinergics. A computed tomography (CT) scan revealed necrosis of the globus pallidus. Smith and Mellick (65) reported four patients with carbon monoxide poisoning, two of whom developed parkinsonism, one with rigidity and tremor 6 weeks postexposure, and the second with confusion and progressive parkinsonism.

There is ample experimental evidence to demonstrate that pallidal necrosis occurs in cats and dogs intoxicated with carbon monoxide, whereas rabbits and guinea pigs also show involvement of the cerebral cortex, hippocampus, and cerebellum (66). Rhesus monkeys subjected to carboxyhemoglobin levels of 72–77% for 60–325 min show abnormalities of globus pallidus and hippocampus, although damage to myelin is the dominant pathological feature (67). The severity of myelin damage may be related to the degree of hypotension, rather than to the duration of carbon monoxide inhalation, level of carboxyhemoglobin, or severity of the attendant acidosis (68,69).

Carbon monoxide, therefore, is a class 1 toxin that primarily acts indirectly to induce global brain energy deficits leading to severe extrapyramidal degeneration.

2. *3-Nitropropionic Acid*

Additional evidence that certain parts of the basal ganglia (other than the substantia nigra pars compacta) are especially susceptible to global brain energy compromise comes from observations of the neurotoxic effects of 3-nitropropionic acid (NPA), a suicide inhibitor of succinate dehydrogenase (a component of complex II of the mitochondrial electron transport chain).

3-Nitropropionic acid has been implicated epidemiologically in an extrapyramidal disorder featured by bilateral putaminal necrosis and delayed dystonia in children after ingestion of sugarcane contaminated with a species of the fungus *Arthrinium*. Within hours of consuming the contaminated material, affected subjects develop gastrointestinal disturbances, followed by acute encephalopathy, with convulsions and coma that may last for up to 20 days. After regaining consciousness, some recover and others develop, up to 6 weeks later, a delayed dystonic movement disorder featured by facial grimacing, sustained athetosis of hands and fingers, torsion spasm, spasmodic torticollis, spasmodic attacks, and uncontrolled coarse movements of the extremities. CT scans reveal bilateral lenticular hypodensities, mainly in the putamen, to a lesser extent in the globus pallidus and, occasionally, in the caudate and claustrum. Diffuse cerebral atrophy is also seen on occasion (13,14).

Controlled studies with mice demonstrate that single or repeated doses of NPA, sufficient to inhibit the enzyme activity of succinic dehydrogenase more or less uniformly throughout the brain (M. I. Sabri, personal communication), cause bilaterally symmetrical lesions of the lateral aspect of the caudate–putamen, the globus pallidus, the endopeduncular nucleus, and the pars reticulata of the anterior substantia nigra, together with abnormalities of myelin in brain and spinal cord (70). Affected regions of the basal ganglia are hallmarked by edematous postsynaptic lesions, dendritic swelling, and nuclear pyknosis, with chromatin clumping, a pattern of lesions comparable with that induced by excessive local concentrations of the excitatory neurotransmitter glutamate. Comparable neuronal abnormalies are found in mouse cortical explants treated with NPA, and these changes are reduced (but not abolished) by pretreatment with glutamate receptor antagonists acting at *N*-methyl-D-aspartate (NMDA) and non-NMDA receptors (71). Likewise, tissue damage associated with anoxia–ischemia is also attenuated by glutamate antagonists (72).

Thus, NPA is a class 1 extrapyramidal agent capable of causing dystonia in severely poisoned subjects who recover from toxin-induced seizures and coma.

3. *Carbon Disulfide and Disulfiram*

Carbon disulfide is used primarily in the production of regenerated rayon and cellophane, and in the manufacture of carbon tetrachloride. As a solvent for resins, rubber, and fats, the agent finds many applications. Carbon disulfide is also used as a preservative for fresh fruit, in semiconductor production, and as a pesticide.

Although the mechanism underlying carbon disulfide neurotoxicity is unknown, the agent reacts with amino acids to form dithiocarbamates, which chelate metal ions of physiological import such as copper and zinc (73). Dithiocarbamates have enjoyed widespread use as agricultural fungicides. Carbon disulfide may also perturb vitamin B_6 metabolism and interfere with dopamine-β-hydroxylase (a copper-containing enzyme), which converts dopamine to norepinephrine.

Long-term exposure to carbon disulfide is associated with systemic disease featured by vascular compromise, serum hypercholesterolemia, atherosclerosis, nephrosclerosis, endocrine dysfunction, and retinal microaneurysms, as well as neurological and psychiatric disturbances (74). Much of this experience comes from the viscose rayon industry, in which workers are exposed to both carbon disulfide and hydrogen sulfide, which inhibits cytochrome oxidase.

The viscose rayon industry has been clearly associated with extrapyramidal and other types of neurological disorders. Disease appears insidiously, with asthenia, paresthesias, and difficulty walking (axonal polyneuropathy), and proceeds to mental deterioration, spastic paraparesis, and pseudobulbar paralysis. Transient hemiplegia may occur. Some subjects develop parkinsonism (75).

Delpech, in papers spanning the years 1856–1863 (26,76), appears to have been the first to mention the peculiar stiffness and trembling of his carbon disulfide patients, and to point out the similarity of their tremor to that of Parkinson's disease (a point later challenged by F. H. Lewy; 77,78). The Italian Quarelli (79,80) insisted that both dystonia and parkinsonism were syndromes or sequelae of carbon disulfide poisoning in almost one-third of his subjects. Raneletti (81) showed that 7% of 100 cases of chronic carbon disulfide poisoning displayed parkinsonism, along with psychoses (52%), polyneuropathy (10%), and a number of characteristic systemic disorders. In 1938, neurologist F. H. Lewy, and other members of the medical staff of the School of Medicine of the University of Pennsylvania, published a survey of 120 subjects in the viscose rayon industry: "Shaking palsy has been found in every seventh individual" with chronic carbon disulfide exposure. On average, parkinsonism appeared in individuals with a mean age of 40, after "10 years of exposure to carbon disulfide." Additionally, one subject who 2 years earlier had been overcome acutely by combined carbon disulfide and hydrogen sulfide fumes showed "a mild degree of parkinsonism," a condition that may reverse, "remain stationary or become progressive" (77,78).

> In CS_2 poisoning, as in lead and manganese intoxication, lesions in the central nervous system show a predilection for the basal ganglia. . . . Disease of this area is followed by parkinsonism (shaking palsy), tremor, choreatic movements (St. Vitus' dance) and unilateral sensory disturbances of central character. . . . Rigidity, tremor, Salbengesicht [greasy face], hyperhydrosis [profuse sweating] of fingers and tremulous handwriting are part of this disease. . . . There is no "pill rolling" movement of the fingers. . . . Parkinson tremor, in contrast to CS_2 tremor, is a repose tremor, which disappears with voluntary movements. In other words, not every tremor in CS_2 intoxication is a Parkinson tremor nor can its isolated appearance be used as evidence of this complication (78).

The same 1938 volume carried B. J. Alpers neuropathological findings of a deceased viscose rayon spinner, with 22 years of exposure to carbon disulfide (82). In addition to neuronal and axonal changes in cortex, brainstem nuclei, cerebellum, spinal cord, and peripheral nerves, he states: "The basal ganglia of the brain show definite changes. The large striatal cells show a decrease in number, and the remainder are diseased. The pallidal cells may be sclerosed . . ."

Megro (83) reported a single case of a young worker exposed to carbon disulfide fumes who developed tremor, cogwheel rigidity, slow speech, micrographia, and impaired convergence. Hamilton and Lewy (84) reported extrapyramidal signs in 16.7% of 120 cases; Gordy and Trumper (85) noted a 55% incidence, but believed the parkinsonian syndrome is seldom complete or pure; and Vigliani (75) reported a frequency of 30%. "That true parkinsonism occurs as a result of carbon disulfide poisoning there can be no doubt," stated Richter (86).

In more recent times, Peters and colleagues (87,88) attributed to carbon disulfide the clinical manifestations of cogwheel rigidity, automaticity, decreased associated movements, resting and intention tremor, peripheral neuropathy, pyramidal tract signs, and neurobehavioral changes they found in grain storage workers occupationally exposed to carbon disulfide and other agents. Two of seven patients showed typical parkinsonian tremors that were resting, pill rolling, and accompanied by cogwheeling and loss of associated movements (87). An additional series of 15 workers revealed widespread cerebellar ataxia, resting and intention tremor, cogwheel rigidity, automaticity, and decreased associated movements. Features distinguishing these patients from Parkinson's disease included young age, preservation of normal voice and vocal strength, infrequent tremor, infrequent bradykinesia, rare disturbances of postural tone and, in one patient, poor response to conventional antiparkinsonian medications (88). A recent report of index finger tremor (5–7 Hz) was linked to exposures to pesticides based on carbon disulfide (89).

Carbon disulfide is also a metabolite of disulfiram (tetraethylthiuram disulfide), a drug used in the treatment of chronic alcoholism. Clinical experience with disulfiram provides further evidence that carbon disulfide acts selectively on basal ganglia. Prolonged treatment with disulfiram sometimes induces reversible or persistent movement disorders with parkinsonism, dystonia, and akinesia (90,91). Brain imaging revealed cystic necrosis of globus pallidus and putamen in a patient who developed a severely disabling dystonia following an acute encephalopathic episode (92).

Richter (86) produced parkinsonism, with degeneration of basal ganglia, in four rhesus monkeys exposed to carbon disulfide by inhalation for periods of 12–21 months. Experimental misadventure led to episodes of acute toxicity, possibly associated with tissue-damaging hypoxia. However, three of the four animals developed a parkinsonism state 6–9 months after the development of an unconscious state. The essential and constant pathological changes consisted of extensive, bilateral, and symmetrical necrosis of the globus pallidus and the zona reticulata of the substantia nigra. The monkeys presented with profound motor disturbances, characterized by reduction and slowness of all types of movement without paralysis, incoordination of locomotion and climbing, plastic cogwheel rigidity of the skeletal muscles, flexor postural attitudes of the trunk and extremities, and severe action tremor. Resting tremor was absent in all but one animal.

Carbon disulfide, therefore, may be a class 1 extrapyramidal agent capable of causing a parkinsonian syndrome with pathological characteristics distinct from those of Parkinson's disease. The distribution of basal ganglia damage is comparable with that found in extrapyramidal disorders resulting from global energy deficits associated with interruption of the electron transport chain. However, the possible role of hypoxia in producing the primate disorder cannot be excluded, nor can a role for hydrogen sulfide in the human occupational disease.

4. Manganese Compounds

Unlike all other substances known to trigger extrapyramidal disease, manganese is required for the maintenance of normal health. Too little manganese increases susceptibility to convulsive states in rodents (93); too much damages the basal ganglia of macaques and humans (94,95). Manganese intoxication is most closely associated with miners extracting manganese-bearing ores. Human exposure to manganese may occur through use of potassium permanganate, a powerful oxidizing agent used industrially to bleach resins, waxes, fats, oils, straws, cotton, silk and other fibers, and chamois skins; to dye wood brown; and in printing of fabrics, exterminating grape mildew, photography, tanning leathers, and purifying water. The fungicide maneb ([ethylene*bis*(dithiocarbamato)]manganese) is another potential source of human exposure to manganese.

Manganese functions in carbohydrate metabolism and gluconeogenesis. Metal ions are taken up by mitochondria for oxidative phosphorylation (succinate dehydrogenase, pyruvate decarboxylase). Manganese replaces Mg^{2+} in many biological reactions of the metal–ATP complex (96).

Unknown is how these functions relate, if at all, to the neurotoxic effects of overexposure to manganese compounds. Judging from the distribution of basal ganglia damage, which is comparable with that seen in global energy-deficient states, a perturbation of energy transformation or of the excitatory amino acid system seems plausible. A direct or indirect mechanism could be envisaged, given that feeding manganese also depresses the serum magnesium concentration (97). Another observation of unknown significance for human health is the depression of hemoglobin formation in pigs, lambs, and rabbits overexposed to manganese (97). Others have emphasized the binding of manganese to melanin and have postulated a related disturbance of dopamine metabolism. Although dopamine drops in the caudate of squirrel monkeys repeatedly injected with manganese, and the degree of reduction correlates well with the extent of extrapyramidal dysfunction, serotonin is also reduced in the caudate, but not in the cerebrum (95). Therefore, it is unclear whether there is a primary disturbance of dopamine metabolism or, more likely, the neurotransmitter changes simply reflect basal ganglia damage from another cause.

The development of manganism is insidious and has been classified in three stages. Onset is marked by apathy, anorexia, asthenia, headache, leg weakness, muscular cramps, joint pain, irritability, and sexual excitement, followed by impotence. The second stage is featured by dysarthria, gait disturbance, and excessive salivation. These signs may be accompanied or preceded by a manganese psychosis, which may disappear when parkinsonism supervenes. Uncontrollable laughter, euphoria, impulsiveness, insomnia, followed by somnolence, may occur. The final stage is characterized by marked rigidity (most pronounced in the lower limbs), muscle pain, and speech disturbances, ranging from slow and difficult articulation to incoherence or complete muteness. Intention, but not resting, tremor is present, and some degree of dystonia may appear. Some rigid and hypokinetic patients are said to respond to L-dopa with improved gait, facial expression, and mental alertness.

Couper (25) was the first to link manganese to a condition resembling paralysis agitans. This conclusion was drawn from observations of five workers employed in a French pyrolusite (manganese dioxide ore) mill for several months:

> During the height of the disease the weakness of the contractile muscles was much greater in the legs than in the arms. It was of such nature that the patient reeled in walking and leaned forward when he wished to walk. The arms were somewhat weak and there was difficulty in speech. He was not able to make himself understood by a person at a little distance. Other sensations and intelligence were unaffected. The trunk muscles had the appearance of a paralytic. Saliva ran from the mouth during speech. There was no trembling of any part of the body, no colic, constipation nor derangement of digestion. . . . As the paralysis increased, manganese was finally suspected to be the cause and the workman moved to another region. After this time there was no augmentation of symptoms and at the end of six years the patient was in good health (Couper; 25).

The disease was rediscovered in 1901 in Austrian workers employed in drying manganese dioxide (96). Over the next 35 years, the medical literature described 152 cases drawn from manganese ore mills, voltaic cell factories, and the iron and steel industry (96). Although Schlocknow, in 1879, described 40–50 cases of walking disorders in zinc miners, and hindsight suggests these were victims of manganism provoked by inhalation of manganese present in the zinc ore, the propensity of miners exposed to manganese dust to develop parkinsonism was not recognized until 50 years had elapsed. Beginning in the 1930s and spanning World War II, manganism was described among miners in Spain, the Sinai, Morocco, Germany, and in Chile, where the association of an extrapyramidal syndrome with cognitive dysfunction (psychomotor hyperkinesis, impulsiveness, euphoria) was studied. Demand for manganese increased with the postwar development of the iron and steel industry, and many additional cases of manganism were recognized in the manganese ore mines of Morocco, Cuba, Mexico, Japan, Rumania, United States, and the former Soviet Union (96).

Significant findings in these cases included the predominant route and agent of intoxication (dust inhalation), the duration of exposure (6 months to 16 years of daily exposure), the age at onset (21–50+ years), the susceptibility of anemic individuals (because the uptake and plasma binding of manganese is linked to that of iron), the prevalence of the occupational disorder (up to 30% of workers), the progressive course of the disease during exposure, the natural regression of the disorder after cessation of exposure to the offending agent, and the association with pneumonia (dust-induced pulmonary inflammation and secondary bacterial infection).

In 1971, Emara and colleagues (98) surveyed dry-battery workers whose job involved mixing a compound of 70% manganese oxide in an unventilated shed. Of 36 workers, 8 had neuropsychiatric disturbances, with 6 of the 8 demonstrating manganese psychosis; 2 workers had signs of parkinsonism. The authors describe 1 worker's clinical picture as follows:

> A male worker aged 30 years, married and with two children, was a previous addict to cannabis and heavy cigarette smoker (40 cigarettes a day for 10 years). He had worked at compressing battery powder for 14 years without any previous occupation. His symptoms started 13 years after the start of exposure with a gradual onset of hallucinations and increased laughter. . . . The course of his disease was progressive. . . . He had uncontrollable laughter and crying, euphoria, and mild amnesia. His speech was slurred and monotonous, his face masked, and he had micrographia (Emara et al.; 98).

There is current widespread use of manganese-based fungicides in agriculture. Ferraz and associates (99) reported on two agricultural workers (ages 27 and 33) who developed parkinsonism following exposure to maneb, an organomanganese compound widely used in market-gardening regions. These two cases of manganese-associated parkinsonism led the investigator to conduct a descriptive study of maneb-exposed workers in Brazil. Of 69 workers, 50 worked either in maneb preparation or fumigation. All subjects were queried on their CNS symptoms and examined by neurologists. The exposed groups differed from nonexposed workers relative to frequency of headache, nervousness, and fatigue; other associations, including tremor, rigidity, and postural instability, were nonsignificant. Despite these clinical findings, serum manganese levels in exposed (7.7 ng/100 ml) and nonexposed (8.8 ng/100 ml) workers were comparable.

Extrapyramidal disease resembling manganism has also been described in individuals drinking well water contaminated with manganese and zinc (100).

The brunt of basal ganglia neuropathology in manganism is in the pallidum, putamen, caudate, and subthalamic nucleus, with relative sparing of the substantia nigra (94,101). The results of fluorodopa positron emission tomography suggest the presence of an intact nigrostriatal pathway (D. B. Calne, personal communication). Cellular damage with glial proliferation in the corpus striatum and cerebral cortex is found in intoxicated rabbits (102).

Manganese, therefore, is a class 1 agent for an extrapyramidal disorder distinct from Parkinson's disease.

5. *Inorganic and Organic Mercurials*

Environmental mercurials occur as elemental mercury (used by dental and thermometer workers), mercurous and mercuric salts, and organic aliphatic (e.g., methyl mercury) or aromatic mercury compounds. Humans with mercury–amalgam dental work are continuously exposed systemically to minute concentrations of inorganic and organic mercury.

Mercury and its inorganic and organic compounds disrupt protein synthesis and energy transformation. Alkyl mercurials perturb glycolysis, Krebs cycle, and the electron transport chain (103). Basal ganglia are affected in mercury intoxication, although the preponderant nervous system targets are elsewhere. Although parkinsonian features may be present in various types of mercury intoxication, mercurialism is usually readily distinguishable from Parkinson's disease.

Severe elemental mercury intoxication is featured by rigidity, chorea, myoclonus, and masked facies, in addition to attention and memory deficits, and an intense generalized static and intentional tremor, aggravated by emotion (104). Swelling and chromatolysis of neurons in the basal ganglia, cerebral cortex, and cerebellum (Purkinje cells), together with involvement of ventrolateral tracts, anterior horn cells, and peripheral nerves, are described (105).

Extrapyramidal signs sometimes occur in methylmercury intoxication, a disorder characterized by neuronal degeneration of dorsal root ganglia (sensory loss), calcarine cortex and adjacent occipital lobes (constricted visual fields), cerebellar cortex (ataxia), and basal ganglia. Epidemiological evidence for the coexistence of parkinsonism and more typical features of methylmercury intoxication has been reported in a small proportion (8.2%) of subjects with Minamata disease:

> The Parkinson's syndrome found in Minamata disease patients consists of mask-like or immobile faces, stooped posture, poverty and slowness of movement, loss of associated movements of the arms and trunk in walking, increased muscular tone, pro- and retropulsions, tremors, occasional salivation and salve-face. On the other hand, they showed constriction of the visual fields, hypoesthesia or anesthesia to all forms of sensation in a glove and stocking-like fashion, impairment of hearing, ataxia and familial incidence of Minamata disease (Tsubaki and Irukayama; 17).

Mercury granules (demonstrated by the Timm method) in the brain of one patient with Minamata disease were plentiful in the caudate and striatum, as well as the calcarine cortex, transverse temporal and postcentral gyri, and cerebellar cortex, brain regions that bear the brunt of the pathological damage in this disease (17). Spongiform degeneration of the claustrum and putamen occurs, and neuropathological changes are found in the caudate and globus pallidus (106,107).

Two epidemiological studies have shown an association between mercury exposure and patients with a diagnosis of Parkinson's disease. Ngim and Devathasan (108) found significantly elevated blood and urinary mercury levels (odds ratios = 21 and 19, respectively) in 54 Singaporean Parkinson's disease patients (diagnosed by a neurologist and responsive to -dopa or bromocriptine) versus 95 controls matched for age, gender, and ethnicity. The difference in mercury levels remained after controlling for fish intake, occupational exposure, amalgam fillings, and use of mercury-containing ethnic medications. The latter appeared to be a significant predictor of disease risk. In a second study, Ohlson and Hogstedt (109) queried 91 Parkinson's disease patients and 75 controls concerning occupational exposure to organic solvents and agricultural chemicals. Six Parkinson's disease patients versus two controls (odds ratio = 2.4, not significant) gave a history of mercury exposure. The lack of significance may have been due to the small sample size and the attendant modest power to detect this modest odds ratio. The authors noted that they were unable to differentiate between organic and inorganic mercury and suggested more detailed exploration of mercury exposure in future studies.

Brain autoradiographs of monkeys 8 days after injection with radiolabeled ethylmercury demonstrate a global brain distribution of the metal, with the highest activity in the occipital pole, cerebellum, substantia nigra, and subthalamus, and appreciable deposition in other parts of the cerebral cortex, olivary nucleus, globus pallidus, putamen, and caudate (106). Pathological evidence of neuronal degeneration occurs in a similar distribution (including claustrum, putamen, globus pallidus, and thalamus) in humans and nonhuman primates (110).

Mercury, therefore, is a class 1 agent for extrapyramidal disease and other types of CNS and PNS damage. The provocative findings of Ngim and Devathasan (108) that mercury is linked to Parkinson's disease require confirmation.

6. *Thallium Salts (Class 2 Extrapyramidal Agent)*

Thallium ions readily enter nerve cells and axons, bind to and inactivate thiol-dependent enzymes, perturb energy transformation, and damage mitochondria (111). Subacute and chronic thallium poisoning is associated with hair loss, a predominantly sensory axonal neuropathy, persistent dementia, and extrapyramidal motor disturbances, such as chorea and tremors. Neuronal degeneration occurs in the cerebral cortex, various hypothalamic nuclei, cerebellar cortex, olivary nucleus, and striatum (112).

7. *Monohalomethanes (Class 2 Extrapyramidal Agent)*

Methyl bromide, a food fumigant, pesticide, delousing agent, refrigerant, fire extinguisher, and methylating agent, inhibits sulfhydryl enzymes, including succinic dehydrogenase. Intoxication is associated with sensorimotor neuropathy, cognitive and memory deficits, cerebellar, pyramidal, and extrapyramidal features (113). Cogwheeling and rigidity may occur (114).

Methyl iodide intoxication has been associated with akinesia, rigidity, and tremor (113,115).

C. Miscellaneous Compounds

1. *Hexachlorobenzene (Class 4 Extrapyramidal Agent)*

Although hexachlorobenzene has been removed from the market for use as a fungicide, it continues to be produced as a by-product in the manufacture of pesticides and hydrocarbons, with over 2 million pounds produced in the United States in 1975 (116).

Between 1955 and 1959, seed grain treated with the fungicide hexachlorobenzene was diverted for bread production and eaten during a famine in southeastern Turkey. The contaminated grain led to an epidemic of porphyria cutanea tarda; over 3000 persons were affected and mortality was estimated at 10%. Peters and colleagues (117) reported on the cutaneous, hepatic, arthritic, urinary, and neurological manifestations of hexachlorobenzene poisoning in 1966. This group returned to the area 25 years later to reexamine a small number of the original cohort (116). Of the 161 patients examined on the second visit, all gave a history of photosensitivity with bullae, fragile skin, hyperpigmentation, and porphyrinuria or red urine. Many patients who were exposed to hexachlorobenzene before puberty demonstrated shortened hands and a painless arthritis, characterized by swelling and spindling of the fingers. Neurological manifestations included weakness (73%), nervousness (65%), "sensory shading" (60%), parethesias (55%), and myotonia (46%). The only extrapyramidal finding, cogwheel rigidity, was seen in 34 (27%) of the patients examined.

2. n-*Hexane*

Although the once widely used organic solvent *n*-hexane is a proven cause of axonal neuropathy in humans and animals (20), and comparable changes may be found in hypothalamus and optic nerves of cats chronically treated with its active metabolite 2,5-hexanedione (118), the proposal that *n*-hexane causes parkinsonism is new and unproven.

Pezzoli and associates (22) reported a case of rapidly progressive parkinsonism in a 49-year-old woman employed in the leather products industry. The patient had a 31-year history of exposure to two glues, and the degree of exposure was said to have increased greatly in the last 3 years. The volatile component of the first glue formulation contained 85.5% *n*-hexane (used daily) and a second, used twice weekly, 49% *n*-hexane, 9% ethyl acetate, 7% trichloroethylene, 5% acetone, and 5% 1,2-dichloropropane. The products were used at work as well as in the patient's home. Fourteen months following the onset of the first signs (severe akinesia, moderate hypertonia, and mild resting tremor), the patient had advanced to stage 5 disease and was confined to a chair (22). Electromyography revealed the presence of a mild axonal neuropathy. The unusually malignant progression of the patient's symptoms was considered inconsistent with Parkinson's disease and likely attributable to *n*-hexane.

Pezzoli's group conducted controlled studies in rodents to determine the action of *n*-hexane and its active metabolite (2,5-hexanedione) on striatal dopamine and homovanillic acid levels (21). Although both levels were significantly depressed after 3 weeks of systemic treatment with either hexacarbon, no dose–response data were presented; the effects of equimolar concentrations of *n*-hexane and 2,5-hexanedione (a much more potent compound) were comparable; no check was made for the presence of axonal neuropathy (internal control), and no neurotoxicologically inactive structural analogue of 2,5-hexanedione (e.g., 2,4-hexanedione) was employed as a negative control. More carefully designed studies, therefore, are needed to address the proposal that *n*-hexane triggers L-dopa-responsive parkinsonism.

VI. CHEMICAL MIXTURES AND PROGRESSIVE EXTRAPYRAMIDAL DISEASE

The two conditions considered in this section—Parkinson's disease and western Pacific ALS–P–D—differ markedly from the preceding movement disorders in one crucially important respect: they display an irrepressible, advancing course of clinical deficit. Unlike the largely self-limiting extrapyramidal disorders linked to defects in energy transformation (see Section V)—conditions that perhaps advance slowly with age—the pathological process of these malignantly progressive conditions is set in an irreversible forward motion, terminating in death of the affected subject. Although the underlying mechanisms are unknown, theoretical considerations suggest this effect might be induced by an agent that (1) is sequestered in vivo and slowly released to effect a continuous endogenous exposure (a characteristic of certain metals, chloroquine, and organochlorine pesticides), (2) causes the expression of a preexisting cellular defect (gene susceptibility), or (3) damages a critical cellular site (e.g., DNA) that is poorly repaired in nerve cells. The second and third scenarios currently seem the most plausible possibilities for Parkinson's disease and ALS–P–D, respectively.

A. Idiopathic Parkinson's Disease

Current information on the relation between environmental factors and Parkinson's disease (PD) is meager. Although prospective studies of individuals exposed to specific agents are published for hexachlorobenzene and are underway for MPTP (J. W. Langston, personal communication), the most published studies seek to identify etiological associations retrospectively. Types of data include case reports, descriptions of case series, and epidemiological studies.

The idealized study employs door-to-door community-based surveys; measures disease incidence, not prevalence (to ensure one is studying risk factors for disease not survival); selects only sporadic cases of disease; matches cases and controls for race, gender, age, and education; employs the skills of the neurologist to define cases and controls; and employs numbers of subjects large enough to muster statistical power sufficient to address the questions of interest. Common problems, which are always easier to identify than eradicate, include errors in the classification of disease status and exposure status. Analysis strategies frequently involve computations of crude odds ratios, and these are often not corrected for potential confounding variables (119) (see also Chapters 8,10, and 11).

Confounding factors peculiar to insidiously evolving neurodegenerative diseases require consideration. Prime among these is the long latent period that may intervene between exposure to an agent and the onset of recognizable and broadly accepted signs of the disease under study (120). Although exposure to certain doses of a compound, such as MPTP, may induce florid parkinsonism with extraordinary rapidity, other individuals (presumably with less severe exposure or a lower susceptibility) may develop a *subclinical* lesion of the substantia nigra (6). These subjects might be at risk for parkinsonism later in life if the effects of toxic damage combine with age-related neuronal attrition to overcome the functional reserve of the normal basal ganglia (121). Once expressed clinically, the chemically induced movement disorder on neurological examination might prove to be indistinguishable from Parkinson's disease.

Other evidence that extrapyramidal disorders may appear after a latent period of years or decades comes from observations of Guam ALS–P–D. Filipinos who migrate to Guam and adopt the lifestyle of the indigenous people (Chamorro) may develop clinically apparent disease after 17–26 years of residency (122). In comparable manner, decades may elapse between last exposure to the Guam environment and clinical appearance of disease (123). Since Guam ALS–P–D advances aggressively in young as well as elderly subjects, factors other than age-related neuronal attrition must have a dominant role. One possibility is that individual susceptibility and dose of the unknown agent are related directly to the duration of the latent period (8,121).

Long-latent diseases pose major challenges for epidemiological surveys searching for evidence of past chemical exposures. Exposures in utero and during early childhood may be very relevant if the neuronal pool is compromised. Loss of memory for remote events and recall bias figure prominently (see Chapter 8). Such problems are minimized by selecting a population of patients who develop the disease at an early age, the very same group who, on theoretical grounds, may have experienced especially large (and therefore memorable) exposures to a causal exotoxin. An additional advantage of young patients is the availability of parents to act as historians of the patient's early-life events.

Published epidemiological studies of Parkinson's disease seeking antecedent xenobiotic exposures focus on chemicals added to the environment as a result of human activity. The investigator and patient alike may labor under the subliminal preconception that the chemical trigger will prove to be a "dangerous pesticide" or some other unsavory product of the chemist's genius. Parkinson's disease, however, is not a disease created in the second half of the 20th century or in the Industrial Revolution (124). Many *naturally occurring* substances have toxic potential, and some induce neuronal degeneration. Certain minerals, such as manganese ores, are established causes of extrapyramidal disease (see Section V. B.4). Chemical principles of plants and their fungal contaminants include potent neurotoxins capable of inducing neurodegenerative disorders. Examples include dystonia from the myotoxin NPA (14) and the spastic parapareses associated with cassava and the Grass pea (125). Although these examples are drawn from developing countries, it is a mistake to assume such agents have no role in Western neurological diseases. The recent outbreak on the eastern coast of Canada of hippocampal damage and dementia following ingestion of seafood contaminated with domoic acid underlines the need for an open mind (126).

1. Evaluating Epidemiological Studies of Parkinson's Disease

Many of the epidemiological studies discussed here demonstrate the methodological difficulties encountered in studying the etiology of Parkinson's disease. Imprecise measures of long-term exposure, problems differentiating primary from secondary findings, and small sample sizes, limit the generalizability of study findings. Despite these limitations, epidemiological studies examine the true disorder as manifest in human populations and embedded within the full constellation of environmental agents that may trigger cell death. Because analytic epidemiological studies vary greatly in terms of purpose, scope, and methodological approach, it is important to evaluate qualitatively and quantitatively the weight of evidence for and against disease causation for each category of suspect agent.

Valanis (127) operationally defines *causation* in epidemiological research as factors which vary with that of the disease or condition of interest. Several authors have proposed criteria to assist in the evaluation of epidemiological evidence for disease causation; those outlined by Schlesselman (119) include the following:

1. *Temporal sequence*: Causative factors must precede those events that are considered as their effects.
2. *Consistency*: The repeated observation of an association between agent and effect; the association must be observed under different conditions of study.

3. *Strength of association*: The larger the value of the relative risk, the less the association is likely to be spurious.
4. *Biological gradient*: The existence of a dose–response relationship makes a causal relationship more likely.
5. *Specificity of effect*: Introduction of the putative factor is followed by the occurrence of the effect; removal of the factor is followed by the absence of the effect.
6. *Biological plausibility*: "The presence of a reasonable biological mechanism to explain the physiological process by which an agent could produce the specific disease of interest" (127).

Note that a neurotoxic chemical fulfilling all these criteria would be classified as a class 2 agent, according to the current scheme. No chemical or mixture implicated on epidemiological grounds currently qualifies; indeed, all such agents receive a class-5 rating (see Table 1).

2. *Rural Residency*

A significant body of research has sought a relation between rural residency and Parkinson's disease, the prevailing hypothesis recognizing a positive association between Parkinson's disease and rural living. Although several methodological tacks have been taken, survey and case–control designs are preponderant in the literature; alternative designs include ecologic studies and investigation of clusters. A more unconventional approach was taken by Rajput and colleagues (128), who performed neuronal counts on 48 normal brains to evaluate the effect of residency on neuronal populations in the substantia nigra. Brains were classified as "urban" or "rural" based on years of the individual's residency (80% of life spent in one setting or the other). Those living in rural areas had lower cell counts by aged 20 relative to their urban counterparts, but, by age 75, there was no difference. The authors speculated that pathogenic factors in the development of Parkinson's disease are operative during the early lives of affected persons.

Of six studies employing exposure-history surveys, five (49,129–132) found patients with past rural residency overrepresented in the Parkinson's disease population. Two of these studies focused on young-onset patients. Tanner (131) compared life histories of young-onset (n = 253, aged 47 or younger) with older-onset (n = 259, aged 54 or older) patients; the younger patients were more likely to have lived in a community of fewer than 1000 residents (p = <0.01). Rajput and colleagues (130) examined a subset of young-onset patients (aged 40 or younger) from a cohort of 557 Parkinson's disease patients from Saskatchewan. Of 21 young-onset Parkinson's disease patients, 19 had been born and had lived the first 15 years of life in communities of 169 or fewer. The authors proposed that young-onset Parkinson's disease patients are exposed to an unidentified causative factor(s) primarily operative in rural communities.

In spite of different operational definitions for rural living, four (129,133–135) case–control studies found significantly elevated odds ratio for rural living. Odds ratios ranged from 1.9 from a study of Kansas residents (134) to 4.9 for those Hong Kong patients (129), with 40 or more years of living in a rural area (95% CI, 1.4–18.2). Semchuk and colleagues (136) found no association between rural living and Parkinson's disease in a community-based study of 130 Parkinson's disease subjects and 260 randomly selected controls. Taken together, this group of studies characterizes some of the methodological problems encountered in case–control studies of Parkinson's disease. Inadequate sample size and imprecise measures of long-term exposure limit the generalizability of many studies' findings. Careful case definition, clear ascertainment of exposure status, and sufficient statistical power are exemplified in the work of Koller et al. (134) and Semchuk (136,137).

Two studies have reported significant inverse associations between rural living and Parkinson's disease. The study by Tanner and colleagues (138) of Chinese Parkinson's disease patients found a 0.3 odds ratio ($p < 0.05$) between "village residence" and Parkinson's disease; these findings were similar to those of Zayed and associates (139) (OR = 0.3, $p < 0.05$) in a study of Parkinson's disease patients from southern Quebec, Canada.

These conflicting findings may reflect differences in the way rural living is defined in epidemiological studies of Parkinson's disease; population density alone may not be the most valid reflection of rural lifestyle. Rural residency might be a proxy variable for one or more environmental agents that are prevalent in many, but not all, rural environments. The highly intercorrelated variables of rural residency, water source, and participation in agriculture, make it difficult to elucidate the nature of the true risk factor or factors for Parkinson's disease.

3. *Water Source*

Stimulated by evidence suggesting a preponderance of Parkinson's disease in rural areas, several investigators have explored the possibility that differences in rural water supplies, particularly private or hand-dug wells, provide a vehicle for the transmission of an etiologic agent (131,140,141). Rajput and associates (141) tested the childhood water sources of 18 Parkinson's disease subjects and 36 controls and found no differences between the two groups relative to metal content (Al, As, Ca, Cu, Mn, Mg, Hg, and Zn) of the water.

Seven case–control studies have analyzed water source in relation to Parkinson's disease. Three of the seven (131,134,142) found a significant positive association between well-water consumption and Parkinson's disease. Koller (134) found an odds ratio of 1.7 ($p = 0.03$) between years of well-water consumption and Parkinson's disease; this relation was greatest during the first 40 years of life. The authors noted that well-water consumption was correlated with rural residency. In a design that differentiated young- from older-onset Parkinson's disease patients, Tanner (131) found an association between use of well water as a primary source of drinking water and young-onset Parkinson's disease ($p < 0.01$).

Many of the reports linking well water with Parkinson's disease are based on an analysis of geographic or family clusters of disease and are limited by small sample size. Although such investigations are important from an exploratory perspective, they are not community-based and may cloud, rather than clarify, any relation between water source and Parkinson's disease.

4. *Farming*

Many case reports of Parkinson's disease describe farmers with a history of heavy pesticide exposure, but this method of reporting makes it impossible to analyze separately risk associated with exposure to farming versus exposure to agents that might be used more commonly in farming (e.g., pesticides) or by farmers (e.g., locally grown food items). Barbeau and coinvestigators (143) associated elevated Parkinson's disease prevalence with agricultural industries; of nine rural hydrogeographic regions, the highest prevalence of Parkinson's disease was noted in the area with the highest production of apples and vegetables.

Of eight case–control studies of farming and Parkinson's disease, three (129,144,145) found significantly elevated odds ratios for farming. Tanner and associates (145) reported an odds ratio of 3.0 ($p < 0.05$) in a study of young-onset Parkinson's disease patients (onset younger than aged 51) in Illinois; of 22 patients who had farmed, 18 were exposed before the age of 21. Ho and colleagues (129) found an odds ratio of 5.2 ($p = 0.05$) for longer than 20 years of farming experience in a study of Hong Kong residents; with evidence of a dose–response relation with decreasing exposure.

To examine risks associated with particular farming practices, Tanner and associates (138) queried 100 Parkinson's disease patients in China on specific farm-related exposures and obtained surprising results. Low odds ratios were found for pig raising (0.17; $p < 0.001$), wheat growing (0.40; $p < 0.02$), and chicken raising (0.53, $p < 0.05$). The authors concluded these farm-related exposures represented proxy variables for rural village life in China, rather than specific factors protective against Parkinson's disease. Until recently, most Chinese farmers are unlikely to have been exposed to synthetic fertilizers, pesticides, and other chemicals. These findings demonstrate the complexities of linking exposures with specific farming practices and argue in favor of disease hypotheses that relate Parkinson's disease risk to environmental agents, rather than to farming practices per se.

5. *Pulp, Paper, Planer, and Sawmills*

Workers in wood-related industries are exposed to a wide variety of chemical compounds used in the processing of wood, in addition to the dusts, vapors, and molds that originate from the wood itself. The most hazardous substances found in sawmills include wood dusts, antistain agents, sawing vapors, and fungal spores (146). Salts of chlorophenols (e.g., pentachlorophenol and polychlorinated dibenzo-*para*-dioxins) are the most common antistain agents used in sawmills. Likewise, paper workers are also exposed to a variety of chemical agents, most of which are used in the process of mechanical wood pulping. Exposures in this industry include gaseous sulfur, chlorine, and chlorine dioxide compounds. Pulp vapors may contain turpentine, sodium hydroxide, methanol, ethanol, sulfuric acid, acetic acid, formic acid, gluconic acid, and hydrogen peroxide (146).

Three ecological epidemiology studies (143,147,148) have examined Parkinson's disease risk for persons living near a pulp or paper mill. A Quebec study by Barbeau and colleagues (143) compared Parkinson's disease mortality and L-dopa use in nine hydrogeographic regions; 15 towns were identified with a Parkinson's disease prevalence three times greater than the province average. Of these 15 towns, 10 had pulp- and paper-processing mills, and the other 5 were located immediately downstream from such industries. A similar method of quantifying Parkinson's disease through L-dopa use was employed by Aguilonius and Hartvig (147) to examine disease prevalence in 24 Swedish counties. One county, with an exceptionally high utilization of L-dopa, contained three steel mills and nine paper or sawmills. More recently, Sethi and colleagues (148) investigated county-specific Parkinson's disease mortality in Georgia (1979–1983); their findings revealed that counties with paper mills did not show increased Parkinson's disease death rates when compared with the remainder of Georgia.

Two case–control studies have queried subjects about past employment in wood products' occupations. In a study of 57 subjects and 122 controls, Hertzman and associates (149) found a positive association between Parkinson's disease and past employment in a planer mill (adjusted OR $= 4.1$; $p = 0.07$). Tanner's group (138) found no such relation in a case–control study of residents of Beijing, China; the odds ratio for employment in a paper mill was 1.1.

Similar to the studies of rural residency, the studies addressing paper and sawmills reflect the known challenges of attempting to quantify exposure to an unknown etiologic agent. Occupational exposure to wood products' manufacturing is certainly of a different character and intensity than residential exposure; clear detail in the design of exposure questions will help investigators to know what they are attempting to characterize. The employment of medical records or pharmaceutical data can introduce several types of classification bias into studies, and reliance on such items moves the investigator farther away from, rather than closer to, direct questioning of subjects. Such techniques are appropriate for ecological research but are of limited applicability for more focused studies of environmental exposures.

6. *Pesticides*

Pesticides are cited as possible culprits in a number of case reports and epidemiological studies of Parkinson's disease; others report no association. Pesticides include a large number of disparate chemicals commonly grouped into use (not chemical) categories, namely insecticides, herbicides, fungicides, rodenticides, and fumigants. Before 1940, the primary pesticides were botanical in origin and compounds of heavy metals. There was a rapid proliferation of synthetic organic compounds after World War II. Insecticides formed the leading class of pesticides until the mid-1960s when herbicides began to rise to a dominant position in worldwide sales. At the same time, there was a shift from the preponderant use of organochlorine insecticides to the organophosphate and carbamate classes and, subsequently, to the pyrethroids (150).

Classes of Pesticides. Many insecticides (nicotine, carbamates, and organophosphates) perturb acetylcholine neurotransmission. Overexposure is associated with acute nicotinic and muscarinic toxicity. Although slurred speech, tremor, generalized weakness, ataxia, convulsions, and coma may occur, tardive involvement of the extrapyramidal system is not recognized. Certain organophosphates have the potential to induce an axonal neuropathy, the late effects of which may be spasticity associated with unrepaired pyramidal tract damage and muscle reinnervation. Long-latent effects from anticholinesterase crises triggered by organophosphates have been poorly documented, but the question of parkinsonism has not been raised (1,150). Poisoning by chlorinated hydrocarbon insecticides, including DDT [1,1,-trichloro-2,2-bis-(*p*-chlorophenyl)ethane], is featured by tremor and seizures, whereas the neurotoxic effects of chlordecone include tremor and opsoclonus. Many organochlorine insecticides have a tendency to accumulate in fat and effectively become stored in the body, the rate of metabolism and subsequent excretion determining their half-life in vivo (150). Long-latent health effects of exposure to organochlorine compounds are unexplored.

Synthetic pyrethroids (and DDT) prolong the sodium current and perturb membrane excitability, leading to perverse sensations (paresthesiae) of the tongue, lips, and face. Severe reactions are not reported in humans, but mammals display increased activity, loss of coordination, paralysis, and death (48).

Chemical control of weeds through the use of herbicides has increased markedly during the past 20 years (150). Widely used are the chlorophenoxy compounds 2,4-D (2,4-dichlorphenoxyacetic acid) and 2,4,5-T (2,4,5-trichlorophenoxyacetic acid) that exert their herbicidal action by behaving as growth hormones in plants. Mild dystonia is reported in workers exposed to polychlorinated phenols, including dioxin (7,8-tetrachlorodibenzo-*p*-dioxin) (151), and heavy occupational exposure to 2,4-D has been linked to peripheral neuropathy (152). The dinitrophenol herbicides uncouple oxidative phosphorylation and, thereby, may perturb neurological function. The dinitroaniline, arylaliphatic acid, substituted ureas, triazines, and carbamate herbicides have low acute toxicities, and the latter display weak anticholinesterase activity. Nitrile herbicides, which uncouple oxidative phosphorylation, have been linked to an occupational disorder featured by inordinate sweating, thirst, fever, headache, dizziness, vomiting, asthenia, weight loss, and myalgias. Organoarsenicals, such as arsphenamine (a former antisyphilitic), have been linked to a rapidly ascending neuropathy. The bipyridyl herbicides paraquat and diquat were discussed earlier.

Fungicides include the dicarboximides, which have structural relations with thalidomide, an agent that induces sensory neuropathy. One of the nitrogen heterocyclic herbicides, 1-hydoxy-2-pyridine-thione—a zinc derivative that is used as an antidandruff agent in a popular shampoo—causes a severe axonal neuropathy in rodents (1). Maneb, a manganese-based dithiocarbamate fungicide; disulfiram, a dithiocarbamate with therapeutic utility; and hexachlorobenzene, a substituted aromatic fungicide, have been discussed earlier. Occupational exposure to the diphenyl fungicide has been linked to incompletely defined CNS and PNS abnormalities (150).

The heterogeneous group of chemicals used as rodenticides includes anticoagulants, such as warfarin; the cardiotonic glycoside and centrally acting emetic scilliroside (a potential convulsant); the peripheral vasoconstrictor norbormide; the Krebs cycle inhibitors fluoroacetamide and its metabolite fluoroacetate (acute convulsant); the pulmonary poison β-naphthylthiourea; the glycine inhibitor strychnine (tetanic convulsant); pyriminil (*N*-3-pyridinylmethyl-*N'*-*p*-nitrophenyl urea) and thallium sulfate, which both produce peripheral neuropathy and widespread CNS effects; zinc phosphide, which yields the pulmonary poison phosphine; and the gastrointestinal and hepatic poison phosphorus (1,150). Carbon monoxide, methyl bromide, and hydrogen cyanide have been used as fumigants to kill rodents in confined spaces, and all three have the potential to induce extrapyramidal deficits in severely exposed human subjects (see earlier discussion). Sulfuryl fluoride is now used as a fumigant.

Fumigants are used in gaseous form to control insect, rodents, and soil nematodes (150). Acrylonitrile may cause cyanide-related poisoning; chloropicrin is a sensory irritant; dibromochloropropane and ethylene dibromide show testicular toxicity; and ethylene oxide (epoxyethane) has the potential to cause an axonal neuropathy.

Epidemiological Studies. Most epidemiological studies solicit information about general, rather than product-specific, exposures to pesticides and herbicides. The strongest evidence linking Parkinson's disease prevalence with pesticide exposure comes from the studies of Barbeau and associates (143), who found a correlation of 0.97 between region-specific observed Parkinson's disease prevalence in Quebec and pesticide utilization per region (kg/yr, 1982). Ho and co-workers (129), studying both parkinsonian patients and control subjects, reported a 3.6 odds ratio between previous use of pesticides and herbicides and development of Parkinson's disease (95% CI, 1.0–12.9). However, in a recent case–control study of Chinese residents, Tanner and associates (138) noted a decreased risk of Parkinson's disease associated with wheat growing. Ho's group (129) attributes the contradictory nature of these findings to differences in the study populations and notes that, whereas Tanner's subjects were mostly recruited from the cooler Beijing area, Hong Kong residents are more likely to farm in light clothing and bare feet. Ho speculates that the increased opportunity for dermal exposure, coupled with the extensive use of pesticides in vegetable farming, may explain the risk differences.

Rajput and Uitti (49,153, also see Ref. 154) examined the relation between pesticides and Parkinson's disease by comparing the incidence of young-onset disease with temporal trends in pesticide and herbicide use in Saskatchewan, Canada over a 60-year period. Their data showed no increase in Parkinson's disease incidence corresponding with the introduction into agricultural practice of sulfuric acid/copper sulfate, 2,4-D, 2-methyl-4-chlorophenoxyacetic acid, triallate, paraquat, diclofop, or sethoxydin.

7. *Epidemiologic Studies Using Multivariate Analysis Techniques*

The development of models based on multifactorial analysis of risk optimizes the usefulness of epidemiological data in the search for etiologic triggers of Parkinson's disease. Three recent studies (136,137,149,155) have employed multivariate analysis techniques to examine simultaneously the effects of multiple factors on Parkison's disease risk.

Two Canadian studies by Hertzman (149) and Semchuk (136,137) used logistic regression techniques to model disease risk and control for confounding variables. Hertzman studied occupational and environmental risks in 57 Parkinson's disease patients and 122 controls. In a model designed to identify independent predictors of Parkinson's disease, significant variables included "ever work in an orchard?" (odds ratio = 3.69; $p = 0.012$), and "ever smoke cigarettes?" (odds ratio = 0.40; $p = 0.019$).

The study by Semchuk and associates (137,156) used a population-based sample of 130 Parkinson's disease patients and 260 age- and gender-matched controls to examine exposure patterns for rural living, well-water consumption, agricultural work, and pesticide use. Subjects were queried about exposure to the general categories of herbicides, insecticides, and fungicides, rather than specific trade or product names. Potential confounders and interactions between exposure variables were held constant in conditional logistic regression analyses. The adjusted odds ratio for herbicide exposure was 3.1. In analyses conducted to evaluate the relation between herbicides and other exposures, significant associations between Parkinson's disease and agricultural work and Parkinson's disease and insecticides were not important after accounting for subjects' and controls' exposure to herbicides. The authors concluded that, although farming and insecticide use might serve as a valid marker for high-risk groups, direct exposure to herbicides should be considered a primary risk factor for Parkinson's disease.

Butterfield and colleagues (157) queried 63 young-onset subjects (Parkinson's disease diagnosis at aged 50 or younger) and 68 controls in a study of risk factors for young-onset Parkinson's disease. After adjusting for six potential confounders, Parkinson's disease was significantly associated with the pesticide-related variables of insecticide exposure (odds ratio = 5.75; $p < 0.001$), herbicide exposure (odds ratio = 3.22; $p < 0.03$), and past residency in a commercially fumigated home (odds ratio = 5.25; $p < 0.05$). Other significant findings related to rural residency (odds ratio = 2.72; $p < 0.03$), and nuts and seed eating (odds ratio = 1.49; $p < 0.02$), and in addition an inverse association between cigarette smoking and Parkinson's disease was found (odds ratios ranged from 0.37 to 0.50) (also see Chapter 11).

Several logistic regression models were then developed to examine sets of independent variables predictive for Parkinson's disease. The first model, containing six demographic variables, successfully predicted the disease status of 67% of subjects and controls. Two additional models showed a significant improvement in predictive power when environmental variables were entered into the equation. In these models, independent predictors of Parkinson's disease included a positive association with exposure to insecticides (odds ratio = 7.24; $p = 0.001$) and a negative association with cigarette smoking 15 years before diagnosis (odds ratio = 0.32; $p = 0.002$).

The analysis techniques applied in these multivariate studies are simutaneously able to weigh the effects of several risk factors for Parkinson's disease. This analysis approach is well suited to neuroepidemiological studies of Parkinson's disease because many of the variables identified with Parkinson's disease risk (i.e., rural residency, farming, pesticide exposure) are intercorrelated. Although vulnerable to the same methodological limitations of case–control studies using univariate analyses, multivariate techniques can help investigators identify exposures for more targeted research (also see Chapter 8 and 11).

B. Western Pacific Parkinsonism–Dementia (P–D)

The Chamorro people of Guam and Rota in the Mariana Islands, Japanese residents of the Kii Peninsula, Honshu Island, and the Auyu and Jaqai linguistic groups of New Guinea (now Irian Jaya, Indonesia) are three distinct population groups that have been afflicted by a high incidence of a rapidly progressive neurodegenerative disease, with clinical features comprising various combinations of motor neuron disease, parkinsonism, supranuclear palsy, and dementia (158). Neuropathological studies of P–D have been performed only on Japanese and Guam cases: widespread loss of neurons and gliosis is evident, especially in the hippocampus, cerebral cortex, amygdala, hypothalamus, globus pallidus, thalamus, substantia nigra, and tegmentum. Numerous intraneuronal neurofibrillary tangles, resembling those seen in Alzheimer disease, are a prominent additional feature (159).

Since high-incidence neurodegenerative disease has essentially disappeared among young people in all three affected population groups, and inherited and infectious etiologies have been virtually ruled out (5,160), the search for the cause(s) of this apparently single disease entity is focused on nontransmissible environmental factors that have declined as the affected population groups have acculturated to more modern lifestyles. Deficient nutritional intake of calcium, associated with absorption and neuronal deposition of aluminum and other metals, has been advanced as causal (158,161,162), but on Guam, calcium concentrations in river water and indigenous foods are unremarkable (163). Aluminum is reported (4) to accumulate in affected nerve cells and, conceivably, may play a role in the disease, although experimental animals chronically treated with aluminum fail to develop clinical and neuropathological signs comparable with the western Pacific disease (158).

Epidemiological study on Guam has shown that preference for Chamorro food is the only 1 of 23 tested variables significantly associated with an increased risk for P–D (164). This is consistent with the hypothesis that seed of the neurotoxic cycad plant (*Cycas circinalis*, L.), a traditional, but declining, source of food and medicine for the Chamorro people, plays an important role in the etiology of the disease of Guam (8,165). Flour derived from cycad seed by Chamorro processing methods contains variable concentrations of cycad toxins (2,166). Recent studies of individual Japanese and Auyu families have revealed that subjects who developed ALS in their 20s were engaged as babies or children in the disappearing practice of employing seed of other *Cycas* spp. for medicinal purposes (12,167). These epidemiological observations suggest a role for cycad seed not only for ALS–P–D in Guam (160) (as originally suggested by Whiting; 168) but in all three western Pacific loci (11). Given that the Auyu (a group of hunters–gatherers who were settled by Dutch missionaries in remote riverine villages untouched by synthetic chemicals; 10) have employed only the fresh kernel of cycad seed (as a poultice for large topical ulcers; 12), research attention is focused on the indigenous toxic principles of *Cycas* spp., rather than the noxious products of a contaminating fungus.

Although hindlimb locomotor disease (cycadism), with muscle wasting and long-tract spinal cord degeneration may develop in cows, sheep, and goats that graze on cycads, and the question of basal ganglia involvement was raised in one controlled study of bovine cycadism (see Ref. 8), neuropathological examination of the brains of these animals has not been reported. The culpable neurotoxic principles are unknown, although it is likely one or other of the cycad azoxyglucosides has a major etiologic role in cycadism. In *Cycas*, three species of which are epidemiologically associated with western Pacific ALS–P–D, the azoxyglucoside is cycasin, the glycone of methylazoxymethanol (MAM), a potent alkylating agent with mutagenic, carcinogenic, teratogenic, hepatotoxic, and neurotoxic potential (169). Postnatal administration of MAM acetate to Swiss mice perturbs CNS development, and multinucleated and ectopic cerebellar neurons are reported both in these animals (44) and in Chamorro and Kii-Japanese who developed and died of ALS as adults (170,171). When these observations are considered in concert with epidemiological data showing that clinical disease appears in Chamorros decades after departure from Guam (123), it is plausible to propose that cycad seed harbors one or more chemicals that behave as slow toxins, hypothetical agents that trigger neuronal disease that advances irreversibly after cessation of exposure (8,19).

Cycad seed contains a large number of chemicals, two of which have been incompletely studied and shown to exhibit neurotoxic potential. β-*N*-Methylamino-L-alanine (BMAA), a minor component of some cycads including *Cycas*, is a weak glutamate excitotoxin, with potency increased by physiological concentrations of bicarbonate and decreased by glutamate-receptor antagonists (172,173). In addition to its activity on the surface of nerve cells, BMAA is transported into neurons where it has unknown sites of action (174). Young rats treated intraperitoneally with BMAA develop delayed-onset ataxia, with selective cerebellar degeneration of GABAergic neurons (175). Primates receiving oral BMAA daily for up to 13 weeks gradually develop pyramidal, extrapyramidal, and behavioral dysfunction, with chromatolytic and early degenerative changes of Betz cells in motor cortex and a few large anterior horn cells in the lumbar spinal cord (176). These primate and rodent studies employed doses of BMAA much larger than those encountered by human populations (166), and neurological disease appeared within a relatively short period. The primate disorder shows remarkable parallels with the human disease, although it is not progressive after BMAA termination and lacks some neuropathological features of the human disease.

The neurotoxic properties of cycasin, the major toxin of *Cycas* spp., are little studied. Cycasin (like BMAA) is transported into mouse cortical tissue explants and, after the appearance of MAM as a metabolite, causes selective neuronal degeneration that is attenuated by NMDA receptor antagonists (174). Like MAM, cycasin disrupts cerebellar development in the rodent (44). Goats treated orally with large doses of cycasin develop hepatic necrosis and spongy degeneration of the thalamus, whereas more prolonged exposure with smaller doses causes animals to become inactive, "hunched down," and weak in the hind legs. Pathological examination of the spinal cord (brain not studied) revealed swollen axons throughout the length of the lateral and ventral funiculi (177). Primate studies are inconclusive: One of three rhesus monkeys fed Chamorro-style cycad flour (said to be "cycasin-free"), which contains cycasin (2), developed severe weakness and wasting of one arm, with postmortem evidence of upper and lower motor neuron degeneration (178); however, another primate study (179) of the carcinogenic and hepatotoxic properties of cycasin and MAM did not report neurological abnormalities.

Although there is no doubt that cycasin, MAM, and BMAA have neurotoxic properties, their ability to act as slow toxins is untested, and their relevance to the etiology of ALS–P–D is unproved. The endogenous metabolites of these agents (other than MAM) have not been characterized, and many other potentially neurotoxic chemicals exist in cycad seed. However, MAM is of special interest because it is the aglycone metabolite of the diverse azoxyglucosides of neurotoxic cycads, and relatively high concentrations of cycasin have been found in Chamorro flour samples obtained from regions of Guam historically most affected by P–D (2). MAM (via the methyldiazonium ion) alkylates DNA with the formation of 7-methyl and O^6-methylguanine adducts (see Ref. 174). DNA repair is poor in brain tissue, and O^6-methylguanine disturbs the normal pattern of cytosine methylation, which silences gene expression in several biological systems (180). Decreased cytosine methylation in immortalized neurons treated with MAM has recently been demonstrated (N. R. Cashman, personal communication). Thus, it is possible that nucleic acid alkylation represents an irreversible and slowly lethal epigenetic change that interferes with normal protein expression and eventuates in neuronal degeneration (19,174). A novel mechanism of this type conceivably could underlie the etiology of western Pacific ALS–P–D and, potentially, other sporadic neurodegenerative disorders, including Parkinson's disease.

VII. CONCLUDING REMARKS

The proposal that exposure to exogenous chemicals causes Parkinson's disease is unproved. In humans, no exogenous chemical has been shown to produce a progressive neurodegenerative disease like Parkinson's disease, although an environmental etiologic factor with these properties seems likely in western Pacific P–D. Laboratory studies are urgently needed to follow up epidemiological leads on the possible causes of this prototypical neurodegenerative disorder.

There are strong data to show that certain chemical agents damage the basal ganglia and elicit signs of parkinsonism that are readily mistaken for Parkinson's disease. With the exception of MPTP, which is taken up by dopaminergic neurons, where it disrupts mitochondria metabolism, these agents do not selectively damage the substantia nigra pars compacta. Other compounds linked to human extrapyramidal disease probably disrupt energy function throughout the brain, a condition that may result in damage to regions of the basal ganglia other than the nigrostriatal pathway. Research is needed to determine whether such damage is mediated by a glutamate excitotoxic mechanism.

Whether Parkinson's disease is a syndrome or a single disease entity is a major unresolved problem. Related to this enigma is the extent to which chemically induced extrapyramidal syndromes are misclassified as Parkinson's disease. Resolution of these questions will come in part from the correlation of careful clinical and neuropathological case definition, with a detailed assessment of environmental exposures. Factors, such as genotype, age, dosage, and duration of chemical exposure, are important considerations. Comprehensive studies of this type are rare in medicine.

Retrospective epidemiological studies have had limited success in identifying environmental factors linked to Parkinson's disease. Focus on such items as rural living, water source, and occupation, represents little more than a series of fishing expeditions in oceans teaming with disparate fauna. Although cause-and-effect relations between Parkinson's disease and specific chemical agents are usually impossible to deduce from such studies, the aggregation of data from several independent retrospective epidemiological investigations may point the way forward. Pesticides have figured prominently in several studies, although none has been able to link Parkinson's disease with specific chemical compounds. Further detailed epidemiological research is urgently needed to find a solution to this issue.

Clusters of Parkinson's disease (in space, in time, or by age) represent a valuable focus for intensive research. Although this may not lead rapidly to the identification of causal factors—as experience with western Pacific P–D illustrates—invaluable leads are obtained through detailed longitudinal study, especially if the disease and environment are shown to change in concert. Whereas there is no substitute for the application of standardized epidemiological techniques, clever detective work is often a powerful, rapid, and inexpensive tool in identifying etiologic leads that are testable in the laboratory setting.

Although clusters of Parkinson's disease subjects seem to be rare, young subjects with the disease are sufficiently numerous for formal study. If disease is triggered by environmental chemicals, these patients represent a valuable population for analytical investigation because the duration between exposure and disease onset is relatively short and recall bias is a weaker confounding factor. Moreover, toxicological studies show that early onset of chemical-induced neurological disease correlates with a larger dose of the causal agent, a factor that might also correlate with the patient's ability to recall exposures. In addition, the young subject is more likely to have living parents or siblings with memories stretching back to the conception of the affected subject. Since one is unable to rule out the possibility that chemical exposure early in life has significance for the etiology of Parkinson's disease, the most carefully performed retrospective survey that fails to consider the developmental period and formative years must be seen as compromised. The foregoing notwithstanding, additional retrospective studies of young-onset Parkinson's disease seem to be merited.

ACKNOWLEDGMENTS

This study was supported in part by The National Institute of Neurological Disorders and Stroke (NS NO1-NS-19611). Dr. J. Hammerstad, Dr. J. Nutt, Dr. H. Schaumburg, and Dr. Steven Johnson provided valuable comments. Monica Bischoff-Fenton is thanked for editorial assistance.

REFERENCES

1. Spencer PS, Schaumburg HH. Experimental and clinical neurotoxicology. Baltimore: Williams & Wilkins, 1980.
2. Kisby GE, Ellison M, Spencer PS. Content of the neurotoxins cycasin (methylazoxymethanol β-D-glucoside) and BMAA (β-*N*-methylamino-L-alanine) in cycad flour prepared by Guam Chamorros. Neurology 1992; 42:1336–1340.
3. Spencer PS, Ross S, Kisby G. Western Pacific amyotrophic lateral sclerosis: putative role of cycad toxins. In: Hudson A, ed. Amyotrophic lateral sclerosis: concepts in pathogenesis and etiology. Toronto: University of Toronto Press, 1990:263–295.
4. Perl DP, Gajdusek DC, Garruto RM, Yanagihara RT, Gibbs CT, Jr. Intraneuronal aluminum accumulation in amyotrophic lateral sclerosis and parkinsonism–dementia of Guam. Science 1982; 217:1053–1055.
5. Gibbs CJ Jr, Gajdusek DC. An update on long-term in vivo and in vitro studies designed to identify a virus as the cause of amyotrophic lateral sclerosis, parkinsonism dementia and Parkinson's disease. In: Rowland L, ed. Human motor neuron diseases. Adv Neurol, 1982; 936:343–353.
6. Langston JW, Ballard PA, Tetrud JW, Irwin I. Chronic parkinsonism in humans due to a product of meperidine–analog synthesis. Science 1983; 219:979–980.
7. Green S, Buttrum S, Molloy H, et al. *N*-Methylation of pyridines in Parkinson's disease. Lancet 1991; 338:120–121.
8. Spencer PS. Guam ALS/parkinsonism–dementia: a long-latency neurotoxic disorder caused by "slow toxin(s)" in food. Can J Neurol Sci 1987; 14:347–357.
9. Raffle PAB, Lee WR, McCallum RI, Murray R. Hunter's diseases of occupations. In: Raffle PAB, Lee WR, McCallum RI, Murray R, eds. Boston: Little, Brown & Co, 1987:62–92.
10. Gajdusek DC, Salazar AM. Amyotrophic lateral sclerosis and parkinsonian syndromes in high incidence among the Auyu and Jakai people of west New Guinea. Neurology 1982; 32:107–126.
11. Spencer PS, Palmer V, Ohta M, Herman A. Cycad, a suspect etiological factor for Guam ALS/P–D, is associated with motor neuron disease in Irian Jaya, Indonesia, and Kii Peninsula, Japan. In: Tsubaki T, Yase Y, eds. Amyotrophic lateral sclerosis. New York: Elsevier Science Publishers 1988:35–40.
12. Spencer PS, Palmer VS, Herman A, Asmedi A. Cycad use and motor neurone disease in Irian Jaya. Lancet 1987; 2:1273–1274.
13. He F, Zhang S, Zhang C. Extrapyramidal lesions induced by mildewed sugar cane poisoning. Three case reports. Chin Med J 1987; 67:395–396.

14. Ludolph AC, He F, Spencer PS, Hammerstad J, Sabri MI. 3-Nitropropionic acid—exogenous animal neurotoxin and possible human striatal toxin. Can J Neurol Sci 1991; 18:492–498.
15. Farrell RK, Sande RD, Lincoln SD. Nigropallidal encephalomalacia in a horse. J Am Vet Med Assoc 1971; 58:1201–1204.
16. Wang Y, Hamburger M, Cheng CHK, et al. Neurotoxic sesquiterpenoids from the yellow star thistle. Helv Chim Acta 1991; 74:117–123.
17. Tsubaki T, Irukayama K. Minamata disease. Kodansha: 1977.
18. Haug H, Barmwater R, Eggers D, Fischer S, Kuhl S, Sass N-L. Anatomical changes in aging brain: morphometric analysis of the human prosencephalon neuropharmacology. In: Cervos-Navarro J, Sarkander H-I. Brain aging: neuropathology and neuropharmacology. New York: Raven Press, 1983:1–12.
19. Spencer PS, Kisby G, Ludolph A. Slow toxins, biologic markers, and long-latency neurodegenerative disease in the western Pacific region. Neurology 1991; 41(suppl 2):62–66.
20. Spencer PS, Schaumburg HH, Sabri MI, Veronesi B. The enlarging view of hexacarbon neurotoxicity. CRC Crit Rev Toxicol 1980; 7:279–356.
21. Pezzoli G, Ricciardi S, Masotto C, Mariani CB, Carenzi A. *n*-Hexane induces parkinsonism in rodents. Brain Res 1990; 531:355–357.
22. Pezzoli G, Barbieri S, Ferrante C, Zecchinelli A. Parkinsonism due to *n*-hexane exposure. Lancet 1989; 874–870.
23. Altenkirch H, Stoltenburg G, Wagner HM. Experimental studies on hydrocarbon neuropathies induced by methyl-ethyl-ketone. J Neurol 1978; 219:159.
24. Altenkirch H, Wagner HM, Stoltenberg G, Spencer PS. Nervous system responses of rats to subchronic inhalation of *n*-hexane and *n*-hexane + methyl ethyl ketone mixtures. J Neurol Sci 1982; 57:209–219.
25. Couper J. On the effects of black oxide of manganese when inhaled into the lungs. Br Ann Med Pharm Vit Stat Gen Sci 1837; 1:41–42.
26. Delpech A. Accidents que developpé, chez les ouvriers en caoutchoue, l'inhalation du CS_2 en vapeur. Union Med 1856; 10:265.
27. Grinker RR. Parkinsonism following carbon monoxide poisoning. J Nerv Ment Dis 1926; 64:18–28.
28. Lehninger AL. Biochemistry. New York: Worth Publishers, 1975.
29. Novelli A, Reilly JA, Lysko PG. Glutamate becomes neurotoxic via the *N*-methyl-D-aspartate receptor when intracellular energy levels are reduced. Brain Res 1988; 451:205–212.
30. Reiderer P, Lange KW. Pathogenesis of Parkinson's disease. Curr Opin Neurol Neurosurg 1992; 5:295–300.
31. Olney JW. Excitotoxic mechanisms of neurotoxicity. In: Spencer PS, Schaumburg HH, eds. Experimental and clinical neurotoxicology. Baltimore: Williams & Wilkins, 1980:272–294.
32. Vyas I, Heikkila RE, Nicklas WJ. Studies on the neurotoxicity of 1-methyl-4-phenyl-1,2,3,6-tetrahydropyridine: inhibition of NAD-linked substrate oxidation by its metabolite, 1-methyl-4-phenylpyridinium. J Neurochem 1986; 46:1501–1507.
33. Rosetti ZL, Sotgiu A, Sharp D, Hadjiconstantinou M, Neff MH. 1-Methyl-4-

phenyl-1,2,3,6-tetrahydropyridine (MPTP) and free radicals in vitro. Biochem Pharmacol 1988; 37:4573–4574.
34. Schapira AHV, Cooper JM, Dexter D, Clark JB, Jenner P, Marsden CD. Mitochondrial complex I deficiency in Parkinson's disease. J Neurochem 1990; 54:823–827.
35. Schapira AHV, Mann VM, Cooper JM, et al. Anatomic and disease specificity of NADH CoQ1 reductase (complex I) deficiency in Parkinson's disease. J Neurochem 1990; 55:2142–2145.
36. Buzzard EF, Greenfield JG. Lethargic encephalitis; its sequelae and morbid anatomy. Brain 1919; 42:305–338.
37. Niwa T, Takeda N, Kaneda N, Hashizume Y, Nagatsu T. Presence of tetrahydroisoquinoline and 2-methyl-tetrahydroquinoline in parkinsonian and normal human brains. Biochem Biophys Res Commun 1987; 144:1084–1089.
38. Tasaki Y, Makino Y, Ohta S, Hirobe M. 1-Methyl-1,2,3,4-tetrahydroisoquinoline, decreasing in 1-methyl-4-phenyl-1,2,3,6-tetrahydropyridine-treated mouse, prevents parkinsonism-like behavior abnormalities. J Neurochem 1991; 57:1940–1943.
39. Shiraki H, Suzuki K, Mizyuno Y, Yoshida M. Selective inhibition of complex I of the brain electron transport system by tetrahydroisoquinoline. Biochem Biophys Res Commun 1989; 144:1541–1545.
40. Nagatsu T, Yoshida M. An endogenous substance of the brain, tetrahydroisoquinoline, produces parkinsonism in primates with decreased dopamine, tyrosine hydroxylase and biopterin in the nigrostriatal regions. Neurosci Lett 1988; 8:178–182.
41. Schapira AHV. MPTP and other Parkinson-inducing agents. Curr Sci 1992; 5:396–400.
42. Holmstedt B. beta-Carbolines and tetrahydroisoquinolines: historical and ethnopharmacological background. In: Bloom F, Barchas J, Sandler M, Usdin E, eds. beta-Carbolines and tetrahydroisoquinolines. New York: AR Liss, 1982:3–13.
43. Rommelspacher H, Susilo R. Tetrahydroisoquinolines and beta-carbolines: putative natural substances in plants and animals. In: Jucker E, ed. Progress in Drug Research, vol 29. Basel: Burkhauser-Verlag, 1985:415–459.
44. Jones M, Yang M, Michelsen O. Effects of methylazoxymethanol glucoside and methylazoxymethanol acetate on the cerebellum of the postnatal Swiss albino mouse. Fed Proc 1972; 31:1508–1511.
45. Albores R, Neafsey EJ, Drucker G, Fields JZ, Collins MA. Mitochondrial respiratory inhibition by *N*-methylated β-carboline derivatives structurally resembling *N*-methyl-4-phenylpyridine. Proc Natl Acad Sci USA 1990; 87:9368–9372.
46. Collins MA, Neafsey EJ, Matsubara K, Cobuzzi RJJr, Rollema H. Indole-*N*-methylated β-carbolinium ions as potential brain-bioactivated neurototoxins. Brain Res 1992; 570:154–160.
47. Hayes WJ. Pesticides studied in man. Baltimore: Williams & Wilkins, 1982.
48. Kaloyanova FP, El Batawi MA. Human toxicology of pesticides. Boca Raton: CRC Press, 1991.
49. Rajput AH, Uitti RJ. Neurological disorders and services in Saskatchewan—a report based on provincial health care records. Neuroepidemiology 1988; 7:145–151.

50. Colucci C, Alfano V, Giordano D, Miele G. Poisoning by paraquat and Parkinson's disease [abstract]. Mov Disord 1990; 5:12.
51. Grcevic N, Jardro-Santel D, Jukic S. Cerebral changes in paraquat poisoning. In: Roizin L, Shiraki H, Grcevic N, eds. Neurotoxicology. New York: Raven Press, 1977:469–484.
52. Adams RA, Sidman A. Introduction to neuropathology. New York: McGraw-Hill, 1968.
53. Weller RO, Swash M, McLellan DL, Scholtz CL. Clinical neuropathology. Berlin: Springer-Verlag, 1983.
54. Adams JH, Corsellis JAN, Duchen LW. Greenfield's neuropathology. New York: John Wiley & Son, 1984.
55. Brierly JB, Graham DI. Hypoxia and vascular disorders of the central nervous system. In: Adams JJ, Corsellis JAN, Duchen LW, eds. Hypoxia and vascular disorders of the central nervous system. New York; Raven Press, 1984:125–207.
56. Nicholls P. Formate as an inhibitor of cytochrome *c* oxidase. Biochem Biophys Res Commun 1975; 67:610–616.
57. Hawker K, Lang AE. Hypoxic–ischemic damage of the basal ganglia. Mov Disord 1990; 5:219–224.
58. Carella F, Grassi MP, Savoiardo M, Contri P, Rapuzzi B, Mangoni A. Dystonic–parkinsonian syndrome after cyanide poisoning: clinical and MRI findings. J Neurol Neurosurg Psychiatry 1988; 51:1345–1348.
59. Matuso F, Cummins JW, Anderson RE. Neurological sequelae of massive hydrogen sulfide inhalation. Arch Neurol 1979; 36:451.
60. LeWitt PA, Martin SD. Dystonia and hyperkinesis with putaminal necrosis after methanol intoxication. Clin Neuropharmacol 1988; 11:161–167.
61. Jaffe LS. Sources, characteristics, and fate of atmospheric carbon monoxide. Ann NY Acad Sci 1970; 174:74–76.
62. Gordon EB. Carbon-monoxide encephalopathy. Br Med J 1965; 1:1232.
63. Ginsberg MD. Carbon monoxide. In: Spencer PS, Schaumburg HH, eds. Experimental and clinical neurotoxicology. Baltimore: Williams & Wilkins, 1980:374–394.
64. Klawans HL, Stein RW, Tanner CM, Goetz CG. A pure parkinsonian syndrome following acute carbon monoxide intoxication. Arch Neurol 1982; 39:302–304.
65. Smith JS, Mellick RS. Neuropsychiatric relapse following acute carbon monoxide poisoning—the contribution of electroconvulsive therapy. Med J Aust 1975; 1:465–468.
66. Meyer A. Experimentelle erfahrungen uber die Kohlinoxydvergiftung des Zentral-Nervensystems. Z Gesamte Neurol Psychiatr 1928; 112–187.
67. Ginsberg MD, Myers RE, McDonagh BF. Experimental carbon monoxide encephalopathy in the primate: II Clinical aspects, neuropathology, and physiologic correlation. Arch Neurol 1974; 30:209.
68. Okeda R, Funata N, Takano T, et al. The pathogenesis of carbon monoxide encephalopathy in the acute phase—physical and morphological correlation. Acta Neuropathol 1981; 54:1–10.
69. Preziosi TJ, Lindenberg R, Levy D, Christenson M. An experimental investigation in animals of the functional and morphological effects of single and repeated

exposures of high and low concentrations of carbon monoxide. Ann NY Acad Sci 1970; 174:369–384.
70. Gould DH, Gustine DL. Basal ganglia degeneration, myelin alterations, and enzyme inhibition induced in mice by the plant toxin 3-nitropropionic acid. Neuropathol Appl Neurobiol 1982; 8:377–393.
71. Ludolph AC, Seelig M, Ludolph A, et al. 3-Nitropropionic acid decreases cellular energy levels and causes neuronal degeneration in cortical explants. Neurodegeneration 1992; 1:155–161.
72. Choi DW, Rothman SM. The role of glutamate neurotoxicity in hypoxic–ischemic cell death. Annu Rev Neurosci 1990; 13:171–182.
73. Barbeau A, Pourcher E. New data on the genetics of Parkinson's disease. Can J Neurol Sci 1982; 9:53–60.
74. Seppalainen AM. Carbon disulfide. In: Spencer PS, Schaumburg HH, eds. Experimental and clinical neurotoxicology. Baltimore: Williams & Wilkins, 1980: 356–373.
75. Vigliani EC. Carbon disulphide poisoning in viscose rayon workers. Br J Ind Med 1954; 11:325–344.
76. Delpech A. Industrie du caoutchoue souffle: recherches sur l'intoxication speciale que determine le CS_2. Ann Hyg Ser 1863; 2:19–65.
77. Lewy FH. Diagnosis and differential diagnosis of CS_2 intoxication. In: Bashore RM, Staley AL, eds. Survey of carbon disulphide and hydrogen sulphide hazards in the viscose rayon industry. Bulletin 46. Harrisburg: Commonwealth of Pennsylvania, Dept. of Labor and Industry, 1938:52–53.
78. Lewy FH. Survey of carbon disulphide and hydrogen sulphide hazards in the viscose rayon industry. Bulletin 46. In: Bashore RM, Staley AL, eds. Neurological aspects of CS_2 intoxication. Harrisburg: Commonwealth of Pennsylvania, Dept. of Labor and Industry, 1938:31–37.
79. Quarelli G. L'Intossicazione professionale du CS_2. Ber Int Kongr Berufskrankh. Budapest: 1928.
80. Quarelli G. Solfocarbonismos professionale. Ressegna Previd Sociale 1930; 21:10.
81. Ranelletti A. Die berufliche Schwefelkohlenstoff Vergiftung in Italien. Arch Gewerbepathol Gewerbehyg 1931; 2:664.
82. Ehrich WE, Alpers BJ. Post-mortem findings in CS_2 poisoning. In: Bashore RM, Staley AL, eds. Survey of carbon disulphide and hydrogen sulphide hazards in the viscose rayon industry. Bulletin 46. Harrisburg: Commonwealth of Pennsylvania Dept. of Labor and Industry, 1938:55–57.
83. Megro F. Les syndromes parkinsoniens par intoxication sulfocarbonée. Rev Neurol 1930; 49:518.
84. Hamilton A, Lewy FH. Carbon disulphide and hydrogen sulphide hazards in the viscose rayon industry in the United States. In: Eighth international congress industrial accidents and occupational disease. Leipzig: G Thieme, 1939:1107–1110.
85. Gordy ST, Trumper M. Carbon disulfide poisoning: report of 21 cases. Ind Med 1940; 9:231.
86. Richter R. Degeneration of the basal ganglia in monkeys from chronic carbon disulfide poisoning. J Neuropathol Exp Neurol 1945; 4:324–353.
87. Peters HA, Levine RL, Matthews CG, Sauter SL, Rankin JH. Carbon disulfide-

induced neuropsychiatric changes in grain storage workers. Am J Ind Med 1982; 3:373–391.
88. Peters HA, Levine RL, Matthews CG, Sauter SL, Chapman L. Synergistic neurotoxicity of carbon tetrachloride/carbon disulfide (80/20 fumigants) and other pesticides in grain storage workers. Acta Pharmacol Toxicol 1986; 59:535–546.
89. Chapman LJ, Sauter SL, Henning RA, Levine RL, Matthew CG, Peters HA. Finger tremor after carbon disulfide-based pesticide exposures. Arch Neurol 1991; 48:866–870.
90. Kane FJ. Carbon disulfide intoxication from overdosage of disulfiram. Am J Psychiatry 1970; 127:690–694.
91. Lang AE. Miscellaneous drug-induced movement disorders. In: Lang AE, Weiner WJ, eds. Drug-induced movement disorders. Mt Kisco: Futura Publishing, 1992:339–381.
92. Krauss JK, Mohadjer M, Wakhloo AK, Mundinger F. Dystonia and akinesia due to pallidoputaminal lesions after disulfiram intoxication. Mov Disord 1991; 6:166–170.
93. Hurley LS, Woolley DE, Rosenthal F, Timiras PS. Influence of manganese on susceptibility of rats to convulsions. Am J Physiol 1963; 204:493–496.
94. Mena I. Manganese poisoning. In: Vinken PJ, Bruyn GW, eds. Handbook of clinical neurology, vol 36. Intoxications of the nervous system, part 1. Amsterdam: North-Holland 1979:217–237.
95. Neff NH, Barrett RE, Costa E. Selective depletion of caudate nucleus dopamine and serotonin during chronic manganese dioxide administration to squirrel monkeys. Experientia 1969; 25:1140–1114.
96. National Academy of Sciences. Medical and biologic effects of environmental pollutants. Washington, DC: National Academy of Sciences, 1973.
97. Hewitt EJ, Nicholas DJD. Cations and anions: inhibitions and interactions in metabolism and enzyme activity. In: Hochster RM, Quastel JH, eds. Metabolic inhibitors. Comprehensive treatment. New York: Academic Press, 1963:311–436.
98. Emara AM, El-Ghawabi SH, Madkour OI, El-Samra GH. Chronic manganese poisoning in the dry battery industry. Ind Med 1971; 28:78–82.
99. Ferraz HB, Betolucci PH, Pereira JS, Lima JG, Andrade LA. Chronic exposure to the fungicide maneb may produce symptoms and signs of CNS manganese intoxication. Neurology 1988; 38:550–553.
100. Kawamura R, Ikuta H, Fukuzumi S, et al. Intoxication by manganese in well water. Kitasato Arch Exp Med 1941; 18:145–169.
101. Barbeau A, Inque N, Cloutier T. Role of manganese in dystonia. Adv Neur 1976; 14:339–352.
102. Penalver R. Manganese poisoning. Ind J Med Surg 1955; 14:1–7.
103. Omata S, Sugano H. Methyl mercury: effects on protein synthesis in nervous tissue. In: Blum K, Manzo L, eds. Neurotoxicology. New York: Marcel Dekker, 1985:369–384.
104. Foa V. Neurotoxicity of elemental mercury: occupational aspects. In: Blum K, Manzo L, eds. Neurotoxicology. New York: Marcel Dekker, 1985:343.
105. Kark RAP. Clinical and neurochemical aspects of inorganic mercury intoxication.

In: Vinken PJ, Bruyn GW, eds. Handbook of clinical neurology, vol 36. Intoxications of the nervous system, part 1. Amsterdam: North-Holland, 1979:147–197.
106. Shiraki H. Neuropathological aspects of organic mercury intoxication, including Minamata disease. In: Vinken PJ, Bruyn GW, eds. Handbook of clinical neurology, vol 36. Intoxications of the nervous system, part 1. Amsterdam: North-Holland, 1979:83–145.
107. Takeuchi T. Neuropathology of Minamata disease in Kumanoto: especially at the chronic stage. In: Roizin L, Shiraki H, Grcevic N, eds. Neurotoxicology. New York: Raven Press, 1977:235–260.
108. Ngim CH, Devathasan G. Epidemiologic study on the association between body burden mercury level and idiopathic Parkinson's disease. Neuroepidemiology 1989; 8:128–141.
109. Ohlson CG, Hogstedt C. Parkinson's disease and occupational exposure to organic solvents, agricultural chemicals and mercury—a case referrant study. Scand J Work Environ Health 1981; 7:252–256.
110. Sato T, Ikuta F. Neuropathology of methylmercury intoxication in Niigata and chronic effects in monkeys. In: Roizin L, Shiraki H, Grcevic N, eds. Neurotoxicology. New York: Raven Press, 1977:261–274.
111. Spencer PS, Peterson ER, Madrid RA, Raine CS. Effects of thallium salts on neuronal mitochondria in organotypic cord ganglia–muscle combination cultures. J Cell Biol 1973; 58:79–95.
112. Prick JJG. Thallium poisoning. In: Vinken PI, Bruyn GW, eds. Handbook of clinical neurology, vol 36. Intoxication of the nervous system, part 1. Amsterdam: North-Holland, 1979:239–278.
113. Moses H, Klawans HL. Bromide intoxication. In: Vinken PJ, Bruyn GW, eds. Handbook of clinical neurology, vol 36. Intoxications of the nervous system, part 1. Amsterdam: North-Holland, 1979:291–318.
114. Rathus EM, Landy PJ. Methyl bromide poisoning. Br J Ind Med 1961; 18:53–57.
115. Appel GB, Galen R, O'Brien J, Schonfeldt R. Methyl iodide intoxication. Ann Intern Med 1975; 82:534–536.
116. Peters HA, Goemen A, Cripps DJ, Bryan GT, Dogramaci I. Epidemiology of hexachlorobenzene-induced porphyria in Turkey. Arch Neurol 1982; 39:744–749.
117. Peters HA, Johnson SAM, Cam S. Hexachlorobenzene-induced porphyria: effect of chelation on the disease, porphyrin and mental methabolism. Am J Med Sci New Ser 1966; 251:314–322.
118. Schaumburg HH, Spencer PS. Environmental hydrocarbons produce degeneration in cat hypothalamus and optic tract. Science 1978; 199:199–200.
119. Schlesselman J. Case–control studies: design, conduct, analysis. New York: Oxford University Press, 1982.
120. Koller WC, Langston JW, Hubble JP, et al. Does a long pre-clinical period occur in Parkinson's disease? Neurology 1991; 41(suppl 2):8–13.
121. Calne DB, Eisen A, McGeer E, Spencer P. Alzheimer's disease, Parkinson's disease, and motoneurone disease: abiotrophic interaction between ageing and environment. Lancet 1986; 2:1067–1070.
122. Garruto RM, Gajdusek DC, Chen KM. Amyotrophic lateral sclerosis and parkin-

sonism–dementia among Filipino migrants to Guam. Ann Neurol 1981; 10:341–350.
123. Garruto RM, Gajdusek DC, Chen KM. Amyotrophic lateral sclerosis among Chamorro migrants from Guam. Ann Neurol 1980; 8:612–619.
124. Calne DB, Dubini A, Stern G. Did Leonardo describe Parkinson's disease. N Engl J Med 1989; 320:594.
125. Haimanot RT, Kidane O, Wuhib E, et al. Lathyrism in rural northwestern Ethiopia: a highly prevalent disorder. Int J Epidemiol 1990; 19:664–672.
126. Teitelbaum JS, Zatorre RJ, Carpenter S, Gendron D. Neurologic sequelae of domoic acid intoxication due to the ingestion of contaiminated mussels. N Engl J Med 1990; 322:1781–1787.
127. Valanis B. Epidemiology in nursing and health care. Norwalk: Appleton-Century-Crofts, 1986.
128. Rajput AH, Thiessen B, Munoz D, Laverty D, Desai H. Consideration of age and environments and number of substantia nigra cells. In: Ninth International Symposium on Parkinson's Disease, 1988:11.
129. Ho SC, Woo J, Lee CM. Epidemiologic study of Parkinson's disease in Hong Kong. Neurology 1989; 39:1314–1318.
130. Rajput AH, Uitti RJ, Stern W, Laverty W. Early onset Parkinson's disease in Saskatchewan—environmental considerations for etiology. Can J Neurol Sci 1986; 13:312–316.
131. Tanner CM. Influence of environmental factors on the onset of Parkinson's disease (PD). Neurology 1986; 36:215.
132. Davanipour Z, Will AD. Residential histories in Parkinson's disease patients. Ann Neurol 1990; 28:295.
133. Golbe LI, Farrell TM, Davis PH. Follow-up study of early-life protective and risk factors in Parkinson's disease. Mov Disord 1990; 5:66–70.
134. Koller W, Vetere-Overfield B, Gray C, et al. Environmental risk factors in Parkinson's disease. Neurology 1990; 40:1218–1221.
135. Wong GF, Gray CS, Hassanein RS, Koller WC. Environmental risk factors in siblings with Parkinson's disease. Arch Neurol 1991; 48:287–289.
136. Semchuk KM, Love EJ, Lee RG. Parkinson's disease and exposure to rural environmental factors: a population based case–control study. Can J Neurol Sci 1991; 18:279–286.
137. Semchuk KM, Love ET, Lee RG. Parkinson's disease and exposure to agricultural work and pesticide chemicals. Neurology 1992; 42:1328–1335.
138. Tanner CM, Chen B, Wang WZ, et al. Environmental factors and Parkinson's disease: a case–control study in China. Neurology 1989; 39:660–664.
139. Zayed J, Ducic S, Campanella G, et al. [Environmental factors in the etiology of Parkinson's disease]. Can J Neurol Sci 1990; 17:286–291.
140. Goldsmith JR, Herishanu Y, Abarbanel JM, Weinbaum Z. Clustering of Parkinson's disease points to environment etiology. Arch Environ Health 1990; 45:88–94.
141. Rajput AH, Uitti RJ, Stern W, et al. Geography, drinking water chemistry, pesticides and herbicides and the etiology of Parkinson's disease. Can J Neurol Sci 1987; 14:414–418.

142. Jimenez-Jimenez FJ, Gonzales DM, Gimenez-Roldan S. Exposure to well-water and pesticides in Parkinson's disease. A case–control study from the south east area of Madrid. In: Ninth International symposium on Parkinson's disease, 1988:118.
143. Barbeau A, Roy M, Bernier G, Campanella G, Paris S. Ecogenetics of Parkinson's disease: prevalence and environmental aspects in rural areas. Can J Neurol Sci 1987; 14:36–41.
144. Reed DM,Brody JA. Amyotrophic lateral sclerosis and parkinsonism–dementia on Guam, 1945–1972. I. Descriptive epidemiology. Am J Epidemiol 1975; 101:287–301.
145. Tanner CM, Grabler P, Goetz CG. Occupation and the risk of Parkinson's disease (PD): a case control study in young onset patients. Neurology 1990; 40:422.
146. IARC working group on the evaluation of the carcinogenic risk of chemicals to humans. IARC monographs on the evaluation of the carcinogenic risk of chemicals to humans, wood, leather and some associated industries, vol 25. Lyon: International Agency for Research on Cancer, 1981.
147. Aquilonius SM,Hartvig P. Utilization of antiparkinson drugs in Sweden. Uppsala J Med Sci 1986; 93.
148. Sethi KD, Meador KJ, Loring D, Meador MP. Neuroepidemiology of Parkinson's disease: analysis of mortality data for the U.S.A. and Georgia. Int J Neurosci 1989; 46:87–92.
149. Hertzman C, Wiens M, Bowering D, Snow B, Calne DB. Parkinson's disease: a case–control study of occupational and environmental risk factors. Am J Ind Med 1990; 17:349–355.
150. Murphy SD. Pesticides. In: Doull J, Klaassen CD, Amdur MO, eds. Cassarett and Doull's toxicology. New York: Macmillan, 1980:357–408.
151. Klawans HL. Dystonia and tremor following exposure to 2,3,7,8-tetrachlorobenzo-*p*-dioxin (TCDD dioxin). Proc Int Symp Neurotoxicol 1992; 1987:
152. Schaumburg HH, Berger AR, Thomas PK. Disorders of peripheral nerves. Philadelphia: FA Davis, 1982.
153. Rajput AH,Uitti RJ. Paraquat and Parkinson's disease [letter]. Neurology 1987; 37:1820–1821.
154. Sanchez-Ramos JR, Factor SA, Weiner WJ. Paraquat and Parkinson's disease: reply from the authors [letter]. Neurology 1987; 37:1820–1821.
155. Butterfield PG, Valanis BG, Spencer PS, Lindeman CA, Nutt JG. Environmental antecedents of young-onset Parkinson's disease. Neurology 1993; 43:1150–1158.
156. Semchuk KM, Love EJ, Lee RG. Parkinson's disease: a test of the multifactorial etiologic hypothesis. Neurology 1993; 43:1173–1180.
157. Butterfield PG, Valanis BG, Spencer PS, Lindeman CA, Nutt JG. Environmental antecedents of young-onset Parkinson's disease. Neurology 1993; 43:1150–1158.
158. Garruto RM, Yase Y. Neurodegenerative disorders of the western Pacific: the search for mechanisms of pathogenesis. Trends Neurosci 1986; 9:368–374.
159. Hirano A, Malamud N, Kurland LT. Parkinsonism–dementia complex, an endemic disease on the island of Guam. II. Pathological features. Brain 1961; 84:662–679.
160. Kurland LT, Molgaard CA. Guamanian ALS: hereditary or acquired? In: Roland LP, ed. Human motor neuron disease. New York: Raven Press, 1982:165–177.

161. Chen KM, Yase Y. Parkinsonism–dementia, neurofibrillary tangles and trace elements in the western Pacific. In: Hutton JT, Kenny AD, eds. Senile dementia of the Alzheimer type. New York: AR Liss, 1985:153–173.
162. Garruto RM, Gajdusek DC. Factors provoking the high incidence of amyotrophic lateral sclerosis and parkinsonism–dementia of Guam: deposition and distribution of toxic metals and essential minerals in the central nervous system. In: Gottfries CG, ed. Normal aging, Alzheimer's disease and senile dementia. Aspects of etiology, pathogenesis, diagnosis and treatment. Bruxelles: Editions de l'Universit de Bruxelles, 1985:65–81.
163. Steele JC, Guzman TQ, Driver MG. Nutritional factors in amyotrophic lateral sclerosis on Guam: observations from Umatac. In: Hudson AJ, ed. Concepts in pathogenesis and etiology. Toronto: University of Toronto Press, 1990:193–223.
164. Reed D, Labarthe D, Chen KM, Stallones R. A cohort study of amyotrophic lateral sclerosis and parkinsonism–dementia on Guam and Rota. Am J Epidemiol 1987; 125:92–100.
165. Kurland LT. An appraisal of the neurotoxicity of cycad and the etiology of amyotrophic lateral sclerosis on Guam. Fed Proc 1972; 31:1540–1542.
166. Duncan MW, Steele JC, Kopin IJ, Markey SP. 2-Amino-3-(methylamino)-propionic acid (BMAA) in cycad flour: an unlikely cause of amyotrophic lateral sclerosis and parkinsonism–dementia of Guam. Neurology 1990; 40:767–772.
167. Spencer PS, Ohta M, Palmer VS. Cycad use and motor neurone disease in Kii Peninsula of Japan. Lancet 1987; 1462.
168. Whiting MG. Food practices in ALS foci in Japan, the Marianas and New Guinea. Fed Proc 1964; 23:1343–1345.
169. Matsumoto H. Cycasin. In: Rechcigl M, ed. CRC handbook of naturally occurring food toxicants. Boca Raton: CRC Press, 1985:45–61.
170. Shiraki H, Yase Y. Amyotrophic lateral sclerosis. In: Vinken P, Bruyn G, eds. Handbook of clinical neurology, vol 22. System disorders and atrophies, part 2. Amsterdam: Elsevier, 1975:353–419.
171. Yase Y. The pathogenesis of amyotrophic lateral sclerosis. Lancet 1972; 2:292–296.
172. Nunn PB, Seelig M, Zagoren JC, Spencer PS. Stereospecific acute neuronotoxicity of "uncommon" plant amino acids linked to human motor-system diseases. Brain 1987; 410:375–379.
173. Weiss JH, Choi DW. β-*N*-Methylamino-L-alanine (BMAA) neurotoxicity: requirement for bicarbonate as a cofactor. Science 1988; 241:973–975.
174. Kisby GE, Ross SM, Spencer PS, Gold BG, Nunn PB,Roy DN. Cycasin and BMAA: candidate neurotoxins for western Pacific amyotrophic lateral sclerosis/parkinsonism–dementia complex. Neurodegeneration 1992; 1:73–82.
175. Seawright A, Brown A, Nolan C. Selective degeneration of cerebellar cortical neurons caused by cycad neurotoxin, L-β-methylaminoalanine (1-BMAA), in rats. Neuropathol Appl Neurobiol 1990; 16:153–169.
176. Spencer PS, Nunn PB, Hugon J, et al. Guam amyotrophic lateral sclerosis–parkinsonism–dementia linked to a plant excitant neurotoxin. Science 1987; 237:517–522.

177. Shimizu T, Yasuda N, Kono I. Hepatic and spinal lesions in goats chronically intoxicated with cycasin. Jpn J Vet Sci 1986; 8:1291–1295.
178. Dastur DK. Cycad toxicity in monkeys: clinical, pathological, and biochemical aspects. Fed Proc 1964; 23:1368–1369.
179. Sieber SM, Correa P, Dalgard DW, McIntire RK, Adamson RH. Carcinogenicity and hepatotoxicity of cycasin and its aglycone methylazoxymethanol acetate in non-human primates. J Natl Cancer Inst 1986; 65:177–189.
180. Cedar H. DNA methylation and gene activity. Cell 1988; 53:3-4.

13

MPTP as It Relates to the Etiology of Parkinson's Disease

J. William Langston

The Parkinson's Institute, Sunnyvale, California

I. INTRODUCTION

There are several reasons why an entire chapter is reserved for 1-methyl-4-phenyl-1,2,3,6-tetrahydropyridine (MPTP) in this book. First, this compound, which induces most, if not all, of the features of Parkinson's disease in human and nonhuman primates (1–4), represents a prototype neurotoxin, serving as a model of how a toxin might induce a human neurodegenerative disease. Second, the discovery of this compound and its parkinsonogenic effects is one of the principal reasons that there has been such a renaissance of interest in the possibility that Parkinson's disease, and possibly other neurodegenerative diseases, might be caused by an environmental toxin (5). Third, studies on the mechanism of action of MPTP have proved a means to study the neurodegenerative process at the neurochemical and molecular level. These investigations have provided new insights into the role and function of the nigrostriatal system, and could eventually lead to important new ways to diagnose, monitor, and treat the disease. For example, the identification of risk factors or a biomarker for Parkinson's disease could enormously benefit epidemiological studies and lay the foundation for new therapeutic approaches directed toward prevention of the disease (6).

Areas covered in this chapter include a review of the biological effects of MPTP, a summary of what is known about its biodisposition, and a critique of the current theories on its mechanism of action. The impact of the discovery of MPTP on epidemiological studies will be considered, followed by a look at the future, with particular emphasis on promising avenues for new research.

II. BEHAVIORAL EFFECTS OF MPTP

One of the many ironies of the discovery of MPTP (7) is that the effects of this compound were first clearly recognized not in experimental animals, but in humans (3). This occurred when MPTP was widely distributed on the streets in northern California as a "new synthetic heroin" (3,8). At least seven of the young addicts who self-injected this compound developed a very striking complex of both acute and chronic symptoms (9). Typically, MPTP caused a severe burning at the site of injection. Individuals using it then experienced a variety of acute symptoms, including a "dreamy or spacey" feeling, hallucinations, dimming of vision, a metallic taste in the mouth (which was often described as similar to that experienced with cocaine), and "jerky" movements of the extremities (9). Most of these symptoms cleared within hours, although the muscle jerks occasionally continued for 1 or 2 days.

Subjects who used the compound repeatedly (over days to weeks) developed a series of motor abnormalities that evolved more gradually, usually over several days to 1–2 weeks (8,9). Typically, these subacute effects, which in all but a few cases became chronic, were characterized by increasing stiffness of the muscles and slowness of movement. Several patients developed a resting tremor of the hands and arms. In one, this was so severe that it was disabling. Other symptoms experienced by these subjects included flexion of posture, oiliness of skin, and a decrease in size of handwriting (a symptom known as micrographia, which is almost unique to parkinsonism) (10).

Physical examination in these individuals was striking. As a group, our original cohort of seven patients demonstrated virtually all of the typical features of Parkinson's disease (3,8). Physical findings included bradykinesia, rest tremor, a fine action tremor, increased tone in the extremities, a loss of blinking, seborrhea, hypophonia, shuffling gait, and marked rigidity of the extremities. In addition, although these subjects were not demented, careful neuropsychological testing revealed subtle abnormalities in mental status activity similar to that seen in nondemented patients with Parkinson's disease (11,12). Careful testing did not reveal a significant abnormality of olfaction in these subjects, however (13).

The similarities to Parkinson's disease continued in response to treatment. These subjects, as a group, have demonstrated virtually all of the side effects of therapy that one typically encounters with long-term treatment of Parkinson's disease (14). These include "wearing-off" of the medications effects, fluctuations (so-called on-and-off effects), dyskinesias, hallucinations, and a gradually closing of therapeutic window, such that a number of subjects reached the point that they now have no good "on" time in response to levodopa or carbidopa (whereas earlier several of them had been nearly normal for 3–4 hr after each dose of these agents).

Although none of our original cohort of subjects with MPTP-induced parkinsonism has died, there is one such report in the literature (15). In the mid-1970s, a college student, who had been making and self-administering a synthetic opiate, developed a parkinsonian syndrome after making what appeared to be a "bad batch." When his case was originally reported, it was unclear which compound had induced his parkinsonism, but in retrospect, with the addition of the California cohort, it seems virtually certain that this subject was yet another example of MPTP toxicity (3). This young man eventually committed suicide, and one-half of the brain was available for pathological examination. Histological studies revealed a striking loss of cells in the substantia nigra, quite similar to that seen in Parkinson's disease. However, other features, such as classic Lewy bodies and involvement of extranigral sites, were not seen. Thus, from a neuropathological view, MPTP appeared to have produced a pure nigrostriatal degeneration.

Spinal fluid examinations in several of our original cohort of subjects also suggest that MPTP induces a relatively pure nigrostriatal dopaminergic deficit, at least in young subjects. The results of these studies demonstrated very low concentrations of homovanillic acid (HVA), a major dopamine metabolite, but normal levels of serotonin, norepinephrine metabolites (5-hydroxyindole acetic acid [HIAA] and 3-methoxy-4-hydroxyphenylethyleneglycol [MHPG]) (16). In accord with these spinal fluid data, two of our original subjects have had positron emission tomography (PET) scans, which revealed a marked loss of ^{18}F-labeled dihydroxyphenylalanine (DOPA) uptake (unpublished observations). We have also used this technique to evaluate a group of MPTP-exposed subjects who have little or no parkinsonism (17,18). Interestingly, ^{18}F-labeled DOPA uptake in these subjects was, as a group, lower than that seen in normals, but higher than in patients with Parkinson's disease, suggesting that PET scanning may be useful for a marker for presymptomatic striatal dopamine deficiency.

III. ANIMAL MODELS

One of the major problems with most animal models of human disease is that one is uncertain exactly how closely the animal model would pattern the disease *in humans*. As tragic as the MPTP experience was for the young drug abusers, who remain severely disabled, the accidental experiment of which they were a part has provided a crucial scientific insight by making it possible to extrapolate the effects of this compound from animal models to the human. For MPTP, we know precisely what the effects of the compound are in humans and just how closely it resembles Parkinson's disease.

Because MPTP has been given to a wide variety of animals, ranging from the medicinal leech to monkeys (19), a comprehensive review will not be attempted here. Rather, this overview will concentrate on two of the most widely used experimental models, primates and rodents.

A. MPTP-Induced Parkinsonism in Nonhuman Primates

Although MPTP clearly affects the nigrostriatal dopaminergic system in a wide variety of animal species (19), nowhere are behavioral changes more evident than in the primate. In fact, most investigators agree that MPTP-induced parkinsonism in primates represents the best animal model now available for Parkinson's disease. However, similar to humans, these animals first develop a wide variety of acute effects after MPTP administration before a parkinsonian syndrome is manifest (2,4). Many of these suggest a serotonergic syndrome, with myoclonus, retropulsion, salivation, and hints that the animals are hallucinating (looking wildly about, at times apparently grasping at objects in the air that do not exist). As in humans, these acute symptoms subside rapidly. Usually, after two to three doses of MPTP, monkeys begin to show a wide variety of parkinsonian signs, including bradykinesia, postural abnormalities, and a tendency to freeze (2,4,20–23).

The issue of resting tremor has been somewhat more controversial in monkeys than in humans (24). Most monkeys appear to develop a tremor, but it occurs more with posture or action than at rest. The one exception to this may be the African green monkey, which does appear to develop a more characteristic resting tremor (25). The parkinsonism in these animals also responded dramatically to levodopa (similar to the humans) (2,4). Furthermore, they develop many of the same side effects to levodopa that occur in humans, including clear-cut dyskinesias and fluctuations (26–34).

In monkeys, as opposed to humans, there are abundant neurochemical data on the effect of MPTP on the nigrostriatal dopaminergic system. When given in maximum, sublethal doses, MPTP produces a profound dopamine depletion in the striatum (2,22,23,35,36). There is some debate whether the putamen is more or less affected than the caudate. This debate is of some importance because of the observation that the putamen appears to be more affected in idiopathic Parkinson's disease than the caudate (37). Although some studies have found that the caudate is more sensitive to MPTP neurotoxicity (as judged by dopamine depletion or mazindol binding; 38,39), others have not (40,41). Whether these differences are due to species differences, dosage schedule, age of the animals, or some other factor(s) is not yet clear (39). However, this will be important to determine, since the issue of selective vulnerability within the nigrostriatal system may be an important clue to the pathophysiology of Parkinson's disease. Should it become clear that MPTP is capable of replicating this more complex pattern of dopamine depletion, this experimental tool can be used to explore even more subtle aspects of the pathophysiology of Parkinson's disease.

Although dopamine depletion in the striatum is the most consistent and dramatic effect of MPTP, there are numerous reports of involvement of other neurotransmitter systems (19,23,42–46). Although initial reports suggested that the nucleus accumbens and ventral tegmental areas were spared, there have now been several reports of depletion of striatal dopamine in the ventral tegmental–accumbens area (23,42–47). Some investigators have also observed changes in the serotonergic, opiate, GABAergic, and noradrenergic systems, but again the results have been variable (see Ref. 23 for review).

These neurochemical findings have, at least to some degree, been reflected at the neuropathological level. Virtually every study of MPTP neurotoxicity has shown that, when adequate doses are given to monkeys, there is clear-cut evidence of cell death in the substantia nigra, primarily in the zona compacta (23). Several studies have suggested that there is even some degree of selectivity within the substantia nigra, although no consistent pattern has emerged (23). In our own studies, acute lesions have induced damage primarily to the medial third of the substantia nigra (48). This differs from Parkinson's disease, in which the lateral third tends to be more severely involved (49). However, in more chronically treated animals or in animals allowed to survive for larger periods after MPTP exposure, a pattern of cell loss more typical of Parkinson's disease is seen (48).

Cell loss in monkeys given MPTP has also been reported in the locus ceruleus (50–54). This is important, since this structure is typically affected in Parkinson's disease. In our experience, at least 50% of animals given adequate doses of MPTP will have unequivocal cell loss in this area (48). Various studies have also suggested abnormalities in the ventral tegmental area and possibly the hypothalamus, both of which are also known to be affected in the idiopathic disease (51,54–56).

Interestingly, inclusions that are somewhat reminiscent of the intraneuronal inclusions seen in idiopathic Parkinson's disease (where they are known as Lewy bodies) have been reported in old squirrel monkeys given MPTP (50). These round eosinophilic intraneuronal bodies are seen in very much the same distribution that has been observed in human Parkinson's disease. However, at electron microscopic level, the MPTP-induced inclusions appear to lack the dense core seen with Lewy bodies (57). One possibility is that these inclusions represent an immature form of Lewy bodies, or "pre-Lewy bodies." At the moment, one can only say that they clearly warrant further study. The potential importance of these observations is that changes in the cytoskeleton are an essential feature of most neurodegenerative diseases. Whether or not such investigations will yield a complete model of the cytoarchitectural changes in Parkinson's disease remains to be seen. But, if so, it could provide a whole new dimension to the use of this model for the study of Parkinson's disease.

B. The Effects of MPTP in Rodents

Even though both rats and mice are widely used as experimental models in the laboratory, the focus here will be on mice, since they appear to be much more sensitive to the compound than rats, which are notoriously insensitive to MPTP

(19,58–67). In fact, most investigators have found it necessary to carry out direct intranigral injection of MPTP or its metabolites to produce cell damage in rats. On the other hand, certain strains of mice, particularly C57BL/6 mice, appear to be quite sensitive to MPTP (68–70). However, even in these animals, exposure to high doses of MPTP does not cause overt parkinsonism, although it is possible to bring out certain behavioral deficits with stress tests (71). Therefore, most of the studies in mice have focused on neurochemical and neuropathological changes.

Virtually any route of administration is effective in producing dopamine depletion in mice, although higher doses of MPTP are required after intraperitoneal and oral administration (72). Interestingly, after intravenous exposure, subcutaneous doses are the most effective (72). At the neuropathological level, MPTP appears to preferentially damage the nerve terminals; nerve cell degeneration is much more difficult to induce, at least with systemic injections of the compound. Perhaps for this reason, a number of studies have shown that there is recovery of striatal dopamine in mice, although this may take months to become complete (73). Although frank nerve cell loss has been more difficult to document after systemic administration of MPTP, the compound clearly induces degeneration in old mice (74).

One problem that has led to confusion in the literature relates to the use of immunostaining for tyrosine hydroxylase (TH) as a marker for dopaminergic nerve cells. There is now little doubt that MPTP can suppress TH immunostaining, without killing cells, at least in primates (75); therefore, one cannot infer that MPTP has induced neuronal degeneration when using this technique alone, although this is frequently done. Use of the Fink–Heimer stain, or the use of Nissl stains, with cell counts, is more appropriate for this purpose, although these are done all too infrequently.

In summary, the MPTP mouse model can be used for a wide variety of studies, particularly those on the mechanism of action of MPTP. However, the mouse does not appear to represent the best model of MPTP neurotoxicity when it comes to behavioral or neuropathological features. On the other hand, since there appears to be considerable recovery in the mouse, this model may be well suited for studies of neuronal plasticity and regeneration.

IV. THE BIODISPOSITION OF MPTP

The sequence of events that occurs after the systemic administration of MPTP has been the focus of intensive investigation over the last decade. During this time, a great deal has been learned about the biological steps that lead to MPTP neurotoxicity. After systemic administration, MPTP can be found in virtually all peripheral organs and tissues (76,77). Its concentrations begin to decline soon thereafter, although the eye appears to represent an exception to this rule (76).

There is now abundant evidence that MPTP is not toxic, but rather must be biotransformed before toxicity occurs. After systemic administration, it is rapidly oxidized both peripherally and in the brain to its pyridinium metabolite, 1-methyl-4-phenylpyridinium ion (MPP^+) (76–78). This oxidation process appears to take place by an intermediate, 2,3-dihydropyridinium ($MPDP^+$) (79–88). The exact mechanism by which the dihydropyridinium is converted to MPP^+ is unclear, but the process may occur nonenzymatically. A key enzyme in this sequence of events is monoamine oxidase (MAO), which is responsible for the transformation of MPTP to $MPDP^+$ (89). MPTP is the substrate for both the A and B forms of the enzyme, but it is preferentially metabolized by MAO B (90).

Most studies indicate that MPP^+ is the ultimate mediator of toxicity (76,78,91,92), since (1) the compound is clearly toxic, (2) it does not appear to be further biotransformed in the brain, and (3) preventing its formation with MAO inhibitors has repeatedly been shown to prevent MPTP neurotoxicity (20,21,78,93–95). It is somewhat of a biochemical irony that the production of MPP^+ probably represents part of a standard detoxification process that has literally backfired, at least in the brain. The detoxification process is probably working systemically, since a standard way to remove potentially harmful xenobiotics is to convert them into water-soluble metabolites that can then be removed by the kidneys. However, for MPTP, it is clear that (1) the metabolite is more toxic than the parent compound, and (2) when this process takes place in the brain, there are several dire consequences.

After the discovery that MPP^+ was generated in the brain, as well as systemically, most investigators assumed that this process was taking place at the target sites (i.e., within dopaminergic neurons) (78). However, this hypothesis was quickly questioned when it was found that MPP^+, but not MPTP, was a substrate for the catecholaminergic uptake system (96–98), because this observation raised serious questions about how MPTP could get into dopaminergic neurons to be biotransformed into MPP^+. Since that time, there has been increasing evidence that the biotransformation of MPTP to MPP^+ takes place in glial cells and not in neurons. The lines of evidence are as follows. First, various studies have shown that primary glial cultures rapidly convert MPTP to MPP^+ (99–101) and that this biotransformation can be blocked by inhibiting MAO. Second, there is increasing evidence that MAO B is located primarily in glia and serotonergic neurons, but not in nigrostriatal dopaminergic neurons (102,103). Although these observations raised the possibility that the biotransformation of MPTP to MPP^+ might be taking place in serotonergic neurons, neurochemical ablation of these neurons does not block neurotoxicity (104,105). By a process of exclusion, then, glial cells appear to be key players in terms of the biotransformation of MPTP to MPP^+.

We have recently completed a series of studies using primary cultures of astrocytes designed to provide a comprehensive picture of the role played by glia (88,101,106,107). Specifically, we hoped to determine the fate of MPP^+ after its generation within these cells and to characterize the toxic consequences resulting from exposure of astrocytes to MPTP. These experiments clearly confirmed the role of MAO in the bioactivation of MPTP. However, whereas MAO B is likely to be primarily involved in the conversion of MPTP to MPP^+ in adult brain, our studies also showed that MAO A may also be important if present in high enough concentrations, compared with MAO B, as it is in the astrocytes harvested from neonatal animals (106).

These studies also showed that astrocytes convert MPTP to MPTP *N*-oxide, probably by flavin monooxygenase (FMO) (106). However, the relevance of this observation to the in vivo situation could be questioned, because MPTP *N*-oxide has not been observed after incubation of MPTP with microsomes isolated from whole brains of adult mice (108). Furthermore, although small amounts of MPTP *N*-oxide are present in the CNS of rats after MPTP administration, it could be argued that these might have reached the brain after being produced in the liver (109). On the other hand, FMO activity is detectable in microsomal fractions prepared from the corpus striatum (110). Since our data indicate that MPTP *N*-oxide is mostly excreted after it is produced within astrocytes, this metabolic pathway may represent a successful detoxification route for MPTP (106).

One of the puzzles for the formation of MPP^+ within astrocytes has been the difficulty in explaining how it gets out of these cells to the extracellular space, where it can be taken up by dopaminergic neurons. In vitro studies have shown that MPTP is converted to $MPDP^+$ by MAO within the astrocytes, and that $MPDP^+$ crosses the plasma membranes of these cells, possibly in the form of the lipophilic free base 1,2-MPDP (88). Once MPDP reaches the extracellular space, it generates MPP^+, most likely by autoxidation. However, there appears to be at least one other mechanism by which it is able to exit cells. Despite its charged chemical structure, MPP^+ itself appears to cross cell membranes from the intracellular to the extracellular compartment. Indeed, after initial exposure to MPTP, the MPP^+ accumulated within astrocytes can be recovered in the extracellular space when MPTP is removed and cell incubations are carried on in fresh medium (88).

There may be an interesting precedent buried within these scientific data. In essence, astrocytes appear to be activating and discharging a neurotoxin into the extracellular space. In other words, "the brain produces its own neurotoxin." Therefore, one can raise the question of whether or not this represents a broader principle for the interaction of environmental substances and the brain. Might there be a whole family of compounds in the environment that, although nontoxic themselves, are subject to toxic activation by the brain?

Once MPP^+ has gained entrance into the extracellular space, most investigators believe that it is then taken up into dopaminergic neurons by the dopamine-uptake system (96). This has been referred to as the "Trojan horse" phenomenon, since the cells apparently are recognizing MPP^+ as a "friendly substrate," but in fact, are accumulating a substance that, in adequate concentrations, will kill them. Since many other neurotoxins appear to gain entrance into nerve cells through their uptake system, this may represent an "Achilles heel" of the nervous system, and probably accounts for the critical importance of the blood–brain barrier (111).

Although the selective uptake of MPP^+, which is actually a relatively nonselective toxin capable of killing everything from liver cells to astrocytes themselves, may explain its effect on dopaminergic neurons, there are still some unsolved puzzles. For example, it is still somewhat of a mystery why dopaminergic cells are particularly susceptible, since one might expect any neurons with catecholaminergic uptake sites to be affected. This represents an important area of future research, since it could provide important clues about the selective vulnerability of dopaminergic systems, both in terms of sensitivity to neurotoxins and relative to their particular vulnerability in a neurodegenerative process such as Parkinson's disease.

As would be predicted if MPP^+ gains entrance into dopaminergic neurons through their own uptake system, several studies in rodents have shown that dopamine blockers prevent MPTP-induced striatal dopamine depletion in mice (112–118). The data are less clear in primates, although at least one group has pursued this question unflaggingly and has provided fairly convincing evidence that dopamine uptake blockers can indeed prevent neurotoxicity in monkeys, at least partially (119,120). One of the reasons that it may have been difficult to protect monkeys with these agents probably relates to the prolonged half-life of MPP^+ in the primate brain. Since most uptake blockers have a relatively short half-life, technically, it may be more difficult to block MPP^+ uptake over an adequate period in these animals. Alternatively, there may be differences in the mechanism by which MPP^+ gains access to dopaminergic neurons in primates, perhaps entering neurons by dendrites on the cell bodies as well as their terminals. Additional experiments will be necessary to clarify this question.

One of the most fascinating findings concerning the biodistribution of MPTP and MPP^+ relates to the elimination of these compounds from the brain. In rodents, MPP^+ appears to disappear quite rapidly, with a half-life of about 4 hr; after 24 hr, little if any MPP^+ can be found in the brain (121). In striking contrast to this, high concentrations of MPP^+ are maintained for days in the primate brain, particularly in dopaminergic areas (122). Although the reason for this difference remains a complete mystery, it does raise the intriguing question of whether or not there may be some essential difference in the primate brain that impairs the ability to handle neurotoxins, particularly charged substances such as MPP^+. The inability to eliminate environmental toxins from the brain certainly could represent a major susceptibility factor to neurotoxic disease.

Since primates (i.e., humans) are the only species to develop Parkinson's disease, this might provide a new avenue for research into the reason(s) for their vulnerability to the disease.

This difference in the ability to eliminate MPP^+ from the brain may be one of the reasons monkeys are so much more susceptible to the effects of MPTP, but there is another intriguing observation that may be as or more important. Kalaria and colleagues (123) were the first to report that there are striking differences in the concentrations of MAO B in the cerebral cerebrocapillary endothelial (CCE), which constitutes the blood–brain barrier. These investigators found that the levels of MAO B are much higher in the CCE of rats than in primates or humans. This intriguing observation may actually represent a protective mechanism against a compound such as MPTP (65,67,124,125). This is because MAO rapidly converts MPTP to MPP^+ in the CCE, which, as a charged substance, may then be unable to gain access to the brain. Rather, MPP^+ is likely to become "trapped" in the CCE, rather than entering the brain as a lipophilic compound (such as MPTP) would do. Supporting this concept is that, when MPP^+ is administered systemically, it does not enter the brain. Once again, a biological observation on MPTP may be providing some potentially interesting insights into mechanisms underlying neurodegenerative disease, suggesting that different characteristics in the blood–brain barrier could explain the vulnerability of primate species to MPTP-like compounds in the environment.

Although MPP^+ appears to be the major metabolite of MPTP, a number of other metabolites have been identified including its *N*-oxide (126), three pyridinones—(1-methyl-4-phenyl-5,6-dihydro-2(1*H*)-pyridinone (MPPyrH2), 1-methyl-4-phenyl-2-(1*H*)-pyridinone, and 1-methyl-4-phenyl-2-piperidinone) —as well as the demethylated form of MPTP (PTP) (109). These metabolites have not been studied in great detail, but they likely represent detoxification pathways (127,128). Since this area has not been studied extensively, it may represent fertile ground for further understanding MPTP toxicity as well as other pathways for xenobiotics in terms of the way toxins are handled by the body and the central nervous system.

In summary, although much has been learned about the biotransformation and biodistribution of MPTP, a great deal still remains to be determined. For example, there is the very interesting work of Rollema and colleagues using intracerebral microdialysis to better understand its effects at the nerve terminal level, which has opened up a whole new area of investigation (129–134). We still do not understand why MPP^+ is eliminated so differently in primates compared with rodents, and why the cell bodies seem to be so much more susceptible to MPTP in monkeys. The nature of the inclusions seen in older monkeys needs to be further elucidated, and the whole question of whether or not there is selective vulnerability within the nigrostriatal system remains to be answered. Answers to each of these questions could provide important new insights into the neurodegenerative process that underlies Parkinson's disease.

V. NEUROMELANIN

Neuromelanin is given its own heading in this chapter because it has been a subject of intense interest both in Parkinson's disease and in the investigation of MPTP. This complex substance has been of great interest for over a century, in part because it is visible to the naked eye in certain areas of the brain, particularly the substantia nigra, which bears its name because of the presence of neuromelanin. It is thought to arise from the spontaneous oxidation of dopamine to various polymers, including DOPA and dopamine quinones (135,136).

The function of neuromelanin is unclear (137). It may simply be an unavoidable by-product of catecholamine metabolism, representing little more than intracellular waste. Since it accumulates throughout much of life, many have postulated that its accumulation may ultimately be damaging to the very neurons that produce it (135). Thus, it has often been suggested that neuromelanin might play a role in causing Parkinson's disease (138). On the other hand, others have argued that it could be a protective agent, since it binds to many agents (139), some of which may be toxic, and may also function as a free radical scavenger. The role of neuromelanin in Parkinson's disease is further dealt with in Chapter 7.

The relation of neuromelanin to MPTP neurotoxicity has been no less controversial. Both MPTP and MPP^+ bind with high affinity to both synthetic dopamine melanin, as well as melanized areas of the central nervous system in vivo (140–144). These observations have led to the suggestion that this substance might be responsible for the sequestering of MPTP or MPP^+ which, in turn, could lead to its selectively toxic effects. If this were so, it should be possible to protect animals from the selective effects of MPTP by blocking the binding of MPTP–MPP^+ to neuromelanin. And indeed, a substance that does this, chloroquine, at least partially protects primates from MPTP neurotoxicity (145). Furthermore, Melamed and colleagues (146) have been able to show that injections of synthetic dopamine melanin may exacerbate toxicity.

In spite of these observations, many investigators have been cautious in accepting neuromelanin as a critical element in neurotoxicity (147). Animals that do not have neuromelanin, such as the mouse, are also susceptible to the effects of MPTP. Furthermore, other areas of the brain that are melanized do not appear to be consistently affected by MPTP.

At the very least, the connection between MPTP and neuromelanin has led to the formulation of new hypotheses to explain an old epidemiological observation. Lerner and Goldman (149) have put forth the intriguing hypothesis that could explain the observation in some studies that the prevalence of Parkinson's disease is lower in blacks than in whites (for further discussion of this issue, see Chapter 10). If an MPTP-like substance played a role in Parkinson's disease, they speculated that, after systemic exposure, cutaneous melanin might bind to MPP^+, serving as a protective "sink," thus preventing access of MPTP or MPP^+ to the CNS. Whether or not such a mechanism will really prove to be at work in

Parkinson's disease remains far from clear. However, this type of speculation provides an excellent example of how laboratory observations can lead to potential explanations for epidemiological data. It is very likely to be this type of interplay between "the field" and the laboratory that will ultimately unravel the cause of Parkinson's disease.

VI. AGING

Aging is the only unequivocally established risk factor for Parkinson's disease. Consequently, early observations that the effects of MPTP were age-related met with great enthusiasm (149). Several groups first noted that MPTP-induced striatal dopamine depletions were greater in older mice than in younger animals (74,150,151). Gupta and colleagues (152) also observed that while MPTP causes a decline in catechol fluorescence only in the nigra of young animals, in very old animals the locus ceruleus and ventral tegmental areas were also affected (152). However, in these earlier studies young (1–2 month) mice were compared with either fully mature (8–10 month) or truly aged (22–24 month) animals, with no intermediate points; thus, one could not be sure if these changes occurred gradually throughout the life span of animals, or primarily during the first half of life.

For these reasons, we recently investigated the changes in susceptibility to MPTP during aging in much greater detail. We used four different aged groups of C57BL/6 mice for the studies; young (6–8 weeks), fully mature (8–10 months), middle-aged (16 months), and old (22–24 months) (122). These studies confirmed that the effects of MPTP did indeed increase dramatically between the ages of 2 and 10 months. However, there was little additional increase between 10 and 16 months, and the degree of dopamine depletion caused by MPTP actually declined between the ages of 16 and 24 months.

These studies have also provided an opportunity to further elucidate the role of MAO in MPTP toxicity. The B form of the enzyme has been reported to increase with age in a variety of species, ranging from rats to humans (153–156). Most investigators originally hypothesized that MAO B was responsible for the enhanced MPTP toxicity with aging. In our studies, using the four different aged groups of animals referred to in the foregoing, MAO B activity closely paralleled the degree of MPTP toxicity in each of these age groups, gradually increasing to maximum levels at 16 months, and declining somewhat thereafter (122). Because of this close correlation between neurotoxicity and MAO levels at different ages, these results are strongly supportive of the hypothesis that MAO B is a critical determinant of MPTP neurotoxicity. They also indicate that the increasing susceptibility to MPTP with age is a phenomenon that occurs primarily during development and maturation, rather than during the period that might best be referred to as aging or senility.

There are several possible interpretations of these experiments. First, it may be that a certain degree of aging is required for the nervous system to become susceptible to environmental toxins. Once the nervous system is vulnerable (the MPTP data would suggest that this occurs in early to mid-adulthood), it still may take a considerable time for a neurotoxic insult to mature or evolve into a full-blown neurodegenerative process (157). In this scenario, maturation of the nervous system may represent "an enabler," rather than a part of the causative process. Alternatively, it could be that the rodent is not the best model for the study of the diseases of aging in humans. If so, it may well be necessary to extend these studies to monkeys, which are much closer phylogenetically to humans. For example, it will be very important to find out if MAO does increase throughout the aging process in primates and whether or not these changes are mirrored by a gradual increase in susceptibility to MPTP neurotoxicity as these animals grow older.

Correlating these results with epidemiological studies of Parkinson's disease, one could formulate a biological hypothesis for two different scenarios. If the data on the mice can be extrapolated to humans, then it might suggest that there is a window of susceptibility during adulthood that begins to decline later in life as MAO levels decrease. Some epidemiological data, in fact, suggest that such a decline occurs in Parkinson's disease, with a peak incidence in the late 50s (158). On the other hand, population-based studies suggest that the incidence of Parkinson's disease continues to increase with age, at least through the eighth to ninth decades (159,160). If that were true, and an MPTP-like phenomenon were the biological basis of Parkinson's disease, one would expect to see increasing MAO throughout the lifetime. Human studies of postmortem tissue suggest that this, in fact, is true (156,161–163). It will be very important to see if nonhuman primates mirror this data (there is little published in this area). If so, we may then have an excellent model for the study of the interrelations between MAO, aging, and MPTP neurotoxicity.

VII. MECHANISMS OF CELL DEATH

The precise mechanism by which MPTP actually kills cells has yet to be fully elucidated. At least three possible mechanisms have been entertained (19). Not surprisingly, these parallel those that have been postulated to cause the process of nigral cell degeneration that underlies Parkinson's disease. In the following section, each of these will be reviewed with a critical discussion of merits of each, as well as a review of their relevance to Parkinson's disease.

A. The Free Radical Hypothesis

Soon after the discovery of MPTP, there was great interest in the possibility that it might kill cells through a process of free radical generation. There were several reasons for this speculation. First, MPP^+ has a number of structural similarities to paraquat, a well-known herbicide. Paraquat generates highly reactive oxygen species in biological systems by a process known as redox cycling (164). However, the reduction potential required for redox-cycling of MPP^+ was much higher than that of paraquat, exceeding that for any known biological system in the brain (165). Furthermore, detailed experiments using oxidatively stressed hepatocytes (the same model that has been widely used to study paraquat), suggested that MPTP–MPP^+ did not act in a manner similar to paraquat; in fact, if anything, MPTP showed mild antioxidant properties in this system (166,167).

A second reason for the great attention paid to the free radical hypothesis of MPTP neurotoxicity relates to the current interest in the possibility that the cause of Parkinson's disease may be the result of oxidative stress. Many researchers currently believe that the oxidation of dopamine, a process that generates hydrogen peroxide and possibly other free radicals, may eventually lead to unacceptable levels of oxidative stress and cell death (168,169). This hypothesis has gained increasing attention in recent years because of the presence of iron in the substantia nigra (170,171). In its ferrous (Fe^{2+}) state, iron may enhance oxygen-mediated reactions (172). Thus, the combination of dopamine and high levels of iron might provide fertile ground for excessive oxidative stress. Youdim and associates have emphasized that this combination, in the presence of neuromelanin, could be an even more potent combination, since neuromelanin might facilitate this reaction (173–175).

In spite of the beauty of these theories, there is as yet little direct evidence that this process is really at work in Parkinson's disease. The situation is not much different when it comes to the studies that have been carried out on MPTP. To date, most studies that have been directed toward determining the role of free radical generation in MPTP neurotoxicity have failed to yield a consistent or convincing picture. Attempts to ameliorate MPTP toxicity by using antioxidants, such as vitamin E, to reduce MPTP toxicity have occasionally been successful (176–178), but an equal number of studies have failed to show that antioxidants or free radical scavengers block or even ameliorate MPTP toxicity (179–181). One piece of evidence that was at first thought to support the free radical hypothesis was that diethyldithiocarbamate (DDC) dramatically enhanced MPTP toxicity; this compound is known to suppress superoxide dismutase (182). However, additional experiments have shown that DDC enhances the MAO-mediated conversion of MPTP and MPP^+ and also appears to retard the elimination of MPP^+ from the brain (183). Thus, there may well be an alternative explanation to the DDC experiments.

In summary, although the free radical hypothesis is no longer the leading theory on the mechanism of action of MPTP, it would be premature to close the door on this area of investigation. As noted, there is great interest in this explanation of cell death in Parkinson's disease, and it still seems possible that MPTP acts, at least partially, by this mechanism. Certainly, further experiments in this area are warranted. This is particularly important, since definitive work in an in vivo setting has yet to be reported.

B. The Mitochondrial Hypothesis

In 1985 Nicklas and colleagues reported that MPTP interfered with mitochondrial respiration (184). This action appeared to be selective for NADH-linked substrates. Their report set off a flurry of research that has since led to a detailed picture of the way in which MPTP and MPP^+ affect mitochondrial function (185). It now appears that, once MPP^+ has gained entrance to cells, it is accumulated by the mitochondria; this process is dependent on the mitochondrial membrane gradient and, therefore, appears to be driven by the mitochondrial membrane potential. Once in mitochondria, MPP^+ inhibits complex I of the electron transport chain (184,186–190) (this is the same site of action of the herbicide rotenone; 191), thereby interrupting the process of cellular energy production. Thus, one of the earliest events that is seen in MPTP toxicity is a rapid depletion of ATP. Although definitive evidence is still lacking, most investigators believe that this energy depletion is the ultimate mediator of cell death (184,186–190). Although most of this work had been done in tissue culture preparations, it has recently been shown that an early depletion of ATP can be detected in vivo after MPTP administration (192). To accomplish this, it was necessary to use high-energy microwave irradiation to stop metabolic activity at the time of sacrifice, since ATP is rapidly depleted in the postmortem state.

These observations have led to an attempt to attenuate or prevent neurotoxicity by enhancing anaerobic metabolism. This was first achieved by DiMonte and colleagues (193), who found that MPTP toxicity in isolated hepatocytes could be overcome by providing alternative substrates for energy production; since fructokinase is preponderant in the liver, they found that fructose was the most effective substrate for providing an alternative source of energy production. Since glucose is a primary substrate for energy metabolism in the brain, one might expect that it would be possible to protect against neurotoxicity with glucose, although attempts to do this have not yet been reported. Interestingly, there is at least some epidemiological evidence that the prevalence of Parkinson's disease may be lower in diabetics, as would be expected if excessive glucose levels were protective (194).

These findings are of interest for a variety of reasons. First, they are timely in view of the increasing interest in the relation between neurodegenerative disease and energy production. MPTP provides a potential bridge between these two phenomena and, therefore, should be useful as an experimental tool for the study of this potential relation. Second, and perhaps one of the most tantalizing recent developments in Parkinson's disease, is the discovery that there are abnormalities in complex I in patients with idiopathic Parkinson's disease (195–199). This abnormality has been identified in a variety of tissues, including striatum, substantia nigra, muscle, and platelets. The finding in platelets is particularly exciting, since it could provide a biomarker for Parkinson's disease (197). The discovery of a biomarker would greatly enhance early detection and epidemiological studies in the disease (6). However, considerable controversy has already developed concerning the selectivity of this deficit. Although most investigators have found abnormalities of complex I in the nigrostriatal system, others have failed to find them in extranigral tissues. For the moment, it appears that it will be necessary to await additional studies to resolve the extent of mitochondrial dysfunction in Parkinson's disease.

Various groups have also been investigating the possibility that changes in mitochondrial DNA might orchestrate this complex I abnormality (185,199–206), but, although a variety of abnormalities have been found, none yet appear to be specific for Parkinson's disease (185,207). However, should it be possible to find an abnormality in mitochondrial DNA (or even nuclear DNA for that matter), it would be extraordinarily useful, since one could apply the technique of polymerase chain reaction (PCR) to detect this abnormality (6). Since only very small amounts of tissue would be needed to determine the presence or absence of such defects, if they are present in an accessible tissue, such as hair, buccal mucosa, or platelets, this could be used as a tool for screening the general population. Such a tool could be enormously useful for detection of preclinical disease and for a much more accurate determination of disease prevalence in epidemiological studies.

In summary, the mitochondrial hypothesis now appears to be the most viable candidate to explain how MPTP–MPP^+ kills cells. Furthermore, this hypothesis has provided a new research direction that offers a model to study basic deficits in energy production that could either cause or predispose neuronal populations to neurodegeneration. The demonstration of a similar deficit in a neurodegenerative disease, such as Parkinson's disease, has provided an even more compelling reason to aggressively pursue research in this area.

C. Excitatory Amino Acids

In the last several years, there has been an explosion of interest in the role of excitatory amino acids (EAAs) in neurological diseases, ranging from stroke and epilepsy, to human neurodegenerative disease (208). Not surprisingly, these studies have quickly invaded the field of MPTP neurotoxicity. This began rather abruptly with a report by Turski et al. (209) that indicated it was possible to block the loss of TH-positive neurons, caused by MPP^+ injected directly into the substantia nigra in rats, by using the NMDA antagonists such as dizocilpine maleate (MK-801). This was somewhat surprising, since Sonsalla and colleagues

(210) had earlier failed to find such an effect using striatal dopamine depletion as a marker of toxicity in mice after systemic administration of MPTP, even though they had been able to show, for the first time, that NMDA antagonists could prevent methamphetamine neurotoxicity. Unfortunately, additional studies have failed to clarify the exact role of EAAs in MPTP neurotoxicity. Those studies that have shown a protective effect of NMDA antagonists against MPTP–MPP^+ neurotoxicity have focused primarily on the substantia nigra and used TH immunohistochemistry as a marker of neuronal damage (209,211,212). Furthermore, Westerink (213) and Carboni (214), two groups using cerebral microdialysis in rats, have reported an increase in the extracellular levels of glutamate and aspartate in the striatum. On the other hand, MPTP–MPP^+-induced striatal dopamine depletion is either not prevented, or only partially blocked, by NMDA antagonists (210,215–218). Moreover, two recent studies with primary cultures of mesencephalic dopamine neurons found that MK-801 failed to protect dopaminergic neurons from MPP^+ toxicity in vitro (219,220).

Given the diverse results, it is quite probable that investigations into this question are likely to continue. Additional work on the effects of NMDA antagonists on the biodisposition of MPTP–MPP^+, and on the differential effects of MPTP–MPP^+ on nigrostriatal nerve terminals versus cell bodies, may help to further elucidate these differences. Such studies could be particularly important in view of the increasing interest in the role of excitatory amino acids in neurodegenerative disease (208). It is possible that the field may be moving toward a global concept in which energy depletion and excitatory amino acids are woven into the cascade of events that lead to neurodegeneration, not only in experimental models, but in human neurodegenerative disease as well (208,221). Should excitatory amino acids be found to represent a link in the chain of events that lead to MPTP neurotoxicity, this selective neurotoxin may become an experimental tool that bridges all of these elements, thereby providing an excellent experimental model for their investigation.

VIII. MPTP IN THE ENVIRONMENT

Before concluding this chapter on MPTP neurotoxicity, an overview of the effect that the discovery of this compound has had on the "environmental hypothesis" of Parkinson's disease is fitting. This review will be relatively brief, since many of the epidemiological investigations that MPTP has spawned are reviewed in Chapters 8 and 12. First, it should be noted that, in spite of a great deal of interest in the possibility of a parkinsongenic agent in the environment, little if any evidence has been produced that MPTP or similar substances may reside in the natural environment (the possible exception to this may the tetrahydroisoquinolines; 222–224). However, the task of finding such compounds in the environment is likely to be extraordinarily difficult.

On the other hand, in man-made environments, there is some evidence that MPTP can produce parkinsonism from environmental exposure. We have reported a chemist who used MPTP in his laboratory in the process of synthesizing new pharmaceutical compounds (225). He was exposed repeatedly to MPTP in the laboratory by inhalation and cutaneous contact. Several years later he developed Parkinson's disease. A survey of employees at a chemical supply plant where MPTP was made revealed no fewer than six employees with subtle signs of parkinsonism (226). Finally, a Danish chemist has been described who developed a severe parkinsonism while working with MPTP (16). All of these anecdotal observations suggest that environmental exposure to MPTP may induce a parkinsonian syndrome, but they do little to further the search for environmental agents that might cause the disease.

Perhaps the most effort in searching for an MPTP-like substance has been directed toward exposure to pesticides and herbicides. The reasons for this are severalfold. The major stimulus was the previously mentioned similarity of MPP^+ to the herbicide paraquat. From this observation, Barbeau and colleagues correlated the prevalence of Parkinson's disease in Quebec Province with a number of environmental factors, including the sales of pesticides and herbicides; he found a striking correlation between the two, as well as an association with paper and pulp mills (227). These observations were presented at approximately the same time that a second Canadian group found a striking correlation between rural living and young-onset Parkinson's disease (228). A more detailed analysis of these results implicated drinking well water as a potential source for an "environmental agent" (228).

Although all of these observations are tantalizing, it has not yet been possible to confirm or identify an agent, or group of environmental agents, that can be clearly linked to Parkinson's disease. Nonetheless, the search for such agents persists and, in my opinion, must still be viewed as being in its infancy.

IX. CONCLUSIONS

There is little doubt that the discovery of MPTP has had a bracing influence on Parkinson's disease research. Not only has the compound provided a very useful animal model for the disease, but it has provided a neurochemical tool to study mechanisms of cellular degeneration and has led to a renaissance of interest in the environmental hypothesis of Parkinson's disease. Each of these has led to new investigations on the possible causes or pathophysiological processes that might lead to Parkinson's disease. This research is likely to continue at an intensive pace, much of it having been generated by the discoveries of a mechanism of action of MPTP. I hope that this chapter has provided an adequate overview of why this might be true, as well as some insights into potential directions for future research. Given the numerous areas of new research directions highlighted in this review, it seems reasonable to hope that a great deal more will be learned in the decade to come, as we continue to use MPTP as a tool to explore the mysteries of Parkinson's disease.

REFERENCES

1. Bossi L, Caffaratti E. [Juvenile parkinsonian hemi-syndrome in a case of extracranial arteriovenous aneurysm of the vertebral artery. Clinical and radiological study]. Minerva Radiol 1967; 12:533–538.
2. Burns RS, Chiueh CC, Markey SP, Ebert MH, Jacobowitz DM, Kopin IJ. A primate model of parkinsonism: selective destruction of dopaminergic neurons in the pars compacta of the substantia nigra by *N*-methyl-4-phenyl-1,2,3,6-tetrahydropyridine. Proc Natl Acad Sci USA 1983; 80:4546–4550.
3. Langston JW, Ballard PA, Tetrud JW, Irwin I. Chronic parkinsonism in humans due to a product of meperidine-analog synthesis. Science 1983; 219:979–980.
4. Langston JW, Forno LS, Rebert CS, Irwin I. Selective nigral toxicity after systemic administration of 1-methyl-4-phenyl-1,2,3,6-tetrahydropyridine (MPTP) in the squirrel monkey. Brain Res 1984; 292:390–394.
5. Tanner CM, Langston JW. Do environmental toxins cause Parkinson's disease? A critical review. Neurology 1990; 40(suppl 3):17–30.
6. Langston JW, Koller W. The next frontier in Parkinson's disease: presymptomatic detection. Neurology 1991; 41(suppl 2):5–7.
7. Lewin R. Trail of ironies to Parkinson's disease [news]. Science 1984; 224:1083–1085.
8. Ballard PA, Tetrud JW, Langston JW. Permanent human parkinsonism due to 1-methyl-4-phenyl-1,2,3,6-tetrahydropyridine (MPTP): seven cases. Neurology 1985; 35:949–956.
9. Langston JW, Irwin I, Langston EB, DeLanney LE, Ricaurte GA. MPTP-induced parkinsonism in humans: a review of the syndrome and observations relating to the phenomenon of tardive toxicity. In: Markey SP, Castagnoli N Jr, Trevor AJ, Kopin IJ, eds. MPTP: a neurotoxin producing a parkinsonian syndrome. New York: Academic Press, 1986:9–21.
10. Langston JW. MPTP-induced parkinsonism: how good a model is it? In: Fahn S, Marsden CD, Teychenne PS, Jenner P, eds. Recent developments in Parkinson's disease. New York: Raven Press, 1986:119–126.
11. Stern Y, Langston JW. Intellectual changes in patients with MPTP-induced parkinsonism. Neurology 1985; 35:1506–1509.
12. Stern Y, Tetrud JW, Martin WRW, Kutner SJ, Langston JW. Cognitive change following MPTP exposure. Neurology 1990; 40:261–264.
13. Doty RL, Singh A, Tetrud JW, Langston JW. Lack of olfactory dysfunction in MPTP-induced parkinsonism. Ann Neurol 1992; 32:97–100.
14. Langston JW, Ballard PA. Parkinsonism induced by 1-methyl-4-phenyl-1,2,5,6-tetrahydropyridine: implications for treatment and the pathophysiology of Parkinson's disease. Can J Neurol Sci 1984; 11:160–165.

15. Davis GC, Williams AC, Markey SP, et al. Chronic parkinsonism secondary to intravenous injection of meperidine analogues. Psychiatry Res 1979; 1:249–254.
16. Burns RS, LeWitt PA, Ebert MH, Pakkenberg H, Kopin IJ. The clinical syndrome of striatal dopamine deficiency: parkinsonism induced by 1-methyl-4-phenyl-1,2,3,6-tetrahydropyridine (MPTP). N Engl J Med 1985; 312:1418–1421.
17. Calne DB, Langston JW, Martin WR, et al. Positron emission tomography after MPTP: observations relating to the cause of Parkinson's disease. Nature 1985; 317:246–248.
18. Martin WRW, Stoessel AJ, Adam MJ, et al. Imaging of dopamine systems in human subjects exposed to MPTP. In: Markey SP, Castagnoli N Jr, Trevor AJ, Kopin IJ, eds. MPTP: a neurotoxin producing a parkinsonian syndrome. New York: Academic Press, 1986:315–325.
19. Langston JW, Irwin I. MPTP: current concepts and controversies. Clin Neuropharmacol 1986; 9:485–507.
20. Langston JW, Irwin I, Langston EB, Forno LS. Pargyline prevents MPTP-induced parkinsonism in primates. Science 1984; 225:1480–1482.
21. Cohen G, Pasik P, Cohen B, Leist A, Mytilineou C, Yahr MD. Pargyline and deprenyl prevent the neurotoxicity of 1-methyl-4-phenyl-1,2,3,6-tetrahydropyridine (MPTP) in monkeys. Eur J Pharmacol 1985; 106:209–210.
22. Jenner P, Marsden CD, Costall B, Naylor RJ. MPTP and MPP^+ induced neurotoxicity in rodents and the common marmoset as experimental models for investigating Parkinson's disease. In: Markey SP, Castagnoli N Jr, Trevor AJ, Kopin IJ, eds. MPTP; a neurotoxin producing a parkinsonian syndrome. Orlando, FL: Academic Press, 1986:45–68.
23. Di Monte DA, Langston JW. MPTP-induced parkinsonism in non-human primates. In: Schneider JS, Gupta M, eds. Current Concepts in Parkinson's Research. Frankfurt: Hogrefe/Hans Huber Science Publishing, 1993:159–179.
24. Tetrud JW, Langston JW. Tremor in MPTP-induced parkinsonism. Neurology 1992; 42:407–410.
25. Tetrud JW, Langston JW. Early parkinsonism in humans due to MPTP exposure [abstract]. Neurology 1986; 36(suppl 2):308.
26. Mitchell IJ, Sambrook MA, Crossman AR. Subcortical changes in the regional uptake of [^{3}H]-2-deoxyglucose in the brain of the monkey during experimental choreiform dyskinesia elicited by injection of a gamma-aminobutyric acid antagonist into the subthalamic nucleus. Brain 1985; 108:405–422.
27. Bedard PJ, Di Paolo T, Falardeau P, Boucher R. Chronic treatment with L-dopa, but not bromocriptine induces dyskinesia in MPTP–parkinsonian monkeys. Correlation with [^{3}H]spiperone binding. Brain Res 1986; 379:294–299.
28. Clarke CE, Boyce S, Robertson RG, Sambrook MA, Crossman AR. Drug-induced dyskinesia in primates rendered hemiparkinsonian by intracarotid administration of 1-methyl-4-phenyl-1,2,3,6-tetrahydropyridine (MPTP). J Neurol Sci 1989; 90:307–314.
29. Schneider JS. Levodopa-induced dyskinesias in parkinsonian monkeys: relationship to extent of nigrostriatal damage. Pharmacol Biochem Behav 1989; 34:193–196.
30. Boyce S, Rupniak NMJ, Steventon MJ, Iversen SD. Characterisation of dyskine-

sias induced by L-dopa in MPTP-treated squirrel monkeys. Psychopharmacology 1990; 102:21–27.
31. Boyce S, Rupniak NMJ, Steventon MJ, Iversen SD. Nigrostriatal damage is required for induction of dyskinesias by L-DOPA in squirrel monkeys. Clin Neuropharmacol 1990; 13:448–458.
32. Kanazawa I, Kimura M, Murata M, Tanaka Y, Cho F. Choreic movements in the macaque monkey induced by kainic acid lesions of the striatum combined with L-dopa. Pharmacological, biochemical and physiological studies on neural mechanisms. Brain 1990; 113:509–535.
33. Rouillard C, Bédard PJ, Di Paolo T. Effects of chronic treatment of MPTP monkeys with bromocriptine alone or in combination with SKF 38393. Eur J Pharmacol 1990; 185:209–215.
34. Bedard PJ, Gomez-Mancilla B, Blanchette P, Gagnon C, Di Paolo T. Levodopa-induced dyskinesia: facts and fancy. What does the MPTP monkey model tell us? Can J Neurol Sci 1992; 19:134–137.
35. Jenner P, Marsden CD. The actions of 1-methyl-4-phenyl-1,2,3,6-tetrahydropyridine in animals as a model of Parkinson's disease. J Neural Transm [Suppl] 1986; 20:11–39.
36. Pifl C, Schingnitz G, Hornykiewicz O. The neurotoxin MPTP does not reproduce in the rhesus monkey the interregional pattern of striatal dopamine loss typical of human idiopathic Parkinson's disease. Neurosci Lett 1988; 92:228–233.
37. Kish SJ, Shannak K, Hornykiewicz O. Uneven pattern of dopamine loss in the striatum of patients with idiopathic Parkinson's disease. N Engl J Med 1988; 318:876–880.
38. Irwin I, DeLanney LE, Forno LS, Finnegan KT, Di Monte DA, Langston JW. The evolution of nigrostriatal neurochemical changes in the MPTP-treated squirrel monkey. Brain Res 1990; 531:242–252.
39. Moratalla R, Quinn B, DeLanney LE, Langston JW, Graybiel AM. Differential vulnerability of primate caudate–putamen and striosome–matrix dopamine systems to the neurotoxic effect of MPTP. Proc Natl Acad Sci USA 1992; 89:3859–3863.
40. Elsworth JD, Deutch AY, Redmond DE Jr, Sladek JR Jr, Roght RH. Differential responsiveness to 1-methyl-4-phenyl-1,2,3,6-tetrahydropyridine toxicity in subregions of the primate substantia nigra and striatum. Life Sci 1987; 40:193–202.
41. Pifl C, Schingnitz G, Hornykiewicz O. Effect of 1-methyl-4-phenyl-1,2,3,6-tetrahydropyridine on the regional distribution of brain monoamines in the rhesus monkey. Neuroscience 1991; 44:591–605.
42. Pifl C, Bertel O, Schingnitz G, Hornykiewicz O. Extrastriatal dopamine in symptomatic and asymptomatic rhesus monkeys treated with 1-methyl-4-phenyl-1,2,3,6-tetrahydropyridine (MPTP). Neurochem Int 1990; 17:263–270.
43. Robertson RG, Clarke CA, Boyce S, Sambrook MA, Crossman AR. The role of striatopallidal neurones utilizing gamma-aminobutyric acid in the pathophysiology of MPTP-induced parkinsonism in the primate: evidence from [^{3}H] flunitrazepam autoradiography. Brain Res 1990; 531:95–104.
44. Elsworth JD, Deutch AY, Redmond DE Jr, Sladek JR Jr, Roth RH. MPTP-induced parkinsonism: relative changes in dopamine concentration in subregions

of substantia nigra, ventral tegmental area and retrorubral field of symptomatic and asymptomatic vervet monkeys. Brain Res 1990; 513:320–324.
45. Dacko S, Schneider JS. Met-enkephalin immunoreactivity in the basal ganglia in symptomatic and asymptomatic MPTP-exposed monkeys: correlation with degree of parkinsonian symptoms. Neurosci Lett 1991; 127:49–52.
46. Porrino LJ, Viola JJ, Crane AM, Pontieri FE. Alterations in opiate receptor binding in MPTP-induced hemiparkinsonian monkeys. Neurosci Lett 1991; 127:155–159.
47. Schneider JS. Chronic exposure to low doses of MPTP. II. Neurochemical and pathological consequences in cognitively-impaired, motor asymptomatic monkeys. Brain Res 1990; 534:25–36.
48. Forno LS, DeLanney LE, Langston JW. Similarities and differences between MPTP-induced Parkinson's disease. Neuropathologic considerations. In: Narabayshi H, Nagatsu T, Yanagisawa N, Mizuno Y, eds. Parkinson's disease: from basic research to treatment. Proceedings of the 10th international symposum on Parkinson's disease. Raven Press, 1993:600–608.
49. Forno LS. Pathology of Parkinson's disease. In: Marsden SD, Fahn S, eds. Movement disorders. London: Butterworth Scientific, 1982:25–40.
50. Forno LS, Langston JW, DeLanney LE, Irwin I, Ricaurte GA. Locus ceruleus lesions and eosinophilic inclusions in MPTP-treated monkeys. Ann Neurol 1986; 20:449–455.
51. Mitchell IJ, Cross AJ, Sambrook MA, Crossman AR. Sites of the neurotoxic action of 1-methyl-4-phenyl-1,2,3,6-tetrahydropyridine in the macaque monkey include the ventral tegmental area and the locus coeruleus. Neurosci Lett 1985; 61:195–200.
52. Hyman C, Hofer M, Barde YA, et al. BDNF is a neurotrophic factor for dopaminergic neurons of the substantia nigra. Nature 1991; 350:230–232.
53. Tanaka J, Nakamura H, Honda S, Takada K, Kato S. Neuropathological study on 1-methyl-4-phenyl-1,2,3,6-tetrahydropyridine of the crab-eating monkey. Acta Neuropathol 1988; 75:370–376.
54. Mavridis M, Degryse A-D, Lategan AJ, Marien MR, Colpaert FC. Effects of locus coeruleus lesions on parkinsonian signs, striatal dopamine and substantia nigra cell loss after 1-methyl-4-phenyl-1,2,3,6-tetrahydropyridine in monkeys: a possible role for the locus coeruleus in the progression of Parkinson's disease. Neuroscience 1991; 41:507–523.
55. German DC, Durach A, Askari S, Speciale SG, Bowden DM. 1-Methyl-4-phenyl-1,2,3,6-tetrahydropyridine-induced parkinsonian syndrome in *Macaca fascicularis:* which midbrain dopaminergic neurons are lost? Neuroscience 1988; 24:161–174.
56. Gibb WRG, Terruli M, Lees AJ, Jenner P, Marsden CD. The evolution and distribution of morphological changes in the nervous system of the common marmoset following the acute administration of 1-methyl-4-phenyl-1,2,3,6-tetrahydropyridine. Mov Disord 1989; 4:53–74.
57. Forno LS, Langston JW, DeLanney LE, Irwin I. An electron microscopic study of MPTP-induced inclusion bodies in an old monkey. Brain Res 1988; 448:150–157.
58. Boyce S, Kelly E, Reavill C, Jenner P, Marsden CD. Repeated administration

of *N*-methyl-4-phenyl-1,2,5,6-tetrahydropyridine to rats is not toxic to striatal dopamine neurons. Biochem Pharmacol 1984; 33:1747–1752.
59. Chiueh CC, Markey SP, Burns RS, Johannessen JN, Pert A, Kopin IJ. Neurochemical and behavioral effects of systemic and intranigral administration of *N*-methyl-4-pheynl-1,2,3,6-tetrahydropyridine in the rat. Eur J Pharmacol 1984; 100:189–194.
60. Enz A, Hefti F, Frick W. Acute administration of 1-methyl-4-phenyl-1,2,3,6-tetrahydropyridine (MPTP) reduces dopamine and serotonin but accelerates norepinephrine metabolism in the rat brain, effect of chronic pretreatment with MPTP. Eur J Pharmacol 1984; 101:37–44.
61. Sahgal A, Andrews JS, Biggins JA, et al. *N*-Methyl-4-phenyl-1,2,3,6-tetrahydropyridine (MPTP) affects locomotor activity without producing a nigrostriatal lesion in the rat. Neurosci Lett 1984; 48:179–184.
62. Rub H, Henning K, Ekhardt H, Przuntek H. The influence of *N*-methyl-4-phenyl-1,2,3,6-tetrahydropyridine on the levels of dopamine, serotonin and their metabolites in the caudate nucleus of the rat. Arzneimittelforschung 1985; 35:481.
63. Bradbury AJ, Costall B, Domeney AM, et al. 1-Methyl-4-phenylpyridine is neurotoxic to the nigrostriatal dopamine pathway. Nature 1986; 319:56–57.
64. Donnan GA, Kaczmarczyk SJ, Solopotias T, et al. The neurochemical and clinical effects of 1-methyl-4-phenyl-1,2,3,6-tetrahydropyridine in small animals. Clin Exp Neurol 1986; 22:155–164.
65. Riachi NJ, Harik SI, Kalaria RN, Sayre LM. On the mechanisms underlying 1-methyl-4-phenyl-1,2,3,6-tetrahydropyridine neurotoxicity. II. Susceptibility among mammalian species correlates with the toxin's metabolic patterns in brain microvessels and liver. J Pharmacol Exp Ther 1988; 244:443–448.
66. Jarvis MF, Wagner GC. 1-Methyl-4-phenyl-1,2,3,6-tetrahydropyridine-induced neurotoxicity in the rat: characterization and age-dependent effects. Synapse 1990; 5:104–112.
67. Riachi NJ, Behmand RA, Harik SI. Correlation of MPTP neurotoxicity in vivo with oxidation of MPTP by the brain and blood–brain barrier in vitro in five rat strains. Brain Res 1991; 555:19–24.
68. Heikkila RE, Hess A, Duvoisin RC. Dopaminergic neurotoxicity of 1-methyl-4-phenyl-1,2,5,6-tetrahydropyridine in mice. Science 1984; 224:1451–1453.
69. Wallace RA, Boldry R, Schmittgen T, Miller D, Uretsky N. Effect of 1-methyl-4-phenyl-1,2,3,6-tetrahydropyridine (MPTP) on monoamine neurotransmitters in mouse brain and heart. Life Sci 1984; 35:285–291.
70. Sonsalla PK, Heikkila RE. Neurotoxic effects of 1-methyl-4-phenyl-1,2,3,6-tetrahydropyridine (MPTP) and methamphetamine in several strains of mice. Prog Neuropsychopharmacol Biol Psychiatry 1988; 12:345–354.
71. Weihmuller FB, Hadjiconstantinou M, Bruno JP. Acute stress or neuroleptics elicit sensorimotor deficits in MPTP-treated mice. Neurosci Lett 1988; 85:137–142.
72. Langston JW, Irwin I, DeLanney LE. Factors that affect the expression of neurotoxicity: lessons from MPTP. In: Rose FC, Norris FH, eds. ALS: new advances in toxicology and epidemiology. New York: Smith-Gordon, 1990:247–255.
73. Ricaurte GA, DeLanney LE, Irwin I, Langston JW. Older dopaminergic neurons do not recover from the effects of MPTP. Neuropharmacology 1987; 26:97–99.

74. Ricaurte GA, Irwin I, Forno LS, DeLanney LE, Langston EB, Langston JW. Aging and MPTP-induced degeneration of dopaminergic neurons in the substantia nigra. Brain Res 1987; 403:43–51.
75. Kitt CA, Cork LC, Eidelberg F, Joh TH, Price DL. Injury of nigral neurons exposed to 1-methyl-4-phenyl-1,2,3,6-tetrahydropyridine: a tyrosine hydroxylase immunocytochemical study in monkey. Neuroscience 1986; 17:1089–1103.
76. Langston JW, Irwin I, Langston EB, Forno LS. 1-Methyl-4-phenyl-pyridinium ion (MPP^+): identification of a metabolite of MPTP, a toxin selective to the substantia nigra. Neurosci Lett 1984; 48:87–92.
77. Irwin I, Langston JW. Selective accumulation of MPP^+ in the substantia nigra: a key to neurotoxicity? Life Sci 1985; 36:207–212.
78. Markey SP, Johannessen JN, Chiueh CC, Burns RS, Herkenham MA. Intraneuronal generation of a pyridinium metabolite may cause drug-induced parkinsonism. Nature 1984; 311:464–467.
79. Chiba K, Peterson LA, Castagnoli KP, Trevor AJ, Castagnoli N Jr. Studies on the molecular mechanism of bioactivation of the selective nigrostriatal toxin 1-methyl-4-phenyl-1,2,3,6-tetrahydropyridine. Drug Metab Dispos 1985; 13:342–347.
80. Peterson LA, Caldera PS, Trevor AJ, Chiba K, Castagnoli N Jr. Studies on the 1-methyl-4-phenyl-2,3-dihydropyridinium species 2,3-$MPDP^+$, the monoamine oxidase catalyzed oxidation product of the nigrostriatal toxin 1-methyl-4-phenyl-1,2,3,6-tetrahydropyridine (MPTP). J Med Chem 1986; 28:1432–1436.
81. Sayre LM, Arora PK, Iacofano LA, Harik SI. Comparative toxicity of MPTP, MPP^+ and 3,3-dimethyl-$MPDP^+$ to dopaminergic neurons of the rat substantia nigra. Eur J Pharmacol 1986; 124:171–174.
82. Wu EY, Chiba K, Trevor AJ, Castagnoli N Jr. Interactions of the 1-methyl-4-phenyl-2,3-dihydropyridinium species with synthetic dopamine–melanin. Life Sci 1986; 39:1695–1700.
83. Trevor AJ, Castagnoli N Jr, Caldera PS, Ramsay RR, Singer TP III. Bioactivation of MPTP: reactive metabolites and possible biochemical sequelae. Life Sci 1987; 40:713–719.
84. Wilson JA, Wilson JS, Weight FF. $MPDP^+$ causes a non-reversible decrease in neostriatal synaptic transmission in mouse brain slice. Brain Res 1987; 425:376–379.
85. Korytowski W, Felix CC, Kalyanaraman B. Evidence for the one-electron oxidation of 1-methyl-4-phenyl-2,3-dihydropyridinium ($MPDP^+$). Biochem Biophys Res Commun 1987; 147:354–360.
86. Trevor AJ, Castagnoli N Jr Singer TP. The formation of reactive intermediates in the MAO-catalyzed oxidation of the nigrostriatal toxin 1-methyl-4-phenyl-1,2,3,6-tetrahydropyridine (MPTP). Toxicology 1988; 49:513–519.
87. Chacon JN, Chedekel MR, Land EJ, Truscott TG. Chemically induced Parkinson's disease II: intermediates in the oxidation and reduction of the 1-methyl-4-phenyl-2,3-dihydropyridinium ion and its depronated form. Biochem Biophys Res Commun 1989; 158:63–71.
88. Di Monte DA, Wu EY, Irwin I, DeLanney LE, Langston JW. Production and

disposition of 1-methyl-4-phenylpyridinium in primary cultures of mouse astrocytes. Glia 1992; 5:48–55.
89. Chiba K, Trevor AJ, Castagnoli N Jr. Metabolism of the neurotoxic tertiary amine, MPTP, by brain monoamine oxidase. Biochem Biophys Res Commun 1984; 120:574–578.
90. Singer TP, Salach JI, Castagnoli N Jr, Trevor AJ. Interactions of the neurotoxic amine 1-methyl-4-phenyl-1,2,3,6- tetrahydropyridine with monoamine oxidases. Biochem J 1986; 235:785–789.
91. Johannessen JN, Kelner L, Hanselman D, Shih MC, Markey SP. In vitro oxidation of MPTP by primate neural tissue: a potential model of MPTP neurotoxicity. Neurochem Int 1985; 7:169–176.
92. Sanchez-Ramos JR, Barrett JN, Goldstein M, Weiner WJ, Hefti F. 1-Methyl-4-phenylpyridinium (MPP^+) but not 1-methyl-4-phenyl-1,2,3,6-tetrahydropyridine (MPTP) selectively destroys dopaminergic neurons in cultures of dissociated rat mesencephalic neurons. Neurosci Lett 1986; 72:215–220.
93. Heikkila RE, Manzino L, Cabbat FS, Duvoisin RC. Protection against the dopaminergic neurotoxicity of 1-methyl-4-phenyl-1,2,5,6-tetrahydropyridine by monoamine oxidase inhibitors. Nature 1984; 311:467–469.
94. Heikkila RE, Duvoisin RC, Finberg JPM, Youdim MBH. Prevention of MPTP-induced neurotoxicity by AGN-1133 and AGN-1136, selective inhibitors of monoamine oxidase-B. Eur J Pharmacol 1985; 116:313–317.
95. Fuller RW, Hemrick-Leucke SK. Influence of selective, reversible inhibitors of monoamine oxidase on the prolonged depletion of striatal dopamine by 1-methyl-4-phenyl-1,2,3,6-tetrahydropyridine in mice. Life Sci 1985; 37:1089–1096.
96. Javitch JA, Snyder SH. Uptake of MPTP ($^+$) by dopamine neurons explains selectivity of parkinsonism-inducing neurotoxin, MPTP. Eur J Pharmacol 1984; 104:455–456.
97. Javitch JA, D'Amato RJ, Strittmatter SM, Snyder SH. Parkinsonism-inducing neurotoxin, *N*-methyl-4-phenyl-1,2,3,6-tetrahydropyridine: uptake of the metabolite *N*-methyl-4-phenylpyridine by dopamine neurons explains selective toxicity. Neurobiology 1985; 82:2173–2177.
98. Chiba K, Trevor AJ, Castagnoli N Jr. Active uptake of MPP^+, a metabolite of MPTP, by brain synaptosomes. Biochem Biophys Res Commun 1984; 128:1229–1232.
99. Ransom BR, Kunis DM, Irwin I, Langston JW. Astrocytes convert the parkinsonism-inducing neurotoxin, MPTP, to its active metabolite, MPP^+. Neurosci Lett 1987; 75:323–328.
100. Schinelli S, Zuddas A, Kopin IJ, Barker JL, Di Porzio U. 1-Methyl-4-phenyl-1,2,3,6-tetrahydropyridine metabolism and 1-methyl-4-phenylpyridinium uptake in dissociated cell cultures from the embryonic mesencephalon. J Neurochem 1988; 50:1900–1907.
101. Di Monte DA, Wu EY, Irwin I, DeLanney LE, Langston JW. Biotransformation of 1-methyl-4-phenyl-1,2,3,6-tetrahydropyridine in primary cultures of mouse astrocytes. J Pharmacol Exp Ther 1991; 258:594–600.
102. Westlund KN, Denney RM, Kochersperger LM, Rose RM, Abell CW. Distinct

monoamine oxidase A and B populations in primate brain. Science 1985; 230:181–183.
103. Levitt P, Pintar JE, Breakefield XO. Immunocytochemical demonstration of monoamine oxidase B in brain astrocytes and serotonergic neurons. Proc Natl Acad Sci USA 1982; 79:6385–6389.
104. Melamed E, Pikarski E, Goldberg A, Rosenthal J, Uzzan A, Conforti N. Effect of serotonergic, corticostriatal and kainic acid lesions on the dopaminergic neurotoxicity of 1-methyl-4-phenyl-1,2,3,6-tetrahydropyridine (MPTP) in mice. Brain Res 1986; 399:178–180.
105. Brooks WJ, Jarvis MF, Wagner GC. Astrocytes as a primary locus for the conversion MPTP into MPP^+. J Neural Transm 1989; 76:1–12.
106. Di Monte DA, Wy EY, Langston JW. Role of astrocytes in MPTP metabolism and toxicity. Ann NY Acad Sci 1992; 648:219–228.
107. Di Monte DA, Wu EY, DeLanney LE, Irwin I, Langston JW. Toxicity of 1-methyl-4-phenyl-1,2,3,6-tetrahydropyridine in primary cultures of mouse astrocytes. J Pharmacol Exp Ther 1992; 261:1–6.
108. Wu E, Shinka T, Caldera-Munoz P, Yoshizumi H, Trevor A, Castagnoli N Jr. Metabolic studies on the nigrostriatal toxin MPTP and its MAO-B generated dihydropyridinium metabolite $MPDP^+$. Chem Res Toxicol 1988; 1:186–194.
109. Arora PK, Riachi NJ, Harik SI, Sayre LM. Chemical oxidation of 1-methyl-4-phenyl-1,2,3,6-tetrahydropyridine (MPTP) and its in vivo metabolism in rat brain and liver. Biochem Biophys Res Commun 1988; 152:1339–1347.
110. Duffel MW, Gillespie SG. Microsomal flavin-containing monooxygenase activity in rat corpus striatum. J Neurochem 1984; 42:1350–1353.
111. Langston JW, Irwin I, Ricaurte GA. Neurotoxins, parkinsonism, and Parkinson's disease. Pharmacol Ther 1987; 32:19–46.
112. Melamed E, Rosenthal J, Cohen O, Globus M, Uzzan A. Dopamine but not norepinephrine or serotonin uptake inhibitors protect mice against neurotoxicity of MPTP. Eur J Pharmacol 1985; 116:179–181.
113. Ricaurte GA, Langston JW, DeLanney LE, Irwin I, Brooks JD. Dopamine uptake blockers protect against the dopamine depleting effects of 1-methyl-4-phenyl-1,2,3,6-tetrahydropyridine (MPTP) in the mouse striatum. Neurosci Lett 1985; 59:259–264.
114. Mayer RA, Jarvis MF, Wagner GC. Cocaine blocks the dopamine depletion induced by MPTP. Res Commun Chem Pathol Pharmacol 1985; 49:145–148.
115. Melamed E, Rosenthal J, Globus M, Cohen O, Uzzan A. Suppression of MPTP-induced dopaminergic neurotoxicity in mice by nomifensine and L-dopa. Brain Res 1985; 342:401–404.
116. Sundstrom E, Jonsson G. Pharmacological interference with the neurotoxic action of 1-methyl-4-phenyl-1,2,3,6-tetrahydropyridine (MPTP) on central catecholamine neurons in the mouse. Eur J Pharmacol 1985; 110:293–299.
117. Pileblad E, Carlsson A. Catecholamine-uptake inhibitors prevent the neurotoxicity of 1-methyl-4-phenyl-1,2,3,6-tetrahydropyridine (MPTP) in mouse brain. Neuropharmacology 1985; 24:689–692.
118. Mayer RA, Kindt MV, Heikkila RE. Prevention of the nigrostriatal toxicity of 1-

methyl-4-phenyl-1,2,3,6-tetrahydropyridine by inhibitors of 3,4-dihydroxyphenylethylamine transport. J Neurochem 1986; 47:1073–1079.

119. Schultz W, Scarnati E, Sundstrom E, Tsutsumi T, Jonsson G. The catecholamine uptake blocker nomifensine protects against MPTP-induced parkinsonism in monkeys. Exp Brain Res 1986; 63:216–220.

120. Schultz W, Scarnati E, Sundstrom E, Romo R. Protection against 1-methyl-4-phenyl-1,2,3,6-tetrahydropyridine-induced parkinsonism by the catecholamine uptake inhibitor nomifensine: behavioral analysis in monkeys with partial striatal dopamine depletions. Neuroscience 1989; 31:219–230.

121. Johannessen JN, Chiueh CC, Burns RS, Markey SP. Differences in the metabolism of MPTP in the rodent and primate parallel differences in sensitivity to its neurotoxic effects. Life Sci 1985; 36:219–225.

122. Irwin I, Finnegan KT, DeLanney LE, Di Monte D, Langston JW. The relationships between aging, monoamine oxidase, striatal dopamine and the effects of MPTP in C57BL/6 mice: a critical reassessment. Brain Res 1992; 572:224–231.

123. Kalaria RN, Mitchell MJ, Harik SI. Correlation of 1-methyl-4-phenyl-1,2,3,6-tetrahydropyridine neurotoxicity with blood–brain barrier monoamine oxidase activity. Proc Natl Acad Sci USA 1987; 84:3521–3525.

124. Riachi NJ, Harik SI. Strain differences in systemic 1-methyl-4-phenyl-1,2,3,6-tetrahydropyridine neurotoxicity in mice correlate best with monoamine oxidase activity at the blood–brain barrier. Life Sci 1988; 42:2359–2363.

125. Riachi NJ, LaManna JC, Harik SI. Entry of 1-methyl-4-phenyl-1,2,3,6-tetrahydropyridine into the rat brain. J Pharmacol Exp Ther 1989; 249:744–748.

126. Cashman JR, Ziegler DM. Contribution of *N*-oxygenation to the metabolism of MPTP (1-methyl-4-phenyl-1,2,3,6-tetrahydropyridine) by various liver preparations. Mol Pharmacol 1986; 29:163–167.

127. Chiba K, Kubota E, Miyakawa T, Kato Y, Ishizaki T. Characterization of hepatic microsomal metabolism as an in vivo detoxification pathway of 1-methyl-4-phenyl-1,2,3,6-tetrahydropyridine in mice. J Pharmacol Exp Ther 1988; 246:1108–1115.

128. Chiba K, Horii H, Kubota E, Ishizaki T, Kato Y. Effects of *N*-methylmercaptoimidazole on the disposition of MPTP and its metabolites in mice. Eur J Pharmacol 1990; 180:59–67.

129. Rollema H, De Vries JB, Damsma G, et al. The use of in vivo brain dialysis of dopamine, acetylcholine, amino acids and lactic acid in studies on the neurotoxin 1-methyl-4-phenyl-1,2,3,6-tetrahydropyridine (MPTP). Toxicology 1988; 49:503–511.

130. Rollema H, Kuhr WG, Kranenborg GL, De Vries JB, Van Den Berg C. MPP^+-induced efflux of dopamine and lactate from rat striatum have similar time courses as shown by in vivo brain dialysis. J Pharmacol Exp Ther 1988; 245:858–866.

131. Rollema H, Alexander GM, Grothusen JR, Matos FF, Castagnoli N Jr. Comparison of the effects of intracerebrally administered MPP^+ (1-methyl-4-phenylpyridinium) in three species: microdialysis of dopamine and metabolites in mouse, rat and monkey striatum. Neurosci Lett 1989; 106:275–281.

132. Rollema H, Johnson EA, Booth RG, et al. In vivo intracerebral microdialysis studies in rats of MPP^+ analogs and related charged species. J Med Chem 1990; 33:2221–2230.

133. Santiago M, Westerink BHC, Rollema H. Responsiveness of striatal dopamine release in awake animals after chronic 1-methyl-4-phenylpyridinium ion-induced lesions of the substantia nigra. J Neurochem 1991; 56:1336–1342.
134. Santiago M, Rollema H, De Vries JB, Westerink BHC. Acute effects of intranigral application of MPP^+ on nigral and bilateral striatal release of dopamine simultaneously recorded by microdialysis. Brain Res 1991; 538:226–230.
135. Graham DG. Oxidative pathways for catecholamines in the genesis of neuromelanin and cytotoxic quinones. Mol Pharmacol 1978; 14:633–643.
136. Sayre LM. Biochemical mechanism of action of the dopaminergic neurotoxin 1-methyl-4-phenyl-1,2,3,6-tetrahydropyridine (MPTP). Toxicol Lett 1989; 48:121–149.
137. Graham DG. On the origin and significance of neuromelanin. Arch Pathol Lab Med 1979; 103:359–362.
138. Mann DMA, Yates PO. Possible role of neuromelanin in the pathogenesis of Parkinson's disease. Mech Age Dev 1983; 21:193–203.
139. Salazar M, Sokoloski TD, Patil PN. Binding of dopaminergic drugs by the neuromelanin of the substantia nigra, synthetic melanins and melanin granules. Fed Proc 1978; 37:2403–2407.
140. Lyden A, Bondesson U, Larsson BS, Lindquist NG. Melanin affinity of 1-methyl-4-phenyl-1,2,3,6-tetrahydropyridine, and inducer of chronic parkinsonism in humans. Acta Pharmacol 1983; 53:429–432.
141. Hartvig P, Lindquist NG, Aquilonius SM, et al. Distribution of 1-methyl-4-phenyl-1,2,3,6-tetrahydropyridine in experimental animals studied by positron emission tomography and whole body autoradiography. Life Sci 1986; 38:89–97.
142. Lindquist NG, Lyden-Sokolowski A, Larsson BS. Accumulation of a parkinsonism-inducing neurotoxin in melanin-bearing neurons: autoradiographic studies on ^{3}H-MPTP. Acta Pharmacol Toxicol 1986; 59:161–164.
143. D'Amato RJ, Lipman ZP, Snyder SH. Selectivity of the parkinsonian neurotoxin MPTP: toxic metabolite MPP^+ binds to neuromelanin. Science 1986; 231:987–989.
144. D'Amato RJ, Benham DF, Snyder SH. Characterization of the binding of *N*-methyl-4-phenylpyridine, the toxic metabolite of the parkinsonian neurotoxin *N*-methyl-4 phenyl -1,2,3,6-tetrahydropyridine, to neuromelanin. J Neurochem 1987; 48:653–658.
145. D'Amato RJ, Alexander GM, Schwartzman RJ, Kitt CA, Price DL,Snyder SH. Evidence for neuromelanin involvement in MPTP-induced neurotoxicity. Nature 1987; 327:324–326.
146. Melamed E, Soffer D, Rosenthal J, Reches A,Pikarski E. Effect of intrastriatal and intranigral administration of synthetic neuromelanin on the dopaminergic neurotoxicity of MPTP in rodents. Neurosci Lett 1987; 83:41–46.
147. Langston JW. MPTP and Parkinson's disease. Trends Neurosci 1985; 8:79–83.
148. Lerner MR, Goldman RS. Skin colour, MPTP, and Parkinson's disease. Lancet 1987; 1:212.
149. Lewin R. Age factors loom in parkinsonian research. Science 1986; 234:1200–1201.
150. Fields JZ. Aging and a novel neurotoxin, MPTP (1-methyl-4-phenyl-1,2,5,6-

tetrahydropyridine) elicit deficits in brain dopamine tracts and increases in duodenal ulcers. Dig Dis Sci 1985; 30:374.

151. Jarvis MF, Wagner GC. Age-dependent effects of 1-methyl-4-phenyl-1,2,3,6-tetrahydropyridine (MPTP). Neuropharmacology 1985; 24:581–583.
152. Gupta M, Gupta BK, Thomas R, Bruemmer V, Sladek JR Jr, Felten DL. Aged mice are more sensitive to 1-methyl-4-phenyl-1,2,3,6-tetrahydropyridine than young adults. Neurosci Lett 1986; 70:326–331.
153. Samorajski T, Rolsten C. Age and regional differences in the chemical composition of brain of mice, monkeys and humans. Proc Brain Res 1973; 40:253–265.
154. Riederer P, Wuketich S. Time course of nigrostriatal degeneration in Parkinson's disease. J Neural Transm 1976; 38:277–301.
155. Benedetti MS, Keane PE. Differential changes in monoamine oxidase A and B activity in the aging rat brain. J Neurochem 1980; 35:1026–1032.
156. Fowler CJ, Wilberg A, Oreland L, Marcusson J, Winblad B. The effect of age on the activity and molecular properties of human brain monoamine oxidase. J Neural Transm 1980; 49:1–20.
157. Calne DB, Langston JW. Aetiology of Parkinson's disease. Lancet 1983; 2:1457-1459.
158. Koller W, O'Hara R, Weiner W, et al. Relationship of aging to Parkinson's disease. Adv Neurol 1986; 45:317–321.
159. Mutch WJ, Dingwall-Fordyce I, Downie AW, Paterson JG,Roy SK. Parkinson's disease in a Scottish city. Br Med J 1986; 292:534–536.
160. Tanner CM, Thelen JA, Offord KP, Rademacher D, Goetz CG,Kurland LT. Parkinson's disease (PD) incidence in Olmsted County, MN: 1935–1988. Neurology 1992; 42(suppl 3):194.
161. Robinson DS, Davis JM, Nies A, Ravaris CL,Sylwester D. Relation of sex and aging to monoamine oxidase activity of human brain, plasma, and platelets. Arch Gen Psychiatry 1971; 24:536–539.
162. Nies A, Robinson DS, Davis JM, Ravaris CL. Changes in monoamine oxidase with aging. In: Eisdorfer C, Fann WE, eds. Advances in behavioral biology, vol 6. Psychopharmacology and aging. New York: Plenum Press, 1973:41–54.
163. Cote LJ, Kremzner LT. Biochemical changes in normal aging in human brain. In: Mayeux R, Rosen WG, eds. The dementias. New York: Raven Press, 1983: 19–30.
164. Bus JS, Aust SD, Gibson JE. Paraquat: model for oxidant-initiated toxicity. Environ Health Perspect 1984; 55:37–46.
165. Frank DM, Arora PK, Blumer JL,Sayre LM. Model study on the bioreduction of paraquat, MPP^+, and analogs. Evidence against a "redox cycling" mechanism in MPTP neurotoxicity. Biochem Biophys Res Commun 1987; 147:1095–1104.
166. Di Monte D, Sandy MS, Ekstrom G, Smith MT. Comparative studies on the mechanism of paraquat and 1-methyl-4-phenylpyridine (MPP^+) cytotoxicity. Biochem Biophys Res Commun 1986; 137:303–309.
167. Ekstrom G, Di Monte DA, Sandy MS, Smith MT. Comparative toxicity and antioxidant activity of 1-methyl-4-phenyl-1,2,3,6-tetrahydropyridine and its monoamine oxidase B-generated metabolites in isolated hepatocytes and liver microsomes. Arch Biochem Biophys 1987; 255:14–18.

168. Cohen G. The pathophysiology of Parkinson's disease: biochemical aspects of dopamine neuron senescence. J Neural Transm 1983; 19:89–103.
169. Olanow C. Oxidation reactions in Parkinson's disease. Neurology 1990; 40 (suppl 3):32–37.
170. Sofic E, Riederer P, Heinsen H, et al. Increased iron (III) and total iron content in post mortem substantia nigra of parkinsonian brain. J Neural Transm 1988; 74:199–205.
171. Sofic E, Paulus W, Jellinger K, Riederer P,Youdim MBH. Selective increase of iron in substantia nigra zona compacta of parkinsonian brains. J Neurochem 1991; 56:978–982.
172. Halliwell B, Gutteridge JMC. Free radicals in biology and medicine. Oxford: Clarendon Press, 1985.
173. Youdim MBH, Ben-Shachar D, Riederer P. Is Parkinson's disease a progressive siderosis of substantia nigra resulting in iron and melanin induced neurodegeneration? Acta Neurol Scand 1989; 126:47–54.
174. Ben-Shachar D, Youdim MBH. Selectivity to melanized nigra–striatal dopamine neurons to degeneration in Parkinson's disease may depend on iron–melanin interaction. J Neural Transm [Suppl] 1990; 29:251–258.
175. Ben-Shachar D, Riederer P, Youdim MBH. Iron-melanin interaction and lipid peroxidation: implications for Parkinson's disease. J Neurochem 1991; 57:1609–1614.
176. Sershen H, Reith MEA, Hashim A, Lajtha A. Protection against 1-methyl-4-phenyl-1,2,3,6-tetrahydropyridine neurotoxicity by the antioxidant ascorbic acid. Neuropharmacology 1985; 24:1257–1259.
177. Wagner GC, Jarvis MF, Carelli RM. Ascorbic acid reduces the dopamine depletion induced by MPTP. Neuropharmacology 1985; 24:1261–1262.
178. Perry TL, Yong VW, Clavier RM, et al. Partial protection from the dopaminergic neurotoxin *N*-methyl-4-phenyl-1,2,3,6-tetrahydropyridine by four different antioxidants in the mouse. Neurosci Lett 1985; 60:109–114.
179. Baldessarini RJ, Kula NS, Francoeur D, Finklestein SP. Antioxidants fail to inhibit depletion of striatal dopamine by MPTP. Neurology 1986; 36:735.
180. Martinovits G, Melamed E, Cohen O, Rosenthal J, Uzzan A. Systemic administration of antioxidants does not protect mice against the dopaminergic neurotoxicity of 1-methyl-4-phenyl-1,2,3,6-tetrahydropyridine (MPTP). Neurosci Lett 1986; 69:192–197.
181. Perry TL, Yong VW, Jones K, Wright JM. Manipulation of glutathione contents fails to alter dopaminergic nigrostriatal neurotoxicity of *N*-methyl-4-phenyl-1,2,3,6-tetrahydropyridine (MPTP) in the mouse. Neurosci Lett 1986; 70:261–265.
182. Corsini GU, Pintus S, Chiueh CC, Weiss JF, Kopin IJ. 1-Methyl-4-phenyl-1,2,3,6-tetrahydropyridine (MPTP) neurotoxicity in mice is enhanced by pretreatment with diethyldithiocarbamate. Eur J Pharmacol 1985; 119:127–128.
183. Irwin I, Wu EY, DeLanney LE, Trevor AJ, Langston JW. The effect of diethyldithiocarbamate (DDC) on the biodisposition of MPTP: an explanation for enhanced neurotoxicity. Eur J Pharmacol 1987; 141:209–217.
184. Nicklas WJ, Vyas I, Heikkila RE. Inhibition of NADH-linked oxidation in brain

mitochondria by 1-methyl-4-phenyl-1,2,3,6-tetrahydropyridine. Life Sci 1985; 36:2503–2508.
185. Di Monte DA. Mitochondrial DNA and Parkinson's disease. Neurology 1991; 41(suppl 2):38–42.
186. Poirier J, Barbeau A. 1-Methyl-4-phenyl-pyridinium-induced inhibition of nicotinamide adenosine dinucleotide cytochrome *c* reductase. Neurosci Lett 1985; 62:7–11.
187. Ramsay RR, Salach JI, Dadgar J, Singer TP. Inhibition of mitochondrial NADH dehydrogenase by pyridine derivatives and its possible relation to experimental and idiopathic parkinsonism. Biochem Biophys Res Commun 1986; 135:269–275.
188. Vyas I, Heikkila RE, Nicklas WJ. Studies on the neurotoxicity of 1-methyl-4-phenyl-1,2,3,6-tetrahydropyridine: inhibition of NAD-linked substrate oxidation by its metabolite, 1-methyl-4-phenylpyridinium. J Neurochem 1986; 46:1501–1507.
189. Ramsay RR, Kowal AT, Johnson K, Salach JI, Singer TP. The inhibition site of MPP^+ the neuotoxic bioactivation product of 1-methyl-4-phenyl-1-1,2,3,6-tetrahydropyridine is near the Q-binding site of NADH dehydrogenase. Arch Biochem Biophys 1987; 259:645–649.
190. Mizuno Y, Suzuki K, Sone N, Saitoh T. Inhibition of ATP synthesis by 1-methyl-4-phenylpyridinium ion (MPP^+) in isolated mitochondria from mouse brains. Neurosci Lett 1987; 81:204–208.
191. Ramsay RR, Krueger MJ, Youngster SK, Gluck MR, Casida JE, Singer TP. Interaction of 1-methyl-4-phenylpyridinium ion (MPP^+) and its analogs with the rotenone/piericidin binding site of NADH dehydrogenase. J Neurochem 1991; 56:1184–1190.
192. Chan P, DeLanney LE, Irwin I, Langston JW, Di Monte DA. Rapid ATP loss caused by 1-methyl-4-phenyl-1,2,3,6-tetrahydropyridine in mouse brain. J Neurochem 1991; 57:348–351.
193. Di Monte DA, Sandy MS, Blank L, Smith MT. Fructose prevents 1-methyl-4-phenyl-1,2,3,6-tetrahydropyridine (MPTP)-induced ATP depletion and toxicity in isolated hepatocytes. Biochem Biophys Res Commun 1988; 153:734–740.
194. Dikman M, Leibowitz Y. Association of diabetes, hypertension and arteriosclerotic heart disease with Parkinson's disease: a pilot study. Proceedings of the 9th International Symposium on Parkinson's Disease, World Federation of Neurology, 1988:117. (abstract)
195. Bindoff LA, Birch-Machin MA, Cartlidge NEF, Parker WD Jr, Turnbull DM. Mitochondrial function in Parkinson's disease. Lancet 1989; 2:49.
196. Mizuno Y, Ohta S, Tanaka M, et al. Deficiencies in complex I subunits of the respiratory chain in Parkinson's disease. Biochem Biophys Res Commun 1989; 163:1450–1455.
197. Parker WD Jr, Boyson SJ, Parks JK. Abnormalities of the electron transport chain in idiopathic Parkinson's disease. Ann Neurol 1989; 26:719–723.
198. Schapira AHV, Cooper JM, Dexter D, Clark JB, Jenner P,Marsden CD. Mitochondrial complex I deficiency in Parkinson's disease. J Neurochem 1990; 54:823–827.
199. Shoffner JM, Watts RL, Juncos JL, Torroni A, Wallace DC. Mitochondrial oxidative phosphorylation defects in Parkinson's disease. Ann Neurol 1991 30:332–339.
200. Lestienne P, Nelson J, Riederer P, Jellinger K, Reichmann H. Normal mitochon-

drial genome in brain from patients with Parkinson's disease and complex I defect. J Neurochem 1990; 55:1810–1812.

201. Ozawa T, Tanaka M, Ikebe S, Ohno K, Kondo T, Mizuno Y. Quantitative determination of deleted mitochondrial DNA relative to normal DNA in parkinsonian striatum by a kinetic PCR analysis. Biochem Biophys Res Commun 1990; 172:483–489.
202. Lestienne P, Nelson I, Riederer P, Reichmann H, Jellinger K. Mitochondrial DNA in postmortem brain from patients with Parkinson's disease. J Neurochem 1991; 56:1819.
203. Ozawa T, Tanaka M, Ino H, et al. Distinct clustering of point mutations in mitochondrial DNA among patients with mitochondrial encephalomyopathies and with Parkinson's disease. Biochem Biophys Res Commun 1991; 176:938–946.
204. Ozawa T, Tanaka M, Sugiyama S, et al. Patients with idiopathic cardiomyopathy belong to the same mitochondrial DNA gene family of Parkinson's disease and mitochondrial encephalomyopathy. Biochem Biophys Res Commun 1991; 177:518–525.
205. Mann VM, Cooper JM, Schapira AHV. Quantitation of a mitochondrial DNA deletion in Parkinson's disease. FEBS Lett 1992; 299:218–222.
206. Nakagawa-Hattori Y, Yoshino H, Kondo T, Mizuno Y, Horai S. Is Parkinson's disease a mitochondrial disorder. J Neurol Sci 1992; 107:29–33.
207. Moraes CT, DiMauro S, Zeviani M, et al. Mitochondrial DNA deletions in progressive external ophthalmoplegia and Kearns–Sayre syndrome. N Engl J Med 1989; 320:1293–1299.
208. Beal MF. Does impairment of energy metabolism result in excitotoxic neuronal death in neurodegenerative illnesses? Ann Neurol 1992; 31:119–130.
209. Turski L, Bressler K, Rettig K-J, Löschmann P-A, Wachtel H. Protection of substantia nigra from MPP^+ neurotoxicity by *N*-methyl-D-aspartate antagonists. Nature 1991; 349:414–418.
210. Sonsalla PK, Nicklas WJ, Heikkila RE. Role for excitatory amino acids in methamphetamine-induced nigrostriatal dopaminergic toxicity. Science 1989; 243: 398–400.
211. Zuddas A, Oberto G, Vaglini F, Fascetti F, Fornai F,Corsini GU. MK-801 prevents 1-methyl-4-phenyl-1,2,3,6-tetrahydropyridine-induced parkinsonism in primates. J Neurochem 1992; 59:733–739.
212. Srivastava R, Brouillet E, Beal MF, Storey E, Hyman BT. Blockade of 1-methyl-4-phenylpyridinium ion (MPP^+) nigral toxicity in the rat by prior decortication or MK-801 treatment: a sterological estimate of neuronal loss. Neurobiol Aging 1993; 14:295–301.
213. Westerink BHC, Damsma G, Rollema H, De Vries JB, Horn AS. Scope and limitations of in vivo brain dialysis: a comparison of its application to various neurotransmitter systems. Life Sci 1987; 41:1763–1776.
214. Carboni S, Melis F, Pani L, Hadjiconstantinou M, Rossetti ZL. The non-competitive NMDA-receptor antagonist MK-801 prevents the massive release of glutamate and aspartate from rat striatum induced by 1-methyl-4-phenylpyridinium (MPP^+). Neurosci Lett 1990; 117:129–133.
215. Sonsalla PK, Zeevalk GD, Manzino L, Giovanni A, Nicklas WJ. MK-801 fails to

protect against the dopaminergic neuropathology produced by systemic 1-methyl-4-phenyl-1,2,3,6-tetrahydropyridine in mice or intranigral 1-methyl-4-phenyl-pyridinium in rats. J Neurochem 1992; 58:1979–1982.
216. Storey E, Hyman BT, Jenkins B, et al. 1-Methyl-4-phenylpyridinium produces excitotoxic lesions in rat striatum as a result of impairment of oxidative metabolism. J Neurochem 1992; 58:1975–1978.
217. Kupsch A, Löschmann P-A, Sauer H, et al. Do NMDA receptor antagonists protect against MPTP-toxicity? Biochemical and immunocytochemical analyses in black mice. Brain Res 1992; 592:74–83.
218. Tabatabaei A, Perry TL, Hansen S, Krieger C. Partial protective effect of MK-801 on MPTP-induced reduction of striatal dopamine in mice. Neurosci Lett 1992; 141:192–194.
219. Michel PP, Agid Y. The glutamate antagonist, MK-801, does not prevent dopaminergic cell death induced by the 1-methyl-4-phenylpyridinium ion (MPP^+) in rat dissociated mesencephalic cultures. Brain Res 1992; 597:233–240.
220. Finiels-Marlier F, Marini AM, Williams P, Paul SM. The *N*-methyl-D-aspartate antagonist MK-801 fails to protect dopaminergic neurons from 1-methyl-4-phyenylpyridinium toxicity in vitro. J Neurochem 1993; 60:1968–1971.
221. Beal MF. Mechanisms of excitotoxicity in neurologic diseases. FASEB J 1992; 6:3338–3344.
222. Ogawa M, Araki M, Nagatsu I, Nagatsu T, Yoshida M. The effect of 1,2,3,4-tetrahydroisoquinoline (TIQ) on mesencephalic dopaminergic neurons in C57BL/6J mice: immunohistochemical studies—tyrosine hydroxylase. Biogenic Amines 1989; 6:427–436.
223. Kikuchi K, Nagatsu Y, Makino Y, Mashino T, Ohta S, Hirobe M. Metabolism and penetration through blood–brain barrier of parkinsonism-related compounds: 1,2,3,4-tetrahydroisoquinoline and 1-methyl-1,2,3,4-tetrahydroisoquinoline. Drug Metab Dispos 1991; 19:257–262.
224. Niwa T, Takeda N, Yoshizumi H, et al. Presence of 2-methyl-6,7-dihydroxy-1,2,3,4-tetrahydroisoquinoline and 1,2-dimethyl-6,7-dihydroxy-1,2,3,4-tetrahydroisoquinoline, novel endogenous amines, in parkinsonian and normal human brains. Biochem Biophys Res Commun 1991; 177:603–609.
225. Langston JW, Ballard PA. Parkinson's disease in a chemist working with 1-methyl-4-phenyl-1,2,5,6-tetrahydropyridine (MPTP). N Engl J Med 1983; 309:310.
226. Barbeau A, Roy M, Langston JW. Neurological consequence of industrial exposure to 1-methyl-4-phenyl-1,2,3,6-tetrahydropyridine [letter]. Lancet 1985; 1:747.
227. Barbeau A, Roy M, Cloutier T, Plasse L, Paris S. Environmental and genetic factors in the etiology of Parkinson's disease. Adv Neurol 1986; 45:299–306.
228. Rajput AH, Uitti RJ, Stern W, Laverty W. Early onset Parkinson's disease in Saskatchewan—environmental considerations for etiology. Can J Neurol Sci 1986; 13:312-316.

14

Infectious Diseases as They Relate to the Etiology of Parkinson's Disease

Matthew M. Zack

Centers for Disease Control and Prevention, Atlanta, Georgia

Caroline M. Tanner

The Parkinson's Institute, Sunnyvale, California

I. INTRODUCTION

A century after James Parkinson described the disease that now bears his name (1), an apparently infectious disease accompanied by parkinsonian signs and symptoms abruptly appeared (2). This condition was known as encephalitis lethargica, and its appearance has since compelled anyone investigating the cause of Parkinson's disease to consider infection as a potential candidate. In this chapter the evidence for and against infection as a cause of Parkinson's disease will be reviewed, beginning with the story of encephalitis lethargica. In addition to the cohort hypothesis that Parkinson's disease has only one cause (encephalitis lethargica), parkinsonian syndromes accompanying specific infections will be covered, with a section on the search for specific infectious agents as causes of Parkinson's disease. In addition to current knowledge of the relation between parkinsonism and infection, possible new directions to test the hypothesis that infection may cause Parkinson's disease are presented.

To begin with a definition, an *infectious agent* is an organism that replicates and may directly or indirectly cause tissue damage or interfere with cell function. An infectious agent could gain access to and damage the substantia nigra either directly (by extension from a nearby focal infection, through the blood or lymphatics, or along neurons), or indirectly (by toxin elaboration or stimulation of autoantibody production) (3,4).

When considering the evidence for and against an infectious etiology for

Parkinson's disease, it is important to remember that most of the work reviewed in this chapter represents associations between Parkinson's disease and a piece of evidence suggesting a specific infectious agent. Cause and effect cannot be concluded from such an association. In rough order of increasing reliability, the evidence used to link infectious agents with Parkinson's disease has generally included one or more of the following: (1) reasoning from available data without providing new data, (2) clinical reports, (3) epidemiological studies, (4), serological (immunological) studies, (5) pathological studies, and (6) microbial isolation.

These various approaches have been applied to both small and large groups as well as single individuals, with tissue samples coming from serum, spinal fluid, and brain. But even the most specific evidence—repeated isolation of the infectious agent from the affected tissue—still does not necessarily prove that the agent caused the disease (4). Some tissues commonly contain persistent resident virus, without associated clinical signs. Furthermore, replication of an infectious agent may be a secondary phenomenon, if the agent replicates better in damaged tissue (4). Similarly, failure to detect an agent in affected tissue also does not prove that the agent did not cause the disease. The detection methods used may have been too insensitive. Although more recent studies employ sophisticated methods, most of the studies reviewed here employed insensitive methods, when judged by modern standards.

II. ENCEPHALITIS LETHARGICA

Before 1917, infectious agents had not been proposed as a major cause of Parkinson's disease. The few clinical series describing Parkinson's disease before this suggested antecedent infection as an "assigned cause" (e.g., assigned by the patient) of illness in only a minority of cases. In a series of 219 cases seen from 1888 through 1904, for example, 6% of the patients attributed their illness to antecedent acute or chronic infectious diseases (grippe, malaria, typhoid, pneumonia, or syphilis) (5). Other proposed causes in this series included emotion, physical injury, prolonged fatigue, and heredity. Forty percent identified no precipitating factor.

In 1917, however, an apparently new infectious disease that caused parkinsonism was first described in the medical literature among patients in Austria and France (2,6,7). Encephalitis lethargica was characterized acutely by persistent fever, headache, lethargy, changes in the pupils, and paralyses of the limbs and of the cranial nerves (especially those innervating the ocular muscles and the esophagus) (8). Stupor, coma, sleep disturbances, seizures, myoclonus, and chorea occurred either acutely or after recovery. About one-third of those affected died. Parkinsonism developed in from 21 to 78% of the survivors, usually within 10 years of the acute encephalitis (9–14). Unlike Parkinson's disease, these patients had a much earlier age at onset and typically had other associated signs—oculogyric crises, hyperkinetic movement disorders, and psychotic behavior.

Encephalitis lethargica affected children and young adults most often, particularly during the winter. Transmission appeared to be airborne because person-to-person spread was almost never observed (8). The origin of the epidemic is unknown and has been variously attributed to Europe, to China, or to an area near Lake Baikal in the Soviet Union (15,16). By 1919, encephalitis lethargica had spread throughout Europe, North America, and Central America, and had reached Africa, India, and Japan.

The acute onset, the clinical symptoms, the epidemic spread, the pathological characteristics, and the reported ability to experimentally transmit the disease to animals, all suggested an infectious cause for encephalitis lethargica. Autopsied cases showed chronic degenerative inflammation, with perivascular infiltrates of lymphocytes and plasma cells in different parts of the central nervous system; but, unlike other forms of acute meningoencephalitis, encephalitis lethargica always affected the midbrain, especially the substantia nigra (17,18). Although analytic techniques available at the time were limited, contemporary researchers thought the agent was viral, rather than bacterial, because it was infective in animals even after having been passed through a filter (7). In some cases, monkeys inoculated with brain tissue from patients with the disease also developed similar signs (19).

Although the specific agent has never been identified, the two main agents considered at the time were the herpesvirus and the agent causing the concurrent influenza pandemic. Some investigators reported isolating a filtrable agent from the brains of patients at autopsy, and suggested that this might represent a herpesvirus (20,21). Others reported reduced neutralizing capacity toward herpesvirus infection of patient sera (22). However, these findings were not consistently found (23).

Influenza was entertained as the cause of encephalitis lethargica based on epidemiological, rather than laboratory, data (24,25). The temporal coincidence of the influenza pandemic, the epidemic of encephalitis lethargica, and the development of encephalitis lethargica in some of those who had influenza, were thought to suggest the influenza virus as a causative agent. In Seattle, Washington, for example, winter peaks in deaths from encephalitis lethargica followed about 1 year after peaks in influenza–pneumonia deaths. No deaths from encephalitis lethargica had occurred on American Samoa from 1918 through 1925, when a quarantine prevented the occurrence of the pandemic influenza; only 70 km away, however, Western Samoa had both epidemic influenza and "fa-ananiva" (a fatal disease of the head) from 1919 through 1922 (26). Because previous pandemic diseases attributed to influenza had been associated with neurological sequelae, it was suggested that the influenza might have acquired neurovirulence, thus leading to encephalitis lethargica (25,27). This hypothesis was controversial (7,28), however, and has never been proved.

III. THE COHORT HYPOTHESIS

Even though epidemic encephalitis lethargica has not occurred since the late 1920s, the association of encephalitis with parkinsonism influenced thinking concerning the cause of Parkinson's disease for decades to come. The most dramatic example of this came about in 1956, with the articulation of a "unitary hypothesis" (later called the "cohort hypothesis")—that all cases of parkinsonism had a single cause: infection with the agent causing encephalitis lethargica (29,30). The typical latent interval, sometimes as long as 10–15 years, from the time of acute encephalitis to the development of parkinsonism gave credence to this hypothesis. Epidemiological investigations of clinical populations from the 1920s to the late 1950s noted progressive increases in the mean age at the time parkinsonism was diagnosed, and in the birth years of Parkinson's disease patients (29–42). Since the epidemic of encephalitis lethargica occurred during a period of 10 years or less, ending in the 1920s, aging of the "at-risk" cohort exposed to encephalitis lethargica would result in an increase both in age at onset and year of birth of those persons with Parkinson's disease, if, as hypothesized, all cases of Parkinson's disease resulted from this single cause. The preceding observations were, therefore, cited as evidence supporting the cohort hypothesis. It was proposed that parkinsonism should ". . . disappear as a major clinical entity by 1980 . . ." (30,31).

Proponents of the cohort hypothesis ignored clinical signs that might differentiate postencephalitic parkinsonism from Parkinson's disease, such as oculogyric crises, more extensive signs of central nervous system injury, or a history of encephalitis. Either tremor or rigidity alone was considered a sufficient criterion for the diagnosis of parkinsonism (30). Differences in postmortem histopathological studies were also discounted (30,43,44). The cohort of individuals living during the epidemic of encephalitis lethargica was defined a priori as being at high risk for parkinsonism; those without acute symptoms were believed to have suffered subclinical exposure (30). Since postencephalitic parkinsonism occurred primarily in young people (as did encephalitis lethargica), the large number of new cases resulting from this epidemic caused both the age of onset of parkinsonism and the mean age of persons with parkinsonism to be relatively young. Since Parkinson's disease, in contrast, is a disorder of later life, the decline in the incidence of postencephalitic parkinsonism after the 1920s was accompanied by a progressive increase in both the age at the onset of parkinsonism and the birth years of affected persons (43,45–59). Figure 1 presents the theoretical effect of the epidemic of postencephalitic parkinsonism on the age-specific incidence of parkinsonism, assuming the age-specific incidence rates of Parkinson's disease

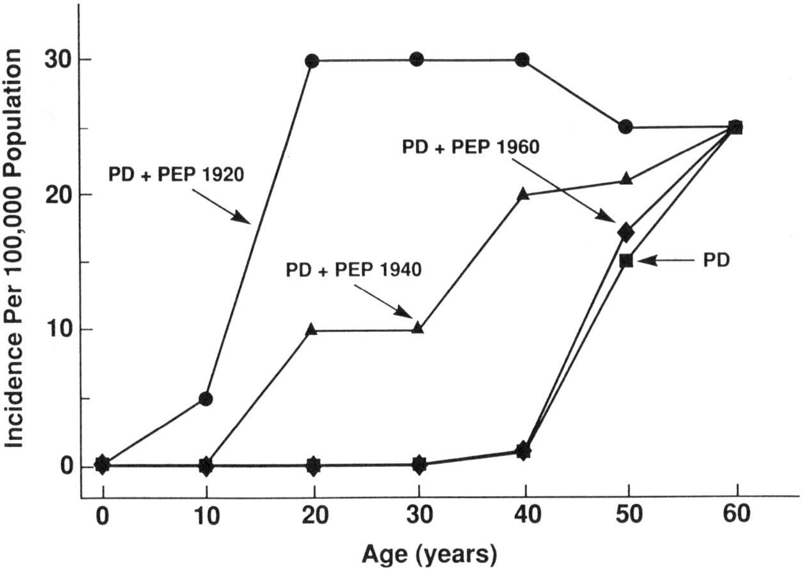

Figure 1 Theoretical effect on age-specific incidence rates, if new cases of Parkinson's disease (PD) and postencephalitic parkinsonism (PEP) are grouped as a single disease, and incidence is observed in 1920, 1940, and 1960. The incidence of Parkinson's disease alone is shown by a solid line. In 1920, parkinsonism incidence (PD + PEP) is increased in all aged groups. The increased incidence is most marked in younger-aged groups, who were most susceptible to encephalitis lethargica. Older persons rarely survived encephalitis lethargica, so at aged 60 there are no new cases of postencephalitic parkinsonism. In 1940, the population exposed to encephalitis lethargica has aged. Many who had severe encephalitis and parkinsonism have not survived. As a result, the overall incidence of parkinsonism is decreased, and mean age at onset has increased. By 1960, the few postencephalitic cases occur in persons aged 50 or older, after a latent interval of nearly 40 years. Mean age at onset of parkinsonism is nearly the same as that for Parkinson's disease. Note that the rates are theoretical for purposes of illustration.

remained constant since the 1920s. Retrospectively, it is easy to see how the assumption that all cases of parkinsonism had a single cause led to a period during which the cohort hypothesis appeared to be correct. In fact, contemporary critics of the cohort hypothesis also put forth this explanation (43,46).

The studies supporting the cohort hypothesis were criticized by contemporary scientists for methodological reasons (43,44,46,60–71). In some studies, one could not be certain that the same person was not counted twice. Age at onset and age at time of study were not distinguished, nor was the interval between age at onset and age at diagnosis. In addition, these studies did not consider the effects of death or admission to a nursing home among those with long-duration disease (61). Others argued that not all contemporary studies showed the expected increase in age at onset of parkinsonism underlying the cohort hypothesis (47,68,69,72). If proponents of the cohort hypothesis had considered the few clinical series published before the encephalitic lethargica epidemic, the error of their analyses may have been avoided. For example, the mean age at onset of parkinsonism observed in clinical populations during the epidemic was much lower than that reported for clinical populations either in the decades preceding 1920 or in those after 1940 (5,44,62,63,66,67,73,74). Interestingly, a similar increase in mean age at disease onset by more recent calendar year has been observed in many diseases affecting the elderly. Such a pattern could be explained by better access to medical care, thus increasing the proportion of elderly persons diagnosed with parkinsonism and, in consequence, mean age at onset (68,72). But by far the most compelling criticism of the cohort hypothesis is the failure to observe the predicted decline in the incidence and prevalence of Parkinson's disease in the 1970s and 1980s as members of the exposed cohort died (71).

IV. OTHER INFECTIOUS CAUSES OF PARKINSONISM

The syndrome of parkinsonism may occasionally be the acute accompaniment of many central nervous system infectious diseases—viral, fungal, and bacterial (Table 1). Such cases are relatively uncommon, however, and are usually reported individually or as a small clinical series. More importantly, the associated parkinsonism is clinically distinct from Parkinson's disease in several ways. First, the parkinsonism occurs acutely or subacutely in relation to the infection. In almost all cases, the parkinsonism is not an isolated phenomenon, but associated with signs of more extensive central nervous system injury. Most often, the reported parkinsonism is transient. If the parkinsonism after these infections is permanent, it is typically less severe and less progressive than postencephalitic parkinsonism or Parkinson's disease. In cases with pathological material available, the lesions generally involve basal ganglia as well as substantia nigra, and the characteristic histopathological changes of Parkinson's disease are not present. Thus, the evidence does not support an etiologic relation between any of the agents causing acute parkinsonism and Parkinson's disease.

Since mortality rates for survivors of encephalitis lethargica were high, likely only a few survivors were alive after 1940 (43). Has encephalitis lethargica occurred since then as sporadic cases? Persons in whom lethargy, eye signs (particularly oculogyric crises), changes in behavior, or parkinsonism developed after a fever or an encephalitis have been reported from time to time as possible cases of encephalitis lethargica (75–83). However, this symptomatic similarity actually only indicates a similar anatomical distribution of abnormalities. In all of these cases, tests for specific antibody or microbial isolation were either not attempted or, when attempted, were not diagnostic of a specific infectious agent

Table 1 Some Infectious Agents Causing Acute or Subacute Parkinsonism

Infectious agents
Viruses
Influenza A (136)
Japanese B encephalitis (137–140)
Western equine encephalitis (141–147)
Eastern equine encephalitis (148)
Le Dantec virus (149)
Measles (150)
Polio (151)
Coxsackie B (84, 152)
HIV (153)
Fungi
Cryptococcus (154)
Aspergillosis (156)
Protazoa
Toxoplasma gondii (155)
Rickettsiae
Central European tick-borne encephalitis (157, 158)
Bacteria
Borrelia burgdorferii (159)
Treponema pallidum (160)
Salmonella typhi (161)

(84). Because the cause of encephalitis lethargica was never convincingly determined, it is unlikely that the relation between these more recent cases and encephalitis lethargica will ever be known.

V. INDICATORS OF SPECIFIC PREVIOUS INFECTIONS

Parkinson's disease is slowly progressive, with an insidious onset. This clinical picture is quite different from that associated with the acute infection-associated parkinsonian syndromes. Others have proposed a postinfectious mechanism as a cause of subsequent parkinsonism. To determine whether or not prior infection with a specific agent increases the risk of Parkinson's disease, both historical (patient self-report) and laboratory investigations have been performed. Some of these have compared controls with patients who have clinically diagnosed postencephalitic parkinsonism, whereas others have compared controls with cases of Parkinson's disease. Some studies have simply not distinguished among different forms of parkinsonism, presenting a serious confounding problem when it comes to interpretation.

Obviously, these different methods of case selection will influence the hypothesis that can be tested. For example, in comparisons of postencephalitic parkinsonism with controls, the causative agent might be inferred from a consistent finding of antibody to a specific infectious agent. In contrast, such a finding in Parkinson's disease patients compared with controls would suggest a different mechanism, such as an immune-mediated postinfectious process, since Parkinson's disease is not associated with signs of an acute infection. Finally, conclusions from studies in which different types of parkinsonism are not distinguished are limited, since it seems unlikely that all types share a common pathogenesis.

A. History of Previous Infection

1. Encephalitis

A self-report of prior encephalitis, or of symptoms suggestive of encephalitis, is often accepted as sufficient evidence of infection in epidemiological investigations. In general, earlier studies frequently found such historical evidence, whereas more recent studies did not. Studies published in 1965 and 1976 reported a history of encephalitis lethargica in 13 and 5% of patients with parkinsonism; there was no such history in controls in either of these investigations (85,86). A history of other encephalitides (diagnosed clinically or serologically) was also more common in cases than in controls in the former study (16 vs. 0%), but not the latter (0.3 vs. 0%). Prior infection with "encephalitis /Spanish flu" was found to be more common among cases of parkinsonism compared with their controls in a Baltimore study that was both hospital-based and community-based. A puzzling aspect of this study is that the increase was statistically significant only for men in the former study (87) but only for women in the latter (88). These conflicting observations may be a result of bias in the selection of the hospital-based sample (see Chapter 11). In a more recent investigation, subjects with an onset of Parkinson's disease before aged 40 were no more likely to report a history of an infection of the central nervous system than Parkinson's disease cases with onset after aged 60 (89).

In case series without comparison groups, the occurrence of the young-onset parkinsonism associated with encephalitis lethargica (or encephalitis) gradually declined over time (43,45–59). The high percentage of self-reported infections in the older studies may reflect the inclusion of many individuals with bona fide exposure to encephalitis lethargica. Whether popular awareness of the proposed association between infection and parkinsonism may also have influenced recall cannot be determined. When the preceding publications are considered, as a whole, a history of prior encephalitis does not appear to constitute a significant risk factor for Parkinson's disease.

2. *Influenza*

The temporal association between encephalitis lethargica and the 1918 pandemic of presumed influenza (90) prompted a search for an association between influenza and Parkinson's disease. In three studies, the percentage of cases with a history of influenza did not differ from that of controls (63,85,86). Severe "flu-like" illness in childhood occurred significantly more often among 72 Parkinson's disease patients than among controls (91). However, other authors have not found a high prevalence of influenza in either case–control studies (92) or case series of parkinsonian patients (49,93).

It has also been suggested that intrauterine exposure to influenza virus during the pandemics from 1890 through 1930 might damage the fetal substantia nigra (94). However, another smaller study did not confirm an association with birth year (95). Furthermore, the low concordance of Parkinson's disease among monozygotic twins suggests that such an intrauterine infection is unlikely (96).

3. *Other Infections*

A large number of studies have searched for evidence of infections preceding the onset of parkinsonism, but differences have not been found between parkinsonian and control subjects. Specific infections that have been evaluated included chickenpox (varicella; 86–88), shingles (herpes zoster; 86–88,97), childhood mumps infection (86–88,92), childhood rubella (German measles) infection (87,88,92), syphilis (87), and tuberculosis (87). Parkinsonism developed in two 69-year-old patients who had poliomyelitis as children (98). However, this association was likely coincidental, since a history of poliomyelitis is no more frequent in Parkinson's disease cases than in controls (99). A case series in which 11 of 21 persons with slowly progressive parkinsonism reported a severe febrile illness occurring 2–28 years before the onset of parkinsonism (100) provides the only positive association yet reported in a larger series, although the significance of such an uncontrolled finding is uncertain.

In one study of men, controls were more likely to report childhood measles with Parkinson's disease, suggesting a protective effect of early measles infection (92), but several other studies found no such effect (86–88,101–103).

B. Serological Investigations of Prior Infections

Serological investigations have generally failed to demonstrate a reproducible association between parkinsonism of any type and evidence of prior infection, despite the investigation of a large number of agents in several different laboratories internationally (Table 2). In fact, only one agent, herpes simplex virus (usually type 1), has been repeatedly associated with any form of parkinsonism.

Table 2 Serological Studies in Parkinsonism versus Controls

Agent	Parkinsonism associated with increased serum serology	Parkinsonism associated with increased CSF serology	Parkinsonism associated with no change or lower serum serology	Parkinsonism associated with no change or lower CSF serology
Influenza A			PEP (110, 162) PD (110, 162) MP (105)	PEP (110) PD (110)
Influenza B			PEP (110) PD (110) MP (105)	PEP (110) PD (110)
Herpes simplex virus type 1	PD (104, 106–108) MP (105, 109)	MP (109)	PEP (110) PD (110, 111, 163)	PEP (110) PD (106, 108, 110, 111, 164)
Herpes simplex virus type 2	PD (106)		PEP (110) PD (110)	PEP (110) PD (106, 110)
Varicella–zoster			PEP (110) PD (110, 111) MP (105)	PEP (110) PD (110, 111)
Cytomegalovirus			PEP (110) PD (106, 110, 111) MP (105)	PEP (110) PD (106, 110, 111)
Measles			PEP (110) PD (108, 110, 111) MP (105, 109)	PEP (110) PD (109, 110, 111) MP (109)
Rubella			PEP (110) PD (110, 111) MP (105)	PEP (110) PD (110, 111)
Coxsackie			PEP (110) PD (110) MP (105)	PEP (110) PD (110)

Parainfluenza 1		PEP (110)	PEP (110)
		PD (109, 110)	PD (110)
Eastern equine encephalitis		PEP (165)	PEP (165)
		PD (165)	PD (165)
Western equine encephalitis		PEP (165)	PEP (165)
		PD (165)	PD (165)
Venezuelan equine encephalitis		PEP (165)	PEP (165)
		PD (165)	PD (165)
Other group A arboviruses		PEP (165)	PEP (165)
(see Ref. 165)		PD (165)	PD (165)
Group B type arboviruses		PEP (165)	PEP (165)
(see Ref. 165)		PD (165)	PD (165)
		MP (85)	
Vaccinia		PD (111)	PD (111)
Epstein–Barr	MP (109)	MP (105)	
Adenoviruses		MP (105)	
Poliovirus		MP (105)	
Echovirus		MP (105)	
Mycoplasma pneumoniae		MP (105)	
Lymphocytic choriomeningitis		PD (166)	
		PEP (166)	
Respiratory syncytial virus		MP (115)	
Mumps		PEP (110)	PEP (110)
		PD (110)	PD (110)
		MP (105)	

PEP, postencephalitic parkinsonism; PD, Parkinson's disease; MP, mixed parkinsonism, Parkinson's disease.

The significance of this association remains uncertain, however. In several studies of a Finnish population, using a variety of methods (complement fixation, immunofluorescence, indirect hemagglutination, and solid-phase radioimmunoassay), Marttila et al. (104–108) found increased antibodies to herpes simplex virus in serum, but not cerebrospinal fluid, of both Parkinson's disease and postencephalitic parkinsonism. Irkec (109) found antibodies to herpes simplex virus type 1 to be greater in both serum and cerebrospinal fluid of 42 cases of parkinsonism, compared with controls. These results were not replicated in other populations (110,111). Since the reported findings provide little evidence for central nervous system involvement, the significance of this finding remains uncertain.

C. Studies of Brain Tissue

In one provocative study, influenza A virus (AO/WSN strain) antigen was detected in the nuclei of cells in the substantia nigra and hypothalamus of all six cases of postencephalitic parkinsonism, but in none of five cases of Parkinson's disease (112,113). This finding was not confirmed in the brain of one person with an acute encephalitis lethargica-like syndrome or of another with longstanding postencephalitic parkinsonism, using antigens to influenza A strains A2/Japan/305/57, A/WS/33, A/swine/1976/31, and A/NWS (114). Similarly, neither brain antigen nor nucleic acid complementary to influenza A strain A/NWS was detected in nine Parkinson's disease patients (115,116). Cases of postencephalitic parkinsonism did not differ from controls relative to the presence of viral antigen in the brain for other kinds of influenza (types B and C) (112–114). Evidence that influenza viruses may trigger immunological responses within the CNS was provided by a study of rabbits immunized with certain H1N1 strains of influenza viruses. These animals produced autoantibodies to a protein specific to the gray matter of rabbit and human brain (117). Nonetheless, the relation of this last finding to parkinsonism is uncertain. When considered together, the proposed association between influenza and postencephalitic parkinsonism is supported only weakly by these studies. None of the reported work suggests an association with Parkinson's disease.

Investigations of other agents have been similarly unrevealing. Searches for herpesviral antigens in the brains of cases of encephalitis lethargica (112,118), postencephalitic parkinsonism (114), and Parkinson's disease (115,119) have been unrewarding. Similarly, nucleic acids complementary to herpes simplex type 1 virus DNA were not detected in the brains of cases with Parkinson's disease (116). Neither were antigens to herpesvirus, cytomegalovirus, mumps, measles, or rubella detected in the brains of a patient who had died acutely with an encephalitis lethargica-like syndrome or of one individual with postencephalitic parkinsonism (114). Nor have measles viral antigens been detected in brains of those who died with Parkinson's disease (112,115) or postencephalitic parkinsonism (112).

VI. RECENT INVESTIGATIONS

Although the more traditional approaches to identifying an association between infection and Parkinson's disease have so far been unrevealing, it is possible that an unusual or previously unrecognized mechanism might explain the cause of this disorder of unknown etiology. Several areas for further investigation are considered here.

Perhaps the first "unusual" mechanism to be considered was the possibility that Parkinson's disease, like kuru and Creutzfeldt–Jakob disease, might be the result of a slow virus infection. Virus-like filaments in juvenile parkinsonism have been interpreted as suggesting "latent" encephalitis (120). Changes in the percentage of purine and pyrimidine bases in the ribonucleic acid (RNA) of neurons and glia in the globus pallidus of Parkinson's disease compared with controls may also suggest a slow virus affecting RNA (121,122). However, antibodies to neurofilaments occur as often in cases of Parkinson's disease and postencephalitic parkinsonism as in age-matched controls (123). Even more importantly, attempts to isolate a slow virus with a long incubation period, leading to slowly progressive disease and death (3,4,124), have been unsuccessful (125–128).

The association between prion proteins and the neurodegenerative disorder Gerstmann–Sraussler–Shencker syndrome prompted the suggestion that these proteins might play a part in other neurodegenerative disorders. In an intriguing review, Prusiner (129) proposed several theoretical mechanisms for the involvement of prion proteins in Parkinson's disease. However, data associating prion proteins and Parkinson's disease have not yet been presented.

Investigation of variations in inborn susceptibility to infection failed to show differences in HLA-associated antigens. For example, in one study, there were no differences between Parkinson's disease cases and ethnically matched controls. In contrast, 44% of cases with postencephalitic parkinsonism had HLA-B14 antigen, compared with only 8% of ethnically matched controls (130). This difference may simply represent better survival for those with this antigen, but the difference may also reflect genetic susceptibility to infections causing parkinsonism.

Indirect evidence for an infectious process is suggested by the finding of larger numbers of reactive microglia in the substantias nigra of Parkinson's disease patients than in controls (131). One interpretation of this finding is that a currently active chronic infection or autoimmune process may cause Parkinson's disease. Further investigation of such a possibility is needed.

Recently, two unusual infectious agents have also been proposed as possibly related to Parkinson's disease. First, enzyme-linked immunoabsorbent assay (ELISA) analyses of spinal fluid from Parkinson's disease patients, those with other neurological diseases, and controls found an elevated antibody response to coronavirus in the spinal fluid of Parkinson's disease patients (132). Coronaviruses typically cause upper respiratory symptoms in humans. However, one coronavirus, a murine hepatitis virus, was observed to cause persistent infection uniquely localized to the substantia nigra and subthalamus (133).

The second proposed association is between a common soil pathogen not thought to cause symptoms of infection in humans—*Nocardia asteroides* (134). This bacteria, like coronavirus, was reported to cause a movement disorder in mice. Postmortem analyses showed loss of nigral neurons and hyaline intracytoplasmic inclusion bodies, suggestive of Lewy bodies, in the absence of detectable organisms. This raised the possibility that a clinically insignificant infection could later cause similar progressive nigral degeneration in humans. This association has been tested in one rural population, for whom antibodies to the organism did not differ in the sera of Parkinson's disease cases and controls (135). However, spinal fluid studies were not performed. Moreover, a high prevalence of antibodies to *Nocardia* would have been expected in both cases and controls, since the organism is ubiquitous in the rural environment from which they were collected. Thus, the power of the study to detect a difference may have been poor.

Finally, an infectious process might increase susceptibility to a subsequent Parkinson's disease-causing insult. In this event, an infectious organism would have damaged substantia nigra neurons, whether or not acute symptoms were detected clinically. Individuals suffering such an infection would then have a smaller complement of functional nigral neurons. If a subsequent insult caused progressive injury to the substantia nigra, such individuals would be at higher risk for progressive parkinsonism. Such cases have yet to be documented, however.

Although all of the foregoing hypotheses deserve further investigation, the body of evidence has yet to strongly support an infectious agent as the single cause of Parkinson's disease. If Parkinson's disease is caused by an infection, current failure to demonstrate this may have a number of explanations. The causative agent may not have been investigated, or current methods may not be sufficiently sensitive to allow its identification. The infectious agent may simply have triggered the progressive neurodegeneration of Parkinson's disease (such as by altering genetic material), and be unidentifiable by the time parkinsonism is clinically present. Alternatively, a systemic infection might cause an autoimmune response that damages the substantia nigra indirectly without direct invasion. Finally, Parkinson's disease may have many different causes, only one of which is infectious. If these causative factors have similar clinical and pathological manifestations, their identification will be difficult. Carefully directed and methodologically sophisticated investigation of these hypotheses will be required to determine their true relevance to Parkinson's disease.

REFERENCES

1. Parkinson J. An essay on the shaking palsy. London: Whittingham and Rowland for Sherwood, Neely, Jones 1817.

2. von Economo C. The sequelae of encephalitis lethargica. In: Newman K, ed. Encephalitis lethargica its sequelae and treatment. London: Oxford University Press, 1931:105–156.
3. Johnson RT, Ter Meulen V. Slow infections of the nervous system. Adv Intern Med 1978; 23:353–383.
4. Mims CA. Viral aetiology of diseases of obscure origin. Br Med Bull 1985; 41:63–69.
5. Hart TS. Paralysis agitans: some clinical observations based on the study of 219 cases seen at the clinic of Professor M. Allen Starr. J Nerv Ment Dis 1904; 31:177–188.
6. Cruchet J, Moutir F, Calmettes A. Quarante cas d'encephalo-myelite subaigue. Soc Med Hop 1917; 41:614–616.
7. Anonymous. Encephalitis lethargica. Lancet 1981; 2:1396–1397.
8. Hall A, Camb M. Epidemiology. In: Epidemic encephalitis. Bristol: John Wright & Sons, 1924:9–43.
9. Souques A. Rapport sur les syndromes parkinsoniens. Rev Neurol 1991; 28:534–573.
10. Hall A. The prognosis and treatment of chronic epidemic encephalitis. Practitioner 1934; 133:26–36.
11. Ziegler L. Follow-up studies on persons who have had epidemic encephalitis. JAMA 1928; July 21:138–141.
12. Holt WL Jr. Epidemic encephalitis: a follow-up study of two hundred and sixty-six cases. Arch Neurol Psychiatry 1937; 38:1135–1144.
13. Leonhard D. Lange Intervalle zwischen akuter Encephalitis Epidemica und dem Parkinsonistischen folegezustand. Nervenarzt 1937; 10:568–572.
14. Tyndel M. Zur Frage des Intervalles zwischen Encephalitis und beginn des postencephalitischen Parkinsonismus. Nervenarzt 1938; 11:305–306.
15. Bender JL. Parkinson's disease—a review. Ill Med J 1975; 148:227–229, 231.
16. Watson A, Yunnanfu B. The origin of encephalitis lethargica. China Med J 1928; 42:427–432.
17. Buzzard EF, Greenfield JG. Lethargic encephalitis; its sequelae and morbid anatomy. Brain 1919; 42:305–338.
18. Hohman L. The histo-pathology of post-encephalitic Parkinson's syndrome. Bull Johns Hopkins Hosp 1925; 36:403–410.
19. Levaditi C, Harvier P. Recherches experimentales dur lencephalite epidemique. CR Sceances 1921; 84:388–390.
20. Zinsser H. The present state of knowledge regarding epidemic encephalitis. Arch Pathol 1928; 6:271–301.
21. Levaditi C. Etiology of epidemic encephalitis its relation to herpes, epidemic poliomyelitis and post-vaccinal encephalopathy. Arch Neurol Psychiatry 1929; 22:767–803.
22. Gay F, Holden M. Loss of viricidal property in serums from patients with herpes and encephalitis. JAMA 1931; 96:2028–2029.
23. Andrewes C, Carmichael E. A note on the presence of antibodies to herpes virus in postencephalitic and other human sera. Lancet 1930; 1:857–858.
24. Crookshank F. Epidemic encephalo-myelitis and influenza [letter]. Lancet 1919; 1:79–80.

25. Jordan E. The influenza epidemic of 1918: I encephalitis and influenza. JAMA 1927; 89:1603–1606.
26. Ravenholt R, Foege W. 1918 influenza, encephalitis lethargica, parkinsonism. Lancet 1982; 2:860–864.
27. Maurizi CP. Why was the 1918 influenza pandemic so lethal? The possible role of a neurovirulent neuraminidase. Med Hypotheses 1985; 16:1–5.
28. Yahr M. Encephalitis lethargica (VonEconomo's disease, epidemic encephalitis. In: Vinken P, Bruyn G, eds. Handbook of clinical neurology. Amsterdam: Excerpta Medica, 1978:451–457.
29. Schwab RS, Doshay LJ, Garland H, Bradshaw P, Garvey E, Crawford B. Shift to older age distribution in parkinsonism: a report on 1,000 patients covering the past decade from three centers. Neurology 1956; 6:783–790.
30. Poskanzer D, Schwab R. Cohort analysis of Parkinson's syndrome; evidence for a single etiology related to subclinical infection about 1920. J Chronk Dis 1963; 16:961–973.
31. Poskanzer DC, Schwab RS. Studies in the epidemiology of Parkinson's disease predicting its disappearance as a major clinical entity by 1980. Trans Am Neurol Assoc 1961; 86:234–235.
32. Poskanzer DC, Schwab RS, Fraser DW. Further observations on the cohort phenomenon in Parkinson's syndrome. In: Barbeau A, Brunette JR, eds. Progress in neuro-genetics: Proceedings of the international congress of neuro-genetics and neuro-opthalmology. Amsterdam: Exerpta Medica, 1969:497–505.
33. Poskanzer DC, Schwab RS, Fraser DW. The cohort phenomenon in Parkinson's syndrome. In: Gillingham FJ, Donaldson I, Fraser J, eds. Third symposium on Parkinson's disease. Edinburgh: F.S. Livingstone, 1969:8–12.
34. Brown EL, Knox EG. Epidemiological approach to Parkinson's disease. Lancet 1972; 1:974–976.
35. Brown EL, Knox EG. Idiopathic parkinsonism as a late complication of encephalitis. Med J Aust 1972; 2:800–801.
36. Brown EL. The epidemiology of Parkinson's disease. Proc R Soc Med 1973; 66:202–203.
37. Leibowitz U, Feldman S. Age shift in parkinsonism. Isr J Med Sci 1973; 9:599–602.
38. Kessler II. Parkinson's disease: perspectives on epidemiology and pathogenesis. Prev Med 1973; 2:88–105.
39. Kaplan SD. Age distribution of patients with Parkinson's disease in 1960 and 1970 in 110 hospitals. Neurology 1974; 24:972–975.
40. Honczarenko K, Kulcyzycki J. [Etiology of Parkinson's syndrome and disease]. Pol Tyg Lek 1975; 30:1069–1070.
41. Kessler II. Parkinson's disease in epidemiologic perspective. In: Neurological epidemiology: principles and clinical applications. Adv Neurol 1978; 19:355–384.
42. Li TM, Swash M, Alberman E. Morbidity and mortality in motor neuron disease: comparison with multiple sclerosis and Parkinson's disease: age and sex specific rates and cohort analyses. J Neurol Neurosurg Psychiatry 1985; 48:320–327.
43. Duvoisin RC, Yahr MD. Encephalitis and parkinsonism. Arch Neurol 1965; 12:227–239.

44. Hoehn MM. Age distribution of patients with parkinsonism. J Am Geriatr Soc 1976; 24:79–85.
45. Gudmundsson KR. A clinical survey of parkinsonism in Iceland. Acta Neurol Scand [Suppl] 1967; 33:9–61.
46. Duvoisin RC, Schweitzer MD. Paralysis agitans mortality in England and Wales 1855–1962. Br J Prev Soc Med 1966; 20:27–33.
47. Rajput AH, Offord KP, Beard CM, Kurland LT. Epidemiology of parkinsonism: incidence, classification, and mortality. Ann Neurol 1984; 16:278–282.
48. Garland HG. Refresher course for general practitioners: parkinsonism. Br Med J 1952; 1:153–155.
49. Martin WE, Loewenson RB, Resch JA, Baker AB. Parkinson's disease. Clinical analysis of 100 patients. Neurology 1973; 23:783–790.
50. Marttila RJ, Rinne U. Epidemiology of Parkinson's disease in Finland. Acta Neurol Scand 1976; 53:81–102.
51. Dupont E. Epidemiology of parkinsonism. The Parkinson investigation, Arhus, Denmark (preliminary results). In: Worm-Peterson J, Bottcher J, eds. Symposium on parkinsonism. New York: Merck, Sharp & Dohme, 1977:65–75.
52. Rosati G, Granieri E, Pinna L, et al. Parkinson's disease. Prevalence and incidence in the Province of Sassari, North Sardinia. Acta Neurol (Naples) 1978; 33:201–207.
53. Lombard A, Gelfand M. Parkinson's disease in the African. Cent Afr J Med 1978; 24:5–8.
54. Rosati G, Granieri E, Pinna L, et al. The risk of Parkinson's disease in Mediterranean people. Neurology 1980; 30:250–255.
55. Marttila RJ, Rinne UK. Epidemiology of Parkinson's disease—an overview. J Neural Transm 1981; 51:135–148.
56. Barbeau A, Pourcher E. New data on the genetics of Parkinson's disease. Can J Neurol Sci 1982; 9:53–60.
57. Harada H, Nishikawa S, Takahashi K. Epidemiology of Parkinson's disease in a Japanese city. Arch Neurol 1983; 40: 151–154.
58. Alonso ME, Otero E, D'Regules R, Figueroa HH. Parkinson's disease: a genetic study. Can J Neurol Sci 1986; 13:248–251.
59. de Pedro Cuesta J. Studies on the prevalence of paralysis agitans by tracer methodology. Acta Neurol Scand [Suppl]1987; 112:1–106.
60. Duvoisin RC. The cause of Parkinson's disease. In: Marsden CD, Fahn S, eds. Movement disorders. London: Butterworth Scientific, 1982:8–24.
61. Kurland LT. Epidemiology: incidence, geographic distribution and genetic considerations. In: Field WS, ed. Pathogenesis and treatment of parkinsonism. Springfield, Il: Charles C Thomas, 1958:5–43.
62. Duvoisin RC, Yahr MD, Schweitzer MR, Merritte HH. Parkinsonism before and since the epidemic of encephalitis lethargica. Arch Neurol 1963; 9:232–236.
63. Hoehn MM, Yahr MD. Parkinsonism: onset, progression and mortality. Neurology 1967; 17:427–442.
64. Nobrega FT, Glattre E, Kurland LT, Okazaki H. Comments on the epidemiology of parkinsonism including prevalence and incidence statistics for Rochester, Minnesota, 1935–1966. In: Barbeau A, Brunette JR, eds. Progress in neuro-genetics.

Proceedings of the international congress of neuro-genetics and neuro-opthalmology. Amsterdam: Exerpta Medica, 1969:474–485.
65. Hull JT. The prevalence and incidence of Parkinson's disease. Geriatrics 1970; 25:128–133.
66. Hoehn MM. The epidemiology of parkinsonism. In: de Ajuriagueffa J, Gauthier G, eds. Monamines noyaux gris centraux et syndrome de Parkinson. Geneva: George et Cie, 1971:281–300.
67. Duvoisin RC, Yahr MD. Epidemiological approach to Parkinson's disease. Lancet 1972; 1:1400–1401.
68. Kurland LT, Kurtzke JF, Goldberg ID, Choi NW, Williams G. Parkinsonism. In: Epidemiology of neurologic and sense organ disorders. Cambridge: Harvard University Press, 1973:41–63.
69. Kurland LT, Brian DD. Contributions to neurology from records linkage in Olmsted County, Minnesota. In: Neurological epidemiology: principles and clinical applications. Adv Neurol 1978; 19:93–105.
70. Yahr MD. Parkinson's disease—overview of its current status. Mt Sinai J Med 1977; 44:183–191.
71. Lipczynska-Lojkowska W. [Etiology of parkinsonism. A verification of Poskanzer's and Schwab's hypothesis]. Neurol Neurochir Pol 1979; 13:593–599.
72. Kurland LT, Hauser W, Okazaki H, Nobrega FT. Epidemiologic studies of parkinsonism with special reference to the cohort hypothesis. In: Gillingham FJ, Donaldson I, Fraser J, eds. Third symposium on Parkinson's disease. Edinburgh: F.S. Livingstone, 1969:12–17.
73. Dimsdale H. Changes in the parkinsonian syndrome in the twentieth century. Q J Med 1946; 15:155–170.
74. Jenkins AC. Epidemiology of parkinsonism in Victoria. Med J Aust 1966; 2:496–502.
75. Rail D, Scholtz C, Swash M. Post-encephalitic parkinsonism: current experience. J Neurol Neurosurg Psychiatry 1981; 44:670–676.
76. Leigh AD. Infection of the nervous system occuring during an epidemic of influenza B. Br Med J 1946; 2:937–939.
77. Bickerstaff ER,Cloake PCP. Mesencephalitis and rhombencephalitis. Br Med J 1951; 2:77–81.
78. Espir MLE, Spalding JMK. Three recent cases of encephalitis lethargica. Br Med J 1956; 1:1141–1144.
79. Nielsen J. Complications of encephalitis of the von Economo type. Bull LA Neurol Soc 1953; 18:84–90.
80. Machetanz E. Postencephalitischer Parkinsonismus mit bickkrampfen im Kindesalter. Z Kinderheilk 1958; 81:555–566.
81. Piechocki DW. [Parkinsonism following lethargic encephalitis]. Neurol Neurochir Pol 1977; 11:603–605.
82. Pruskauer-Apostol B, Popescu-Pretor R, Plaiasu D, Tataru E, Ciobanu I, Voiculescu V. The present status of encephalitis lethargica. Neurol Psihiatr (Buchar) 1977; 15:125–128.
83. Miyasaki K, Takayoshi F. Parkinsonism following encephalitis of unknown etiology. J Neuropathol Exp Neurol 1977; 36:1–8.

84. Poser CM, Huntley CI,Poland ID. Para-encephalitic parkinsonism. Report of an acute case due to Coxsackie virus type B^2 and re-examination of the etiologic concepts of post-encephalitic parkinsonism. Acta Neurol Scand 1969; 45: 199–215.
85. Eadie MJ, Sutherland JM,Doherty RL. Encephalitis in etiology of parkinsonism in Australia. Arch Neurol 1965; 12:240–245.
86. Marttila RJ, Rinne UK. Arteriosclerosis, heredity, and some previous infections in the etiology of Parkinson's disease. A case–control study. Clin Neurol Neurosurg 1976; 79:46–56.
87. Kessler II. Epidemiologic studies of Parkinson's disease. II. A hospital-based survey. Am J Epidemiol 1972; 95:308–318.
88. Kessler II. Epidemiologic studies of Parkinson's disease. III. A community-based survey. Am J Epidemiol 1972; 96:242–254.
89. Dulaney E, Stern M, Hurtig H, et al. The epidemiology of Parkinson's disease: a case–control study of young-onset versus old-onset patients [abstract]. Mov Disord 1990; 5:12.
90. Kilbourne E. History of influenza. New York: Plenum Press, 1987. 3–22.
91. Treves TA, Rabey JM, Korczyn AD. Case–control study, with use of temporal approach, for evaluation of risk factors for Parkinson's disease (PD) [abstract]. Mov Disord 1990; 5:11.
92. Sasco AJ,Paffenbarger RS Jr. Measles infection and Parkinson's disease. Am J Epidemiol 1985; 122:1017–1031.
93. Icannovic H, Stojanovic M, Nikolic M. [Risk factors for the onset of Parkinson's disease]. Srp Arkh Tselok Lek 1988; 116:413–417.
94. Mattock CH, Marmot M,Stern G. Could Parkinson's disease follow intra-uterine influenza? A speculative hypothesis. J Neurol Neurosurg Psychiatry 1988; 51:753–756.
95. Ebmeier KP, Mutch WJ, Calder SA, Crawford JR, Stewart L, Besson JOA. Does idiopathic parkinsonism in Aberdeen follow intrauterine influenza? J Neurol Neurosurg Psychiatry 1989; 52:911–913.
96. Singer C,Weiner W. Could Parkinson's disease follow intra-uterine influenza? A speculative hypothesis. J Neurol Neurosurg Psychiatry 1989; 52:931.
97. Ragozzino MW, Kurland LT, Rajput AH. Investigation of the association between herpes zoster and Parkinson's disease. Neuroepidemiology 1983; 2:89–92.
98. Vincent F, Myers W. Poliomyelitis and parkinsonism. N Engl J Med 1978; 298:688–689.
99. Marttila RJ. Poliomyelitis and arteriosclerosis in the etiology of Parkinson's disease [letter]. N Engl J Med 1978; 299:313.
100. Scott RM, Brody JA. Benign early-onset Parkinson's disease: a syndrome distinct from classic postencephalitic parkinsonism. Neurology 1970; 20:400.
101. Tanner CM, Chen B, Wang WZ, et al. Environmental factors and Parkinson's disease: a case–control study in China. Neurology 1989; 39:660–664.
102. Bharucha NE, Stokes L, Schoenberg BS, et al. A case–control study of twin pairs discordant for Parkinson's disease: a search for environmental risk factors. Neurology 1986 36:284–288.
103. Rajput AH, Offord KP, Beard CM,Kurland LT. A case–control study of smoking

habits, dementia, and other illnesses in idiopathic Parkinson's disease. Neurology 1987; 37:226–232.
104. Marttila RJ, Rinne UK. Herpes simplex virus antibodies in patients with Parkinson's disease. J Neurol Sci 1978; 35:375–379.
105. Marttila RJ, Arstila P, Nikoskelainen J, Halonen PE, Rinne UK. Viral antibodies in the sera from patients with Parkinson disease. Eur Neurol 1977; 15:25–33.
106. Marttila RJ, Rinne UK, Halonen PE, Madden DL, Sever JL. Herpesviruses and parkinsonism. Arch Neurol 1981; 38:19–21.
107. Marttila RJ, Kalimo KOK, Ziola BR, Halonen PE, Rinne UK. Herpes simplex virus subunit antibodies in patients with Parkinson's disease. Arch Neurol 1978; 35:668–671.
108. Marttila RJ, Rinne U, Tiilikainen A. Virus antibodies in Parkinson's disease. Herpes simplex and measles virus antibodies in serum and CSF and their relation to HLA types. J Neurol Sci 1982; 54:227–238.
109. Irkec C. Evaluation of the role of viral antibodies in the pathogenesis of degenerative and demyelinating disease. Mikrobiyol Bul 1989; 23:40–50.
110. Elizan TS, Madden DL, Noble GR, et al. Viral antibodies in serum and CSF of parkinsonian patients and controls. Arch Neurol 1979; 36:529–534.
111. Elizan TS, Duvoisin RC, Madden DL, Smith H. HLA antigens and viral antibody titers in identical twins discordant for Parkinson's disease. Mt Sinai J Med 1982; 49:83–84.
112. Gamboa ET, Wolf A, Yahr MD, et al. Influenza A virus as a possible cause of postencephalitic parkinsonism. Trans Am Neurol Assoc 1973; 98:177–180.
113. Gamboa ET, Wolf A, Yahr MD, et al. Influenza virus antigen in postencephalitic parkinsonism brain: detection by immunofluorescence. Arch Neurol 1974; 31:228–232.
114. Elizan TS, Casals J. No viral antigens detected in brain tissue from a case of acute encephalitis lethargica and another case of post-encephalitic parkinsonism. J Neurol Neurosurg Psychiatry 1989; 52:800–801.
115. Schwartz J, Elizan TS. Search for viral particles and virus-specific products in idiopathic Parkinson disease brain material. Ann Neurol 1979; 6:261–263.
116. Wetmur JG, Schwartz J, Elizan TS. Nucleic acid homology studies of viral nucleic acids in idiopathic Parkinson's disease. Arch Neurol 1979; 36:462–464.
117. Laing P, Knight J, Hill J, et al. Influenza viruses induce autoantibodies to a brain-specific 37-kDa protein in rabbit. Proc Natl Acad Sci USA 1989; 86:1998–2002.
118. Esiri MM, Swash M. Absence of herpes simplex virus antigen in brain in encephalitis lethargica. J Neurol Neurosurg Psychiatry 1984; 47:1049–1050.
119. Mann DMA, Yates PO, Davies JS, Hawkes J. Viruses, parkinsonism and Alzheimer's disease [letter]. J Neurol Neurosurg Psychiatry 1981; 44:651.
120. Waggener J, Beggs J, Sidell A. Virus-like filaments in juvenile parkinsonism. J Neuropathol Exp Neurol 1972; 31:187.
121. Gomirato G, Hyden H. A biochemical glia error in the Parkinson disease. Brain 1963; 86:773–780.
122. Gomirato G, Hyden H. Etiologic problems of so-called idiopathic Parkinson's disease. Ital J Neurol Sci 1981; 2:131–134.

123. Elizan TS, Casals J, Yahr MD. Antineurofilament antibodies in postencephalitic and idiopathic Parkinson's disease. J Neurol Sci 1983; 59:341–347.
124. Horta-Barbosa L, Fuccillo DA, Sever JL. Chronic viral infections of the central nervous system. JAMA 1971; 218:1185–1188.
125. Gajdusek DC, Gibbs CJ. Attempts to demonstrate a transmissible agent in kuru, amyotrophic lateral sclerosis, and other sub-acute and chronic nervous system degenerations of man. Nature 1964; 204:257–259.
126. Gibbs CJ Jr, Gajdusek DC. Amyotrophic lateral sclerosis, Parkinson's disease, and the amyotrophic lateral sclerosis–parkinsonism–dementia complex on Guam: a review and summary of attempts to demonstrate infection as the aetiology. J Clin Pathol [Suppl] (R Coll Pathol) 1972; 25:132–140.
127. Gibbs CJ Jr, Gajdusek DC. An update on long-term in vivo and in vitro studies designed to identify a virus as the cause of amyotrophic lateral sclerosis, parkinsonism dementia and Parkinson's disease. In: Rowland L, ed. Human motor neuron diseases. Adv Neurol 1982; 36:343–353.
128. Merz PA, Rohwer RG, Kascak R, et al. Infection-specific particle from the unconventional slow virus diseases. Science 1984; 225:437–440.
129. Prusiner SB. Prions and neurodegenerative diseases. N Engl J Med 1987; 317:1571–1581.
130. Elizan TS, Terasaki PI, Yahr MD. HLA-B14 antigen and postencephalitic Parkinson's disease: their association in an American–Jewish ethnic group. Arch Neurol 1980; 37:542–544.
131. McGeer PL, Itagaki S, Akiyama H, McGeer G. Rate of cell death in parkinsonism indicates active neuropathological process. Ann Neurol 1988; 24:574–576.
132. Fazzini E, Fleming J,Fahn S. Cerebrospinal fluid antibodies to coronaviruses in patients with Parkinson's disease. Mov Disord 1992; 7:153–158.
133. Fishman PS, Gass JS, Swoveland PT. Infection of the basal ganglia by a murine coronavirus. Science 1985; 229:877–879.
134. Kohbata S, Beaman BL. L-Dopa-responsive movement disorder caused by *Nocardia asteroides* localized in the brains of mice. Infect Immunol 1991; 59:181–191.
135. Hubble J, Kjelstrom J, Beaman B,Koller W. *Nocardia* serology in Parkinson's disease [abstract]. Mov Disord 1992; 7:292–293.
136. Isgreen WP, Chutorian AM, Fahn S. Sequential parkinsonism and chorea following "mild" influenza. Trans Am Neurol Assoc 1976; 101:56–59.
137. Dickerson RB, Newton JR, Hansen JE. Diagnosis and immediate prognosis of Japanese B encephalitis. Am J Med 1952; 12:277–288.
138. Richter R, Shimojyo S. Neurologic sequelae of Japanese B encephalitis. Neurology 1961; 11:553–559.
139. Goto A. A long duration follow-up study of Japanese encephalitis. Psychiatr Neurol Jpn 1962; 64:236–266.
140. Shiraki H, Goto A, Narabayashi H. Etat passe et present de l'encephalite Japonaise au Japon. Rev Neurol 1963; 108:633–696.
141. Mulder D, Parrott M, Thaler M. Sequelae of western equine encephalitis. Neurology 1951; 1:318–327.

142. Palmer R, Finley K. Sequelae of encephalitis: report of a study after the California epidemic. Calif Med 1956; 84:98–100.
143. Fulton JS, Burton AN. After effects of western equine encephalomyelitis infection in man. Can Med Assoc J 1953; 69:268–272.
144. Riggs N, Finley K. Sequelae of western encephalitis and St. Louis encephalitis. Calif Vector Views 1960; 7:35–41.
145. Finley KH. Postencephalitic manifestations of viral encephalitides. In: Field WS, ed. Pathogenesis and treatment of parkinsonism. Springfield, IL: Charles C Thomas, 1958:69–93.
146. Herzon H, Shelton J, Bruyn H. Sequelae of western equine and other arthropod-borne encephalitides. Neurology 1957; 7:535–548.
147. Schultz DR, Barthal JS, Garrett G. Western equine encephalitis with rapid onset of parkinsonism. Neurology 1977; 27:1095–1096.
148. Chambers RA, Levey GS. Studies of eastern encephalitis. Read before the 13th annual meeting of the American Academy of Neurology, Detroit, 1961.
149. Woodruff AW, Ansdell VE, Bowen ETW. Le Dantec virus infection in a patient who had not been to West Africa. Br Med J 1977; 2:1632–1633.
150. Meyer B. Encephalitis after measles with severe parkinsonism rigidity: recovery. Br Med J 1943; 1:508.
151. Warembourg H, Niquet G, Pauchant M, Ducloux G. Syndrome parkinsonien. Sequelle d'une poliomyèlite aiguë a forme d'encephalite lethargique chez un enfant de 20 mois. Sem Hop Paris 1962; 38:2299–2307.
152. Walters J. Postencephalitic Parkinson syndrome after meningoencephalitis due to Coxsackie virus group B, type 2. N Engl J Med 1960; 263:744–747.
153. Nath A, Jankovic J, Pettigrew L. Movement disorders and AIDS. Neurology 1987; 37:37–41.
154. Wszolek Z, Monsour H, Smith P, Pfeiffer R. Cryptococcal meningoencephalitis with parkinsonian features. Mov Disord 1988; 3:271–273.
155. Noel S, Guillaume M-P, Telerman-Toppet N, Cogan E. Movement disorders due to cerebral *Toxoplasma gondii* infection in patients with the acquired immunodeficiency syndrome (AIDS). Acta Neurol Belg 1992; 92:148–156.
156. Adler CH, Stern MB, Brooks ML. Parkinsonism secondary to bilateral striatal fungal abscesses. Mov Disord 1989; 4(4):333–337.
157. Henner K, Hanzal F, Lesny I, et al. Les encephalites Europeennes a tiques. Rev Neurol 1963:697–752.
158. Seitelberger F, Jellinger K. Neuropathologie der Zeckenencephalitis. Neuropathologia 1966; 4:367–400.
159. Viader F, Poncelet AM, Chapon F, et al. Les formes neurologiques de la maladie de Lyme: 12 cas. Rev Neurol (Paris) 1989; 145:362–368.
160. Wilson S, Cobb S. Mesencephalitis syphilitica. J Neurol Psychopathol 1924; 5:44–60.
161. Osuntokun BO, Bademosi O, Ogunremi K, Wright SG. Neuropsychiatric manifestations of typhoid fever in 959 patients. Arch Neurol 1972; 27:7–13.
162. Marttila RJ, Halonen P, Rinne UK. Influenza virus antibodies in parkinsonism. Arch Neurol 1977; 34:99–100.

163. Elizan TS, Yahr MD. The possible role of virus infection in the etiology and pathogenesis of Parkinson's disease [abstract 459], Excerpta Medica Intl Cong Series No. 427, 11th world congress of neurology. Amsterdam: Excerpta Medica, 1977. 154–155.
164. Rinne UK. Recent advances in research on parkinsonism. In: Marttila RJ, ed. Proceedings of the 22nd Scandinavian congress of neurology. Acta Neurol Scand 1978; 57(suppl 67):77–113.
165. Elizan TS, Schwartz J, Yahr MD,Casals J. Antibodies against arboviruses in postencephalitic and idiopathic Parkinson's disease. Arch Neurol 1978; 35:257–260.
166. Elizan TS, Yahr MD, Casals J. Indirect immunofluorescence test against lymphocytic choriomeningitis (LCM) virus in Parkinson's disease [letter]. Mt Sinai J Med 1979; 46:597–598.

15

Bibliography Relating to the Etiology of Parkinson's Disease

Jonas H. Ellenberg

National Institute of Neurological Disorders and Stroke, National Institutes of Health, Bethesda, Maryland

I. INTRODUCTION

The idea for a book on the etiology of Parkinson's disease grew out of a recognition by the Parkinson's Epidemiology Research Committee that concurrent with initiation of an attempt to map out a strategy for searching for the etiology for Parkinson's disease, a thorough review of the past research was in order. As noted in the Introduction, at the outset, this task was incorrectly thought to be a straightforward undertaking, especially in view of the electronic reference services that existed.

Each of the editors, as well as the contributors, were to some degree parochial in their view of what was available in the literature, relying heavily on their own interest or developed perception of what was important and what was published. The resulting mass of research was, therefore, a surprise to us all.

We began our search with the subject index of *Parkinson's Disease and Related Disorders: Cumulative Bibliography 1800–1970* (1). For electronic searches, we used subjects, keywords, text words, and other citations that were as general as possible to capture the widest possible array of literature that could later be culled for relevance, once in hand. We performed electronic searches through 1994, on MEDLINE beginning with 1966, Exerpta Medica beginning with 1974, and BIOS beginning with 1970. These searches netted an enormous array of citations, including journal articles, books, and abstracts from scientific meetings. A major source for citations not retrieved electronically was through citations to books and from books to other books or peer-reviewed journals. This was especially the case for references prior to the mid-1960s.

Each reference was reviewed in most cases through hard-copy examination where possible or otherwise through on-line electronic examination. Papers were included in the bibliography if considered relevant to the etiology of Parkinson's disease. With some exceptions, only those articles were included that were written in English or that had an English summary. This was especially the case for references prior to the mid-1960s.

The citations were reviewed for accuracy against the actual article in all but the few cases where we could not obtain or gain access to the printed work. Electronic storage, reference manipulation, and error checking of the more than 2400 citations was accomplished using Reference Manager (Version 5.2) (2).

Almost all the references cited in the chapters in this book are included in this bibliography, except where they were used only for technical backup to arguments related to the etiology of Parkinson's disease. For example, references to statistical or epidemiological texts or articles in support of methodological approaches are included in the separate chapters, but not in the bibliography. Conversely, many hundreds of articles not included in the chapters are included in the bibliography for the sake of completeness. For example, while an author may have selected a subset of references from several articles providing corroborative data on the same issue, they would all be included in the main bibliography.

We intend this bibliography to be a tool for researchers searching for the etiology of Parkinson's disease and have made it as complete as possible. The references are in alphabetical order by name of first author and use the format of the *New England Journal of Medicine*.

ACKNOWLEDGMENTS

Undertakings such as these require painstaking care, long hours, tedious, and repetitious checking and rechecking for accuracy. We owe a great debt to Ms. Jean Hoffman, in the Biometry Branch at the National Institute of Neurological Disorders and Stroke, for her unstinting patience and meticulous organization skills that made this daunting task possible.

REFERENCES

1. Columbia University New York. Parkinson's disease and related disorders: Cumulative Bibliography 1800–1970 (NTIS-PB-294-456). Springfield, Virginia: U.S. Department of Commerce, National Technical Information Service, 1978.
2. Research Information Systems Inc. Reference Manager. Carlsbad, California: Research Information Systems, Inc., 1990.

BIBLIOGRAPHY

1. Abbott RA, Cox M, Markus H, Tomkins A. Diet, body size and micronutrient status in Parkinson's disease. Eur J Clin Nutr 1992; 46:879–884.
2. Abd El Naby S, Hassanein M. Neuropsychiatric manifestations of chronic manganese poisoning. J Neurol Neurosurg Psychiatry 1965; 28:282–285.
3. Abe S, Miyasaka K, Tashiro K, Takei H, Isu T, Tsuru M. Evaluation of the brainstem with high-resolution CT in cerebellar atrophic processes. Am J Neuroradiology 1983; 4(3):446–449.
4. Abramsky O, Litvin Y. Automimmune response to dopamine-receptor as a possible mechanism in the pathogenesis of Parkinson's disease and schizophrenia. Perspect Biol Med 1978; 22:104–114.
5. Accardi R, Arnetoli G, Ammannati F. Parkinsonism caused by chronic subdural hematoma. A case report. Ital J Neurol Sci 1985; 6:109–111.
6. Acosta J. Epidemiology of Parkinson's disease: record of patients in our rural medium: Verjel de la Frontera. 9th International Symposium on Parkinson's Disease 1988; 57.
7. Adams JH, Corsellis JAN, Duchen LW. Greenfield's neuropathology. New York: Wiley, 1984.
8. Adams RD. Recent observations on normal pressure hydrocephalus. Schewizer Arch Neurol Neurochir Psychiatr 1975; 116:7–15.
9. Adams RD, Adam MJ. Striatonigral degeneration. In: Vinken P, Bruyn G, Klawans H, eds. Handbook of Clinical Neurology, Vol 49 Extrapyamidal disorders. Amsterdam: Elsevier, 1986:205–212.
10. Adams RD, Van Bogaert L, Vander Eecken H. Striatonigral degeneration. J Neuropathol Exp Neurol 1964; 23:584–608.
11. Adler CH, Stern MB, Brooks ML. Parkinsonism secondary to bilateral striatal fungal abscesses. Mov Disord 1989; 4(4):333–337.
12. Agid Y. Conclusions. In: Litvan I, Agid Y, eds. Progressive supranuclear palsy. Clinical and research approaches. New York, Oxford: Oxford University Press, 1992:270–273.
13. Agid Y, Blin J. Nerve cell death in degenerative diseases of the central nervous system: Clinical aspects. Ciba Found Symp 1987; 126:3–29.
14. Agid Y, Cervera P, Hirsch E, et al. Biochemistry of Parkinson's disease 28 years later: a critical review. Mov Disord 1989; 4:S126–S144.
15. Agnoli A, Bruno G, Nappi G, et al. Neurotoxicity and Parkinson's disease: Etiopathogenic role of pesticides. 9th International Symposium on Parkinson's Disease 1988; 10.
16. Agostini L, Piccirilli M, Ricci S. Parkinson's disease and amyotrophic lateral sclerosis. Rivista Di Patologia Nervosa E Mentale 1980; 101:51–66.
17. Airaksinen MM, Kari I. Beta-carbolines, psychoactive compounds in the mammalian body. Med Biology 1981; 59:190–211.
18. Albin RL, Gilman S. Autoradiographic localization of inhibitory and excitatory amino acid neurotransmitter receptors in human normal and olivopontocerebellar atrophy cerebellar cortex. Brain Res 1990; 522 (1):37–45.

19. Albores R, Neafsey EJ, Drucker G, Fields JZ, Collins MA. Mitochondrial respiratory inhibition by N-methylated B-carboline derivatives structurally resembling N-methyl-4-phenylpyridine. Proc Natl Acad Sci 1990; 87:9368–9372.
20. Aldrich M, Foster N, White R, Bluemlein L, Prokopowicz G. Sleep abnormalities in progressive supranuclear palsy. Ann Neurol 1989; 25:577–581.
21. Allan W. Inheritance of the Shaking Palsy. Arch Intern Med 1937; 60:424–436.
22. Alonso ME, Otero E, D'Regules R, Figueroa HH. Parkinson's disease: a genetic study. Can J Neurol Sci 1986; 13:248–251.
23. Altenkirch H, Stoltenburg G, Wagner HM. Experimental studies on hydrocarbon neuropathies induced by methly-ethyl-ketone. J Neurol 1978; 219:159.
24. Altenkirch H, Wagner HM, Stoltenberg G, Spencer PS. Nervous system responses of rats to subchronic inhalation of n-hexane and n-hexane + methyl ethyl ketone mixtures. J Neurol Sci 1982; 57:209–219.
25. Alter M. Environmental toxins: Their possible role in inducing parkinsonism. 9th Iternational Symposium on Parkinson s Disease 1988; 56.
26. Alter M, Schaumann B. A family with amyotrophic lateral sclerosis and Parkinsonism. J Neurol 1976; 212:281–284.
27. Alvord EC, Forno LS. Pathology. In: Koller WC, ed. Handbook of Parkinson's disease. Second Edition. New York: Marcel Dekker, Inc., 1992:255-284.
28. Alvord EC Jr. The pathology of parkinsonism: Etiologic, pathogenetic and prognostic implications. Trans Am Neurol Assoc 1965; 90:167-170.
29. Alvord EC Jr. The pathology of Parkinsonism. II. An interpretation with special reference to other changes in the aging brain. Contemp Neurol Ser 1971; 8:131-161.
30. Amato L, Cuffaro F, Lupo I, Nava L, Rizzo M. Discussion of a clinical case of associated amyotrophic lateral sclerosis-parkinsonism-dementia. Acta Neurol Scand 1986; 8:310–313.
31. Ambani LM. Genetics of Parkinson's disease: Biochemical epidemiologic and neuropathologic correlation. Indian J Med Sci 1977; 31:21–29.
32. Ambani LM, Van Woert MH, Murphy S. Brain peroxidase and catalase in Parkinson's disease. Arch Neurol 1975; 32:114–118.
33. Ambrosetto P. CT in progressive supranuclear palsy. Am J Neuroradiology 1987; 8(5):849–851.
34. Amenomori M, Nagao Y, Ogino K, Banba M, Shigeta Y. [Parkinsonism caused by chronic subdural hematoma. A case report]. Nippon Naika Gakkai Zasshi 1989; 78:708–709.
35. Aminoff M, Wilcox C, Workes M, Kremer M. Levodopa therapy for parkinsonism in the Shy-Drager syndrome. J Neurol Neurosurg Psychiatry 1973; 36:350–353.
36. Anand P, Bannister R, McGregor GP, Chatei MA, Mulderry PK, Bloom SR. Marked depletion of dorsal spinal cord substance P and calcitonin gene-related peptide with intact skin flare responses in multiple system atrophy. J Neurol Neurosurg Psychiatry 1988; 51(2):192–196.
37. Anden NE, Carlsson A, Dahlstrom A, Fuxe K, Hillarp NA, Larsson K. Demonstration and mapping out of nigro-neostriatal dopamine neurons. Life Sci 1964; 3:523–530.

38. Anderson DW, Schoenberg BS, Haerer AF. Prevalence surveys of neurologic disorders: methodologic implications of the Copiah County Study. J Clin Epidemiol 1988; 41:339–345.
39. Anderson F, Richardson E, Okazaki H. Neurofibrillary degeneration of Guam: Frequency in Chamorros and non-Chamorros with no known neurologic disease. Brain 1975; 102:65–77.
40. Andrewes C, Carmichael E. A note on the presence of antibodies to herpes virus in postencephalitic and other human sera. Lancet 1930; 1:857–858.
41. Andrews JM. Neurological disease on Guam. A review of past and present investigations. Bull L A Neurol Soc 1967; 32:30–42.
42. Anonymous. Encephalitis Lethargica. Lancet 1981; December 19/26:1396–1397.
43. Anonymous. Parkinson's disease: One illness or many syndromes? Lancet 1992; 339:1263–1264.
44. Ansari KA, Johnson A. Olfactory function in patients with Parkinson's disease. J Chron Dis 1975; 28:493–497.
45. Ansher SS, Cadet JL, Jakoby WB, Baker JK. Role of N-methyltransferases in the neurotoxicity associated with the metabolites of 1-methyl-4-phenyl-1,2,3,6-tetrahydropyridine (MPTP) and other 4-substituted pyridines in the environment. Biochem Pharmacol 1986; 35:3359–3363.
46. Ansley D. Aging twins offer clues to late-onset diseases. Science 1993; 259:1826–1828.
47. Antunes JL, Fahn S, Cote L. Normal pressure hydrocephalus and Parkinson's disease. J Neurol Transm Suppl 1983; 19:225–231.
48. Anzil A. Progressive supranuclear palsy: Case report with pathological findings. Acta Neuropathol (Berlin) 1969; 14:72–76.
49. Appel GB, Galen R, O'Brien J, Schonfeldt R. Methyl iodide intoxication. Ann Intern Med 1975; 82:534–536.
50. Appel SH. A unifying hypothesis for the cause of amyotrophic lateral sclerosis, parkinsonism, and Alzheimer disease. Ann Neurol 1981; 10:499–505.
51. Aquilonius SM. Parkinson's disease—etiology and smoking. In: Nordberg A, Fuxe K, Holmstedt B, Sundwall A, eds. Progress in Brain Research. Uppsala, Sweden: Elsevier Science Publishers B.V. (Biomedical Division), 1989:329–333.
52. Aquilonius SM, Hartvig P. Utilization of Antiparkinson Drugs in Sweden. Uppsala J Med Sci 1986; 93.
53. Aquilonius SM, Hartvig P. A Swedish county with unexpectedly high utilization of anti-parkinsonian drugs. Acta Neurol Scand 1986; 74:379-382.
54. Araki S, Iwasaki Y, Kuroiwa Y. Epidemiological study of amyotrophic lateral sclerosis and allied disorders in the Kii Penisula (Japan). J Neurol Sci 1967; 4:279-287.
55. Armon C, Miller P, Carwile S, et al. Valproate-induced parkinsonism-dementia syndrome: A potential model for acquired chronic degenerative diseases. Ann Neurol 1991; 30:41-42.
56. Armon C, Kurland LT, Daube JR, O'Brien PC. Epidemiologic correlates of sporadic amyothrophic lateral sclerosis. Neurology 1991; 41:1077-1084.
57. Armstrong M, Daly AK, Cholerton S, Bateman DN, Idle JR. Mutant debrisoquine hydroxylation genes in Parkinson's disease. Lancet 1992; 339:1017-1018.

58. Arnoud B. [Etiology of Parkinson's disease]. Soins 1986; 7–8.
59. Arora PK, Riachi NJ, Harik SI, Sayre LM. Chemical oxidation of 1-methyl-4-phenyl-1,2,3,6-tetrahydropyridine (MPTP) and its in vivo metabolism in rat brain and liver. Biochem Biophys Res Commun 1988; 152:1339–1347.
60. Ashok PP, Radhakrishnan K, Sridharan R, Mousa ME. Epidemiology of Parkinson's disease in Benghazi, North-East Libya. Clin Neurol Neurosurg 1986; 88(2):109–113.
61. Atadzhanov M. [The role of heredity in Parkinson's disease]. Zh Nevropatol Psikhiatr 1973; 73:195–199.
62. Atadzhanov M. [Hereditary aspects of Parkinson's disease (review of the literature)]. Zh Nevropatol Psikhiatr 1973; 73:919–926.
63. Atadzhanov M. [Diabetes mellitus in families with Parkinson's disease]. Klin Med (Mosk) 1973; 51:87–91.
64. Atadzhanov M. [Modeling parkinsonism (review)]. Zh Nevropatol Psikhiatr 1982; 82:110–119.
65. Atadzhanov M, Tret'iakova KA, Shavolina VA. [Catecholamine excretion in patients with parkinsonism and their relatives]. Klin Med (Mosk) 1972; 50:48–51.
66. Aubby D, Saggu HK, Jenner P, Quinn NP, Harding AD, Marsden CD. Leukocyte glutamate dehydrogenase activity in patients with degenerative neurological disorders. J Neurol Neurosurg Psychiatry 1988; 51(7):893–902.
67. Aubert I, Araujo DM, Cécye D, Robitaille Y, Gauthier S, Quirion R. Comparative alterations of nicotinic and muscarinic binding sites in Alzheimer's and Parkinson's diseases. J Neurochem 1992; 58(2):529–541.
68. Aw TY, Nicotera N, Manzo L, Orrenius S. Tributyltin stimulates apoptosis in rat thymocytes. Arch Biochem Biophys 1990; 283:46–50.
69. Axt KJ,Commins DL, Vosmer G, Seiden LS. A-Methyl-p-tyrosine pretreatment partially prevents methamphetamine-induced endogenous neurotoxin formation. Brain Res 1990; 515:269–276.
70. Ayd F. A Survey of drug-induced extrapyramidal reactions. JAMA 1961; 175:1054–1060.
71. Azevedo I, Osswald W. Adrenergic nerve degeneration induced by condensation products of adrenaline and acetaldehyde. Arch Pharmacol 1977; 300:139–144.
72. Bademosi O, Al-Rajeh IH, Awada A, et al. Prevalence of Parkinson's disease (PD) in an Arab community: The Thugbah study. In: Congrés de neurologie tropicale. September 26–28, 1991. Limoges: Recherche en Neurologie Tropicale Press, 1991:27.
73. Bahiga LM, Kotb NA, El-Dessoukey EA. Neurological syndromes produced by some toxic metals encountered industrially or environmentally. Z Ernahrungswiss 1978; 17:84–88.
74. Baldessarini RJ, Kula NS, Francoeur D, Finklestein SP. Antioxidants fail to inhibit depletion of striatal dopamine by MPTP. Neurology 1986; 36:735.
75. Ball B. About the insanity in paralysis agitans. Encephale 1882; 2:22–32.
76. Ballard PA, Tetrud JW, Langston JW. Permanent human parkinsonism due to 1-methyl-4-phenyl-1,2,3,6-tetrahydropyridine (MPTP): Seven cases. Neurology 1985; 35:949–956.

77. Bannister R. Degeneration of the autonomic nervous system. Lancet 1971; 2:175–179.
78. Bannister R, Mowbray J, Sidgwick A. Genetic control of progressive autonomic failure: evidence for association with an HLA antigen. Lancet 1983; 1:1017.
79. Bannister R, Oppenheimer DR. Degenerative disease of the nervous system associated with autonomic failure. Brain 1972; 95:457–474.
80. Bannon MJ, Goedert M, Williams B. The possible relation of glutathione, melanin and 1-methyl-4-phenyl-1,2,5,6-tetrahydropyridine (MPTP) to Parkinson's disease. Biochem Pharmacol 1984; 33:2697–2698.
81. Barbeau A. Etiology and pathogenesis—recent developments. Appl Ther 1967; 9:448–450.
82. Barbeau A. Parkinson's disease as a systemic disorder. In: Gillingham FJ, Donaldson IML, eds. Third symposium on Parkinson's disease. Edinburgh: Livingstone Ltd., 1969:66–73.
83. Barbeau A. Six years of high-level levodopa therapy in severely akinetic parkinsonian patients. Arch Neurol 1976; 33:333–338.
84. Barbeau A. Parkinson's disease: Etiological considerations. Res Publ Assoc Res Nerv Ment Dis 1976; 55:281–292.
85. Barbeau A. Peptides in Parkinson's disease. Adv Exp Med Biol 1978; 113:101–110.
86. Barbeau A. Etiology of Parkinson's disease: A research strategy. Can J Neurol Sci 1984; 11:24–28.
87. Barbeau A. Parkinson's disease: Clinical features and etiopathology. In: Vinken PJ, Bruyn GW, Klawans HL, eds. Handbook of clinical neurology, Vol.5. Extrapyramidal disorders. Amsterdam: Elsevier Science Publishers, 1986:87–152.
88. Barbeau A, Cloutier T, Roy M, Plasse L, Paris S, Poirier J. Ecogenetics of Parkinson's disease: 4-hydroxylation of debrisoquine. Lancet 1985; 2:1213–1216.
89. Barbeau A, Inque N, Cloutier T. Role of manganese in dystonia. In: Eldridge R, Fahn S, eds. Advances in Neurology, Vol.14. New York: Raven Press, 1976:339–352.
90. Barbeau A, Pourcher E. New data on the genetics of Parkinson's disease. Can J Neurol Sci 1982; 9:53–60.
91. Barbeau A, Pourcher E. Genetics of early onset Parkinson's disease. Excerpta Medica 1983; 1–16.
92. Barbeau A, Roy M. Familial subsets in idiopathic Parkinson's disease. Can J Neurol Sci 1984; 11:144–150.
93. Barbeau A, Roy M. Uneven prevalence of Parkinson's disease in the Province of Quebec. Can J Neurol Sci 1985; 12:169–170.
94. Barbeau A, Roy M. Genetic susceptibility, environmental factors and Parkinson's disease. VIII International Symposium on Parkinson's disease 1985; 13.
95. Barbeau A, Roy M, Bernier G, Campanella G, Paris S. Ecogenetics of Parkinson's disease: Prevalence and environmental aspects in rural areas. Can J Neurol Sci 1987; 14:36–41.
96. Barbeau A, Roy M, Boyer L. Genetic studies in Parkinson's disease. In: Parkin-

son-specific motor and mental disorders, role of the pallidum: pathophysiological, biochemical, and therapeutic aspects—Advances in Neurology, Vol 40. New York: Raven Press, 1984:333–339.

97. Barbeau A, Roy M, Cloutier T. Smoking, cancer, and Parkinson's disease. Ann Neurol 1986; 20:105–106.
98. Barbeau A, Roy M, Cloutier T, Plasse L, Paris S. Environmental and genetic factors in the etiology of Parkinson's disease. In: Yahr MD, Bergmann KJ, eds. Parkinson's disease-Advances in Neurology, Vol 45. New York: Raven Press, 1986:299–306.
99. Barbeau A, Roy M, Langston JW. Neurological consequence of industrial exposure to 1-methyl-4-pheny1-1,2,3,6-tetrahydropyridine [letter]. Lancet 1985; 1:747.
100. Barden H. Relationship of Golgi thaiminepyrophosphatase and lyososomal acid phosphatase to neuromelanin and lipofuscin in cerebral neurons of the aging rhesus monkey. J Neuropathol Exp Neurol 1970; 29:225–240.
101. Barinaga M. Amino acids: How much excitement is too much? Science 1990; 247:20-22.
102. Barker R. Substance P and Parkinson's disease: A causal relationship. J Theor Biol 1986; 120:353–362.
103. Barker R. Environmental toxins and Parkinson's disease [letter]. TINS 1989; 12:82.
104. Barker R. Substance P and neurodegenerative disorders. A speculative review. neuropeptides 1991; 20:73–78.
105. Barker SA, Harrison REW, Monti JA, Brown GB, Christian ST. Identification and quantification of 1,2,3,4-tetrahydro-beta-carboline, 2-methyl-1,2,3,4-tetrahydro-beta-carboline, and 6-methoxy-1,2,3,4-tetrahydro-beta-carboline as in vivo constituents of rat brain and adrenal gland. Biochem Pharmacol 1981; 30:9–17.
106. Barnes NJG, Bradbury AJ, Costall B, Domeney AM, Kelly ME, Naylor RJ. Neuropharmacological manipulations with MPTP. J Neural Transm 986; 47–63.
107. Barolin GS, Hornykiewicz O. Zur diagnostischen Wertigkeit der Homovanillinsaure im Liquor cerebrospinalis. Wein Klin Wochenschr 1967; 79:85–88.
108. Baron JA. Cigarette smoking and Parkinson's disease. Neurology 1986; 36:1490–1496.
109. Barr A. Progressive supranuclear palsy. In: Vinken P, Bryun G, Klawans H, eds. Handbook of clinical neurology, Vol 49. Amsterdam: 1986:239–254.
110. Barrass BC, Coult DB, Pinder RM. 3-Hydroxy-4-methoxyphenethylamine: the endogenous toxin of parkinsonism. J Pharm Pharmacol 1972; 24:499–501.
111. Bauer RB, Stevens Ç, Reveno WS, Rosenbaum H. L-Dopa treatment of Parkinson's disease: a ten-year follow-up study. J Am Geriatr Soc 1982; 30:322–325.
112. Baumann RJ, Jameson HD, McKean HE, Haack DG, Weisberg LM. Cigarette smoking and Parkinson disease: I. A comparison of cases with matched neighbors. Neurology 1980; 30:839–843.
113. Baust W. [Assessment of the correlation between accidental and non-traumatic nervous diseases]. Med Welt 1976; 27:6–63.

114. Beal MF. Does impairment of energy metabolism result in excitotoxic neuronal death in neurodegenerative illnesses? Ann Neurol 1992; 31:119–130.
115. Beal MF. Mechanisms of excitotoxicity in neurologic diseases. FASEB J 1992; 6:3338–3344.
116. Beal MF, Hyman BT, Koroshetz W. Do defects in mitochondrial energy metabolism underlie the pathology of neurodegenerative diseases? TINS 1993; 16:125–131.
117. Bebin EM, Bebin J, Currier RD, Smith EE, Perry TL. Morphometric studies in dominant olivopontocerebellar atrophy. Comparison of cell losses with amino acid decreases. Arch Neurol 1990; 47(2):188–192.
118. Beck O, Repke DB, Faull KF. 6-Hydroxymethtryptoline is naturally occurring in mammalian urine: identification by combined chiral capillary gas chromatography and high resolution mass spectrometry. Biomed Environ Mass Spectrom 1986; 13:469–472.
119. Bedard PJ, Di Paolo T, Falardeau P, Boucher R. Chronic treatment with L-Dopa, but not bromocriptine induces dyskinesia in MPTP-parkinsonian monkeys. Correlation with [^{3}H]spiperone binding. Brain Res 1986; 379:294–299.
120. Bedard PJ, Gomez-Mancilla B, Blanchette P, Gagnon C, Di Paolo T. Levodopa-induced dyskinesia: facts and fancy. What does the MPTP monkey model tell us? Can J Neurol Sci 1992; 19:134–37.
121. Behrman S, Carroll J, Mathews W. Progressive supranuclear palsy: clinico-pathological study of four cases. Brain 1969; 92:663–678.
122. Bekkelund SI, Selseth B, Mellgren SI. [Parkinson's disease in a population group in northern Norway]. Tidsskr Nor Laegeforen 1989; 109:561–563.
123. Bell J, Clark AJ. A pedigree of paralysis agitans. Ann Eugenics 926; 455–462.
124. Ben-Shachar D, Eshel G, Finberg JP, Youdim MB. The iron chelator desferrioxamine (Desferal) retards 6-hydroxydopamine-induced degeneration of nigrostriatal dopamine neurons. J Neurochem 1991; 56(4): 1441–1444.
125. Ben-Shachar D, Eshel G, Riederer P, Youdim MBH. Role of iron and iron chelation in dopaminergic-induced neurodegeneration: Implication for Parkinson's disease. Ann Neurol 1992; 32 Suppl.:S105–S110.
126. Ben-Shachar D, Riederer P, Youdim MBH. Iron-melanin interaction and lipid peroxidation: Implications for Parkinson's disease. J Neurochem 1991; 57:1609–1614.
127. Ben-Shachar D, Youdim MBH. Selectivity to melanized nigra-striatal dopamine neurons to degeneration in Parkinson's disease may depend on iron-melanin interaction. J Neural Transm 1990; Supplement 29:251–258.
128. Ben-Shachar D, Youdim MBH. Intranigral iron injection induces behavioural and biochemical "parkinsonism" in rats. J Neurochem 1991; 57:2133–2135.
129. Bender JL. Parkinson's disease-a review. Ill Med J 1975; 148:227–229, 231.
130. Benedetti MS, Dostert P, Dedieu M. Ratio of enantiomers of salsolinol in human urine and effect of food. 15th CINP Congress, Puerto Rico, 12/14–17, book of abstracts 1986; 56. (abstract)
131. Benedetti MS, Keane PE. Differential changes in monoamine oxidase A and B activity in the aging rat brain. J Neurochem 1980; 35:1026–1032.

132. Benitez J, Ladero JM, Jiminez-Jiminez FJ, et al. Oxidative polymorphism of debrisoquine in Parkinson's disease. J Neurol Neurosurg Psychiatry 1990; 53:289–292.
133. Berciano J. Olivopontocerebellar atrophy. A review of 7 cases. J Neurol Sci 1982; 53(2):253–272.
134. Berciano J. Olivopontocerebellar atrophy. In: Jankovic J, Tolosa E, eds. Parkinson's disease and movement disorders. Baltimore-Munich: Urban & Schwarzenberg, 1988:131–151.
135. Berger L, Gauthier S, Leblanc R. Akinetic mutism and parkinsonism associated with obstructive hydrocephalus. Can J Neurol Sci 1985; 12:255–258.
136. Bergeron C, Pollanen M. Lewy bodies in Alzheimer disease - one or two diseases. Alzheimer Dis Assoc Disord 1989; 3:97–204.
137. Bergeron C, Steele JC. Guam Parkinson-dementia complex and amyotrophic lateral sclerosis: Clinic-pathological correlation of seven cases. Int ALS-MND Update 1989; 2Q:13–14.
138. Bergevin P, Patwardhan V, Weissman J. Neurotoxicity of 5-fluorouracil. Lancet 1975; i:410.
139. Beringer K. Uber ein neues, auf das extrapyramidal-motorische system wirkendes alkaloid (Banisterin). Der Nervenarzt 1928; 1:265–275.
140. Beringer K. Zur banisterin und harminfrage. Der Nervenarzt 1929; 2:548–549.
141. Bernheimer H, Birkmayer W, Hornykiewicz O, Jellinger K, Seitelberger F. Brain dopamine and the syndromes of Parkinson and Huntington. J Neurol Sci 1973; 20:415–455.
142. Bethlem J, Den Hartog Jager WA. The incidence and characteristics of Lewy bodies in idiopathic paralysis agitans (Parkinson's disease). J Neurol Neurosurg Psychiatry 1960; 23:74–80.
143. Betti OO, Franke E, Ottino CA, Mendieta NR, Hana VJ. [Traumatic encephalopathy]. Prensa Med Argent 1970; 57:976–979.
144. Betti OO, Ottino CA. Pugilistic encephalopathy. Acta Neurol Latinoam 1969; 15:47–51.
145. Bharucha EP, Bharucha NE. Epidemiological study of Parkinson's disease in Parsis in India. In: Narabayashi H, Nagatsu T, Yanagisawa N, Mizuno Y, eds. From basic research to treatment. Advances in Neurology, Vol. 60. New York: Raven Press, 1993:352–354.
146. Bharucha NE, Bharucha EP, Bharucha AE, Bhise AV, Schoenberg BS. Prevalence of Parkinson's disease in the Parsi community of Bombay, India. Arch Neurol 1988; 45:1321–1323.
147. Bharucha NE, Bharucha EP, Dastur HD, et al. Pilot survey of the prevalence of neurologic disorders in the Parsi community of Bombay. Am J Prev Med 1987; 3:293–299.
148. Bharucha NE, Stokes L, Schoenberg BS, et al. A case-control study of twin pairs discordant for Parkinson's disease: A search for environmental risk factors. In:. Neurology, 1986:284–288.
149. Bhatia KP, Daniel SE, Marsden CD. Familial parkinsonism with depression; A clinicopathological study. Ann Neurol 1993; 34:842–847.

150. Bhatt MH, Snow BJ, Martin WR, Cooper S, Calne DB. Positron emission tomography in Shy-Drager syndrome. Ann Neurol 1990; 28(1):101–103.
151. Bhatt MH, Snow BJ, Martin WR, Peppard R, Calne DB. Positron emission tomography in progressive supranuclear palsy. Arch Neurol 1991; 48(4):389–391.
152. Bickerstaff ER, Cloake PCP. Mesencephalitis and rhombencephalitis. Br Med J 1951; 2:77–81.
153. Biemond A, Beck W. Neural muscel atrophy with degeneration of the substantia nigra. Confin Neurol 1955; 15:142–153.
154. Biemond A, Sinnege JLM. Tabes of Friedreich with degeneration of the substantia nigra, a special type of hereditary parkinsonism. Confin Neurol 1955; 15: 129–142.
155. Bindoff LA, Birch-Machin MA, Cartlidge NEF, Parker WD Jr, Turnbull DM. Mitochondrial function in Parkinson's disease. Lancet 1989; ii:49.
156. Bindoff LA, Birch-Machin M, Cartlidge NEF, Parker WDJr, Turnbull DM. Mitochondrial function in Parkinson's disease (Letter). Lancet 1989; ii:49.
157. Bindoli A, Rigobello MP, Galzigna L. Toxicity of aminochromes. Toxicol Lett 1989; 48:3–20.
158. Bird ED, Iversen LL. Huntington's chorea. Post-mortem measurement of glutamic acid decarboxylase, choline acetyltransferase and dopamine in basal ganglia. Brain 1974; 97:457–472.
159. Bird M, Paulson G. The rigid form of Huntington's chorea. Neurology 1971; 21:271–276.
160. Bird TD. Medical genetics and clinical neurology: the common ground. Prog Med Genet 1985; 6:1–8.
161. Birkmayer W. Distinction between benign and malignant type of Parkinson's disease. Clin Neurol Neurosurg 1979; 81:158–164.
162. Bjorklund A. Fluorescence histochemistry of biogenic monoamines. In: Bjorklund A, Hokfelt T, eds. Handbook of chemical neuroanatomy, volume 1: methods in chemical neuroanatomy. Amsterdam: Elsevier Science Publishers, 1983:50–121.
163. Blair JA, Parveen H, Barford PA, Leeming RJ. Aetiology of Parkinson's disease. Lancet 1984; 1:167.
164. Blake NM, Kirk RL, Wilson SR, et al. Search for a red cell enzyme or serum protein marker in amyotrophic lateral sclerosis and parkinsonism-dementia of Guam. Am J Med Genet 1983; 14:299–305.
165. Blin J, Bonnet AM, Agid Y. Does levodopa aggravate Parkinson's disease. In: Fahn S, Marsden CD, Goldstein M, Calne DB, eds. Recent developments in Parkinson's disease, Volume II. Florham Park, New Jersey: Macmillan Healthcare Information, 1987:165–181.
166. Blin J, Bonnet AM, Agid Y. Does levodopa aggravate Parkinson's disease. Neurology 1988; 38:1410–1416.
167. Blocq P, Marinesco G. Sur un cas de tremblement parkinsonien hémiplégique symptomatique d'une tumeur du peduncule cérébral. Mem Soc Biol 1893; 45:105–111.
168. Bloom F, Barchas J, Sandler M, Usdin E. Beta-carbolines and tetrahydroisoquinolines-Proceedings of a workshop held at the Salk Institute, La Jolla, California,

December 12 and 13, 1981. Progress in clinical and biological research; v. 90. New York: Alan R. Liss, 1982.

169. Blunt SB, Jenner P, Marsden CD. The effect of chronic L-DOPA treatment on the recovery of motor function in 6-hydroxydopamine-lesioned rats receiving ventral mesencephalic grafts. Neuroscience 1991; 40:453–464.
170. Bocchetta A, Bernardi F, Piccardi MP, Zuddas A, Del Zompo M, Corsini GU. MPTP Model: Renewed interest in environmental factors in Parkinson's disease. In: Nappi G, ed. beurodegenerative Disorders: The role played by endotoxins and xenobiotics. 1988: 121–127.
171. Bocchetta A, Corsini GU. Aetiology of Parkinson's disease [letter]. Lancet 1985; 1:112–113.
172. Bocchetta A, Corsini GU. Parkinson's disease and pesticides [letter]. Lancet 1986; 2:1163.
173. Bodis-Wollner I. Visual deficits related to dopamine deficiency in experimental animals and Parkinson's disease patients. TINS 1990; 13:296–302.
174. Bodis-Wollner I. The visual system in Parkinson's disease. Res Publ Assoc Res Nerv Ment Dis 1990; 67:297–316.
175. Bodmer WF. Population genetics of the HLA system: retrospect and prospect. In: Dausset J, Colombani J, eds. Histocompatibility testing 1972. Copenhagen: Munksgaard, 1973:611–667.
176. Bogerts B. A brainstem atlas of catecholaminergic neurons in man, using melanin as a natural marker. J Comp Neurol 1981; 197:63–80.
177. Bojinov S. Encephalitis with acute Parkinsonian syndrome and bilateral inflammatory necrosis of the substantia nigra. J Neurosurg Sci 1971; 12:383–415.
178. Boller F, Mizutani T, Roessmann U, Gambetti P. Parkinson disease, dementia, and Alzheimer disease: Clinicopathological correlations. Ann Neurol 1980; 7:329–335.
179. Bonduelle M, Bouygues P, Escourolle R, Lormeau G. Simultaneous development of amyotrophic lateral sclerosis, Parkinson's syndrome and progressive dementia. Apropos of 2 anatomoclinical cases. Attempted interpretation. J Neurol Sci 1968; 6:315–332.
180. Bonuccelli O, Piccini P, Del Dotto P, Rossi G, Corsini GU, Muratorio A. Apomorphine test for dopaminergic responsiveness: A dose assessment study. Mov Disord 1993; 8:158–164.
181. Bonuccelli U, Piccini P, Del Dotto P, Pacifici GM, Corsini GU, Muratorio A. Platelet monoamine oxidase B activity in parkinsonian patients. J Neurol Neurosurg Psychiatry 1990; 53:854–855.
182. Booth RG, Castagnoli NJ, Rollema H. Intracerebral microdialysis neurotoxicity studies of quinoline and isoquinoline derivatives related to MPTP/MPP+. Neurosci Lett 1989; 100:306–312.
183. Booth RG, Trevor AJ, Singer TP, Castagnoli NJ. Studies on semirigid tricyclic analogues of the nigrostriatal toxin 1-methyl-4-phenyl-1,2,3,6-tetrahydropyridine. J Med Chem 1989; 32:473–477.
184. Boranic M, Raci F. A parkinson-like syndrome as side effect of chemotherapy with vincristine and adriamcycin in a child with acute leukaemia. Biomedicine 1979; 31:124–125.

185. Borit A, Rubinstein LJ, Urich H. The striatonigral degnerations. Putaminal pigments and nosology. Brain 1975; 98(1):101–112.
186. Borm PJ, Van Vliet C. Susceptibility in Parkinson's disease. 'Of mice and men'. Med Hypotheses 1988; 27:205–207.
187. Bosin TR, Borg S, Faull KF. Harman in rat brain, lung and human CSF: Effect of alcohol consumption. Alcohol 1989; 5:505–511.
188. Bosin TR, Faull KF. Indole derivatization procedures for electron capture negative chemical ionization mass spectrometry: identification of 1-methyl-1,2,3,4-tetrahydro-beta-carboline in rat brain and lung. Biomed Environmental Mass Spectrometry 1989; 18:247–252.
189. Bossi L, Caffaratti E. [Juvenile parkinsonian hemi-syndrome in a case of extracranial arteriovenous aneurysm of the vertebral artery. Clinical and radiological study]. Minerva Radiol 1967; 12:533–538.
190. Bostantjopoulou S, Logothetis J, Katsarou Z, Mentenopoulos G. Clinical observations in early and late onset Parkinson's disease. Functional neurology 1991; 6(2):145–149.
191. Bostroem A. Psychische Veranderungen. Monogr Neurol Psychiat 1922; 33:166–170.
192. Botez MI, Bertrand G, Leveille J, Marchand L. Parkinsonism—dementia complex, hydrocephalus and Paget's disease. Can J Neurol Sci 1977; 4:139–142.
193. Boudouresques J, Toga M, Roger J, et al. Maladie de Hallervorden-Spatz tardive avec importante participation reticulaire et cerebelleuse. Rev Neurol (Paris) 1967; 116:693–704.
194. Boyce S, Kelly E, Reavill C, Jenner P, Marsden CD. Repeated administration of N-methyl-4-phenyl-1,2,5,6-tetrahydropyridine to rats is not toxic to striatal dopamine neurons. Biochem Pharmacol 1984; 33:1747–1752.
195. Boyce S, Rupniak NMJ, Steventon MJ, Iversen SD. Characterisation of dyskinesias induced by L-dopa in MPTP-treated squirrel monkeys. Psychopharmacology (Berlin) 1990; 102:21–27.
196. Boyce S, Rupniak NMJ, Steventon MJ, Iversen SD. Nigrostriatal damage is required for induction of dyskinesias by L-DOPA in squirrel monkeys. Clin Neuropharmacol 1990; 13:448–458.
197. Boyson SJ. Parkinson's disease and the electron transport chain. Ann Neurol 1991; 30:330–331.
198. Bradbury AJ, Costall B, Domeney AM, et al. 1-Methyl-4-phenylpyridine is neurotoxic to the nigrostriatal dopamine pathway. Nature 1986; 319:56–57.
199. Braestrup C, Schmiechen R, Neef G, Nielsen M, Petersen EN. Interaction of convulsive ligands with benzodiazepine receptors. Science 1982; 216:1241–1243.
200. Braham J. [Parkinson's disease: new clues to the etiology (editorial)]. Harefuah 1985; 108:103–104.
201. Brait K, Fahn S, Schwarz G. Sporadic and familial parkinsonism and motor neuron disease. Neurology 1973; 23:990–1002.
202. Bramble MG. Dopamine and duodenal ulcer [letter]. Lancet 1979; 2:1191–1192.
203. Brazin ME, Epstein LG. Reversible parkinsonism from shunt failure. Pediatr Neurol 1985; 1:306–307.
204. Brett EM. Juvenile Parkinsonism. Dev Med Child Neurol 1972; 14:391–393.

205. Brewis M, Poskanzer DC, Rolland C, Miller H. Neurological disease in an English city. Acta Neurol Scand 1966; 42:Suppl 24:1–89.
206. Briebach T, Baas H, Fischer PA. [Orthostatic dysregulation in Parkinson syndrome. Results of a study of 250 patients]. Der Nervenarzt 1990; 61:491–494.
207. Brierly JB, Graham DI. Hypoxia and vascular disorders of the central nervous system. In: Adams JJ, Corsellis JAN, Duchen LW, eds. Hypoxia and vascular disorders of the central nervous system. New York: Raven Press, 1984:125–207.
208. Briskin JG, Lehrman K, Guilleminault C. Shy-Drager syndrome and sleep apnea. In: Guilleminault C, Dement W, eds. Sleep Apnea Syndromes. New York: Alan R. Liss, 1978:317–322.
209. Brissaud E. Leçons sur les maladies nerveuses. Paris: Masson et Cie, 1895.
210. Brizzee KR. Risk factors for senility. In: Rothschild H, ed. Pathophysiology of aging. New York: Oxford University Press, 1984:44–62.
211. Brody JA, Chase TN, Gordon EK. Depressed monoamine catabolite levels in cerebrospinal fluid of patients with parkinsonism dementia of Guam. N Engl J Med 1970; 282:947–950.
212. Brody JA, Chen KM. Recent studies of amyotrophic lateral sclerosis and parkinsonism-dementia on Guam. Proc Aust Assoc Neurol 1968; 5:331–334.
213. Brody JA, Hirano A, Scott RM. Recent neuropathologic observations in amyotrophic lateral sclerosis and parkinsonism-deme of Guam. Neurology 1971; 21:528–536.
214. Broe GA, Akhtar AJ, Andrews GR, Caird FI, Gilmore AJ, McLennan WJ. Neurological disorders in the elderly at home. J Neurol Neurosurg Psychiatry 1976; 39:361–363.
215. Broman T. Parkinson's syndrome, prevalence and incidence in Goteborg. Acta Neurol Scand 1963; suppl 4:95–101.
216. Brooks DJ. Detection of preclinical Parkinson's disease with PET. Neurology 1991; 41(suppl 2):24—28.
217. Brooks DJ, Ibanez V, Sawle GV, et al. Differing patterns of striatal 18F-dopa uptake in Parkinson's disease, multiple system atrophy, and progressive supranuclear palsy. Ann Neurol 1990; 28:547–555.
218. Brooks DJ, Playford ED, Ibanez V, et al. Isolated tremor and disruption of the nigrostriatal dopaminergic system: An 18F-dopa PET study. Neurology 1992; 42:1554–1560.
219. Brooks DJ, Salmon EP, Mathias CJ, et al. The relationship between locomotor disability, autonomic dysfunction, and the integrity of the striatal dopaminergic system in patients with multiple system atrophy, pure autonomic failure, and Parkinson's disease, studied with PET. Brain 1990; 113:1539–1552.
220. Brooks WJ, Jarvis MF, Wagner GC. Attenuation of MPTP-induced dopaminergic neurotoxicity by a serotonin uptake blocker. J Neural Transm 1988; 71:85–90.
221. Brooks WJ, Jarvis MF, Wagner GC. Astrocytes as a primary locus for the conversion MPTP into MPP+. J Neural Transm 1989; 76:1–12.
222. Brown EL. The epidemiology of Parkinson's disease. Proc R Soc Med 1973; 66:202–203.
223. Brown EL, Knox EG. Idiopathic Parkinsonism as a late complication of encephalitis. Med J Aust 1972; 2:800–801.

224. Brown EL, Knox EG. Epidemiological approach to Parkinson's disease. Lancet 1972; i:974–976.
225. Brown EL, Knox EG. Epidemiological approach to Parkinson's disease. Lancet 1972; ii:48–49.
226. Brown GL, Wilson WP. Parkinsonism and depression. South Med J 1972; 65:540–545.
227. Brown RG, Marsden CD. How common is dementia in Parkinson's disease? Lancet 1984; 2:1262–1265.
228. Brucke TR, Riederer P. Neurobiological and pharmacological examinations on the pathogenesis of Parkinson's Disease. Wien Med Wochenschr 1986; 136:401–408.
229. Bruetsch WL, DeArmond M. The parkinsonian syndrome due to trauma. J Nerv Ment Dis 1935; 81:531–541.
230. Brunori M, Rotilio G. Biochemistry of oxygen radical systems. In: Packer L, ed. Methods in Enzymology, Volume 105: Oxygen Radicals in Biological Systems. New York: Academic Press, 1984:22–31.
231. Buchman AS, Goetz C, Klawans H. Hemiparkinsonism with hemiatrophy. Neurology 1988; 38:527–530.
232. Burch PR. Cigarette smoking and Parkinson disease [letter]. Neurology 1981; 31:500–501.
233. Burchinskii SG. [Study of the problem of parkinsonism and aging (review of the literature)]. Vrach Delo 1987; 72–76.
234. Burn DJ, Mark MH, Playford ED, et al. Parkinson's disease in twins studied with 18F-dopa and positron emission tomography. Neurology 1992; 42:1894–1900.
235. Burnell G. X Disease. Med J Aust 1922; 126–127.
236. Burns RS, Chiueh CC, Markey SP, Ebert MH, Jacobowitz DM, Kopin IJ. A primate model of Parkinsonism: Selective destruction of dopaminergic neurons in the pars compacta of the substantia nigra by N-methyl-4-phenyl-1,2,3,6-tetrahydropyridine. Proc Natl Acad Sci 1983; 80:4546–4550.
237. Burns RS, LeWitt P, Ebert M, Pakkenberg H, Kopin IJ. The clinical syndrome of striatal dopamine deficiency. Parkinsonism induced by 1-Methyl-4-phenyl-1,2,3,6-tetrahydropydidine (MPTP). N Engl J Med 1985; 312:1418–1421.
238. Burns RS, Markey SP, Phillips JM, Chiueh CC. The Neurotoxicity of 1-Methyl-4-phenyl-1,2,3,6-tetrahydropyridine in the Monkey and Man. Can J Neurol Sci 1984; 11:166–168.
239. Burns RS, Phillips JM, Chiueh CC, Parisi JE. The MPTP-treated monkey model of Parkinson's disease. In: MPTP: A neurotoxin producing a parkinsonian syndrome. Orlando: Academic Press, 1986:23–42.
240. Burton K, Calne DB. Aetiology of Parkinson's disease. In: Stern GM, ed. Parkinson's disease. Baltimore: The Johns Hopkins University Press, 1990: 269–293.
241. Bus JS, Aust SD, Gibson JE. Paraquat:Model for oxidant-initiated toxicity. Environ Health Perspect 1984; 55:37–46.
242. Busenbark KL, Huber SJ, Greer G, Pahwa R, Koller WC. Olfactory function in essential tremor. Neurology 1992 42:1631–1632.
243. Busse EW. The brain and aging. Clin Obstet Gynecol 1986; 29:374–383.

244. Butterfield PG, Valanis BG, Spencer PS, Lindeman CA, Nutt JG. Environmental antecedents of young-onset Parkinson's disease. Neurology 1993; 43:1150–1158.
245. Butterfield PG, Valanis BG, Spencer PS, Lindeman CA, Nutt JG. Environmental antecedents of young-onset Parkinson's disease. Neurology 1993; 43:1150–1158.
246. Button JC. Causes of Parkinson's Disease. In: Hope and help in Parkinson's disease. Norman Oklahoma: The Transcript Press, 1953:36–47.
247. Buzzard EF, Greenfield JG. Lethargic encephalitis; its sequelae and morbid anatomy. Brain 1919; 42:305–338.
248. Byrne E, Thomas PK, Zilkha KJ. Familial extrapyramidal disease with peripheral neuropathy. J Neurol Neurosurg Psychiatry 1982; 45:372–374.
249. Byrne EJ, Lennox G, Lowe J, Godwin-Austen RB. Diffuse Lewy body disease: Clinical features in 15 cases. J Neurol Neurosurg Psychiatry 1989; 52:709–717.
250. Cadet JL. A unifying theory of movement and madness: involvement of free radicals in disorders of the isodendritic core of the brainstem. Med Hypotheses 1988; 27:59–63.
251. Cain M, Weber RW, Guzman F. Beta-carbolines: Synthesis and neurochemical and pharmacological actions on brain benzodiazepine receptors. J Med Chem 1982; 25:1081–1091.
252. Calne DB. Current views on Parkinson's disease. Can J Neurol Sci 1983; 10:11–15.
253. Calne DB. Options for the etiology of Parkinson's disease: the association with dementia. Mt Sinai J Med 1988; 55:58–61.
254. Calne DB. Is ''Parkinson's disease'' one disease? J Neurol Neurosurg Psychiatry 1989; 18–21.
255. Calne DB. Current concepts on the etiology of Parkinson's disease. Mov Disord 1989; 4:S11–S14.
256. Calne DB. Early markers of Parkinson's disease (Abstract). Mov Disord 1990; 5:1.
257. Calne DB. The free radical hypothesis in idiopathic parkinsonism: Evidence against it. Ann Neurol 1992; 32:799-803.
258. Calne DB. Is idiopathic parkinsonism the consequence of an event or a process? Neurology 1994; 44:5-10.
259. Calne DB, Calne JS. Normality and disease. Can J Neurol Sci 1988; 15:3-4.
260. Calne DB, Dubini A, Stern G. Did Leonardo describe Parkinson's disease. N Engl J Med 1989; 320:594.
261. Calne DB, Duvoisin RC, McGeer E. Speculations on the etiology of Parkinson's disease. In: Hassler RG, Christ JF, eds. Parkinson-specific motor and mental disorders, role of the pallidum: pathophysiological, biochemical, and therapeutic aspects—Advances in neurology, Vol 40. New York: Raven Press, 1984:353–360.
262. Calne DB, Eisen A. Pathogenesis of Idiopathic Parkinsonism (abstract). Meeting of the American Neurological Association 1989; 10.
263. Calne DB, Eisen A, McGeer E, Spencer P. Alzheimer's disease, Parkinson's disease, and motorneurone disease: Abiotrophic interaction between ageing and environment. Lancet 1986; ii:1067–1070.
264. Calne DB, Eisen A, Meneilly G. Normal aging of the nervous system. Ann Neurol 1991; 30:206–207.

265. Calne DB, Hochberg FH, Snow BJ, Nygaard T. Theories of neurodegeneration. Ann N Y Acad Sci 1992; 648:1–5.
266. Calne DB, Kebabian JK. Parkinson's disease: Unanswered questions. J Neural Transm Suppl 1980; 1–5.
267. Calne DB, Langston JW. Aetiology of Parkinson's disease. Lancet 1983; ii:1457–1459.
268. Calne DB, Langston JW, Martin WR, et al. Positron emission tomography after MPTP: Observations relating to the cause of Parkinson's disease. Nature 1985; 317:246–248.
269. Calne DB, Lees A. Late progression of post-encephalitic Parkinson's syndromee. Can J Neurol Sci 1988; 15:135-138.
270. Calne DB, Peppard RF. Aging of the nigrostriatal pathway in humans. Can J Neurol Sci 1987; 14:424-427.
271. Calne DB, Snow BJ, Lee C. Criteria for diagnosing Parkinson's disease. Ann Neurol 1992; 32, (Supp.):125-127.
272. Calne S, Schoenberg BS, Martin W, Uitti RJ, Spencer P, Calne DB. Familial Parkinson's disease: Possible role of environmental factors. Can J Neurol Sci 1987; 14:303-305.
273. Camerlingo M, Casto L, Gazzaniga GC, Ferraro B, Viscardi M, Mamoli A. Normal copper, iron and manganese in the CSF of Parkinson's disease (Abstract). Mov Disord 1990; 5:30.
274. Camp CD. Pathology of Paralysis Agitans. JAMA 1907; 48:1230–1239.
275. Campanella G, Filla A, Michele GD, Zayed J, Roy M, Barbeau A. Etiology of Parkinson's Disease: Results of two case-control studies (Abstract). Mov Disord 1990; 5:11.
276. Campanella G, Idone M, De Michele G, Filla A. Paternal preponderance in familial Parkinson's disease [letter]. Neurology 1984; 34:1398–1400.
277. Campanella G, Roy M, Masson H, et al. A case-control study of Parkinson's disease in Southern Quebec: Exposure to metals and pesticides. 9th International Symposium on Parkinson's Disease 1988; 57.
278. Caradoc-Davies TH, Weatherall M, Dixon GS, Caradoc-Davies G, Hantz P. Is the prevalence of Parkinson's disease in New Zealand really changing. Acta Neurol Scand 1992; 86:40–44.
279. Carboni S, Melis F, Pani L, Hadjiconstantinou M, Rossetti ZL. The non-competitive NMDA-receptor antagonist MK-801 prevents the massive release of glutamate and aspartate from rat striatum induced by 1-methyl-4-phenylpyridinium (MPP+). Neurosci Lett 1990; 117:129–133.
280. Carella F,, Grassi MP, Savoiardo M, Contri P, Rapuzzi B, Mangoni A. Dystonic-parkinsonian syndrome after cyanide poisoning: Clinical and MRI findings. J Neurol Neurosurg Psychiatry 1988; 51:1345–1348.
281. Carlen PL, Lee MA, Jacob M. Parkinsonism provoked by alcoholism. Ann Neurol 1981; 9:84–86.
282. Carlier G, Dubru JM. Familial juvenile Parkinsonism. Acta Paediatr Belg 1979; 32:123–127.
283. Carlsson A, Fornstedt B. Catechol metabolites in the cerebrospinal fluid as possible markers in the early diagnosis of Parkinson's disease. Neurology 1991; 40(suppl 2):50–52.

284. Carlsson A, Nyberg P, Winblad B. The influence of age and other factors on concentrations of monoamines in the human brain. In: Nyberg P, ed. Brain monoamines in normal aging and dementia. Sweden: Umea University Medical dissertations, 1984:53–84.
285. Carlsson A, Winblad B. Influence of age and time interval between death and autopsy on dopamine and 3-methoxytramine levels in human basal ganglia. J Neural Transm 1976; 38:271–276.
286. Carstam R, Brinck C, Hindemith-Augustsson A, Rorsman H, Rosengren E. The neuromelanin of the human substantia nigra. Biochim Biophysi Acta 1991; 1097:152–160.
287. Carvey PM, McRae A, Flint TF, et al. The potential use of a dopamine neuron antibody and a striatal-derived neurotrophic factor as diagnostic markers in Parkinson's disease. Neurology 1991; 41(suppl 2):53–60.
288. Casetta I, Granieri E, Govoni V, et al. Epidemiology of Parkinson's disease in Italy. A descriptive survey in the U.S.L. of Cento, province of Ferrara, Emilia-Romagna. Acta Neurol (Napoli) 1990; 12:284–291.
289. Cashman JR, Ziegler DM. Contribution of N-oxygenation to the metabolism of MPTP (1-methly-4-phenyl-1,2,3,6-tetrahydropyridine) by various liver preparations. Mol Pharmacol 1986; 29:163–167.
290. Caskey CT, Pizzuti A, Fu YH, Fenwick RG, Nelson DL. Triple repeat mutations in human disease. Science 1992; 256:784–789.
291. Cazzato G, Capus L, Monti F, Carraro N. [Smoking and Parkinson's disease]. Riv Neurol 1985; 55:79–87.
292. Ceballos I, Javoy-Agid F, Delacourte A. Neuronal localization of copper-zinc superoxide dismutase protein and mRNA within the human hippocampus from control and Alzheimer's disease brains. Free Radic Res Commun 1991; 12–13 PT 2:571–580.
293. Ceballos I, Lafon M, Javoy-Agid F, et al. Superoxide dismutase and Parkinson's disease (Letter). Lancet 1990; 335:1035–1036.
294. Cedar H. DNA Methylation and gene activity. Cell 1988; 53:3–4.
295. Cedarbaum JM, Sheu KF, Harding BJ, Blass JP, Javoy-Agid F, Agid Y. Deficiency of glutamate dehydrogenase in postmortem brain samples from parkinsonian putamen [letter; comment]. Ann Neurol 1990; 28:111–112.
296. Cedarbaum JM, Sheu KFR, Blass JP, Agid Y, Javoy-Agid F. Deficiency of glutamate dehydrogenase in Parkinson's disease putamen (Abstract). Mov Disord 1990; 5:30.
297. Celesia G, Wanamaker W. Psychiatric disturbances in Parkinson's disease. Dis Nerv Syst 1972; 33:577–583.
298. Chacon JN, Chedekel MR, Land EJ, Truscott TG. Chemically induced Parkinson's disease II: Intermediates in the oxidation and reduction of the 1-methyl-4-phenyl-2,3-dihydropyridinium ion and its depronated form. Biochem Biophys Res Commun 1989; 158(1):63–71.
299. Chacon JN, Truscott TG. Chemically induced Parkinson's disease III: a study of a possible role of singlet molecular oxygen in Parkinson's disease. J Photochem Photobiol B: Biol 1991; 11:261–267.
300. Chalfie M, Wolinsky E. The identification and suppression of inherited neurodegeneration in Caenorhabditis elegans. Nature 1990; 345:410–416.

301. Chalmanov VN. Epidemiological studies of parkinsonism in Sofia. Neuroepidemiology 1986; 5:171–177.
302. Chambers RA, Levey GS. Studies of eastern encephalitis, read before the 13th Annual Meeting of the American Academy of Neurology, Detroit, 1961.
303. Chan P, DeLanney LE, Irwin I, Langston JW, Di Monte DA. Rapid ATP loss caused by 1-methyl-4-phenyl-1,2,3,6-tetrahydropyridine in mouse brain. J Neurochem 1991; 57:348–351.
304. Chandra V, Bharucha E, Schoenberg BS. Mortality Data for the US for deaths due to and related to twenty neurologic diseases. Neuroepidemiology 1984; 3:149–168.
305. Chapman LJ, Sauter SL, Henning RA, Levine RL, Matthew CG, Peters HA. Finger tremor after carbon disulfide-based pesticide exposures. Arch Neurol 1991; 48:866–870.
306. Charcot JM. Lectures on diseases of the nervous system. London: New Sydenham Society, 1987:
307. Charcot JM, Vulpian A. De la paralysie agitante. Gazette Hebdomadaire de Medecin et de Chirurgie 1861; 8:765–767.
308. Charlton CG. Excessive biological methylation may cause Parkinson's disease. FASEB 73rd Meeting 1989.
309. Chase TN, Schnur JA, Brody JA, Gordon EK. Parkinsonism-dementia and amyotrophic lateral sclerosis of Guam. Effect of probenecid on monoamine catabolte levels in cerebrospinal fluid. Arch Neurol 1971; 25:9–13.
310. Chebotarev DF. [Biology of aging and diseases in man]. Vestn Akad Med Nauk SSSR 1980; 3–7.
311. Chen K, Brody JA, Kurland LT, Elizan TS. Clinical and genetic patterns of neurological diseases other than amyotrophic lateral sclerosis on Guam. Neurology 1970; 20:954–964.
312. Chen K, Chase TN. Parkinsonism-dementia. In: Vinken P, Bruyn G, Klawans HL, eds. Handbook of Clinical Neurology. Amsterdam: Elsevier Science, 1986:167–183.
313. Chen KM. Dementias other than ALS/PDC occurring on Gaum. Proceedings of International Symposium on Neurodegenerative Disorders in the Western Pacific Region, on Guam, February 17–18, 1992.
314. Chen KM, Brody JA, Kurland LT. Patterns of neurologic diseases on Guam. Arch Neurol 1968; 19:573–578.
315. Chen KM, Yase Y. Parkinsonism-dementia, neurofibrillary tangles and trace elements in the Western Pacific. In: Hutton JT, Kenny AD, eds. Senile dementia of the Alzheimer type. New York: Alan R Liss, 1985:153–173.
316. Chiba K, Horii H, Kubota E, Ishizaki T, Kato Y. Effects of N-methylmercaptoimidazole on the disposition of MPTP and its metabolites in mice. Eur J Pharmacol 1990; 180:59–67.
317. Chiba K, Kubota E, Miyakawa T, Kato Y, Ishizaki T. Characterization of hepatic microsomal metabolism as an in vivo detoxication pathway of 1-methyl-4-phenyl-1,2,3,6-tetrahydropyridine in mice. J Pharmacol Exp Ther 1988; 246(3):1108–115.
318. Chiba K, Peterson LA, Castagnoli KP, Trevor AJ, Castagnoli N, Jr.. Studies on

the molecular mechanism of bioactivation of the selective nigrostriatal toxin 1-methyl-4-phenyl-1,2,3,6-tetrahydropyridine. Drug Metab Dispos 1985; 13:342–347.

319. Chiba K, Trevor AJ, Castagnoli N, Jr.. Active uptake of MPP+, a metabolite of MPTP, by brain synaptosomes. Biochem Biophys Res Commun 1984; 128:1229–1232.

320. Chiba K, Trevor AJ, Castagnoli N,Jr. Metabolism of the neurotoxic tertiary amine, MPTP, by brain monoamine oxidase. Biochem Biophys Res Commun 1984; 120:574–578.

321. Chien KR, Pfau RG, Farber JL. Ischemic myocardial cell injury. Prevention by chlorpromazine of an accelerated phospholipid degradation and associated membrane dysfunction. Am J Pathol 1979; 97:505–530.

322. Chiueh CC, Markey SP, Burns RS, Johannessen JN, Pert A, Kopin IJ. Neurochemical and behavioral effects of systemic and intranigral administration of N-methyl-4-pheynl-1,2,3,6-tetrahydropyridine in the rat. Eur J Pharmacol 1984; 100:189–194.

323. Choi DW. Calcium-mediated neurotoxicity: relationship to specific channel types and role in ischemic damage. TINS 1988; 11(10):465–469.

324. Choi DW, Rothman SM. The role of glutamate neurotoxicity in hypoxic-ischemic cell death. Annu Rev Neurosci 1990; 13:171–182.

325. Chokroverty S. Autonomic dysfunction in olivopontocerebellar atrophy. In: Duvoisin R, Plaitakis A, eds. The olivopontocerebellar atrophies - Advances in neurology, Vol 41. New York: Raven Press, 1984:104–141.

326. Chokroverty S, Nicklas W, Miller D, et al. Multiple system degeneration with glutamate dehydrogenase deficiency: pathology and biochemistry. J Neurol Sci 1990; 53:1099–1101.

327. Chouza C, Caamano J, Aljanati R, Scaramelli A, DeMedina O, Romero S. Parkinsonism, tardive dyskinesia, akathisia, and depression induced by flunarizine. Lancet 1986; i:1303–1304.

328. Chui HC, Teng EL, Henderson VW, Moy AC. Clinical subtypes of dementia of the Alzheimer type. Neurology 1985; 35:1544–1550.

329. Clarke CE, Boyce S, Robertson RG, Sambrook MA, Crossman AR. Drug-induced dyskinesia in primates rendered hemiparkinsonian by intracarotid administration of 1-methyl-4-phenyl-1,2,3,6-tetrahydropyridine (MPTP). J Neurol Sci 1989; 90:307–314.

330. Cleeves L, Findley LJ, Koller W. Lack of association between essential tremor and Parkinson's disease. Ann Neurol 1988; 24:23–26.

331. Cleeves L, Findley LJ, Koller W. Essential tremor and Parkinson's disease—Reply to letter. Ann Neurol 1989; 25:211.

332. Clough CG. A case of normal pressure hydrocephalus presenting as levodopa responsive parkinsonism [letter]. J Neurol Neurosurg Psychiatry 1987; 50:234.

333. Cobb WA, Marshall J, Scaravilli F. Long survival in subacute sclerosing panencephalitis. J Neurol Neurosurg Psychiatry 1984; 47:176–183.

334. Cohan S, Redmond D. Flunarizine inhibits depolarization-induced calcium uptake by gerbil synaptosomes. Neurology 1990; 40 suppl 1:384.

335. Cohen G. The pathophysiology of Parkinson's disease: Biochemical aspects of dopamine neuron senescece. J Neural Transm 1983; 19:89–103.

336. Cohen G, Collins MA. Alkaloids from catecholamines in adrenal tissue: Possible role in alcoholism. Science 1970; 167:1749–1751.
337. Cohen G, Heikkila RE. The generation of hydrogen peroxide, superoxide radical, and hydroxyradical of 6-hydroxydopamine, dialuric acid, and related cytotoxic agents. J Biol Chem 1974; 249:2447–2452.
338. Cohen G, Heikkila RE. Mechanisms of action of hydroxylated phenylethylamine and indoleamine neurotoxins. Ann N Y Acad Sci 1978; 305:74–84.
339. Cohen G, Pasik P, Cohen B, Leist A, Mytilineou C, Yahr MD. Pargyline and deprenyl prevent the neurotoxicity of 1-methyl-4-phenyl-1,2,3,6-tetrahydropyridine (MPTP) in monkeys. Eur J Pharmacol 1985; 106:209–210.
340. Cohn DF. The Parkinsonian syndrome induced by intracranial space occupying lesions. Nervenarzt 1977; 48:383–385.
341. Colebatch JG, Findley LJ, Frackowiak RS, Marsden CD, Brooks DJ. Preliminary report: Activation of the cerebellum in essential tremor. Lancet 1990; 336:1028–1030.
342. Collins MA. Acetaldehyde and its condensation products as markers in alcoholism. In: Galanter M, ed. Recent developments in alcoholism, Volume 6. New York: Plenum Press, 1988:387–403.
343. Collins MA, Hannigan JJ, Weiner C. Effects of catecholic tetrahydroisoquinolines on endogenous catecholamines. In: Galanter M, ed. Currents in Alcholism, Volume V. Biomedical Issues and Clinical Effects of Alcholism. New York: Grune & Stratton, 1979:53–59.
344. Collins MA, Neafsey EJ. Beta-carboline analogues of N-methyl-4-phenyl-1,2,5,6-tetrahydropyridine (MPTP): Endogenous factors underlying idiopathic parkinsonism. Neurosci Lett 1985; 55:179–184.
345. Collins MA, Neafsey EJ, Cheng By. Endogenous analogs of N-methyl-4-phenyl-1,2,3,6-tetrahydropyridine: Indoleamine derived tetrahydro-beta-carbolines as potential causative factors in Parkinson's disease. In: Yahr MD, Bergmann KJ, eds. Advances in Neurology, Volume 45. New York: Raven Press, 1986:179–182.
346. Collins MA, Neafsey EJ, Matsubara K, Cobuzzi RJJr, Rollema H. Indole-N-methylated B-barbolinium ions as potential brain-bioactivated neurototoxins. Brain Res 1992; 570:154–160.
347. Collins MA, Neafsey EJ, Matsubara K, et al. Indole-N-methylation of B-carbolines: The brain's bioactivation route to toxins in Parkinson's disease. Ann N Y Acad Sci 1992; 648:263–265.
348. Collins MA, Weiner CD. Studies on the effects of tetrahydroisoquinoline derivatives of catecholamines and aldehydes on tyrosine hydroxylase. In: Thurman R, Williamson J, Drott H, eds. Alcohol and Aldehyde Metabolizing Systems III. New York: Academic Press, 1977:511–526.
349. Colucci C, Alfano V, Giordano D, Miele G. Poisoning by Paraquat and Parkinson's disease (Abstract). Mov Disord 1990; 5:12.
350. Columbia University New York. Parkinson's disease and related disorders: Cumulative bibliography 1800–1970 (NTIS-PB-294–456). Springfield, Virginia: U.S. Department of Commerce, National Technical Information Service, 1978.
351. Comella CL, Tanner CM, Goetz GC, Gans S, Rapp D, Fischer J. Debrisoquine metabolism in Parkinson's disease. Neurology 1987; 37:261–262.

352. Compin O. Clinical study of abnormal kinds of Parkinson's disease—These de Lyon. 1902.
353. Conte-Devoix B, Pfister B, Viallet F, Rey M, Conte-Devoix J. La fonction endocrine anté-hypophysaire dans la maladie de Parkinson. La Presse Médicale 1987; 16:566–568.
354. Cooper B. The epidemiology of primary degenerative dementia and related neurological disorders. Eur Arch Psychiatry Clin Neurosci 1991; 240:223–233.
355. Corrodi H, Hillarp NA. Fluoreszenzmethoden zur histochemischen sichtbarmachung von monoaminen. I. Identifizierung fluoreszierenden produkte aus modellversuchen mit 6,7-dimethoxyisochinolinderivaten und formaldehyd. Helv Chimica Acta 1963; 46:2425–2430.
356. Corrodi H, Hillarp NA. Fluoreszenzmethoden zur histochemischen sichtbarmachung von monoaminen. 2. Identifizierung des fluoreszierenden produktes aus dopamin und formaldehyd. Helv Chimica Acta 1964; 47:911–918.
357. Corsellis JAN, Bruton CJ, Freeman-Browne D. The aftermath of boxing. Psychological Medicine 1973; 3:270–303.
358. Corsini GU, Pintus S, Chiueh CC, Weiss JF, Kopin IJ. 1-Methyl-4-phenyl-1,2,3,6-tetrahydropyridine (MPTP) neurotoxicity in mice is enhanced by pretreatment with diethyldithiocarbamate. Eur J Pharmacol 1985; 119:127–128.
359. Cortopassi GA, Arnheim N. Detection of a specific mitochondrial DNA deletion in tissues of older humans. Nucleic Acids Research 1990; 18(23):6927–6933.
360. Coscia CJ, Burke W, Jamroz G. Occurrence of a new class of tetrahyroisoquinoline alkaloids in L-dopa-treated parkinsonian patients. Nature 1977; 269: 617–619.
361. Cote L, Yahr M, Duvoisin R, Wolf A, Marksbery W. Analysis of deaths in Parkinson patients on long-term levodopa therapy. Trans Am Neurol Assoc 1970; 95:73–77.
362. Cote LJ, Kremzner LT. Biochemical changes in normal aging in human brain. In: Mayeux R, Rosen WG, eds. The Dementias—Advances in neurology—Vol 38. New York: Raven Press, 1983:19–30.
363. Cotman CW, Iversen LL. Excitatory amino acids in the brain—focus on NMDA receptors. TINS 1987; 10(7):263–265.
364. Cotzias GC. Manganese in health and disease. Physiol Rev 1958; 38:503–529.
365. Cotzias GC, Miller ST, Papavasiliou PS, Tang LC. Interactions between manganese and brain dopamine. Medical Clinics of North America 1976; 60(4):729-738.
366. Cotzias GC, Miller ST, Tang LC, Papavasiliou PS. Levodopa, fertility, and longevity. Science 1977; 200:549–551.
367. Cotzias GC, Papavasiliou PS, Ginos J, Steck A, Duby S. Metabolic modification of Parkinson's disease and of chronic manganese poisoning. Ann Rev Med 1971; 22:305–326.
368. Cotzias GC, Van Woert MH, Schiffer LM. Aromatic amino acids and modification of Parkinsonism. N Engl J Med 1967; 276:374–379.
369. Coughlin S, Pincus J, Karstaedt P, Chiazze L. An international comparison of dietary protein consumption and mortality from Parkinson's disease (Abstract). Mov Disord 1990; 5:12.

370. Couper J. On the effects of black oxide of manganese when inhaled into the lungs. Br Ann Med Pharm Vit Stat Gen Sci 1837; 1:41–42.
371. Coutinho P, Andrade C. Autosomal dominant system degeneration in Portuguese families of the Azores Island. A new genetic disorder involving cerebellar, pyramidal, extrapyramidal and spinal cord motor functions. Neurology 1978; 28(7):703–709.
372. Cowen PJ, Green AR, Nutt DJ. Ethyl beta-carboline carboxylate lowers seizure threshold and antagonizes flurazepam-induced sedation in rats. Nature 1981; 290:54–55.
373. Cox TA, McDarby JV, Lavine L, Steele JC, Calne DB. A retinopathy on Guam with high prevalence in Lytico-Bodig. Ophthalmology 1989; 96:1731–5.
374. Crane GE, Smeets RA. Tardive dyskinesia and drug therapy in geriatric patients. Arch Gen Psychiatry 1974; 30:341–343.
375. Creveling CR, Morris N, Shimizu H, Ong HH, Daly J. Catechol-O-methyltransferase. Mol Pharmacol 1972; 8:398–403.
376. Critchley M. Arteriosclerotic parkinsonism. Brain 1929; 52:23–83.
377. Critchley M. Medical aspects of boxing, particularly from a neurological standpoint. Br Med J 1957; 1:357–362.
378. Critchley M. Observations on essential (heredofamilial) tremor. Brain 1949; 72:111–140.
379. Crookshank F. Epidemic encephalo-myelitis and influenza [Letter]. Lancet 1919; i:79–80.
380. Croucher M, de Sarro G, Jensen LH, Meldrum BS. Behavioural and convulsant actions of two methyl esters of beta-carboline-3-carboxylic acid in photosensitive baboons and in DBA/2 mice. Eur J Pharmacol 1984; 104:55–60.
381. Crouzon O, Justin-Besancon L. Le parkinsonisme traumatique. Presse med 1929; 37:1325–1327.
382. Crowley T, Rutledge C, Hohen M. Low urinary dopamine and prediction of phenothiazine induced parkinsonism: A preliminary report. Am J Psychiatry 1976; 133:703–706.
383. Cruchet J, Moutir F, Calmettes A. Quarante cas d'encephalo-myelite subaigue. Societe Medicale Des Hopitaux 1917; 41:614–616.
384. Cummings JL. The dementias of Parkinson's disease: Prevalence, characteristics, neurobiology, and comparison with dementia of the Alzheimer type. Eur Neurol 1988; 28(Suppl 1):15–23.
385. Cummings JL. Depression and Parkinson's disease: A review. Am J Psychiatry 1992; 149:443–454.
386. Currier R, Glover G, Jackson J, Tipton A. Spinocerebellar ataxia, Study of a large kindred. Part 1 (general information and genetics). Neurology 1972; 22:1040–1043.
387. D'Alessandro R, Bennassi G, Morganti G. Side-effects of flunarizine. Lancet 1986; i:463.
388. D'Alessandro R, Gamberini G, Granieri E, Benassi G, Naccarato S, Manzaroli D. Prevalence of Parkinson's disease in the Republic of San Marino. Neurology 1987; 37:1679–1682.
389. D'Amato RJ, Alexander GM, Schwartzman RJ, Kitt CA, Price DL, Snyder SH.

Evidence for neuromelanin involvement in MPTP-induced neurotoxicity. Nature 1987; 327:324–326.

390. D'Amato RJ, Benham DF, Snyder SH. Characterization of the binding of N-methyl-4-phenylpyridine, the toxic metabolite of the parkinsonian neurotoxin N-methyl-4-1,2,3,6-tetrahydropyridine, to neuromelanin. J Neurochem 1987; 48:653–658.
391. D'Amato RJ, Lipman ZP, Snyder SH. Selectivity of the parkinsonian neurotoxin MPTP: Toxic metabolite MPP+ binds to neuromelanin. Science 1986; 231:987–989.
392. D'Amato RJ, Zweig RM, Whitehouse PJ, et al. Aminergic systems in Alzheimer's disease and Parkinson's disease. Ann Neurol 1987; 22:229–236.
393. Da Prada M, Cesura AM, Launay JM, Richards JG. Platelets as a model for neurones. Experientia 1988; 44:115–126.
394. Dacko S, Schneider JS. Met-enkephalin immunoreactivity in the basal ganglia in symptomatic and asymptomatic MPTP-exposed monkeys: Correlation with degree of parkinsonian symptoms. Neurosci Lett 1991; 127:49–52.
395. Dada TO. The nigerian neurological profile. Dis Nerv Syst 1970; 31:746–755.
396. Dagani F, Anderson JJ, Chase TN. Mitochondrial function in Parkinson's disease. Ann Neurol 1992; 32:226–227.
397. Danielczyck W, Streifler M, Konradi C, Reiderer P, Moll G. Platelet MAO-B activity and the psychopathology of Parkinson's disease, senile dementia and multi-infarct dementia. Acta Psychiatr Scand 1988; 78:730–736.
398. Dastur D, Palekar R. The experimental pathology of cycad toxicity with special reference to oncogenic effects. Indian J Cancer 1974; 2:33–49.
399. Dastur DK. Cycad toxicity in monkeys: Clinical, pathological, and biochemical aspects. Fed Proc 1964; 23:1368–1369.
400. Dastur DK, Palekar RS, Manhani DK. Toxicity of various forms of cycas circinalis in rhesus monkeys. Pathology of brain, spinal cord and liver. In: Rose C, Norris F, eds. ALS: New advances in toxicology and epidemiology. London: Smith-Gordon, 1990:129–141.
401. Date I, Felten DL, Felten SY. Long-term effect of MPTP in the mouse brain in relation to aging: Neurochemical and immunocytochemical analysis. Brain Res 1990; 519:266–276.
402. Davanipour Z, Will AD. Residential histories in Parkinson's disease patients. Ann Neurol 1990; 28:295.
403. David N, Mackey E, Smith J. Further observations in progressive supranuclear palsy. Neurology 1968; 18:349–356.
404. Davis GC, Williams AC, Markey SP, et al. Chronic Parkinsonism secondary to intravenous injection of meperidine analogues. Psychiatry Res 1979; 1:249–254.
405. Davis P, Globe L, Schoenberg BS, Duvoisin R. The natural history and prevalence of progressive supranuclear palsy. Neurology 1987; 37 (suppl):121.
406. Davis PH, Golbe LI, Duvoisin RC, Schoenberg BS. Risk factors for progressive supranuclear palsy. Neurology 1988; 38:1546–1552.
407. Davis VE, Cashaw JL. Metabolism of tetrahydroisoquinolines and related alkaloids. Prog Clin Biol Res 1982; 90:99–111.

408. Davis VE, Walsh MJ. Alcohol, amines, and alkaloids: A possible biochemical basis for alcohol addiction. Science 1970; 167:1005–1007.
409. de Pedro Cuesta J. Tracers for paralysis agitans in epidemiological research V. Prevalence of the disease in Swedish counties. Neuroepidemiology 1986; 5:207–219.
410. de Pedro Cuesta J. Studies on the prevalence of paralysis agitans by tracer methodology. Acta Neurol Scand Suppl 1987; 112:1–106.
411. de Pedro Cuesta J. Epidemiological evidence for a causal hypothesis for parkinsonism (Abstract). 9th International Symposium on Parkinson's Disease 1988; 56–50.
412. de Pedro Cuesta J. Parkinson's disease occurrence in Europe. Acta Neurol Scand 1991; 84:357–365.
413. de Pedro Cuesta J, Stawiarz L. Parkinson's disease incidence: Magnitude, comparability, time trends. Acta Neurol Scand 1991; 84:382–388.
414. de Pedro Cuesta J, Stawiarz L. Evaluation of how age modifies the risk for Parkinson's disease, based on stratified comparisons of descriptive data. Acta Neurol Scand 1991; 84:295–302.
415. de Smet Y, Ruberg M, Serdaru M, Dubois B, Lhermitte F, Agid Y. Confusion, dementia and anticholinergics in Parkinson's disease. J Neurol Neurosurg Psychiatry 1982; 45:1161–1164.
416. de Vera Reyes JA. Parkinsonian-like syndrome caused by posterior fossa tumor. Case report. J Neurosurg 1970; 33:599–601.
417. de Yebenes JG, Gervas JJ, Iglesias J, Mena MA, Martin del Rio R, Somoza E. Biochemical findings in a case of parkinsonism secondary to brain tumor. Ann Neurol 1982; 11:313–316.
418. Deapen DM, Henderson BE. A case-control study of amyotrophic lateral sclerosis. Am J Epidemiol 1986; 123:790–797.
419. Defendini R, Markesbery WR, Mastri AR, Duffy PE. Hallervorden-Spatz disease and infantile neuroaxonal dystrophy. J Neurol Sci 1973; 20:7–23.
420. Degl'Innocenti F, Maurello MT, Marini P. A parkinsonian kindred. Ital J Neurol Sci 1989; 10:307–310.
421. Deitrich R, Erwin V. Biogenic amine-aldehyde condensation products: Tetrahydroisoquinolines and tryptolines (beta-carbolines). Ann Rev Pharmacol Toxicol 1980; 20:55–80.
422. Dejerine J, Thomas A. L'atrophie olivo-ponto-cerebelleuse. Nouv Iconogr Salpet 1900; 13:330–370.
423. DeJong D. Parkinson's Disease—V.A.—D.V.A. Study Group. Part I. Biostatistics and case reporting. Med Ser J Canada 1960; 3–12.
424. DeJong JD, Burns BD. Parkinson's disease—A random process. Can Med Assoc J 1967; 97:49–56.
425. Delay J, Deniker P. Drug-induced extrapyramidal syndromes. In: Vinken P, Bruyn G, eds. Handbook of clinical neurology. Amsterdam: North-Holland, 1968:248–266.
426. Delpech A. Accidents que developpe, chez les ouvriers en caoutchoue, l'inhalation du CS2 en vapeur. Union Med 1856; 10:265.

427. Delpech A. Industie du caoutchoue souffle: Recherches sur l'intoxication speciale que determine le CS2. Ann d'Hygiene Series 1863; 2:19–65.
428. Den Hartog Jager WA, Bethlem J. The distribution of Lewy bodies in the central and autonomic nervous systems in idiopathic paralysis agitans. J Neurol Neurosurg Psychiatry 1960; 23:283–290.
429. Desaiah D, Vig PJ, Subramony SH, Curier RD. Inositol 1,4,5-trisphosphate receptors and protein kinase C in olivopontocerebellar atrophy. Brain Res 1991; 552(1):36–40.
430. Deschamps E. Paralysie agitante de cause traumatique. Bull Soc Clin Paris 1885; 9:240–243.
431. Destunis G. Olivopontocerebellar atrophy. Neurol Psychiatry 1944; 188:683–699.
432. Devlin AJ, Bhatti AR, Williams AC, Ramsden DB. Inhibition of human benzylamine oxidase (BzAO) by analogues of 1-methyl-4-phenyl-1,2,3,6-tetrahydropyridine (MPTP). Toxicol Lett 1990; 54:135–142.
433. DeVolder AG, Francart J, Laterre C, et al. Decreased glucose utilization in the striatum and frontal lobe in probable striatonigral degeneration. Ann Neurol 1989; 26(2):239–247.
434. Dexter D, Carter C, Agid F, et al. Lipid peroxidation as cause of nigral cell death in Parkinson's disease [letter]. Lancet 1986; 2:639–640.
435. Dexter DT, Carayon A, Javoy-Agid F. Alterations in the levels of iron, ferritin and other trace metals in Parkinson's disease and other neurodegenerative diseases affecting the basal ganglia. Brain 1991; 114:1953–1975.
436. Dexter DT, Carayon A, Vidailhet M, et al. Decreased ferritin levels in Parkinson's disease. J Neurochem 1990; 55:16–20.
437. Dexter DT, Carter CJ, Wells FR, et al. Basal lipid peroxidation in substantia nigra is increased in Parkinson's disease. J Neurochem 1989; 52:381–389.
438. Dexter DT, Jenner P, Schapira AHV, Marsden CD. Alterations in levels of iron, ferritin, and other trace metals in neurodegenerative diseases affecting the basal ganglia. Ann Neurol 1992; 32 Suppl.:S94–S100.
439. Dexter DT, Sian J, Jenner P, Marsden CD. Implications of alterations in trace element levels in brain in Parkinson's disease and other neurological disorders affecting the basal ganglia. In: Narabayashi H, Nagatsu T, Yanagisawa N, Mizuno Y, eds. Parkinson's disease: From basic research to treatment. Advances in Neurology, Vol. 60. New York: Raven Press, 1993:273–281.
440. Dexter DT, Wells FR, Agid FJ. Increased nigral iron content in postmortem parkinsonian brain. Lancet 1987; 2:1219–1220.
441. Dexter DT, Wells FR, Lees AJ, et al. Increased nigral iron content and alterations in other metal ions occurring in brain in Parkinson's disease. J Neurochem 1989; 52:1830–1836.
442. deYebenes JG, Jimenez A, Morales B, et al. Familial Parkinsonism in Spain. Meeting of the American Neurological Association 15.
443. Di Monte D, Sandy MS, Ekstrom G, Smith MT. Comparative studies on the mechanism of paraquat and 1-methyl-4-phenylpyridine (MPP+) cytotoxicity. Biochem Biophys Res Commun 1986; 137:303–309.

444. Di Monte DA. Mitochondrial DNA and Parkinson's disease. Neurology 1991; 41 Suppl. 2:38–42.

445. Di Monte DA, Chan P, Sandy MS. Glutathione in Parkinson's disease: A link between oxidative stress and mitochondrial damage. Ann Neurol 1992; 32(Supplement):S111–S115.

446. Di Monte DA, Langston JW. MPTP-induced parkinsonism in non-human primates. In: Schneider, Gupta M, eds. Current Concepts in Parkinson's Research. Frankfurt: Hogrefe/Hans Huber Science Publishing, 1993:159–179.

447. Di Monte DA, Sandy MS, Blank L, Smith MT. Fructose prevents 1-methyl-4-phenyl-1,2,3,6-tetrahydropyridine (MPTP)-induced ATP depletion and toxicity in isolated hepatocytes. Biochem Biophys Res Commun 1988; 153:734–740.

448. Di Monte DA, Wu EY, DeLanney LE, Irwin I, Langston JW. Toxicity of 1-methyl-4-phenyl-1,2,3,6-tetrahydropyridine in primary cultures of mouse astrocytes. J Pharmacol Exp Ther 1992; 261:1–6.

449. Di Monte DA, Wu EY, Irwin I, DeLanney LE, Langston JW. Biotransformation of 1-methyl-4-phenyl-1,2,3,6-tetrahydropyridine in primary cultures of mouse astrocytes. J Pharmacol Exp Ther 1991; 258:594–600.

450. Di Monte DA, Wu EY, Irwin I, DeLanney LE, Langston JW. Production and disposition of 1-methyl-4-phenylpyridinium in primary cultures of mouse astrocytes. Glia 1992; 5:48–55.

451. Di Monte DA, Wy EY, Langston JW. Role of astrocytes in MPTP metabolism and toxicity. Ann N Y Acad Sci 1992; 648:219–228.

452. Diamond SG, Markham CH. Present mortality in Parkinson's disease: The ratio of observed to expected deaths with a method to calculate expected deaths. J Neural Transm 1976; 38:259–269.

453. Diamond SG, Markham CH, Hoehn MM, McDowell FH, Muenter MD. Effect of age at onset on progression and mortality in Parkinson's disease. Ann Neurol (Abstract) 1988; 24:180.

454. Diamond SG, Markham CH, Hoehn MM, McDowell FH, Muenter MD. Effect of age at onset on progression and mortality in Parkinson's disease. Neurology 1989; 39:1187-1190.

455. Diamond SG, Markham CH, Hoehn MM, McDowell FH, Muenter MD. Does Parkinson's disease differ in men and women. Ann Neurol 1989; 26:141–140.

456. Diamond SG, Markham CH, Hoehn MM, McDowell FH, Muenter MD. An examination of male-female differences in progression and mortality of Parkinson's disease. Neurology 1990; 40:763–766.

457. Diamond SG, Markham CH, Treciokas LJ. Long-term experience with L-dopa: Efficacy, progression and mortality. In: Birkmayer W, Hornykiewicz O, eds. Advances in Parkinsonism. Basel: Roche, 1976:444–455.

458. Dick RS, Barold SS. Diltiazem-induced parkinsonism. Am J Med 1989; 87:95–96.

459. Dickerson RB, Newton JR, Hansen JE. Diagnosis and immediate prognosis of Japanese B encephalitis. Am J Med 1952; 12:277–288.

460. Difazio MC, Hollingswoth Z, Young AB, Penney JBJ. Glutamate receptors in the substantia nigra of Parkinson's disease brains. Neurology 1992; 42:402–406.

461. Dikman M, Leibowitz Y. Association of diabetes, hypertension and arteriosclerotic heart disease with Parkinson's disease: A pilot study. Book of abstracts, 9th International Symposium on Parkinson's disease, 1988.
462. DiMonte D. Mitochondrial DNA and Parkinson's disease. Neurology 1991; 41 (Suppl 2):38–42.
463. DiMonte DA, Sandy MS, Jewell SA, Adornato B, Tanner CM, Langston JW. Oxidative phosphorylation by intact muscle mitochondria in Parkinson's disease. Neurodegeneration 1993; 2:275–281.
464. Dimsdale H. Changes in the parkinsonian syndrome in the twentieth century. Quart J Med 1946; 15:155–170.
465. Dipasquale B, Marini AM, Youle RJ. Apoptosis and DNA degradation induced by 1-methyl-4-phenylpyridinium in neurons. Biochem Biophys Res Commun 1991; 181, No.3:1442–1448.
466. Ditter SM, Mirra SS. Neuropathologic and clinical features of Parkinson's disease in Alzheimer's disease patients. Neurology 1987; 37:754–760.
467. Dix M, Harrison M, Lewis P. Progressive supranuclear palsy: The Steele-Richardson-Olszewski syndrome: A report of 9 cases with particular reference to the mechanism of the oculomotor disorder. J Neurol Sci 1971; 13:237–256.
468. Doi H, Chen K, Chase T. Effect of L-dopa on clinical duration and quality of life in parkinsonism-dementia of Guam. Clin Neurol 1983; 23:935–942.
469. Doll R, Peto R. Mortality in relation to smoking: 20 years' observations on male British doctors. Br Med J 1976; 1525–1536.
470. Donnan GA, Kaczmarczyk SJ, Solopotias T, et al. The neurochemical and clinical effects of 1-methyl-4-phenyl-1,2,3,6-tetrahydropyridine in small animals. Clin Exp Neurol 1986; 22:155–164.
471. Dormandy TL. An approach to free radicals. Lancet 1983; 2:1010–1014.
472. Doshay LJ. Problem situations in the treatment of paralysis agitans. JAMA 1954; 156:680–684.
473. Dostert P, Benedetti MS, Bellotti V, Allievi C, Dordain G. Biosynthesis of salsolinol, a tetrahydroisoquinoline alkaloid, in healthy subjects. J Neural Transm 1990; 81:215–223.
474. Dostert P, Benedetti MS, Dedieu M. Ratio of enantiomers of salsolinol in human urine. Pharmacol Toxicol 1987; 60(Supplement 1):13.
475. Dostert P, Benedetti MS, Dordain G. Dopamine-derived alkaloids in alcoholism and in Parkinson's and Huntington's diseases. J Neural Transm 1988; 74:61–74.
476. Doty RL, Deems D, Stellar S. Olfactory dysfunction in parkinsonism: A general deficit unrelated to neurologic signs, disease stage, or disease duration. Neurology 1988; 38:1237–1244.
477. Doty RL, Perl DP, Steele JC, et al. Odor identification deficit of the parkinsonism-dementia complex of Guam: Equivalence to that of Alzheimer's and idiopathic Parkinson's disease. Neurology 1991; 41(suppl 2):77–80.
478. Doty RL, Riklan M, Deems DA, Reynolds C, Stellar S. The olfactory and cognitive deficits of Parkinson's disease: Evidence for independence. Ann Neurol 1989; 25:166–171.
479. Doty RL, Singh A, Tetrud JW, Langston JW. Lack of olfactory dysfunction in MPTP-induced parkinsonism. Ann Neurol 1992; 32:97–100.

480. Dougan D, Wade D, Mearrick P. Effects of L-dopa metabolites at a dopamine receptor suggest a basis for "on-off" effect in Parkinson's disease. Nature 1975; 254:70–72.
481. Drayer BP, Olanow W, Burger P, Johnson GA, Herfkens R, Riederer S. Parkinson plus syndrome: diagnosis using high field MR imaging of brain iron. Radiology 1986; 159:493–498.
482. Drucker G, Raikoff K, Neafsey EJ, Collins MA. Dopamine uptake inhibitory capacities of B-carboline and 3,4-dihydro-B-carboline analogs of N-methyl-4-phenyl-1,2,3,6-tetrahydropyridine (MPTP) oxidation products. Brain Res 1990; 509:125–133.
483. Dubinsky R, Jankovic J. Progressive supranuclear palsy and a multi-infarct state. Neurology 1987; 37:570–576.
484. Duckett S, Galle P, Escourolle R, Grey F. Presence of aluminum and magnesium in the cerebral arteries and parenchyma of patients with striatonigral syndrome: study by Castaing's microprobe. D Sciences Naturelles 1976; 282(23):2115–2117.
485. Duffel MW, Gillespie SG. Microsomal flavin-containing monooxygenase activity in rat corpus striatum. J Neurochem 1984; 42:1350–1353.
486. Duffy PE, Tennyson VM. Phase and electron microscopic observations of Lewy bodies and melanin granules in the substantia nigra and locus coeruleus in Parkinson's disease. J Neuropathol Exp Neurol 1965; 24:398–414.
487. Duke RC, Cohen JJ. IL-2 addiction: Withdrawal of growth factor activates a suicide program in dependent T cells. Lymphokine Res 1986; 5:289–299.
488. Dulaney E, Stern M, Hurtig H, et al. The epidemiology of Parkinson's disease: A case-control study of young-onset versus old-onset patients (Abstract). Mov Disord 1990; 5:12.
489. Dumas M, Munoz M, Boutros-Toni F, et al. Neuroepidemiological study in Limousin (France). J Neurol 1985; 232 (suppl):76.
490. Duncan C, Deitrich RA. A critical evaluation of tetrahydroisoquinoline induced ethanol preference in rats. Pharmacol Biochem Behavior 1980; 13:265–281.
491. Duncan M, Kopin IJ, Lavine L, Garruto R, Markey S. The putative neurotoxin BMAA in cycad-derived foods is an unlikely cause of ALS-PD. Lancet 1988; 2:631–632.
492. Duncan MW, Marini AM, Watters R, Kopin IJ, Markey SP. Zinc, a neurotoxin to cultured neurons, contaminates cycad flour prepared by traditional Guamanian methods. J Neurosci 1992; 12:1523–1537.
493. Duncan MW, Steele JC, Kopin IJ, Markey SP. 2-Amino-3-(methylamino)-propionic acid (BMAA) in cycad flour: An unlikely cause of amyotrophic lateral sclerosis and parkinsonism-dementia of Guam. Neurology 1990; 40:767–772.
494. Dupont E. Epidemiology of Parkinsonism. The Parkinson investigation, Arhus, Denmark (Preliminary Results). In: Worm-Peterson J, Bottcher J, eds. Symposium on Parkinsonism. New York: Merck, Sharp & Dohme, 1977:65–75.
495. Durrieu G, Senard JM, Rascol O, et al. Blood pressure and plasma catecholamines in never-treated parkinsonian patients: effect of a selective D1 agonist (CY 208–243). Neurology 1990; 40:707–709.
496. Duvoisin R. History of Parkinsonism. Pharmac Ther 1987; 32:1–17.

497. Duvoisin R. Epidemiological and genetic aspects of Parkinson's disease. In: Nappi C, ed. Focus on Parkinson's Disease. Milan: 1991:79–93.
498. Duvoisin RC. Parkinsonism. Clin Symp 1976; 28:1–29.
499. Duvoisin RC. Problems in the treatment of parkinsonism. Adv Exp Med Biol 1977; 90:131–135.
500. Duvoisin RC. The cause of Parkinson's disease. In: Marsden CD, Fahn S, eds. Movement Disorders. London: Butterworth Scientific, 1982:8–24.
501. Duvoisin RC. Is Parkinson's disease acquired or inherited. Can J Neurol Sci 1984; 2:151–155.
502. Duvoisin RC. Parkinson's disease: Intrauterine influence in twins? [letter]. Neurology 1985; 35:774–775.
503. Duvoisin RC. The genetics of Parkinson's disease. VIII International Symposium on Parkinson's disease 1985; 12.
504. Duvoisin RC. Etiology of Parkinson's disease: Current concepts. Clin Neuropharmacol 1986; 9:S3–21.
505. Duvoisin RC. On heredity, twins, and Parkinson's disease [editorial]. Ann Neurol 1986; 19:409–411.
506. Duvoisin RC. Genetics of Parkinson's disease. In: Parkinson's disease - Advances in neurology, Vol 45. New York: Raven Press, 1987:307–312.
507. Duvoisin RC, Chokroverty S, Lepore F. Glutamate dehydrogenase in patients with olivopontocerebellar atrophy. Neurology 1983; 33:1322–1326.
508. Duvoisin RC, Gearing FR, Schweitzer MD, Yahr MD. A family study of parkinsonism. In: Barbeau A, Brunette JR, eds. Proceedings of the 2nd International Congress of Neuro-Genetics and Neuro-Opthalmology, Montreal, 1967, International Congress Series. Amsterdam: Excerpta Medica Foundation, 1969:492–496.
509. Duvoisin RC, Golbe L, Lepore F. Progressive supranuclear palsy. Can J Neurol Sci 1987; 14:547–554.
510. Duvoisin RC, Golbe LI. Toward a definition of Parkinson's disease. Neurology 1989; 39:746.
511. Duvoisin RC, Nichlas WJ, Ritchie V, Agae J, Chokroverty S. Low leukocyte glutamate dehydrogenase activity does not correlate with a particular type of multiple system atrophy. J Neurol Neurosurg Psychiatry 1988; 51(12):1508–1511.
512. Duvoisin RC, Schweitzer MD. Paralysis agitans mortality in England and Wales 1855–1962. Brit J Prev Soc Med 1966; 20:27–33.
513. Duvoisin RC, Yahr MD. Encephalitis and parkinsonism. Arch Neurol 1965; 12:227–239.
514. Duvoisin RC, Yahr MD. Epidemiological approach to Parkinson's disease. Lancet 1972; 1:1400–1401.
515. Duvoisin RC, Yahr MD, Schweitzer MR, Merritte HH. Parkinsonism before and since the epidemic of encephalitis lethargica. Arch Neurol 1963; 9:232–236.
516. Duvoisin RC, Eldridge R, Williams A, Nutt J, Calne DB. Twin study of Parkinson disease. Neurology 1981; 31:77–80.
517. Dwork AJ, Balmaceda C, Fazzini EA, MacCollin M, Côtè L, Fahn S. Dominantly

inherited, early-onset parkinsonism: Neuropathology of a new form. Neurology 1993; 43:69–74.

518. Eadie MJ. Pathology of certain medullary nuclei in parkinsonism. Brain 1963; 86:781–792.
519. Eadie MJ, Sutherland JM, Doherty RL. Encephalitis in etiology of Parkinsonism in Australia. Arch Neurol 1965; 12:240–245.
520. Earle KM. Studies on Parkinson's disease including X-ray fluorescent spectroscopy of formalin fixed brain tissue. J Neuropathol Exp Neurol 1968; 27(1):1–14.
521. Eatough VM, Kempster PA, Stern GM, Lees AJ. Premorbid personality and idiopathic Parkinson's disease. In: Parkinson's disease: anatomy, pathology and therapy—Advances in Neurology—Vol 53. New York: Raven Press, 1990:335–337.
522. Ebmeier KP, Calder S, Crawford J, Stewart L. Parkinson's disease in Aberdeen: survival after 3.5 years. Acta Neurol Scand 1990; 81:294–299.
523. Ebmeier KP, Calder SA, Crawford JR, Stewart L, Besson JOA, Mutch WJ. Mortality and causes of death in idiopathic Parkinson's disease: results from the Aberdeen whole population study. Scott Med J 1990; 35:173–175.
524. Ebmeier KP, Mutch WJ, Calder SA, Crawford JR, Stewart L, Besson JOA. Does idiopathic parkinsonism in Aberdeen follow intrauterine influenza? J Neurol Neurosurg Psychiatry 1989; 52:911–913.
525. Ehrich WE, Alpers BJ. Post-mortem findings in CS2 poisoning. In: Bashore RM, Staley AL, eds. Survey of carbon disulphide and hydrogen sulphide hazards in the viscose rayon industry. Bulletin #46. Harrisburg: Commonwealth of PA Dept. of Labor and Industry, 1938:55–57.
526. Ehringer H, Hornykiewicz O. Verteilung von Noradrenalin und Dopamin (3-Hydroxytyramin) in Gehirn des Menschen und ihr Verhalten bei Erkrankungen des extrapyramidalen Systems. Klinische Wochenschrift 1960; 1236–1239.
527. Eisen A, Calne D. Amyotrophic lateral sclerosis, Parkinson's disease and Alzheimer's disease: Phylogenetic disorders of the human neocortex sharing many characteristics. Can J Neurol Sci 1992; 19 (Suppl 1):117–123.
528. Ekstrom G, Di Monte DA, Sandy MS, Smith MT. Comparative toxicity and antioxidant activity of 1-methyl-4-phenyl-1,2,3,6-tetrahydropyridine and its moanamine oxidase B-generated metabolites in isolated hepatocytes and liver microsomes. Arch Biochem Biophys 1987; 255:14–18.
529. el-Awar M, Kish S, Oscar-Berman M, Robitaille Y, Schut L, Freedman M. Selective delayed alternation deficits in dominantly inherited olivopontocerebellaratrophy. Brain & Cognition 1991; 16(2):121–129.
530. Eldridge R. Parkinson's disease in twins . . . reply from author. Neurology 1984; 34:1399–1400.
531. Eldridge R. Molecular genetics, basal ganglia disorders, and the clinical neurologist. Neurol Clin 1984; 2:581–603.
532. Eldridge R, Ince S. The cause of Parkinson's disease in twins. Am J Hum Genet 1983; 35:88A.
533. Eldridge R, Ince SE. The low concordance rate for Parkinson's disease in twins: a possible explanation. Neurology 1984; 34:1354–1356.

534. Eldridge R, Ince SE. Reply from Authors. Neurology 1985; 35:775.
535. Eldridge R, Rocca WA. The clinical syndrome of striatal dopamine deficiency: Parkinsonism induced by MPTP. N Engl J Med 1985; 313:1159–1160.
536. Eldridge R, Rocca WA. Parkinson disease. In: King R, Rotter J, Motulsky A, eds. The genetic basis of common diseases. New York: McGraw-Hill, 1990:775–791.
537. Eldridge R, Rocca WA, Ince SE. Parkinson's disease; Evidence against a toxic etiology and for an alternative theory. In: Markey SP, Castagnoli NJr, Trevor AJ, Kopin IJ, eds. MPTP: A neurotoxin producing a Parkinsonian syndrome. Orlando: Academic Press, 1986:355–367.
538. Eldridge R, Rosario J, Brody JA. Amyotrophic lateral sclerosis and parkinsonism dementia in a migrant population from Guam. Trans Am Neurol Assoc 1968; 93:204–206.
539. Eldridge R, Ryan E, Rosario J, Brody JA. Amyotrophic lateral sclerosis and parkinsonism dementia in a migrant population from Guam. Neurology 1969; 19:1029–1037.
540. Elizan TS, Casals J. The viral hypothesis in parkinsonism. J Neural Transm 1983; 19:75–88.
541. Elizan TS, Casals J. The viral hypothesis in Parkinson's disease and in Alzheimer's disease: A critique. In: Kurstak E, Lipowski SJ, Morozov PV, eds. Viruses, immunity and mental disorders. New York: Plenum Press, 1987:47–59.
542. Elizan TS, Casals J. No viral antigens detected in brain tissue from a case of acute encephalitis lethargica and another case of post-encephalitic Parkinsonism. J Neurol Neurosurg Psychiatry 1989; 52:800–801.
543. Elizan TS, Casals J, Yahr MD. Antineurofilament antibodies in postencephalitic and idiopathic parkinson's disease. J Neurol Sci 1983; 59:341–347.
544. Elizan TS, Chen KM, Mathai KV, Dunn D, Kurland LT. Amyotrophic lateral sclerosis and parkinsonism-dementia complex. A study in non-Chamorros of the Mariana and Caroline Islands. Arch Neurol 1966; 14:347–355.
545. Elizan TS, Duvoisin RC, Madden DL, Smith H. HLA antigens and viral antibody titers in identical twins discordant for parkinson's disease. Mount Sinai J Med 1982; 49, No. 1:83–84.
546. Elizan TS, Hirano A, Abrams BM, Need RL, Van Nuis C, Kurland LT. Amyotrophic lateral sclerosis and parkinsonism-dementia complex of Guam. Neurological reevaluation. Arch Neurol 1966; 14:356–368.
547. Elizan TS, Madden DL, Noble GR, et al. Viral antibodies in serum and CSF of Parkinsonian patients and controls. Arch Neurol 1979; 36:529–534.
548. Elizan TS, Schwartz J, Yahr MD, Casals J. Antibodies against arboviruses in postencephalitic and idiopathic Parkinson's disease. Arch Neurol 1978; 35:257–260.
549. Elizan TS, Terasaki PI, Yahr MD. HLA-B14 antigen and postencephalitic Parkinson's disease: Their association in an American-jewish ethnic group. Arch Neurol 1980; 37:542–544.
550. Elizan TS, Yahr MD. The possible role of virus infection in the etiology and pathogenesis of Parkinson's disease. Abstract 459, Excerpta Medica Intl Cong Series No. 427, 11th World Congress of Neurology. Amsterdam: Excerpta Medica, 1977:154–155.

551. Elizan TS, Yahr MD, Casals J. Indirect immunofluorescence test against lymphocytic choriomeningitis (LCM) virus in Parkinson's disease [letter]. Mt Sinai J Med 1979; 46:597–598.
552. Elizan TS, Yahr MD, Moros DA, Mendoza MR, Pang S, Bodian CA. Selegiline use to prevent progression of Parkinson's disease: Experience in 22 de novo patients. Arch Neurol 1989; 46:1275–1279.
553. Ellenberg JH. The extrapolation of attributable risk to new populations. Statistics in Medicine 1988; 7:717–725.
554. Ellenberg JH. Preclinical detection in studies of the etiology, natural history, and treatment of Parkinson's disease. Neurology 1991; 41(suppl 2):14–22.
555. Ellenberg JH. Early life and demographic factors predisposing to Parkinson's disease. In: Ellenberg JH, Koller WC, Langston JW, eds. Etiology of Parkinson's disease. New York: Marcel Dekker, 1994:277–294.
556. Ellenberg JH. Prediction of Parkinson's disease. In: Ellenberg JH, Koller WC, Langston JW, eds. Etiology of Parkinson's disease. New York: Marcel Dekker, 1994:295–317.
557. Ellison G, Eison MS, Huberman HS, Daniel F. Long-term changes in dopaminergic innervation of caudate nucleus after continuous amphetamine administration. Science 1978; 201:276–278.
558. Elsworth JD, Deutch AY, Redmond DE, Jr., Sladek JR, Jr., Roght RH. Differential responsiveness to 1-methyl-4-phenyl-1,2,3,6-tetrahydropyridine toxicity in subregions of the primate substantia nigra and striatum. Life Sci 1987; 40:193–202.
559. Elsworth JD, Deutch AY, Redmond DE,Jr., Sladek JR,Jr., Roth RH. MPTP-induced parkinsonism: Relative changes in dopamine concentration in subregions of substantia nigra, ventral tegmental area and retrorubral field of symptomatic and asymptomatic vervet monkeys. Brain Res 1990; 513:320–324.
560. Emara AM, El-Ghawabi SH, Madkour OI, El-Samra GH. Chronic manganese poisoning in the dry battery industry. Indust Med 1971; 28:78–82.
561. Emery AE, Holloway S. Familial motor neuron diseases. In: Human motor neuron diseases—Advances in neurology, Vol 36. New York: Raven Press, 1982:139–147.
562. Endo A, Hara S, Kano S, Kuriiwa F. Effects of a paraquat containing hericide, Gramoxon, on the central monoamine and acetylcholine in mice. Res Commun Psychia Behav 1988; 13:261–270.
563. Enz A, Hefti F, Frick W. Acute administration of 1-methyl-4-phenyl-1,2,3,6-tetrahydropyridine (MPTP) reduces dopamine and serotonin but accelerates norepinephrine metabolism in the rat brain, effect of chronic pretreatment with MPTP. Eur J Pharmacol 1984; 101:37–44.
564. Escourolle R. [Anatomic lesions in Parkinson's disease and parkinsonian syndromes]. Ann Med Interne (Paris) 1972; 123:349–356.
565. Esiri MM, Swash M. Absence of herpes simplex virus antigen in brain in encephalitis lethargica. J Neurol Neurosurg Psychiatry 1984; 47:1049–1050.
566. Espir MLE, Spalding JMK. Three recent cases of encephalitis lethargica. Br Med J 1956; 1:1141–1144.
567. Evans WE, Relling MV, Rahman A, McLeod HL, Scott EP, Lin J-S. Genetic

basis for a lower prevalence of deficient CYP2D6 oxidative drug metabolism phenotypes in black americans. J Clin Invest 1993; 91:2150–2154.
568. Factor SA. Posttraumatic parkinsonism. In: Stern MB, Koller WC, eds. Parkinsonian syndromes. New York: Marcel Dekker, 1993:95–110.
569. Factor SA, Sanchez-Ramos J, Weiner WJ. Trauma as an etiology of parkinsonism: A historical review of the concept. Mov Disord 1988; 3:30–36.
570. Factor SA, Sanchez-Ramos J, Weiner WJ. Trauma as an etiology of parkinsonism: Opinions in the nineteenth century (Letter). Mov Disord 1989; 4:284–285.
571. Factor SA, Weiner WJ. Head trauma and Parkinson's disease (Abstract). Mov Disord 1990; 5:13.
572. Factor SA, Weiner WJ. Prior History of head trauma in Parkinson's disease. Mov Disord 1991; 6 (3):225–229.
573. Factor SA, Weiner WJ, Hefti F. Acetaminophen metabolism by cytochrome P450 monooxygenases in Parkinson's disease. Ann Neurol 1989; 26:286–288.
574. Fahn S, Greenberg J. Striatonigral degeneration. Trans Am Neurol Assoc 1972; 97:275–277.
575. Falck G, Hillarp NA, Thieme G, Torp A. Fluorescence of catecholamines and related compounds condensed with formaldehyde. J Histochem Cytochem 1962; 10:348–354.
576. Falconer DC. The inheritance of liability to certain diseases, estimated from the incidence among relatives. Am J Hum Genet 1965; 29:51–76.
577. Fanali A, Nardini M, Sorgona F. [Action of amantadine in extrapyramidal syndromes caused by neuroleptics]. Sist Nerv 1970; 22:273–285.
578. Faraj BA, Camp VM, Kutner M. Interrelationship between activation of dopaminergic pathways and cerebrospinal fluid concentration of dopamine tetrahydroisoquinoline metabolite salsolinol in humans: Preliminary findings. Alcoholism (NY) 1991; 15:86–89.
579. Fariello RG, Calabrese V. Oxidative stress and energy transduction defects as causes of selective neuronal degeneration. In: Nappi G, Hornykiewicz O, Fariello RG, Klawans HL, Agnoli A, eds. Neurodegenetive disorders. The role played by endotoxins and xenobiotics. New York: Raven Press, 1988:81–92.
580. Farlow M, Yee R, Clouhy S, Conneally P, Azzarelli B, Ghetti B. Gerstmann-Sträussler-Scheinker disease. 1. Extending the clinical spectrum. Neurology 1989; 39:1446–1452.
581. Farrell RK, Sande RD, Lincoln SD. Nigropallidal encephalomalacia in a horse. J Am Vet Med Assoc 1971; 58:1201–1204.
582. Fawthrop DJ, Boobis AR, Davies DS. Mechanisms of cell death. Arch Toxicol 1991; 65:437–444.
583. Fazzini E, Fleming J, Fahn S. Cerebrospinal fluid antibodies to coronaviruses in patients with Parkinson's disease. Mov Disord 1992; 7(2):153–158.
584. Fearnley JM, Lees AJ. Striatonigral degeneration. A clinicopathological study. Brain 1990; 113:1823–1842.
585. Fearnley JM, Lees AJ. Ageing and Parkinson's disease; substantia nigra regional selectivity. Brain 1991; 114:2283–2301.
586. Feldman RG. Ecoetiological factors in Parkinson's disease: Manganese (Neuro-

toxins and their potential role in neurodegeneration). The New York Academy of Sciences, May 6–8 1991; PI-12. (abstract)
587. Feldman RG. Manganese as possible ecoetiologic factor in Parkinson's disease. Ann N Y Acad Sci 1992; 648:266–267.
588. Felix CC, Hyde JS, Sarna T, Sealy RC. Melanin photoreactions in aereated media: Electron spin resonance evidence for production of superoxide and hydrogen peroxide. Biochem Biophys Res Commun 1978; 84:335–341.
589. Fellman JH, Nutt JN. MPTP-like molecules and Parkinson's disease. Lancet 1985; 1:924.
590. Felten DL, Felten SY, Fuller RW. Chronic dietary pergolide preserves nigrostriatal neuronal integrity in aged-Fischer-344 rats. Neurobiol Aging 1992; 13:339–351.
591. Felten DL, Felten SY, Steece-Collier K, Date I, Clemens JA. Age-related decline in the dopaminergic nigrostriatal system: The oxidative hypothesis and protective strategies. Ann Neurol 1992; 32 Suppl.:S133–S136.
592. Fermaglich J, Chase T. Methyldopa or methyldopahydrazine as levodopa synergists. Lancet 1973; 1:1261–1262.
593. Fermaglich J, Delaney P. Parkinson's disease, melanoma and levodopa. J Neurol 1977; 215:221–224.
594. Ferrari MD, Peeters EA, Haan J, et al. Cytochrome P450 and Parkinson's disease. Poor parahydroxylation of phenytoin. J Neurol Sci 1990; 96:153–157.
595. Ferraz HB, Betolucci PH, Pereira JS, Lima JG, Andrade LA. Chronic exposure to the fungicide maneb may produce symptoms and signs of CNS manganese intoxication. Neurology 1988; 38:550–553.
596. Fields JZ. Aging and a novel neurotoxin, MPTP (1-methyl-4-phenyl-1,2,5,6-tetrahydropyridine) elicit deficits in brain dopamine tracts and increases in duodenal ulcers. Dig Dis Sci 1985; 30:374.
597. Findley L, Cleeves L, Koller W. Is there a relationship between essential tremor and Parkinson's disease? Neurology 1987; 37:122.
598. Findley LJ, Cleeves L. The relation of essential tremor to Parkinson's disease [letter]. J Neurol Neurosurg Psychiatry 1985; 48:192.
599. Findley LJ, Gresty MA, Halmagyi GM. Tremor, the cogwheel phenomenon, and clonus in Parkinson's disease. J Neurol Neurosurg Psychiatry 1981; 44: 534–546.
600. Finiels-Marlier F, Marini AM, Williams P, Paul SM. The N-methyl-D-aspartate antagonist MK-801 fails to protect dopaminergic neurons from 1-methyl-4-phyenylpyridinium toxicity in vitro. J Neurochem 1993; 60:1968–1971.
601. Fink JS, Hotamisligil GS, Girmen aS, et al. Allelic variations in the MAO-A gene mark activity state and may predict vulnerability to Parkinson's disease. Neurology 1992; 42 (Suppl 3):173.
602. Finkelstein MM, Liss GM. Selection bias in occupational case-control studies that use death registries to select subjects: A discussion and demonstration. Am J Ind Med 1987; 12:21–31.
603. Finlayson MH, Superville B. Distribution of cerebral lesions in acquired hepatocerebral degeneration. Brain 1981; 104:79–95.

604. Finley KH. Postencephalitic manifestations of viral encephalitides. In: Field. W.S., ed. Pathogenesis and treatment of parkinsonism. Springfield: Charles C. Thomas, 1958:69–93.

605. Finnegan KT, Karler R. Protein synthesis inhibition blocks the neurotoxic effects of methamphetamine in rats. Soc Neurosci 1991; 17:1277.(abstract)

606. Finocchiaro G, Taroni F, DiDonato S. Glutamate dehydrogenase in olivopontocerebellar atrophies: Leukocytes fibroblasts and muscle mitochondria. Neurology 1986; 36:550–553.

607. Fisher J, Dewald J. Parkinsonism associated with intraventricular amphotericin. B J Antimicrob Therapy 1983; 12:97–99.

608. Fishman PS, Gass JS, Swoveland PT. Infection of the basal ganglia by a murine coronavirus. Science 1985; 229:877–879.

609. Fitzgerald PM, Jankovic J. Lower body parkinsonism: evidence for vascular etiology. Mov Disord 1989; 4:249–260.

610. Fitzgerald PM, Jankovic J, Glaze D, Schultz R, Percy A. Extrapyramidal involvement in Rett's syndrome. Neurology 1990; 40:293–295.

611. Flaten TP. Changing mortality from Parkinson's disease. Neurology 1991; 41:329–330.

612. Foa V. Neurotoxicity of elemental mercury: occupational aspects. In: Blum K, Manzo. L., eds. Neurotoxicology. New York: Marcel Dekker, 1985:343.

613. Foley JM, Baxter D. On the nature of pigment granules in the cells of the locus coeruleus and the substantia nigra. J Neuropathol Exp Neurol 1958; 17:586–598.

614. Fonne-Pfister R, Bargetzi MJ, Meyer UA. MPTP, the neurotoxin inducing Parkinson's disease, is a potent competitive inhibitor of human and rat cytochrome P450 isozymes (P450bufI, P450db1) catalyzing debrisoquine 4-hydroxylation. Biochem Biophys Res Commun 1987; 148(3):1144–1150.

615. Fontan M, Petit H, Delahousse J, Ascher J, Decoulx-Poutignat M. Signes extrapyramidaux d'intoxications aigues ou subaigues par disulfiram ou disulfiram-alcool. Lille Med 1967; 12:814–817.

616. Forno LS. Concentric hyalin intraneuronal inclusions of Lewy type in the brains of elderly persons (50 incidental cases): Relationship to Parkinsonism. J Am Geriatr Soc 1969; 17:557–575.

617. Forno LS. Pathology of Parkinson's Disease. In: Marsden SD, Fahn S, eds. Movement disorders. London: Butterworth Scientific, 1982:25–40.

618. Forno LS. The Lewy Body in Parkinson's Disease. In: Parkinson's disease—Advances in neurology, Vol 45. New York: Raven Press, 1986:35–43.

619. Forno LS. The neuropathology of Parkinson's disease. In: Hefti F, Weiner WJ, eds. Progress in Parkinson research. New York: Plenum Publishing Corporation, 1988:11–21.

620. Forno LS. Pathology of Parkinson's disease, The importance of the substantia nigra and the Lewy bodies. In: Stern G, ed. Parkinson's disease. London: Chapman, Hall, 1990:185–238.

621. Forno LS. Neuropathological features of Parkinson's Huntington's, and Alzheimer's diseases. Ann N Y Acad Sci 1992; 648:6–16.

622. Forno LS, Alford EC,Jr.. The pathology of parkinsonism. Some observations and new correlations. Contemp Neurol 1971; 8:120–130.

623. Forno LS, DeLanney LE, Irwin I, Di Monte D., Langston JW. Astrocytes and Parkinson's disease. In: Yu ACH, Hertz L, Norenberg MA, Sykova E, Waxman SG, eds. Progress in Brain Research, Vol. 94. Amsterdam: Elsevier Science, 1992:429–436.
624. Forno LS, DeLanney LE, Irwin I, Langston JW. Neuropathology of MPTP-treated monkeys: Comparison with the neuropathology of human idiopathic Parkinson's disease. In: Markey SP, Castagnoli N, Jr., Trevor AJ, Kopin IJ, eds. MPTP: A Neurotoxin Producing a Parkinsonian Syndrome. New York: Academic Press, 1986:119–140.
625. Forno LS, DeLanney LE, Irwin I, Langston JW. Similarities and differences between MPTP-induced parkinsonism and Parkinson's disease. In: Narabayashi H, Nagatsu T, Yanagisawa N, Mizuno Y, eds. Parkinson's disease: From basic research to treatment. Advances in neurology, Volume 60. 10th International Symposium on Parkinson's disease. New York: Raven Press, 1993:600–608.
626. Forno LS, Irwin I, DeLanney LE, Langston JW. Neuropathology in MPTP-induced parkinsonism in animals. Neuropathology 1991; (suppl 4):67–76.
627. Forno LS, Langston JW. Lewy bodies and aging: Relation to Alzheimer's and Parkinson's diseases. Neurodegeneration 1993; 2:19–24.
628. Forno LS, Langston JW, DeLanney LE, Irwin I. An electron microscopic study of MPTP-induced inclusion bodies in an old monkey. Brain Res 1988; 448:150–157.
629. Forno LS, Langston JW, DeLanney LE, Irwin I, Ricaurte GA. Locus ceruleus lesions and eosinophilic inclusions in MPTP-treated Monkeys. Ann Neurol 1986; 20:449–455.
630. Forno LS, Murphy GM, Eng LF. Immunocytochemical study of Lewy bodies in sympathetic ganglia. Neurodegeneration 1992; 1:135–144.
631. Forno LS, Norville RL. Ultrastructure of Lewy bodies in the stellate ganglion. Acta Neuropathol (Berlin) 1976; 34:183–197.
632. Forno LS. Pathological considerations in the etiology of Parkinson's disease. In: Ellenberg JH, Koller WC, Langston JW, eds. Etiology of Parkinson's disease. New York: Marcel Dekker, 1994:65–95.
633. Fornstedt B, Rosengren E, Carlsson A. Occurrence and distribution of 5-s-cysteinyl derivatives of dopamine, dopa and dopac in the brains of eight mammalian species. Neuropharmacology 1986; 25:451–454.
634. Foster HD. Disease family trees: The possible roles of iodine in goitre, cretinism, multiple sclerosis, amyotrophic lateral sclerosis, Alzheimer's and Parkinson's diseases and cancers of the thyroid, nervous system and skin. Med Hypotheses 1987; 24:249–263.
635. Fowler CJ, Wilberg A, Oreland L, Marcusson J, Winblad B. The effect of age on the activity and molecular properties of human brain monoamine oxidase. J Neural Transm 1980; 49:1–20.
636. Frank DM, Arora PK, Blumer JL, Sayre LM. Model study on the bioreduction of paraquat, MPP+, and analogs. Evidence against a "redox cycling" mechanism in MPTP neurotoxicity. Biochem Biophys Res Commun 1987; 147:1095–1104.
637. Freeman W. The pathology of paralysis agitans. Ann Clin Med 1925; 4:106–116.
638. Fridovich I. Oxygen free radicals and tissue damage. Excerpta Medica 1979.

639. Friedman JH. Parkinson's disease update. R I Med J 1989; 72:393–398.
640. Friedman JH. Progressive parkinsonism in boxers. South Med J 1989; 82:543–546.
641. Frigyesi TL, Schwartz R, Ige A, Iulo A. 6-hydroxy-dopamine induced chemonigrectomy and resultant sensorimotor impediment. Trans Am Neurol Assoc 1971; 96:238–241.
642. Fruncillo RJ. Toxin-induced parkinsonism: Recent developments. Am Fam Physician 1986; 33:251–254.
643. Fujisawa Y, Tsuji T, Sasaki K. Parkinsonism induced by indeloxazine hydrochloride. Clin Ther 1989; 11:807–811.
644. Fuller RW. Comparison of MPTP and amphetamines as dopaminergic neurotoxins (Neurotoxins and their potential role in neurodegeneration). The New York Academy of Sciences, May 6–8 1991; 12.(abstract)
645. Fuller RW, Hemrick-Leucke SK. Influence of selective, reversible inhibitors of monoamine oxidase on the prolonged depletion of striatal dopamine by 1-methyl-4-phenyl-1,2,3,6-tetrahydropyridine in mice. Life Sci 1985; 37:1089–1096.
646. Fuller RW, Hemrick-Luecke SK. Inability of monoamine oxidase inhibitors to prevent the persistent depletion of striatal dopamine by amphetamine in rats. Res Commun Subst Abuse 1984; 5:247–252.
647. Fulton JS, Burton AN. After effects of western equine encephalomyelitis infection in man. Can Med Assoc J 1953; 69:268–272.
648. Furtado JCS, Mazurek MF. MPTP-Induced neurotoxicity and the quest for a preventative therapy for Parkinson's disease. Can J Neurol Sci 1991; 18 (1):77–82.
649. Furukawa Y, Nishi K, Kondo T, Mizuno Y, Narabayashi H. Juvenile parkinsonism: Ventricular CSF biopterin levels and clinical features. J Neurol Sci 1992; 108:207–213.
650. Gainotti G. [Anatomo-clinical aspects of Parkinson's disease and parkinsonian syndromes]. Riv Neurol 1978; 48:143–192.
651. Gajdusek DC. Motor-neuron disease in natives in New Guinea. N Engl J Med 1963; 268:474–476.
652. Gajdusek DC. Environmental factors provoking physiological changes which induce motor neuron disease and early neuronal aging in high incidence foci in the Western Pacific: Calcium deficiency-induced secondary hyperparathyroidism and resultant CNS deposition of calcium and other metallic cations as the cause of ALS and PD in high incidence foci. In: Rose F, ed. Progress in motor neuron disease. Kent: Pitman Books, 1984:44–69.
653. Gajdusek DC. Sounding Board Hypothesis: Interference with axonal transport of neurofilament as a common pathogenetic mechanism in certain diseases of the central nervous system. N Engl J Med 1985; 312:714–719.
654. Gajdusek DC, Gibbs CJ. Attempts to demonstrate a transmissible agent in Kuru, amyotrophic lateral sclerosis, and other sub-acute and chronic nervous system degenerations of man. Nature 1964; 204:257–259.
655. Gajdusek DC, Salazar AM. Amyotrophic lateral sclerosis and parkinsonian syndromes in high incidence among the Auyu and Jaki people of West New Guinea. Neurology 1982; 32:107–126.

656. Galloway PG, Bergeron C, Perry G. The presence of tau distinguishes Lewy bodies of diffuse Lewy body disease from those of idiopathic Parkinson's disease. Neurosci Lett 1989; 100:6–10.
657. Galloway PG, Mulvihill P, Perry G. Filaments of Lewy bodies contain insoluble cytoskeletal elements. Am J Pathol 1992; 140:809–822.
658. Gamboa ET, Wolf A, Yahr MD, et al. Influenza A virus as a possible cause of postencephalitic parkinsonism. Trans Am Neurol Assoc 1973; 98:177–180.
659. Gamboa ET, Wolf A, Yahr MD, et al. Influenza virus antigen in postencephalitic parkinsonism brain: Detection by immunofluorescence. Arch Neurol 1974; 31:228–232.
660. Gan EV, Haberman HF, Menon IA. Electron transfer properties of melanin. Arch Biochem Biophys 1976; 173:666–672.
661. Gan EV, Lam KM, Haberman HF, Menon IA. Oxidizing and reducing properties of melanins. Br J Dermatol 1977; 96:25–28.
662. Ganrot PO. Metabolism and possible health effects of aluminum. Environ Health Perspect 1986; 65:363–441.
663. Garland HG. Refresher course for general practitioners: Parkinsonism. Br Med J 1952; 1:153–155.
664. Garruto RM. Pacific paradigms of environmentally-induced neurological disorders: Clinical, epidemiological and molecular perspectives. Neurotoxicology 1991; 12:347–378.
665. Garruto RM, Fukatsu R, Yanagihara R. Imaging of calcium and aluminum in neurofibrillary tangle-bearing neurons in parkinsonism-dementia of Guam. Proc Natl Acad Sci 1984; 81:1875–1879.
666. Garruto RM, Gajdusek DC. Factors provoking the high incidence of amyotrophic lateral sclerosis and parkinsonism-dementia of Guam: Deposition and distribution of toxic metals and essential minerals in the central nervous system. In: Gottfries CG, ed. Normal aging, Alzheimer's disease and senile dementia. Aspects of etiology, pathogenesis, diagnosis and treatment. Bruxelles: Editions de l'Universit de Bruxelles, 1985:65–81.
667. Garruto RM, Gajdusek DC, Chen KM. Amyotrophic lateral sclerosis among Chamorro migrants from Guam. Ann Neurol 1980; 8:612–619.
668. Garruto RM, Gajdusek DC, Chen KM. Amyotrophic lateral sclerosis and parkinsonism-dementia among Filipino migrants to Guam. Ann Neurol 1981; 10:341–350.
669. Garruto RM, Plato CC, Myrianthopoulos NC, Schanfield MS, Gajdusek DC. Blood groups, immunoglobulin allotypes and dermatoglyphic features of patients with amyotrophic lateral sclerosis and parkinsonism-dementia of Guam. Am J Med Genet 1983; 14:289–298.
670. Garruto RM, Yanagihara R, Gajdusek DC. Disappearance of high-incidence amyotrophic lateral sclerosis and parkinsonism-dementia on Guam. Neurology 1985; 35:193–198.
671. Garruto RM, Yanagihara R, Gajdusek DC. Cycads and amyotrophic lateral sclerosis/parkinsonism-dementia. Lancet 1988; 2:1079.
672. Garruto RM, Yanagihara R, Gajdusek DC, Arion DM. Concentrations of heavy metals and essential minerals in garden soil and drinking water in the Western

Pacific. In: Chen KM, Yase Y, eds. Amyotrophic lateral sclerosis in Asia and Oceania. Taiwan, Republic of China. National Taiwan University, 1984:265–329.

673. Garruto RM, Yase Y. Neurodegenerative disorders of the Western Pacific: The search for mechanisms of pathogenesis. TINS 1986; 9:368–374.
674. Gaspar P, Gray F. Dementia in idiopathic Parkinson's disease. A neuropathological study of 32 cases. Acta Neuropathol 1984; 64:43–52.
675. Gasser T, Schwarz J, Arnold G, Trenkwalder C, Oertel WH. Apomorphine test for dopaminergic responsiveness in patients with previously untreated Parkinson's disease. Arch Neurol 1992; 49:1131–1134.
676. Gasser T, Wszolek Z, Trofatter J, et al. Genetic linkage studies in autosomal dominantly inherited levodopa-responsive Parkinsonism: Evaluation of seven candidate genes. Mov Disord 1993; 8:408.
677. Gay F, Holden M. Loss of viricidal property in serums from patients with herpes and encephalitis. JAMA 1931; 96:2028–2029.
678. Geerling R. Encephalitis Africana. A preliminary report. S Afr Med J 1950; 24:339–343.
679. Geiger LE. Etiologies of Parkinsonism. Bull L A Neurol Soc 1975; 40:160–164.
680. Geraghty JJ, Jankovic J, Zetusky WJ. Association between essential tremor and Parkinson's disease. Ann Neurol 1985; 17:329–333.
681. German DC, Durach A, Askari S, Speciale SG, Bowden DM. 1-Methyl-4-phenyl-1,2,3,6-tetrahydropyridine-induced parkinsonian syndrome in macaca fascicularis: Which midbrain dopaminergic neurons are lost? Neuroscience 1988; 24:161–174.
682. German DC, Manaye K, Smith WK, Woodward DJ, Saper CB. Midbrain dopaminergic cell loss in Parkinson's disease: Computer visualization. Ann Neurol 1989; 26:507–514.
683. German DC, Manaye KF, Sonsalla PK, Brooks BA. Midbrain dopaminergic cell loss in Parkinson's disease and MPTP-induced parkinsonism. Sparing of Calbindin D-28K-containing cells. Ann N Y Acad Sci 1992; 648:42–62.
684. Gershanik OS. Early-onset Parkinsonism. In: Jankovic J, Tolosa E, eds. Parkinson's disease and movement disorders. 2nd ed. Baltimore: Williams & Wilkins, 1993:235–252.
685. Gershanik OS, Nygaard TG. Parkinson's disease beginning before age 40. In: Parkinson's disease: anatomy, pathology and therapy—Advances in neurology, Vol 53. New York: Raven Press, 1990:251–258.
686. Gerstenbrand F. 2. The symptomatology of the apallic syndrome. Monogr Gesamtgeb Psychiatr (Berlin) 1977; 14:14–21.
687. Gerstenbrand F, Poewe WH. The classification of Parkinson's disease. In: Stern G, ed. Parkinson's disease. London: Chapman & Hall Med Press, 1990:315–331.
688. Ghika J, Tennis M, Hoffman E, Schoenfeld D, Growdon J. Idazoxan treatment in progressive supranuclear palsy. Neurology 1991; 41:986–991.
689. Gibb C, Willoughby J, Glober V, et al. Analoges of 1-methyl-4-phenyl-1.2.3.6-tetrahydropyridine as monoamine oxidase substrates: A second ring is not necessary. Neurosci Lett 1987 76:316–322.

690. Gibb W, Luthert P, Marsden C. Corticobasal degeneration. Brain 1989; 112:1171–1191.
691. Gibb W, Terruli M, Lees A. The significance of the Lewy body in idiophatic parkinson's disease. X Int Cong Neuropathol 1986; 432. (abstract)
692. Gibb WR. Neuropathology of the substantia nigra. European Neurology 1991; 31(suppl 1):48–59.
693. Gibb WRG. Recent developments in Parkinson's disease. Vol.II. In: Fahn S, Marsden CD, Calne DB, Goldstein M, eds. The epidemiology of Lewy bodies. New Jersey: Macmillan Healthcare Information, 1987:1–13.
694. Gibb WRG. The neuropathology of Parkinson's disease. In: Jankovic J, Tolosa E, eds. Parkinson's disease and movement disorders. Baltimore: Urban and Schwarzenberg, 1988:205–223.
695. Gibb WRG, Esiri MM, Lees AJ. Clinical and pathological features of diffuse cortical Lewy body disease (Lewy body dementia). Brain 1985; 110:1131–1153.
696. Gibb WRG, Fearnley JM, Lees AJ. The anatomy and pigmentation of the human substantia nigra in relation to selective neuronal vulnerability. In: Streifler MB, Korczyn AD, Melamed E, Youdim MBH, eds. Parkinson's disease: Antomy, pathology and therapy-Advances in neurology, Vol 53. New York: Raven Press, 1990:31–34.
697. Gibb WRG, Fearnley JM, Lees AJ. The progression of idiopathic parkinson's disease is not explained by age-related changes. Clinical and pathological comparisons with post-encephalitic parkinsonian syndrome. Acta Neuropathol 1987; 73:195–201.
698. Gibb WRG, Lees AJ. A comparison of clinical and pathological features of young-and old-onset Parkinson's disease. Neurology 1988; 38:1402–1406.
699. Gibb WRG, Lees AJ. The relevance of the Lewy body of the pathogenesis of idiopathic Parkinson's disease. J Neurol Neurosurg Psychiatry 1988; 51:745–752.
700. Gibb WRG, Lees AJ. The significance of the Lewy body in the diagnosis of idiopathic Parkinson's disease. Neuropathol Appl Neurobiol 1989; 15:27–44.
701. Gibb WRG, Luthert PJ, Janota I, Lantos PL. Cortical Lewy body dementia: Clinical features and classification. J Neurol Neurosurg Psychiatry 1989; 52:185–192.
702. Gibb WRG, Scott T, Lees AJ. Neuronal inclusions of Parkinson's disease. Mov Disord 1991; 6:2–11.
703. Gibb WRG, Terruli M, Lees AJ, Jenner P, Marsden CD. The evolution and distribution of morphological changes in the nervous system of the common marmoset following the acute administration of 1-methyl-4-phenyl-1,2,3,6-tetrahydropyridine. Mov Disord 1989; 4(1):53–74.
704. Gibberd FB. Aetiology of Parkinson's disease. Lancet 1984; January 21:167.
705. Gibberd FB, Simmonds JP. Neurological Disease in Ex-far-east prisoners of war. Lancet 1980; 135–137.
706. Gibbs C,J.Jr., Gajdusek D. Kuru-A prototype subacute infectious disease of the nervous system as a model for the study of amyotrophic lateral sclerosis. In: Motor Neuron Diseases. New York: Grune & Stratton, 1968:269–279.
707. Gibbs CJ, Jr., Gajdusek DC. Amyotrophic lateral sclerosis, Parkinson's disease,

and the amyotrophic lateral sclerosis-Parkinsonism-dementia complex on Guam: A review and summary of attempts to demonstrate infection as the aetiology. J Clin Pathol Suppl (R Coll Pathol) 1972; 25:132–140.

708. Gibbs CJJr, Gajdusek DC,. An update on long-term in vivo and in vitro studies designed to identify a virus as the cause of amyotrophic lateral sclerosis, parkinsonism dementia and Parkinson's disease. In: Rowland L, ed. Human motor neuron diseases. Advances in Neurology, Vol. 36. New York: Raven Press, 1982:343–353.
709. Giladi N, Burke R, Kostic V. Hemiparkinsonism-hemiatrophy syndrome: Clinical and neuroradiologic features. Neurology 1990; 40:1731–1734.
710. Gilks CF. Cycads and sago [letter]. Lancet 1988; 1:181–182.
711. Gillette JR. A perspective on the role of chemically reactive metabolites of foreign compounds in toxicity—I. Correlation of changes in covalent binding of reactivity metabolites with changes in the incidence and severity of toxicity. Biochem Pharmacol 1974; 23:2785–2794.
712. Gillman M, Sandyk R. Parkinsonism induced by methyldopa. S Afr Med J 1984; 65:194.
713. Gilman S, Markel D, Koeppe R, et al. Cerebellar and brainstem hypometabolism in olivopontocerebellar atrophy detected with positron emission tomography. Ann Neurol 1988; 23:223–230.
714. Gimenez-Roldan S, Martin Moro M, Mateo D, Cardenas A. [Changeable aspects in the epidemiology of Parkinson disease (analysis of 262 cases during a period of 9 years]. Rev Clin Esp 1980; 156:25–30.
715. Gimenez-Roldan S, Mateo D. Cinnarizine-induced parkinsonism. Susceptibility to aging and essential tremor. Clin Neuropharmacol 1991; 14:156–164.
716. Ginsberg MD. Carbon monoxide. In: Spencer PS, Schaumburg HH, eds. Experimental and clinicalneurotoxicology. Baltimore: Williams and Wilkins, 1980:374–394.
717. Ginsberg MD, Myers RE, McDonagh BF. Experimental carbon monoxide encephalopathy in the primate: II Clinical aspects, neuropathology, and physiologic correlation. Arch Neurol 1974; 30:209–XX.
718. Giovannini P, Piccolo I, Genitrini S, et al. Early-onset Parkinson's disease. Mov Disord 1991 6:36–42.
719. Girotti F, Soliveri P, Carella F, et al. Dementia and cognitive impairment in Parkinson's disease. J Neurol Neurosurg Psychiatry 1988; 51:1498–1502.
720. Giroud M, Vincent MC, Thierry A, Binnert D, Marin A, Dumas R. [Parkinsonian syndrome caused by traumatic hematomas in the basal ganglia]. Neurochirurgie 1988; 34:61–63.
721. Giuffre R. [Unilateral Parkinsonian symptomatology caused by a bilateral frontal sagittal meningioma]. Riv Neurol 1965; 11:698–707.
722. Gjerris F. Transitory procaine-induced parkinsonism. J Neurol Neurosurg Psychiatry 1971; 34:20–22.
723. Glatt S, Fine S, Kaplan J. Parkinsonism as a presentation of subdural hematoma. Neurology 1983; 33 (suppl 2):61.
724. Glatt SL, Hubble JP, Karst A, et al. Risk factors for dementia in Parkinson's disease (Abstract). Mov Disord 1993; 8(3):408. (abstract)

725. Glover V, Gibb C, Sandler M. The role of MAO in MPTP toxicity—a review. J Neural Transm Suppl 1986; 20:65–76.
726. Godwin-Austen RB, Lee PN, Marmot MG, Stern GM. Smoking and Parkinson's disease. J Neurol Neurosurg Psychiatry 1982; 45:577–581.
727. Goetz CG. Drug-induced parkinsonism and idiopathic Parkinson's disease (Letter to the Editor). Arch Neurol 1983; 40:325–326.
728. Goetz CG, Klawans HL, Tanner CM. Movement disorders induced by neuroleptic drugs. In: Shah NS, Tanner CM, eds. Movement Disorders. New York and London: Plenum Medical Book Company, 1986:309–321.
729. Goetz CG, Stebbins GT. Effects of head trauma from motor vehicle accidents on Parkinson's disease. Ann Neurol 1991; 29:191–193.
730. Goetz CG, Tanner CM, Stebbins GT, Buchman AS. Risk factors for progression in Parkinson's disease. Neurology 1988; 38:1841–1844.
731. Golbe L. Genetics of Parkinson's disease. In: Ellenberg JH, Koller WC, Langston JW, eds. Etiology of Parkinson's disease. New York: Marcel Dekker, 1994:115–140.
732. Golbe L. Progressive supranuclear palsy. In: Stern MB, Koller WC, eds. Parkinsonian syndromes. New York: Marcel Dekker, 1993:227–247.
733. Golbe LI. The genetics of Parkinson's disease: A reconsideration. Neurology 1990; 40(Supplement):7–14.
734. Golbe LI. Young-onset Parkinson's disease: A clinical review. Neurology 1991; 41:168–173.
735. Golbe LI. A kindred with juvenile/young-onset Lewy body parkinsonism. Neurology 1992; 42(Suppl 3):472. (abstract)
736. Golbe LI. The genetics of Parkinson's disease. Rev Neurosciences 1993; 4:1–16.
737. Golbe LI, Cody RA, Duvoisin RC. Smoking and Parkinson's disease. Search for a dose-response relationship. Arch Neurol 1986; 43:774–778.
738. Golbe LI, Di Iorio G, Bonavita V, Miller DC, Duvoisin RC. A large kindred with autosomal dominant Parkinson's disease. Ann Neurol 1990; 27:276–282.
739. Golbe LI, Di Iorio G, Lazzarini AM, Bonavita V, Duvoisin RC. A large kindred with Parkinson's disease: Onset age, segregation ratios, and anticipation. Mov Disord 1993; 8:406.
740. Golbe LI, Duvoisin RC. Smoking and Parkinson's disease. Neurology 1985; 35:275.
741. Golbe LI, Duvoisin RC, Miller DC. A large kindred with autosomal dominanat Parkinson's disease. Ann Neurol 1988; 24:151–152.
742. Golbe LI, Farrell TM, Davis PH. Case-control study of early life dietary factors in Parkinson's disease. Arch Neurol 1988; 45:1350–1353.
743. Golbe LI, Farrell TM, Davis PH. Follow-up study of early-life protective and risk factors in Parkinson's disease. Mov Disord 1990; 5:66–70.
744. Golbe LI, Langston JW. The etiology of Parkinson's disease: New directions for research. In: Jankovic J, Tolosa E, eds. Parkinson's disease and movement disorders. 2nd ed. Baltimore: Williams & Wilkins, 1993:93–101.
745. Golbe LI, Lazzarini AM, Schwarz KO, Mark MH, Dickson DW, Duvoisin RC. Autosomal dominant parkinsonism with benigh course and typical Lewy-body pathology. Neurology 1993; 43:2222–2227.
746. Golbe LI, Miller DC, Duvoisin RC. Autosomal dominant Lewy-body Parkinson's

disease. In: Parkinson's disease: anatomy, pathology and therapy - Advances in neurology, Vol 53. New York: Raven Press, 1990:287–292.

747. Golbe LI, Pae J. Validity of a mailed epidemiological questionnaire and physical self-assessment in Parkinson's disease. Mov Disord 1988; 3:245–254.

748. Goldberg ID, Kurland LT. Mortality in 33 countries from diseases of the nervous system. World Neurology 1972; 3:444–463.

749. Goldman JE, Yen SH, Chiu FC, Peress NS. Lewy bodies of Parkinson's disease contain neurofilament antigen. Science 1983; 221:1082–1084.

750. Goldsmith JR, Herishanu Y, Abarbanel JM, Weinbaum Z. Clustering of Parkinson's disease points to environmental etiology. Archives of Environmental Health 1990; 45:88–94.

751. Gomirato G, Hyden H. A biochemical glia error in Parkinson disease. Brain 1963; 86:773–780.

752. Gomirato G, Hyden H. Etiologic problems of so-called idiopathic Parkinson's disease. Ital J Neurol Sci 1981; 2:131–134.

753. Gonzalez FJ. The molecular biology of cytochrome P450s. Pharmacol Rev 1989; 40(4):243–288.

754. Gonzalez FJ, Skoda RC, Kimura S, et al. Characterisation of the common genetic defect in humans deficient in debrisoquine metabolism. Nature 1988; 331:442–446.

755. Good PF, Olanow CW, Perl DP. Neuromelanin-containing neurons of the substantia nigra accumulate iron and aluminum in Parkinson's disease: a LAMMA study. Brain Res 1992; 593:343–346.

756. Gordon EB. Carbon-monoxide encephalopathy. Br Med J 1965; 1:1232.

757. Gordy ST, Trumper M. Carbon disulfide poisoning: Report of 21 cases. Indust Med 1940; 9:231.

758. Goto A. A long duration follow-up study of Japanese encephalitis. Psychiatria Neurologia Japonica 1962; 64:236–266.

759. Gottlieb D, Melamed E. Is there a relationship between Parkinson's disease and stroke (Abstract). 9th Iternational Symposium on Parkinson's Disease 1988; 117–110.

760. Gotz ME, Freyberger A, Riederer P. Oxidative stress: A role in the pathogenesis of Parkinson's disease. J Neural Transm Suppl 1990; 29:241–249.

761. Gould DH, Gustine DL. Basal ganglia degeneration, myelin alterations, and enzyme inhibition induced in mice by the plant toxin 3-nitropropionic acid. Neuroipathol Appl Neurobiol 1982; 8:377–393.

762. Gourie-Devi M, Ramu MG, Venkataram BS. Treatment of Parkinson's disease in 'Ayurveda' (ancient India system of medicine): Discussion paper. J Roy Soc Med 1991; 84:491–492.

763. Govoni S, Battaini F, Magnoni M, Trabucchi M. Non-vascular central nervous system effects of calcium entry blockers. Cephalalgia 1985; 5(supp 2):115–118.

764. Gowers WR. A manual of diseases of the nervous system. Philadelphia: Blakiston, Son & Co, 1888:

765. Gowers WR. Paralysis agitans. In: A manual of disease of the nervous system II. London: J&A Churchill, 1893:636–639.

766. Gowers WR. A lecture on abiotrophy. Lancet 1902; ii:1003–1007.

767. Graham DG. Oxidative pathways for catecholamines in the genesis of neuromelanin and cytotoxic quinones. Mol Pharmacol 1978; 14:633–643.

768. Graham DG. On the origin and significance of neuromelanin. Arch Pathol Lab Med 1979; 103:359–362.

769. Graham DG. Catecholamine toxicity: a proposal for the molecular pathogenesis of manganese neurotoxicity and Parkinson's disease. Neurotoxicology 1984; 5:83–96.

770. Graham DG. Commentary on "Toxicity of aminochromes." Toxicol Lett 1989; 48:1–2.

771. Graham DG, Szakal-Quin GY, Priest JW, Anthony DC. In vitro evidence that covalent cross-linking of neurofilament occurs in gamma-diketone neuropathy. Proc Natl Acad Sci 1984; 81:4979–4982.

772. Graham DG, Tiffany SM, Bell WRJ, Gutknecht WF. Autoxidation versus covalent binding of quinones as the mechanism of toxicity of dopamine, 6-hydroxydopamine, and related compounds toward C1300 neuroblastoma cells in vitro. Mol Pharmacol 1978; 14:644-653.

772a. Grandinetti A, Morens DM, Reed D, MacEachern D. Prospective study of cigarette smoking and the risk of developing idiopathic Parkinson's disease. Am J Epidemiol 1994; 139:1129–1138.

773. Granerus AK, Mellstrom D. (smoking and Parkinson's disease). Lakartidningen 1987; 84:2025-2026.

774. Granieri E, Carreras M, Casetta I, et al. Parkinson's disease in Ferrara, Italy, 1967 through 1987. Arch Neurol 1991; 48:854–857.

775. Grant FC. The parkinsonian syndrome and brain tumor: Report of a case. Arch Neurol Psychiatry 1953; 69:450–451.

776. Grant WT. Brain Tumor with parkinsonian manifestations. Report of a case. Bull L A Neurol Soc 1948; 8:139–143.

777. Graybiel AM, Hirsch EC, Agid Y. The nigrostriatal system in Parkinson's disease. In: Streifler MD, Korczyn AD, Melamed E, Youdim MBH, eds. Parkinson's disease: Anatomy, pathology & therapy—Advances in neurology—Vol.53. New York: Raven Press, 1990:17–29.

778. Grcevic N, Jardro-Santel D, Jukic S. Cerebral changes in paraquat poisoning. In: Roizin L, Shiraki H, Grcevic N, eds. Neurotoxicology. New York: Raven Press, 1977:469–484.

779. Green MJ, Hill HAO. Chemistry of dioxygen. In: Packer L, ed. Methods in Enzymology, Volume 105: Oxygen radicals in biological systems. New York: Academic Press, 1984: 3–21.

780. Green S, Buttrum S, Molloy H, et al. N-Methylation of pyridines in Parkinson's disease. Lancet 1991; 338:120–121.

781. Greenamyre JT, Higgins DS, Eller RV. Quantitative autoradiography of dihydrorotenone binding to complex I of the electron transport chain. J Neurochem 1992; 59:746–749.

782. Greenfield JG, Bosanquet PD. The brainstem lesion in parkinsonism. J Neurol Neurosurg Psychiatry 1953; 16:213–226.

783. Greenwald I. The supposed relation between paralysis agitans and insufficiency of the parathyroid glands. Am J Med Sci New Series 1914; 147:225–227.

784. Greiner B, Rommelspacher H. Urinary metabolites of tetrahydronoharmane in the rat. Prog Clin Biol Res 1982; 90:201–208.
785. Grimberg L. Paralysis agitans and trauma. J Nerv Ment Dis 1934; 49:14–42.
786. Grimes JD, Hassan MN, Trent G, Halle D, Armstrong GW. Clinical and radiographic features of scoliosis in Parkinson's disease. In: Parkinson's disease—Advances in Neurology, Vol 45. New York: Raven Press, 1987: 353–355.
787. Grinker RR. Parkinsonism following carbon monoxide poisoning. J Nerv Ment Dis 1926; 64:18–28.
788. Groppetti A, Rusconi L, Parati E, Cappabianca V, Parenti M. Degeneration of nigro-striatal dopaminergic neurons by manganese in rats: A model for Parkinson's disease? In: Nappi G, ed. Neurodegenerative disorders: The role played by endotoxins and xenobiotics. New York: Raven Press, 1988:111-119.
789. Grossman A, Rosenberg R, Warmoth L. Glutamate and malate dehydrogenase activities in Joseph disease and olivopontocerebellar atrophy. Neurology 1987; 37:106-111.
790. Grufferman S, Cohen HJ, Delzell ES, Morrison MC, Schold SC, Jr., Moore JO. Familial aggregation of multiple myeloma and central nervous system diseases. J Am Geriatr Soc 1989; 37:303–309.
791. Grunitzky KE, Dumas M, Tatagan-agbi K, et al. Prevalence et distribution des principles affections neurologiques au Togo. In: Congrés de neurologie tropicale. September 26–28, 1991. Limoges: Groupe Francophone d'étude et de Recherche en Neurologie Tropicale Press, 1991:16.
792. Gudjonsson O, Sanz E, Alvan G, Aquilonius SM, Reviriego J. Poor hydroxylator phenotypes of debrisoquine and S-mephenytoin are not over-represented in a group of patients with Parkinson's disease [letter]. Br J Clin Pharmacol 1990; 30:301–302.
793. Gudmundsson KR. A clinical survey of parkinsonism in Iceland. Acta Neurol Scand 1967; Suppl 33:9–61.
794. Gunn JA. The pharmacological actions of tetrahydroharmine. Q J Pharm Pharmacol 1930; 3:1–20.
795. Gunn JA. Relations between chemical constitution, pharmacological actions, and therapeutic uses, in the harmine group of alkaloids. Arch Int Pharmacodynam 1935; 50:379–396.
796. Gupta M, Felten DL, Gash DM. MPTP alters central catecholamine neurons in addition to the nigrostriatal system. Brain Res 1984; 13:737–742.
797. Gupta M, Gupta BK, Thomas R, Bruemmer V, Sladek JR, Jr., Felten DL. Aged mice are more sensitive to 1-methyl-4-phenyl-1,2,3,6-tetrahydropyridine than young adults. Neurosci Lett 1986; 70:326–331.
798. Guterman A, Smith RW. Neurological sequelae of boxing. Sport Medicine 1987; 4:194–210.
799. Haack DG, Baumann RJ, McKean HD, Jameson HD, Turbek JK. Nicotine exposure and parkinson disease. Am J Epidemiol 1981; 114:191–200.
800. Haber F, Weiss J. Uber die katalyse des hydroperoxydes. Naturwissenschaften 1932; 20:948–950.

801. Haberlandt WF. Amyotrophic lateral sclerosis, a clinicopathologic and genetic-demographic study. Stuttgart: Gustav-Fischer, 1964.
802. Habermann-Little B. An analysis of the prevalence and etiology of depression in Parkinson's disease. J Neurosci Nurs 1991; 23 (3):165–169.
803. Hadberg B, Aicardi J, Dias K, Ramos O. A progressive syndrome of autism, dementia, ataxia, and loss of purposeful hand use in girls: Rett's syndrome: report of 35 cases. Ann Neurol 1983; 14:471–479.
804. Haddad R, Rabe A, Dumas R. Comparison of the effects of methylazoxymethanol on brain development in different species. Fed Proc 1972; 31:1520–1523.
805. Haddad R, Rabe A, Dumas R. Neuroteratogenicity of methylazoxymethanol acetate: Behavioral deficits of ferrets with transplacentally induced lissencephaly. Neurotoxicity 1979; 1:171–189.
806. Haerer AF, Anderson DW, Schoenberg BS. Prevalence of essential tremor. Results from the Copiah County study. Arch Neurol 1982; 39:750–751.
807. Haerer AF, Anderson DW, Schoenberg BS. Survey of major neurologic disorders in a biracial United States population: the Copiah County Study. South Med J 1987; 80:339–343.
808. Haimanot RT. Parkinson's disease in Ethiopia: A prospective study of 70 patients. East Afr Med J 1985; 62:571–579.
809. Haimanot RT, Kidane, Wuhib E, et al. Lathyrism in rural northwestern Ethiopia: A highly prevalent disorder. Int J Epidemiol 1990; 19:664–672.
810. Hakim AM, Mathieson G. Dementia in Parkinson disease: a neuropathologic study. Neurology 1979; 29(9 Pt 1):1209–1214.
811. Hakim S, Adams RD. The special clinical problem of symptomatic hydrocephalus with normal cerebrospinal fluid pressure. J Neurol Sci 1963; 2:307–327.
812. Hall A. The prognosis and treatment of chronic epidemic encephalitis. Practitioner 1934; 133:26–36.
813. Hall A, Camb M. Later manifestations or residua. In: Epidemic encephalitis. Bristol: John Wright & Sons Ltd, 1924:109–138.
814. Hall A, Camb M. Epidemiology. In: Epidemic encephalitis. Bristol: John Wright & Sons Ltd, 1924:9–43.
815. Hall R, Jackson R, Swan J. Neurotoxic reactions resulting from chlorpromazine administration. JAMA 1956; 161:214–218.
816. Hallervorden J, Spatz H. Eigenartige erkiankung in extrapyramidalen system mit besonderer Beteilgung des globus pallidus and der substantia nigra. Z Ges Neurol Psychiatry 1922; 79:259–268.
817. Halliday AM. The clinical incidence of myoclonus. Mod Trends Neurol 1967; 4:69–105.
818. Halliwell B. Oxidants and the central nervous system: some fundamental questions. Is oxidant damage relevant to Parkinson's disease, Alzheimer's disease, traumatic injury or stroke. Acta Neurol Scand Suppl 1989; 126:23–33.
819. Halliwell B, Gutteridge JMC. Oxygen radicals and the nervous system. TINS 1985; 7(1):22–26.
820. Halliwell B, Gutteridge JMC. Free radicals in biology and medicine. Oxford: Clarendon Press, 1985.
821. Hamilton A, Lewy FH. Carbon disulphide and hydrogen sulphide hazards in the

viscose rayon industry in the United States. 8th Internat Cong Indust Accid Occupat Dis Leipzig G Thieme 1939; 1107–1110.
822. Hamilton MG, Blum K, Hirst M. Identification of an isoquinoline alkaloid after chronic exposure to ethanol. Alcohol Clin Exp Res 1978; 2(2):133–137.
823. Hammond E. Smoking in relation to the death rates of one million men and women. Natl Cancer Inst monograph no 19 166; 127–204.
824. Hansen L, Salmon D, Galasko D, et al. The Lewy body variant of Alzheimer's disease: A clinical and pathological entity. Neurology 1990; 40:1–8.
825. Hara K, Tohyama I, Kimura H, Fukuda H, Nakamura S, Kameyama M. Reversible serotoninergic neurotoxicity of N-methyl-4-phenyl-1,2,3,6-tetrahydropyridine (MPTP) in mouse striatum studied by neurochemical and immunohistochemical approaches. Brain Res 1987; 410:371–374.
826. Harada H, Nishikawa S, Takahashi K. An epidemiological study of Parkinson's disease in the Sanin district, Sanin, Japan. 12 World Congress of Neurology 1981; series 548:30.
827. Harada H, Nishikawa S, Takahashi K. Epidemiology of Parkinson's disease in a Japanese city. Arch Neurol 1983; 40:151–154.
828. Hardie RJ, Lees AJ. Neuroleptic-induced Parkinson's syndrome: Clinical features and results of treatment with levodopa. J Neurol Neurosurg Psychiatry 1988; 51:850–854.
829. Harding BN, Dunger DB, Grant DB, Erdohazi M. Familial olivonpontocerebellar atrophy with neonatal onset: A recessively inherited syndrome with systemic and biochemical abnormalities. J Neurol Neurosurg Psychiatry 1988; 51(3):385–390.
830. Harik SI, Schmidley JW, Iacofano LA, Blue P, Arora PK, Sayre LM. On the mechanisms underlying 1-methyl-4-phenyl-1,2,3,6-tetrahydropyridine neurotoxicity: The effect of perinigral infusion of 1-methyl-4-phenyl-1,2,3,6-tetrahydropyridine, its metabolite and their analogs in the rat. J Pharmacol Exp Ther 1987; 241:669–676.
831. Harnois C, Di Paolo T. Decreased dopamine in the retinas of patients with Parkinson's disease. Invest Ophthalmol Vis Sci 1990; 31:2473–2475.
832. Harper PS, Harley HG, Reardon W, Shaw DJ. Anticipation in myotonic dystrophy: New light on an old problem. Am J Hum Genet 1992; 51:10–16.
833. Harrison PJ. Neurodegeneration and the nose [editorial]. Clin Otolaryngol 1990; 15:289–291.
834. Hart TB. Parkinson's disease and pesticides [letter]. Lancet 1987; 1:38.
835. Hart TS. Paralysis agitans: Some clinical observations based on the study of 219 cases seen at the clinic of Professor M. Allen Starr. J Nerv Ment Dis 1904; 31:177–188.
836. Hartvig P, Lindquist NG, Aquilonius SM, et al. Distribution of 1-methyl-4-phenyl-1,2,3,6-tetrahydropyridine in experimental animals studied by positron emission tomography and whole body autoradiography. Life Sci 1986; 38:89–97.
837. Hassler R. Zur Pathologie der Paralysis agitans und des postenzephalitischen Parkinsonismus. J fur Psychologie und Neurologie 1938; 48:387–476.
838. Hattori N, Tanaka M, Ozawa T, Mizuno Y. Immunohistochemical studies on complexes I,II,III,and IV of mitochondria in Parkinson's disease. Ann Neurol 1991; 30:563–571.

839. Hatziefthimiou A, Mitsacos A, Mitsaki E, Plaitakis A, Kouvelas ED. Quantitative autoradiographic study of L-glutamate binding sites in normal and atrophic human cerebellum. J Neurosci Res 1991; 28(3):367–375.
840. Haug H, Barmwater R, Eggers D, Fischer S, Kuhl S, Sass N-L. Anatomical changes in aging brain: Morphometric analysis of the human prosencephalon neuropharmacology. In: Cervos-Navarro J. Sarkander H-I. Brain agina: Neuropathology and neuropharmacology. New York: Raven Press, 1983:1–12.
841. Hawker K, Lang AE. Hypoxic-ischemic damage of the basal ganglia. Mov Disord 1990; 5:219–224.
842. Hayes WJ. Pesticides studied in man. Baltimore: Williams & Wilkins, 1982:
843. He F, Zhang S, Zhang C. Extrapyramidal lesions induced by mildewed sugar cane poisoing. Three case reports. Chin Med J 1987; 67:395–396.
844. Heacock RA. The chemistry of adrenochrome and related compounds. Chem Rev 1959; 59:181–237.
845. Heacock RA, Mattock GL. The reaction of adrenochrome with glutathione. Arch Biochem Biophys 1964; 107:352–353.
846. Heacock RA, Powell BS. Adrenochrome and related compounds. In: Ellis GP, West GB, eds. Progress in medicinal chemistry 9. Amsterdam: North-Holland Publishing Company, 1973:275–339.
847. Heafield MT, Fearn S, Steventon GB, Waring RH, Williams AC, Sturman SG. Plasma cysteine and sulphate levels in patients with motor neurone, Parkinson's and Alzheimer's disease. Neurosci Lett 1990; 110:216–220.
848. Hedin CA. Smoker's melanosis may explain the lower hearing loss and lower frequency of Parkinson's disease found among tobacco smokers—a new hypothesis. Med Hypotheses 1991; 35:247–249.
849. Hefti F, Melamed E, Bhawan J, Wurtman RJ. Long-term administration of L-dopa does not damage dopaminergic neurons in the mouse. Neurology 1981; 31:1194–1195.
850. Heikkila RE, Duvoisin RC, Finberg JPM, Youdim MBH. Prevention of MPTP-induced neurotoxicity by AGN-1133 and AGN-1136, selective inhibitors of monoamine oxidase-B. Eur J Pharmacol 1985; 116:313–317.
851. Heikkila RE, Hess A, Duvoisin RC. Dopaminergic neurotoxicity of 1-methyl-4-phenyl-1,2,5,6-tetrahydropyridine in mice. Science 1984; 224:1451–1453.
852. Heikkila RE, Manzino L, Cabbat FS, Duvoisin RC. Protection against the dopaminergic neurotoxicity of 1-methyl-4- pheynl-1,2,5,6-tetrahydropyridine by monoamine oxidase inhibitors. Nature 1984; 311:467–469.
853. Heikkila RE, Winston B, Cohen G, Barden H. Alloxan-induced diabetes—evidence for hydroxyl radical as a cytotoxic intermediate. Biochem Pharmacol 1976; 25:1085–1092.
854. Heilig CW, Knopman DS, Mastri AR, Frey W 2d. Dementia without Alzheimer pathology. Neurology 1985; 35:762–765.
855. Henner K, Hanzal F, Lesny I, et al. Klinicky obraz uzdravenych, kteri prodelali roznavskou Encefalituidu Na Jare Roku 1951. Podle vysetreni v obdobi od unora 1952 Do LEdna 1953. Prognosticke a Epikriticke Zavery. In: Unknown, ed. Epidemia Encefalidty v Roznavskom Prirodnom ohnisku Nakaz. Bratislava: Slovenska Akademia Vied, 1954:64–83.

856. Henner K, Hanzal F, Lesny I, et al. Les encephalites europeennes a tiques. In: Revue Neurologique. 1963:697–752.
857. Henriksson T, Barbour RM, Braa S, et al. Analysis and quantitation of the beta-amyloid precursor protein in the cerebrospinal fluid of Alzheimer's disease patients with a monoclonal antibody-based immunoassay. J Neurochem 1991; 56:1037–1042.
858. Herishann Y, Noah Z. On acute encephalitic parkinsonian syndrome: Case report and review of the recent literature. Eur Neurol 1973; 10:117–124.
859. Herishanu YO, Goldsmith JR, Abarbanel JM, Weinbaum Z. Clustering of Parkinson's disease in southern Israel. Can J Neurol Sci 1989; 16:402–405.
860. Herkenham M, Little MD, Bankiewicz K, Yang SC, Markey SP, Johannessen JN. Selective retention of MPP+ within the monoaminergic systems of the primate brain following MPTP administration: An in vivo autoradiographic study. Neuroscience 1991; 40:133–158.
861. Hershon HI, Kennedy PF, McGuire RJ. Persistence of extra-pyramidal disorders and psychiatric relapse after withdrawal of long-term phenothiazine therapy. Br J Psychiatry 1972; 120:41–50.
862. Herskey L, Gift T, Rivera-Calminlin L. Not Parkinson's disease. Lancet 1982; ii: 49.
863. Herskovits E, Micheli F, Fernandez-Pardal M, et al. Development of parkinsonism after transient ischemic attacks. Medicina (B Aires) 1989; 49:573–576.
864. Hertzman C, Wiens M, Bowering D, Snow B, Calne DB. Parkinson's disease: a case-control study of occupational and environmental risk factors. Am J Ind Med 1990; 17:349–355.
865. Herzon H, Shelton J, Bruyn H. Sequelae of western equine and other arthropod-borne encephalitides. Neurology 1957; 7:535–548.
866. Hesselink JMK. [Parkinson's disease: Neuropathology and pathogenesis in conflict in the period 1817–1953]. Ned Tijdschr Geneeskd 1988; 132:2367–2371.
867. Hesselink JMK. Trauma as an etiology of parkinsonism: Opinions in the nineteenth century (Letter). Mov Disord 1989; 4:283–285.
868. Heston LL. Dementia associated with Parkinson's disease: A genetic study. J Neurol Neurosurg Psychiatry 1980; 43: 846–848.
869. Hewitt EJ, Nicholas DJD. Cations and anions: Inhibitions and interactions in metabolism and enzyme activity. In: Hochster RM, Quastel JH, eds. Metabolic inhibitors. Comprehensive treat is. New York: Academic Press, 1963:311–436.
870. Heyde W. Zur frage des traumatischen parkinsonismus, zugleich ein Beitrag zur Kenntnis extrapyramidal-motorischer Storungen nach Hirnverletzungen. Arch Psychiatry 1932; 97:600–643.
871. Hill JM. Comments on "Putatitive biological mechanisms of the effect of iron deficiency on brain chemistry and behavior." Am J Clin Nutr 1989; 50:616–617.
872. Hill WD, Arai M, Cohen JA, Trojanowski JQ. Neurofilament mRNA is reduced in Parkinson's disease substantia nigra pars compacta neurons. J Comp Neurol 1993; 329:328–336.
873. Hill WD, Lee VM-Y, Hurtig HI, Murray JM, Trojanowski JQ. Epitopes located in spatially separate domains of each neurofilament subunit are present in Parkinson's disease Lewy bodies. J Comp Neurol 1991; 309:150–160.

874. Hinchliffe JR. Cell death in embryogenesis. In: Bowen ID, Lockshin RA, eds. Cell death in biology and pathology. London: Chapman and Hall, 1981:35–78.
875. Hirai S, Tanaka M, Sotomatsu A. [Free radicals and degenerative diseases of the nervous system]. Nippon Ronen Igakkai Zasshi 1990; 27:171–176.
876. Hirano A, Kurland L, Krooth B, Lesseil S. Parkinsonism-dementia complex, an endemic disease on the island of Guam I. Clinical features. Brain 1961; 84:642–661.
877. Hirano A, Malamud N, Kurland LT. Parkinsonism-dementia complex, an endemic disease on the island of Guam. II. Pathological features. Brain 1961; 84:662–679.
878. Hirano A. Cytopathology of amyotrophic lateral sclerosis. Adv Neurol 1991; 56:91–101.
879. Hirano A, Malamud N, Elizan TS, Kurland LT. Amyotrophic lateral sclerosis and parkinsonism-dementia complex of Guam: Further pathologic studies. Arch Neurol 1966; 15:35–51.
880. Hirata Y, Sugimura H, Takei H, Nagatsu T. The effects of pyridinium salts, structurally related compounds of 1-methyl-4-phenylpridinium Ion (MPP+), on tyrosine hydroxylation in rat striatal tissue slices. Brain Res 1986; 397:341–344.
881. Hirsch EC, Brandel JP, Galle P, Javoy-Agid F, Agid Y. Iron and aluminum increase in the substantia nigra of patients with Parkinson's disease: An X-ray microanalysis. J Neurochem 1991; 56:446–451.
882. Hirsch EC, Graybiel AM, Agid Y. Selective vulnerability of pigmented dopaminergic neurons in Parkinson's disease. Acta Neurol Scand Suppl 1989; 126:19–22.
883. Hirsch EC, Mouatt A, Thomasset M, Javoy-Agid F, Agid Y, Graybiel AM. Expression of Calbindin D28K-like immunoreactivity in catecholaminergic cell groups in the human midbrain. Normal distribution and distribution in Parkinson's disease. Neurodegeneration 1992; 1:83–93.
884. Ho BT, McIsaac WM, Walker KE, Estevez V. Inhibitors of monoamine oxidase. Influence of methyl substitution on the inhibitory activity of beta-carbolines. J Pharm Sci 1968; 57(2):269–274.
885. Ho SC, Woo J, Lee CM. Epidemiologic study of Parkinson's disease in Hong Kong. Neurology 1989; 39:1314–1318.
886. Hoehn MM. The epidemiology of parkinsonism. In: de Ajuriagueffa J, Gauthier G, eds. Monamines noyaux gris centraux et syndrome de Parkinson. Geneva: George et Cie, 1971:281–300.
887. Hoehn MM. Age distribution of patients with Parkinsonism. J Am Geriatr Soc 1976; 24:79–85.
888. Hoehn MM. Parkinsonism treated with levodopa: Progression and mortality. J Neural Transm 1983; Supplement 19:253–264.
889. Hoehn MM. Result of chronic levodopa therapy and its modification by bromocriptine in Parkinson's disease. Acta Neurol Scand 1985; 71:97–106.
890. Hoehn MM. Parkinson's disease: Progression and mortality. In: Yahr MD, Bergmann KJ, eds. Parkinson's disease. Advances in Neurology, Vol. 45. New York: Raven Press, 1986:457–461.

891. Hoehn MM. Natural history of the untreated pre-levodopa disease. In: Stern G, ed. Parkinson's disease. London: Chapman & Hall Medical, 1990:307–314.
892. Hoehn MM, Yahr MD. Parkinsonism: Onset, progression and mortality. Neurology 1967; 17:427–442.
893. Hoffman PM, Robbins DS, Gibbs CJ, Jr., Gajdusek DC, Garruto RM, Terasaki OI. Histocompatibility antigens in amyotrophic lateral sclerosis and parkinsonism-dementia on Guam (letter). Lancet 1977; 2:717.
894. Hofman A, Collette HJA, Bartelds AIM. Incidence and Risk Factors of Parkinson's Disease in The Netherlands. Neuroepidemiology 1989; 8:296–299.
895. Hofman A, Schulte W, Tanja RA, et al. History of dementia and Parkinson's disease in 1st-degree relatives of patients with Alzheimer's disease. Neurology 1989; 39:1589–1592.
896. Hohman L. The Histo-pathology of post-encephalitic parkinson's syndrome. Bull Johns Hopkins Hosp 1925; 36:403–410.
897. Holmstedt B. Betacarbolines and tetrahydroisoquinolines: Historical and ethnopharmacological background. Progress in Clinical Biological Research 1982; 90:3–13.
898. Holmstedt B. Beta-carbolines and tetrahydroisoquinolines: Historical and ethnopharmacological background. In: Bloom F, Barchas J, Sandler M, Usdin E, eds. Beta-carbolines and tetrahydroisoquinolines. 2nd ed. New York: Alan R Liss, 1982:3–13.
899. Holt WL Jr. Epidemic encephalitis: A follow-up study of two hundred and sixty-six cases. Arch Neurol Psychiatry 1937; 38:1135–1144.
900. Honczarenko K, Kulcyzycki J. [Etiology of Parkinson's syndrome and disease]. Pol Tyg Lek 1975; 30:1069–1070.
901. Hoogenraad TU. Dithiocarbamates and Parkinson's disease. Lancet 1988; i:767.
902. Hoppel CL, Greenblatt D, Kwok HK, Arora PK, Singh MP, Sayre LM. Inhibition of mitochondrial respiration by analogs of a 4-phenylpyridine and 1-methyl-4-phenylpyridinium cation (MPP+), the neurotoxic metabolite of MPTP. Biochem Biophys Res Commun 1987; 148:684–693.
903. Hornabrook RW, Nagurney J. Essential tremor in Papua New Guinea. Brain 1976; 99:659–672.
904. Hornsby PJ. Parkinson's disease, vitamin E, and mitochondrial energy metabolism [letter]. Arch Neurol 1989; 46:840–841.
905. Hornykiewicz O. Parkinson's disease: From brain homogenate to treatment. Fed Proc 1973; 32:183–190.
906. Hornykiewicz O. The mechanisms of action of L-dopa in Parkinson's disease. Life Sci 1974; 15:1249–1259.
907. Hornykiewicz O. Parkinsonism induced by dopaminergic agonists. In: Calne D, Barbeau A, eds. Dopaminergic mechanisms - Advances in neurology, Vol 9. New York: Raven Press, 1975:155–164.
908. Hornykiewicz O. Parkinson's disease and its chemotherapy. Biochem Pharmacol 1975; 24:1061–1065.
909. Hornykiewicz O. Dopamine changes in the aging human brain: Functional considerations. In: Agnoli A, ed. Aging: Aging brain and ergot alkaloids. 23rd ed. New York: Raven Press, 1983:9–13.

910. Hornykiewicz O. Dopamine deficiency and dopamine substitution in Parkinson's disease. In: Winlow W, Markstein R, eds. The neurobiology of dopamine systems. Manchester: Manchester University Press, 1986:321–328.
911. Hornykiewicz O. Neurochemical pathology and the etiology of Parkinson's disease: Basic facts and hypothetical possibilities [published erratum appears in Mt Sinai J Med (NY) 1988 Mar; 55(2): inside back cover]. Mt Sinai J Med 1988; 55:11–20.
912. Hornykiewicz O. Ageing and neurotoxins as causative factors in idiopathic Parkinson's disease—a critical analysis of the neurochemical evidence. Prog Neuropsychopharmacol Biol Psychiatry 1989; 13:319–328.
913. Hornykiewicz O. The primary site of dopamine neuron damage in Parkinson's disease: Substantia nigra or striatum. Mov Disord 1992; 7:288.
914. Hornykiewicz O, Kish SJ. Biochemical pathophysiology of Parkinson's disease. In: Yahr MD, Bergmann KJ, eds. Parkinson's disease - Advances in neurology, Vol 45. New York: Raven Press, 1986:19–34.
915. Hornykiewicz O, Pifl C, Schingnitz G, Kish SJ. The cause of Parkinson's disease: MPTP, ageing and the striatal dopamine loss. In: Nappi G, ed. Neurodegenerative disorders: The role played by endotoxins and xenobiotics - Advances in neurology. New York: Raven Press, 1988:73–80.
916. Horrobin DF. Letter: Parkinsonism, growth hormone and prolactin. N Engl J Med 1976; 294:1347.
917. Horslen SP, Clayton PT, Harding BN, Hall NA, Keir G, Winchester B. Olivopontocerebellar atrophy of neonatal onset and disialotransferrin developmental deficiency syndrome. Arch Dis Child 1991; 66(9):1027–1032.
918. Horta-Barbosa L, Fuccillo DA, Sever JL. Chronic viral infections of the central nervous system. JAMA 1971; 218:1185–1188.
919. Huang C, Chu N, Lu C, et al. Chronic manganese intoxication. Arch Neurol 1989; 46:1104–1106.
920. Huang Di. Huang Di Nei Jing plain question. Beijing: People's Health Press, 1963:538–539.
921. Hubble J, Kjelstrom J, Beaman B, Koller W. Nocardia serology in Parkinson's disease (Abstract). Mov Disord 1992; 7:292–293.
922. Hubble JP. Drug-induced parkinsonism. In: Stern MB, Koller WC, eds. Parkinsonian syndromes. New York: Marcel Dekker, 1993:111–122.
923. Hubble JP, Hassanein R, Cao T, Neuberger J, Koller W. Herbicide-pesticide exposure independent of rural living as a risk factor for Parkinson's disease. Neurology 1992; 42 (Suppl 3):174.
924. Huber S, Shuttleworth E, Freidenberg D. Neuropsychological differences in the dementia of Alzheimer's and Parkinson's disease. Arch Neurol 1989; 46:1287–1291.
925. Huber SJ, Shuttleworth EC, Christy JA, Chakeres DW, Curtin A, Paulson GW. Magnetic resonance imaging in dementia of Parkinson's disease. J Neurol Neurosurg Psychiatry 1989; 52:1221–1227.
926. Hudson A, Rice G. Similarities of Guamanian ALS/PD to post-encephalitic parkinsonism/ALS: Possible viral cause. Can J Neurol Sci 1990; 17:427–433.
927. Hudson AJ. Amyotrophic lateral sclerosis and its association with dementia,

parkinsonism and other neurological disorders: A review. Brain 1981; 104:217–247.
928. Hudson AJ. Amyotrophic lateral sclerosis/parkinsonism/dementia: Clinico-pathological correlations relevant to Guamanian ALS/PD. Can J Neurol Sci 1991; 18 (3 Suppl):387–389.
929. Hughes AJ, Ben-Shlomo Y, Daniel SE, Lees AJ. What features improve the accuracy of clinical diagnosis in Parkinson's disease: A clinicopathologic study [published erratum appears in Neurology 1992 42:1436]. Neurology 1992; 42:1142–1146.
930. Hughes AJ, Daniel SE, Blankson S, Lees AJ. A clinicopathologic study of 100 cases of Parkinson's disease. Arch Neurol 1993; 50:140–148.
931. Hughes AJ, Daniel SE, Kilford L, Lees AJ. Accuracy of the clinical diagnosis of idiopathic Parkinson's disease: A clinicopathological study of 100 cases. J Neurol Neurosurg Psychiatry 1992; 55:181–184.
932. Hughes AJ, Lees AJ, Stern GM. Apomorphine in the diagnosis and treatment of parkinsonian tremor. Clin Neuropharmacol 1990; 13:312–317.
933. Hughes AJ, Lees AJ, Stern GM. Challenge tests to predict the dopaminergic response in untreated Parkinson's disease. Neurology 1991; 41(11):1723–1725.
934. Hull JT. The prevalence and incidence of Parkinson's disease. Geriatrics 1970; 25:128–133.
935. Humfrey CDN, Steventon GB, Sturman SG, Waring RH, Griffiths B, Williams AC. Monoamine oxidase substrates in Parkinson's disease. Biochem Pharmacol 1990; 40:2562–2564.
936. Hunskåar S. [Pethidine and parkinsonism 1-methyl-4-phenyl-1,2,3,6-tetrahydroxypyridine, a new neurotoxin]. Tidsskr Nor Laegeforen 1986; 106: 219–220.
937. Hunt EL, Lisa JR. Frontal lobe tumor. A case simulating epidemic encephalitis with Parkinson's syndrome. JAMA 1927; 89:1674–1676.
938. Hunt J. Progressive atrophy of the globus pallidus (primary atrophy of the pallidal system): A system disease of the motor cells of the corpus striatum. Brain 1917; 40:58–148.
939. Hunter D, Raffle PAB. Hunter's diseases of occupations. Boston: Little, Brown, 1987.
940. Hunter H. A controlled study of the psychopathology and physical measurements of Klinefelter's syndrome. Br J Psychiatry 1969; 115:443–448.
941. Hurley LS, Woolley DE, Rosenthal F, Timiras PS. Influence of manganese on susceptibility of rats to convulsions. Am J Physiol 1963; 204:493–496.
942. Hurtig H. Vascular parkinsonism. In: Stern MB, Koller WC, eds. Parkinsonian syndromes. New York: Marcel Dekker, 1993:81–92.
943. Hurtig HI. What causes Parkinson's disease? [letter]. Lancet 1984; 1:336–337.
944. Hussels I. [A family with sex-linked retinitis pigmentosa, Parkinson's disease and other neuro-psychiatric disorders]. J Genet Hum 1967; 16:106–155.
945. Hyman C, Hofer M, Barde YA, et al. BDNF is a neurotrophic factor for dopaminergic neurons of the substantia nigra. Nature 1991; 350:230–232.
946. Iacono RP, Sandyk R, Consroe PF, Bamford CR. A cortical vs. subcortical

distinction of dementia contrasts with the unifying pathoetiology of Alzheimer's and Parkinson's disease [letter]. Int J Neurosci 1987; 32:983–985.
947. Iacopino A, Christakos S, German D, Sonsalla PK, Altar CA. Calbindin-D28K-containing neurons in animal models of neurodegeneration: Possible protection from excitotoxicity. Mol Brain Res 1992; 13:251–261.
948. Iacopino AM, Christakos S. Specific reduction of calcium-binding protein (28-kilodalton calbindin-D) gene expression in aging and neurodegenerative diseases. Proc Natl Acad Sci 1990; 87:4078–4082.
949. Icannovic H, Stojanovic M, Nikolic M. [Risk factors for the onset of Parkinson's disease]. Srp Arh Celok Lek 1988; 116:413–417.
950. Ikebe S, Hattori N, Mizuno Y, Tanaka M, Ozawa T. Point mutation of mitochondrial DNA in Parkinson's disease. Mov Disord 1992; 7(Suppl 1):71.
951. Ikebe S, Tanaka M, Ohno K, et al. Increase of deleted mitochondrial DNA in the striatum in Parkinson's disease and senescence. Biochem Biophys Res Commun 1990; 170:1044–1048.
952. Ince P, Irving D, MacArthur F, Perry RH. Quantitative neuropathological study of Alzheimer-type pathology in the hippocampus: Comparison of senile dementia of Alzheimer type, senile dementia of Lewy body type, Parkinson's disease and non-demented elderly control patients. J Neurol Sci 1991; 106:142–152
953. Indakoetxea B, de Munain AL, Marti-Masso JF, Linazasoro G. Parkinsonism after methyl alcohol poisoning. Neurologia 1990; 5:238–241.
954. Indo T, Ando K. Metoclopramide induced parkinsonism. Arch Neurol 1982; 39:494–496.
955. Inose T, Miyakawa M, Miyakawa K, Mizushima S, Oyanagi S, Ando S. Clinical and neuropathological study of a familial case of juvenile parkinsonism. Jpn J Psychiatry Neurol 1988; 42:265–276.
956. Inoue N, Tsukada Y, Barbeau A. Behavioral effects in rats following intrastriatal microinjection of manganese. Brain Res 1975; 95:103–124.
957. Irkec C. [Virologic and immunologic considerations in Parkinson's disease]. Mikrobiyol Bul 1982; 16:293–296.
958. Irkec C. Evaluation of the role of viral antibodies in the pathogenesis of degenerative and demyelinating disease. Mikrobiyol Bul 1989; 23:40–50.
959. Irwin I, Langston JW. Mechanism of cell death. In: Ellenberg JH, Koller WC, Langston JW, eds. Etiology of Parkinson's disease. New York: Marcel Dekker, 1994:97–113.
960. Irwin I, Langston JW. Endogenous toxins as potential etiologic agents in Parkinson's disease. In: Ellenberg JH, Koller WC, Langston JW, eds. Etiology of Parkinson's disease. New York: Marcel Dekker, 1994:153–201.
961. Irwin I, DeLanney LE, Forno LS, Finnegan KT, Di Monte DA, Langston JW. The evolution of nigrostriatal neurochemical changes in the MPTP-treated squirrel monkey. Brain Res 1990; 531:242–252.
962. Irwin I, DeLanney LE, Langston JW. MPTP and aging: Studies in the C57BL/6 mouse. In: Narabayashi H, Nagatsu T, Yanagisawa N, Mizuno Y, eds. Parkinson's disease: From basic research to treatment. Advances in Neurology, Volume 60. Proceedings of the 10th International Symposium on Parkinson's disease. New York: Raven Press, 1992:197–206.

963. Irwin I, Finnegan KT, DeLanney LE, Di Monte D, Langston JW. The relationships between aging, monoamine oxidase, striatal dopamine and the effects of MPTP in C57BL/6 mice: A critical reassessment. Brain Res 1992; 572:224–231.
964. Irwin I, Langston JW. Selective accumulation of MPP+ in the substantia nigra: A key to neurotoxicity? Life Sci 1985; 36:207–212.
965. Irwin I, Langston JW. The fate of MPTP in mice and squirrel monkeys. In: Nagatsu T, Yoshida M, Kanazawa I, Ogawa N, eds. Brain and Parkinson's disease. Tokyo: Heibonsha, 1988:71–79.
966. Irwin I, Langston JW, Delanney E. 4-phenylpyridine(4PP) and MPTP: The relationship between striatal MPP+concentrations and neurotoxicity. Life Sci 1987; 40(8):731–740.
967. Irwin I, Wu EY, DeLanney LE, Trevor AJ, Langston JW. The effect of diethyldithiocarbamate (DDC) on the biodisposition of MPTP: An explanation for enhanced neurotoxicity. Eur J Pharmacol 1987; 141:209–217.
968. Isgreen WP, Chutorian AM, Fahn S. Sequential parkinsonism and chorea following "mild": influenza. Trans Am Neurol Assoc 1976; 101:56–59
969. Ishino H, Higashi H, Kuroda S, Yabuki S, Hayahara T, Otsuki S. Motor nuclear involvement in progressive supranuclear palsy. J Neurol Sci 1974; 22:235–244.
970. Ishino H, Otsuki S. Contribution to clinical pathology of progressive supranuclear palsy: Subcortical argyrophilic dystrophy. J Neurol Sci 1975; 24:471–481.
971. Ito K. [Effects and side effects of levodopa in parkinsonism-results of a collaborative study. (1) Therapeutic responses in relation to the etiology and clinical types]. Rinsho Shinkeigaku 1976; 16:869–870.
972. Iwasaki Y, Kinoshita M, Ikeda K, Takamiya K. Human T-Lymphotrophic virus type-I associated myleopathy presenting as spinocerebellar syndrome. Ann Neurol 1989; 25:419–420.
973. Iwatsubo T, Nakano I, Fukunaga K, Miyamoto E. CA2+/calmodddulin-dependent protein kinase II immunoreactivity in Lewy bodies. Acta Neuropathol 1991; 82:159–163.
974. Jackson J, Jankovic J, Ford J. Progressive supranuclear palsy: Clinical features and responses to treatment in sixteen patients. Ann Neurol 1983; 13:273–278.
975. Jaeken J. Disalotransferrin developmental deficiency syndrome and olivopontocerebellar atrophy. Arch Dis Child 1989; 64(5):764–765.
976. Jaffe LS. Sources, characteristics, and fate of atmospheric carbon monoxide. Ann N Y acad Sci 1970; 174:74–76.
977. Jankovic J. Progressive supranuclear palsy. Clinical and pharmacologic update. Neurol Clin 1984; 2:473–486.
978. Jankovic J. Essential tremor and Parkinson's disease [letter]. Ann Neurol 1989; 25:211–212.
979. Jankovic J. Parkinsonism-plus syndromes. Mov Disord 1989; 4:S95–119.
980. Jankovic J, Beach J, Schwartz K. Tremor and longevity in relatives of patients with Parkinson's disease, essential tremor and control subjects (Abstract). Neurology 1994; (in press)
981. Jankovic J, Kirkpatrick J, Blomquist K, Langlais P, Bird E. Late-onset Hallervorden-Spatz disease presenting as familial parkinsonism. Neurology 1985; 35:227–234.

982. Jankovic J, McDermott M, Carter J, et al. Variable expression of Parkinson's disease: A base-line analysis of the DATATOP cohort. Neurology 1990; 40:1529–1534.
983. Jankovic J, Newmark M, Peter P. Case report. Parkinsonism and acquired hydrocephalus. Mov Disord 1986; 1:59–64.
984. Jankovic J, Reches A. Parkinson's disease in monozygotic twins. Ann Neurol 1986; 19:405–408.
985. Jansson B, Jankovic J. Low cancer rates among patients with Parkinson's disease. Ann Neurol 1985; 17:505–509.
986. Jarman J, Glover V, Sandler M, Turjanski N, Stern G. Platelet monoamine oxidase B activity in Parkinson's disease: A re-evaluation. J Neural Transm 1993; 5:1–4.
987. Jarvis MF, Wagner GC. Age-dependent effects of 1-methyl-4-phenyl-1,2,3,6-tetrahydropyridine (MPTP). Neuropharmacology 1985; 24:581–583.
988. Jarvis MF, Wagner GC. 1-Methyl-4-phenyl-1,2,3,6-tetrahydropyridine-induced neurotoxicity in the rat: Characterization and age-dependent effects. Synapse 1990; 5:104–112.
989. Javitch JA, D'Amato RJ, Strittmatter SM, Snyder SH. Parkinsonism-inducing neurotoxin, N-methyl-4-phenyl-1,2,3,6-tetrahydropyridine: Uptake of the metabolite N-methyl-4-phenylpyridine by dopamine neurons explains selective toxicity. Neurobiology 1985; 82:2173–2177.
990. Javitch JA, Snyder SH. Uptake of MPTP(+) by dopamine neurons explains selectivity of parkinsonism-inducing neurotoxin, MPTP. Eur J Pharmacol 1984; 104:455–456.
991. Javoy-Agid F, Agid Y. Is the Mesocortical dopaminergic system involved in Parkinson Disease? Neurology 1980; 30:1326–1330.
992. Javoy-Agid F, Hirsch EC, Dumas S, Duyckaerts C, Mallet J, Agid Y. Decreased tyrosine hydroxylase messenger RNA in the surviving dopamine neurons of the substantia nigra in Parkinson's disease: An in situ hybridization study. Neuroscience 1990; 38:245–253.
993. Jellinger K. [Prolonged post-traumatic encephalopathy]. Wien Med Wochenschr 1968; 118:747–753.
994. Jellinger K. Trauma as an etiologic agent in Parkinson disease [letter]. Mov Disord 1989; 4:90–92.
995. Jellinger K. Morphology of Alzheimer's disease and related disorders. In: Maurer K, Riederer P, Beckman H, eds. Epidemiology, neuropathology, neurochemistrry, and clinics. Wien, New York: Springer Verlag, 1990:61–77.
996. Jellinger K. New developments in the pathology of Parkinson's disease. In: Parkinson's disease: anatomy, pathology and therapy - Advances in neurology, Vol 53. New York: Raven Press, 1990:1–16.
997. Jellinger K. Progressive pallidum atrophie. J Neurol Sci 1991; 6:19–44.
998. Jellinger K, Kienzl E, Rumpelmair G. Iron-melanin complex in substantia nigra of parkinsonian brains: An x-ray microanalysis. J Neurochem 1992; 59:1168–1171.
999. Jellinger K, Paulus W, Grundke-Iqbal I, Riederer P, Youdim MB. Brain iron and ferritin in Parkinson's and Alzheimer's diseases. J Neural Transm Park Dis Dement Sect 1990; 2:327–340.

1000. Jellinger K, Riederer P. Dementia in Parkinson's disease and (pre)senile dementia of Alzheimer type: Morphological aspects and changes in intracerebral MAO activity. In: Hassler RG, Christ JF, eds. Parkinson-specific motor and mental disorders. Role of the pallidum: Pathophysiological, biochemical and therapeutic aspects. Advances in Neurology, Vol.40. 40th ed. New York: Raven Press, 1984:199–210.

1001. Jellinger KA. Pathology of Parkinson's disease changes other than the nigrostriatal pathway. Mol Chem Neuropathol 1991; 14:153–197.

1002. Jellinger KA, Bancher C. Neuropathology. In: Litvan I, Agid Y, eds. Progressive supranuclear palsy. Clinical and research approaches. New York, Oxford: Oxford University Press, 1992:44–88.

1003. Jellinger KA, Kienzl E, Rumpelmaier G, et al. Iron and ferritin in substantia nigra in Parkinson's disease. In: Narabayashi H, Nagatsu T, Yanagisawa N, Mizuno Y, eds. Parkinson's disease: From basic research to treatment. Advances in Neurology, Vol. 60. New York: Raven Press, 1993:267–272.

1004. Jenkins AC. Epidemiology of parkinsonism in Victoria. Med J Aust 1966; 2:496–502.

1005. Jenkyn C, Reeves A. Neurologic signs in uncomplicated aging (senescence). Semin Neurol 1981; 7:21–30.

1006. Jenner P. Clues to the mechanism underlying dopamine cell death in Parkinson's disease. J Neurol Neurosurg Psychiatry 1989; 22–28.

1007. Jenner P. Oxidative stress as a cause of Parkinson's disease. Acta Neurol Scand 1991; 84 (suppl 136):6–15.

1008. Jenner P. What process causes nigral cell death in Parkinson's disease? Neurol Clin 1992; 10:387–403.

1009. Jenner P, Marsden C. Neurochemical basis of parkinsonian tremor. In: Findley LT, Capideo R, eds. Movement disorders: Tremor. London: MacMillan, 1984:305–320.

1010. Jenner P, Marsden CD. The actions of 1-methyl-4-phenyl-1,2,3,6-tetrahydropyridine in animals as a model of Parkinson's disease. J Neural Transm Suppl 1986; 20:11–39.

1011. Jenner P, Marsden CD. MPTP-induced parkinsonism in primates and its use in the assessment of novel strategies for the treatment of Parkinson's disease. In: Rose FC, ed. Current problems in neurology (6): Parkinson disease:clinical and experimental advances. London: John Libbey, 1988:149–162.

1012. Jenner P, Marsden CD. MPTP-induced Parkinsonism: A model of Parkinson's disease and its relevance to the disease process. In: Jankovic J, Tolosa E, eds. Parkinson's disease and movement disorders. 2nd ed. Baltimore: Williams & Wilkins, 1993:55–75.

1013. Jenner P, Marsden CD, Costall B, Naylor RJ. MPTP and MPP+ induced neurotoxicity in rodents and the common marmoset as experimental models for investigating Parkinson's disease. In: Markey SP, Castagnoli N, Jr., Trevor AJ, Kopin IJ, eds. MPTP; A neurotoxin producing a parkinsonian syndrome. Orlando, FL: Academic Press, 1986:45–68.

1014. Jenner P, Schapira AHV, Marsden CD. New insights into the cause of Parkinson's disease. Neurology 1992; 42:2241–2250.

1015. Jenner P, Sian J, Dexter DT, Schapira AHV, Marsden CD. Decreased reduced glutathione levels are an early pathological marker of Parkinson's disease. Mov Disord 1992; 7(3):288–289.

1016. Jimenez-Jimenez FJ, Gonzales DM, Gimenez-Roldan S. Exposure to well-water and pesticides in Parkinson's disease. A case-control study from the South East area of Madrid. 9th Iternational Symposium on Parkinson's Disease 1988; 118.

1017. Jimenez-Jimenez FJ, Mateo D, Gimenez-Roldan S. Premorbid smoking, alcohol consumption, and coffee drinking habits in Parkinson's disease: A case-control study. Mov Disord 1992; 7:339–344.

1018. Joachim CL, Morris JH, Selkoe DJ. Clinically diagnosed Alzheimer's disease: autopsy results in 110 cases. Ann Neurol 1988; 24:50–56.

1019. Johannessen JN, Chiueh CC, Burns RS, Markey SP. Differences in the metabolism of MPTP in the rodent and primate parallel differences in sensitivity to its neurotoxic effects. Life Sci 1985; 36:219–225.

1020. Johannessen JN, Kelner L, Hanselman D, Shih MC, Markey SP. In vitro oxidation of MPTP by primate neural tissue: A potential model of MPTP neurotoxicity. Neurochem Int 1985; 7:169–176.

1021. Johnsen JA, Miller VT. Tobacco intolerance in multiple system atrophy. Neurology 1986; 36(7):986–988.

1022. Johnson RT, Price DL. Chronic neurological diseases: Their societal burdens and potential solutions. J Chron Dis 1980; 33:129–133.

1023. Johnson RT, Ter Meulen V. Slow infections of the nervous system. Adv Intern Med 1978; 23:353–383.

1024. Johnson W, Davidson M, Yoshidome H, Lustenberger A, Stenroos S. Genetics of Parkinson's Disease (PD), The Multifactorial/Threshold (MF/T) Model (Abstract). Mov Disord 1990; 5:92.

1025. Johnson WG. The clinical spectrum of hexosaminidase deficiency diseases. Neurology 1981; 31(11):1453–1456.

1026. Johnson WG. Genetic susceptibility to Parkinson's disease. Neurology 1991; 41 (Suppl 2):82–87.

1027. Johnson WG, Hodge SE, Duvoisin R. Twin studies and the genetics of Parkinson's disease—A reappraisal. Mov Disord 1990; 5:187–194.

1028. Jones M, Yang M, Michelsen O. Effects of methylazoxymethanol glucoside and methylazoxymethanol acetate on the cerebellum of the postnatal Swiss albino mouse. Fed Proc 1972; 31:1508–1511.

1029. Jonsson G, Sundstrom E. [New clues to the etiology of Parkinson disease: Parkinsonism induced by the neurotoxin MPTP]. Lakartidningen 1986; 83:215–218.

1030. Jordan BD. Neurologic aspects of boxing. Arch Neurol 1987; 44:453–459.

1031. Jordan E. The influenza epidemic of 1918: Encephalitis and influenza. JAMA 1927; 89:1603–1606.

1032. Joseph C, Chassan J, Koch M. Levodopa in Parkinson disease: A long-term appraisal of mortality. Ann Neurol 1978; 3:116–118.

1033. Jovicic A. [Parkinson's syndrome. Etiopathogenesis and possibilities of treatment]. Vojnosanit Pregl 1985; 42:206–210.

1034. Juncos J, Hirsch E, Malessa S, Duyckaets C, Hersh L, Agid Y. Mesencephalic cholinergic nulei in progressive supranuclear palsy. Neurology 1991; 41:25–30.
1035. Juncos RA, Abdala J, Celis DO. [Parkinsonism due to manganese intoxication]. Rev Fac Cienc Med Cordoba 1968; 26:57–63.
1036. Jurna I, Nell T, Schreyer I. Motor disturbance induced by tremorine and oxotremorine. Naunyn Schmiedebergs Arch Pharmacol 1970; 267:80–98.
1037. Kaakkola S, Marnela KM, Oja SS, Icen A, Palo J. Leukocyte glutamate dehydrogenase and CSF amino acids in late onset ataxias. Acta Neurol Scand 1990; 82(5):292–296.
1038. Kahler SG, Riley E. Inherited parkinsonism [letter]. Clin Genet 1979; 15:110–111.
1039. Kahn HA. The Dorn study of smoking and mortality among U.S. veterans: Report on eight and one-half years of observation. In: Haenszel W, ed. Epidemiological approaches to the study of cancer and other chronic diseases. Bethesda, Maryland: Health, Education and Welfare, National Cancer Institute, Monograph 19, U.S., 1966:1–27.
1040. Kak VK, Gordon DS. ABO blood groups and Parkinson's disease. Ulster Med J 1970; 39:132–134.
1041. Kakulas BA, Tan N, Ojeda VJ. The neuropathology of progressive autonomic failure of central origin (the Shy-Drager syndrome). Clin Exp Neurol 1986; 22:103–111.
1042. Kalaria RN, Mitchell MJ, Harik SI. Correlation of 1-methyl-4-phenyl-1,2,3,6-tetrahydropyridine neurotoxicity with blood-brain barrier monoamine oxidase activity. Proc Natl Acad Sci 1987; 84:3521–3525.
1043. Kallio J, Marttila RM, Rinne UK, Sonninen V, Syvalahti E. Debrisoquine oxidation in Parkinson's disease. Acta Neurol Scand 1991; 83:194–197.
1044. Kaloyanova FP, El Batawi MA. Human toxicology of pesticides. Boca Raton: CRC Press, 1991:
1045. Kan AE. Striatonigral degeneration. Pathology 1978; 10(1):45–52.
1046. Kanazawa I. [Internal neurology—b. Degenerative nerve diseases—approach to etiology]. Nippon Rinsho 1987; 45:2133–2143.
1047. Kanazawa I, Kimura M, Murata M, Tanaka Y, Cho F. Choreic movements in the macaque monkey induced by kainic acid lesions of the striatum combined with L-Dopa. Pharmacological, biochemical and physiological studies on neural mechanisms. Brain 1990; 113:509–535.
1048. Kane FJ. Carbon disulfide intoxication from overdosage of disulfiram. Am J Psychiatry 1970; 127:690–694.
1049. Kane J, Rifkin A, Quitkin F, Klein D. Extrapyramidal side effects with lithium treatment. Am J Psychiatry 1078; 135:851–853.
1050. Kaneda N, Nagatsu T. [Pathogenesis of Parkinson's disease, a molecular genetic approach]. Rinsho Shinkeigaku 1989; 29:1510–1513.
1051. Kano M, Mitsuhata Y, Kishida S, Yano Y, Muro T. Shy-Drager syndrome and human T-Lymphyotrophic virus type I infection. Ann Neurol 1989; 25:420–421.
1052. Kaplan SD. Age distribution of patients with Parkinson's disease in 1960 and 1970 in 110 hospitals. Neurology 1974; 24:972–975.
1053. Kark RAP. Clinical and neurochemical aspects of inorganic mercury intoxication.

In: Vinken PJ, Bruyn GW, eds. Handbook of clinical neurology, Vol 36, Intoxication of the nervous system, pt. 1. Amsterdam: North-Holland, 1979:147–197.
1054. Kass GEN, Wright JM, Nicotera P, Orrenius S. The mechanism of 1-methyl-4-phenyl-1,2,3,6-tetrahydropyridine toxicity: Role of intracellular calcium. Arch Biochem Biophys 1988; 260:789–797.
1055. Kato S, Nakamura H. Cytoplasmic argyrophilic inclusions in neurons of pontine nuclei in patients with olivopontocerebellar atrophy: Immunohistochemical and ultranstructural studies. Acta Neuropathol 1990; 79(6):584–594.
1056. Katzman R, Terry R. Normal aging of the nervous system. In: Katzman R, Rowe JW, eds. Principles of geriatric neurology. Philadelphia: Davis, 1992:18–58.
1057. Katzman R, Terry R, DeTeresa R, et al. Clinical, pathological, and neurochemical changes in dementia: A subgroup with preserved mental status and numerous neocortical plaques. Ann Neurol 1988; 23:138–144.
1058. Kawamura R, Ikuta H, Fukuzumi S, et al. Intoxication by manganese in well water. Kitasato Arch Exp Med 1941; 18:145–169.
1059. Kehrer F. Der Ursachenkreis des Parkinsonismus (Erblichkeit, Trauma, Syphilis). Arch Psychiatr Nervenkr 1930; 187:268.
1060. Kehrer F. Uber das erbliche Zittern und und die Bedeutung von Langlebigkeit, Kinderreichtum und Zwillingsgeburten in Sippen mit heredodegenerativen Nervenleiden. Dtsch Z Nervenheilk 1930; 114:165–208.
1061. Kemp BE, Pearson RB. Protein kinase recognition sequence motifs. Trends in Biochemical Sciences 1990; 15:342–346.
1062. Kennedy PG, Duchen LW. A quantitative study of intermediolateral column cells in motor neuron disease and the Shy-Drager syndrome. J Neurol Neurosurg Psychiatry 1985; 48(11):1103–1106.
1063. Kenyhercz TM, Kissinger PT. High-performance liquid chromatographic assay of isoquinoline alkaloid formation from reaction of biogenic amines and aldehydes. J Pharm Sci 1978; 67(1):112–113.
1064. Kerr JFR, Wyllie AH, Currie AR. Apoptosis: A basic biological phenomenon with wide-ranging implications in tissue kinetics. Br J Cancer 1972; 26:239–257.
1065. Keshavarzian A, Wibowo A, Gordon JH, Fields JZ. MPTP-induced duodenal ulcers in rat: Prevention by reuptake blockers for serotonin and norepinephrine, but not dopamine. Gastroenterology 1990; 98:554–560.
1066. Kessler II. Epidemiologic studies of Parkinson's disease. III. A community-based survey. Am J Epidemiol 1972; 96:242–254.
1067. Kessler II. Epidemiologic studies of Parkinson's disease. II. A hospital-based survey. Am J Epidemiol 1972; 95:308–318.
1068. Kessler II. Parkinson's disease: Perspectives on epidemiology and pathogenesis. Prev Med 1973; 2:88–105.
1069. Kessler II. Parkinson's disease in epidemiologic perspective. In: Neurological epidemiology: Principles and clinical applications - Advances in Neurology, Vol 19. New York: Raven Press, 1978:355–384.
1070. Kessler II, Diamond EL. Epidemiologic studies of Parkinson's disease. I. Smoking and Parkinson's disease: A survey and explanatory hypothesis. Am J Epidemiol 1971; 94:16–25.
1071. Khandogina EK, Mutovin GR, Filiushkin IV, Akif'ev AP. [Radiation injuries

of the chromosomes in the lymphocytes of hereditary disease patients]. Med Radiol (Mosk) 1980; 25:53–58.

1072. Khurana R, Nelson E, Azzarelli B. Shy-Drager syndrome: Dignosis and treatment of cholinergic dysfunction. Neurology 1980; 30:805–809.

1073. Kikuchi K, Nagatsu Y, Makino Y, Mashino T, Ohta S, Hirobe M. Metabolism and penetration through blood-brain barrier of Parkinsonism-related compounds: 1,2,3,4-Tetrahydroisoquinoline and 1-methyl-1,2,3,4-tetrahydroisoquinoline. Drug Metab Dispos 1991; 19:257–262.

1074. Kilbourne E. History of influenza. New York: Plenum, 1987:3–22.

1075. Kindt MV, Youngster SK, Sonsalla PK, Duvoisin RC, Heikkila RE. Role for monoamine oxidase-A (MAO-A) in the bioactivation and nigrostriatal dopaminergic neurotoxicity of the MPTP analog, 2'Me-MPTP. Eur J Pharmacol 1988; 146:313–318.

1076. Kinemuchi H, Fowler CJ, Tipton KF. The Neurotoxicity of 1-Methyl-4-Phenyl-1,2,3,6,-Tetrahydropyridine (MPTP) and its relevance to Parkinson's disease. Neurochem Int 1987; 11:(4):359–(4):373.

1077. Kirch DG, Alho A, Wyatt JW. Hypothesis: A nicotine-dopamine interaction linking smoking with Parkinson's disease and tardive dyskinesia. Cellular and Molecular Neurobiology 1988; 8:285–291.

1078. Kirchner C. [Some psychodiagnostic aspects of Parkinson's syndrome with regard to different etiology and various degrees of severity]. Z Psychol 1970; 177:91–111.

1079. Kisby G, Gold B, Spencer P. Neurotoxic effects of cycasin in murine organotypic cultures. Soc Neurosci Abstr 1990; 16:1113.

1080. Kisby GE, Ellison M, Spencer PS. Content of the neurotoxins cycasin (methylazoxymethanol B-D-glucoside) and BMAA (B-N-methylamino-L-alanine) in cycad flour prepared by Guam Chamorros. Neurology 1992; 42:1336–1340.

1081. Kisby GE, Ross SM, Spencer PS, Gold BG, Nunn PB, Roy DN. Cycasin and BMAA: Candidate neurotoxins for western Pacific amyotrophic lateral sclerosis/parkinsonism-dementia complex. Neurodegeneration 1992; 1:73–82.

1082. Kish S, Chang L, Mirchandani L, Shannak K, Hornykiewicz O. Progressive supranuclear palsy: Relationship between extrapyramidal disturbances, dementia, and brain neurotransmitter markers. Ann Neurol 1985; 18:530–536.

1083. Kish SJ, Currier RD, Schut L, Perry TL, Morito CL. Brain choline acetyltransferase reduction in dominantly inherited olivopontocerebellar atrophy. Ann Neurol 1987; 22(2):272–275.

1084. Kish SJ, Distefano LM, Dozic S, et al. [3H]Vesamicol binding in human brain cholinergic deficiency disorders. Neurosci Lett 1990; 117(3):347–352.

1085. Kish SJ, Du F, Parks DA, et al. Quinolinic acid catabolism is increased in cerebellum of patients with dominantly inherited olivopontocerebellar atrophy. Ann Neurol 1991; 29(1):100–104.

1086. Kish SJ, el-Awar M, Schut L, Leach L, Oscar-Berman M, Freedman M. Cognitive deficits in olivopontocerebellar atrophy: Implications for the cholinergic hypothesis of Alzheimer's dementia. Ann Neurol 1988; 24(2):200–206.

1087. Kish SJ, Morito C, Hornykiewicz O. Glutathione peroxidase activity in Parkinson's disease brain. Neurosci Lett 1985; 58:343–346.

1088. Kish SJ, Morito CL, Hornykiewicz O. Brain glutathione peroxidase in neurodegenerative disorders. Neurochem Pathol 1986; 4(1):23–28.
1089. Kish SJ, Rajput A, Gilbert J, et al. Elevated gamma-aminobutyric acid level in striatal but not extrastriatal brain regions in Parkinson's disease: Correlation with striatal dopamine loss. Ann Neurol 1986; 20:26–31.
1090. Kish SJ, Robitaille Y, Ball M, et al. Glycerophosphoethanolomine concentration is elevated in brain of patients with dominantly inherited olivopontocerebellar atrophy. Neurosci Lett 1990; 120:209–211.
1091. Kish SJ, Robitaille Y, el-Awar M, et al. Non-Alzheimer-type pattern of brain cholineacetyltransferase reduction in dominantly inherited olivopontocerebellar atrophy. Ann Neurol 1989; 26(3):362–367.
1092. Kish SJ, Schut L, Simmons J, Gilbert J, Chang LJ, Rebbetory M. Brain acetylcholinesterase activity is markedly reduced in dominantly-inherited olivopontocerebellar atrophy. J Neurol 1988; 51(4):544–548.
1093. Kish SJ, Shannak K, Hornykiewicz O. Uneven pattern of dopamine loss in the striatum of patients with idipathic Parkinson's disease: Pathophysiologic and clinical implications. N Engl J Med 1988; 318(14):876–880.
1094. Kish SJ, Shannak K, Rajput A, Deck JHN, Hornykiewicz O. Aging produces a specific pattern of striatal dopamine loss: Implications for the etiology of idiopathic Parkinson's disease. J Neurochem 1992; 58:642–648.
1095. Kissel P, Andre JM. [Parkinson's disease and anosmia in monozygotic twin sisters (author's transl)]. J Genet Hum 1976; 24:113–117.
1096. Kitani M, Kobayashi S, Yamaguchi S. Computerized tomography with longitudinal follow-up of brain atrophy in patients with Parkinson's disease. Gerontology 1990; 36:361–368.
1097. Kitt CA, Cork LC, Eidelberg F, Joh TH, Price DL. Injury of nigral neurons exposed to 1-methyl-4-phenyl-1,2,3,6-tetrahydropyridine: A tyrosine hydroxylase immunocytochemical study in monkey. Neuroscience 1986; 17(4): 1089–1103.
1098. Klaue V. Parkinsonsche Krankheit (paralysis agitans) und postencephalitischer Parkinsonismus. Arch Psychiatr Nervenkr 1940; 111:251–321.
1099. Klawans HL,Jr.. Hemiparkinsonism as a late complication of hemiatrophy. A new syndrome. Neurology 1981; 31:625–628.
1100. Klawans HL. Dystonia and tremor following exposure to 2,3,7,8-tetrachlorobenzo-p-dioxin (TCDD Dioxin). Proc Int Symp Neurotox 1992; 1987.
1101. Klawans HL, Lupton M, Simon L. Calcification of the basal ganglia as a cause of levodopa-resistant parkinsonism. Neurology 1976; 26:221–225.
1102. Klawans HL, Stein RW, Tanner CM, Goetz CG. A pure parkinsonian syndrome following acute carbon monoxide intoxication. Arch Neurol 1982; 39:302–304.
1103. Klawans HLJr, Bergen D, Bruyn G. Prolonged drug-induced parkinsonism. Contemp Neurol 1973; 35:368–377.
1104. Klawans HLJr, Cohen MM. Diseases of the extrapyramidal system. Dis Mon 1970; 1–52.
1105. Klawans HLJr, Zeithin B. L-dopa in parkinsonism associated with cerebellar dysfunction probable olivopontocerebellar degeneration. J Neurol Neurosurg Psychiatry 1971; 34:14–19.

1106. Kluin KJ, Gilman S, Markel DS, Koeppe RA, Rosenthal G, Junck L. Speech disorders in olivopontocerebellar atrophy correlate with positron emission tomography findings. Ann Neurol 1988; 23(6):547–554.
1107. Kluyskens Y, Bossaert L, Snoeck J, Martin JJ. Idiopathic orthostatic hypotension and the Shy-Drager syndrome. Physiological studies in four cases, pathological report of one case. Acta Cardiol 1977; 32(5):317–335.
1108. Knoll J. Extension of life span of rats by long-term (-) deprenyl treatment. Mt Sinai J Med 1988; 55(1):67–74.
1109. Kobayashi A. Cycasin in cycad materials used in Japan. Fed Proc 1972; 31:1476–1477.
1110. Koch MJ, Hoffman P, Brody JA, Edgar AH. Neurologic disorders following surgery for peptic ulcer disease. Arch Neurol 1975; 32:206–207.
1111. Koerner D. Amyotrophic lateral sclerosis on Guam. Ann Intern Med 1952; 37:1204.
1112. Kohbata S, Beaman BL. L-dopa-responsive movement disorder caused by Nocardia asteroides localized in the brains of mice. Infect Immunol 1991; 59:181–191.
1113. Kohno M, Ohta S, Hirobe M. Tetrahydroisoquinoline and 1-methyl-tetrahydroisoquinoline as novel endogenous amines in rat brain. Biochem Biophys Res Commun 1986; 140(1):448–454.
1114. Koller W, O'Hara R, Weiner W, et al. Relationship of aging to Parkinson's disease. In: Yahr MD, Bergmann KJ, eds. Parkinson's disease—Advances in neurology, Vol 45. New York: Raven Press, 1986:317–321.
1115. Koller W, Vetere-Overfield B, Gray C, et al. Environmental risk factors in Parkinson's disease. Neurology 1990; 40:1218–1221.
1116. Koller WC. Essay on the shaking palsy: James Parkinson's description compared to current concepts. Neurology 1983; 33 (suppl II):150.
1117. Koller WC. Alcohol and Parkinson disease [letter]. Ann Neurol 1983; 13:467.
1118. Koller WC. The diagnosis of Parkinson's disease. Arch Intern Med 1984; 144:2146–2147.
1119. Koller WC. Sensory symptoms in Parkinson's disease. Neurology 1984; 34:957–959.
1120. Koller WC. Paraquat and Parkinson's disease [letter]. Neurology 1986; 36:1147.
1121. Koller WC. Paraquat and Parkinson's Disease: Reply from the Author (Letter). Neurology 1987; 37:728.
1122. Koller WC. How accurately can Parkinson's disease be diagnosed? Neurology 1992; 42 (suppl. 1):6–16.
1123. Koller WC. When does Parkinson's disease begin? Neurology 1992; 42(suppl 4):27–31.
1124. Koller WC, Busenbark K, Miner K, Essential Tremor Study group. The relationship of essential tremor to other movement disorders: Report on 678 patients. Ann Neurol 1994; (in press)
1125. Koller WC, Glatt S, Wilson R, Fox J. Motor signs are infrequent in dementia-Alzheimer type. Ann Neurol 1984; 16:514–516.
1126. Koller WC, Hubble JP. Classification of Parkinsonism. In: Koller WC, ed. Handbook of Parkinson's Disease. Marcel Dekker, 1992:59–104.

1127. Koller WC, Lang AE. Age of onset of Parkinson's disease [letter]. Can J Neurol Sci 1987; 14:179.
1128. Koller WC, Langston JW. Preclinical detection of Parkinson's disease. Neurology 1991; 41 (suppl. 2):1–92.
1129. Koller WC, Langston JW, Hubble JP, et al. Does A Long Pre-Clinical Period Occur in Parkinson's Disease? Neurology 1991; 41(5) (Suppl 2):8–13.
1130. Koller WC, O'Hara R, Nutt J, Young J, Rubino F. Monozygotic twins with Parkinson's disease. Ann Neurol 1986; 19:402–405.
1131. Koller WC, Rope SD, Huber SJ, Blumenthal DC, Blumenthal HJ. Metabolism of glucurolactone to glucarate in Parkinson's disease. Neurology 1992; 42:1807–1808.
1132. Koller WC, Trimble J. The gait abnormality of Huntington's disease. Neurology 1985; 35:1450–1455.
1133. Koller WC, Wong GF, Lang A. Post traumatic movement disorders: a review. Mov Disord 1989; 4:20–36.
1134. Kondo I, Kanazawa I. Debrisoquine hydroxylase and Parkinson's disease. In: Narabayashi H, Nagatsu T, Yanakisawa N, Mizuno Y, eds. Parkinson's disease: From basic research to treatment. Advances in Neurology, Vol.60. New York: Raven Press, 1993:338–342.
1135. Kondo I, Kanazawa I. Association of Xba I allele (Xba I 44kb) of the human cytochrome P-450dbI (CYP2D6) gene in Japanese patients with idiopathic Parkinson's disease. In: Yoshida M, Nagatsu T, Narabayashi H, eds. Key topics in brain research: Parkinson's disease. From clinical aspects to molecular basis. New York: Springer-Verlag, 1991:111–117.
1136. Kondo K. A genetic analysis of Parkinson's disease. Trans Am Neurol Assoc 1971; 96:261–262.
1137. Kondo K. Motor neuron disease: Changing population patterns and clues for etiology. In: Neurological epidemiology: Principles and clinical applications - Advances in Neurology, Vol 19. New York: Raven Press, 1978:509–543.
1138. Kondo K. Motor neuron disease and Parkinson's disease are not associated with other disorders in autopsy. Neuroepidemiology 1984; 3:182–194.
1139. Kondo K. Epidemiological clues for the etiology of Parkinson's disease. In: Hassler RG, Christ F, eds. Parkinson-specific motor and mental disorders, role of the pallidum: Pathophysiological, biochemical, and therapeutic aspects—Advances in neurology, Vol. 40. New York: Raven Press, 1984:345–351.
1140. Kondo K. Epidemiological evaluations of risk factors in Parkinson's disease. In: Yahr Md, Bergmann KJ, eds. Parkinson's disease—Advances in neurology, Vol 45. New York: Raven Press, 1986:289–293.
1141. Kondo K, Kurland LT, Schull WJ. Parkinson's disease. Genetic analysis and evidence of a multifactorial etiology. Mayo Clin Proc 1973; 48:465–475.
1142. Kondo K, Shibasaki H. Epidemiology of Parkinson's disease: clues for etiology. Excerpta Medica 1981; 548:233.
1143. Kondo K, Sobue I. Genetic and clinical patterns of heritable cerebellar ataxias in adults. I. Genetic analyses. J Med Genet 1980; 17:416–423.
1144. Kondo K, Watanabe K. Lifestyles, risk factors, and inherited predispositions in

Parkinson's disease. Preliminary report of a case-control study. In: Narabayashi H, Nagatsu T, Yanakisawa N, Mizuno Y, eds. Parkinson's disease. From basic research to treatment. Advances in Neurology, Vol. 60. New York: Raven Press, 1993:346–351.

1145. Konig H. Aus der kgl. psychiatrischen und Nervenklinik zu Kiel. Arch Psychiatr Nervenkr 1912; 50:285–305.

1146. Koningsmark B, Weiner J. The olivopontocerebellar atrophies. A review. Medicine 1970; 49:227–241.

1147. Konno H, Yamamoto T, Iwasaki Y, Iizuka H. Shy-Drager syndrome and amyotrophic lateral sclerosis. Cytoarchitectonic and morphometric studies of sacral autonomic neurons. J Neurol Sci 1986; 73(2):193–204.

1148. Kopin IJ. Toxins and Parkinson's Disease. VIII International Symposium on Parkinson's disease 1985; 11–10.

1149. Kopin IJ. Toxins and Parkinson's Disease: MPTP Parkinsonism in Humans and Animals. In: Parkinson's disease—Advances in neurology, Vol 45. New York: Raven Press, 1986:137–144.

1150. Kopin IJ. MPTP: An industrial chemical and contaminant of illicit narcotics. Environ Health Perspect 1987; 75:45–51.

1151. Kopin IJ, Burns RS, Chiueh CC, Markey SP. MPTP-induced parkinsonian syndromes in humans and animals. In: Fisher A, Hanin I, Lachman C, eds. Alzheimer's and Parkinson's Diseases: Strategies for Research and Development. 29th ed. New York and London: Plenum Press, 1986:519–530.

1152. Korten JJ, Ketterings K. [Anthropologic aspects of Parkinson's disease]. Nervenarzt 1972; 43:201–205.

1153. Korytowski W, Felix CC, Kalyanaraman B. Evidence for the one-electron oxidation of 1-methyl-4-phenyl-2,3-dihydropyridinium (MPDP+). Biochem Biophys Res Commun 1987; 147(1):354–360.

1154. Korytowski W, Hintz P, Sealy RC, Kalyanaraman B. Mechanism of dismutation of superoxide produced during auto-oxidation of melanin pigments. Biochem Biophys Res Commun 1985; 131:659–665.

1155. Kosaka K. Diffuse Lewy body disease in Japan. J Neurol 1990; 237:197–204.

1156. Kosaka K, Yoshimura M, Ikeda K, Budka H. Diffuse type of Lewy body disease: Progressive dementia with abundant cortical Lewy bodies and senile changes of varying degree—A new disease? Clinical Neuropathol 1984; 3:185–192.

1157. Kosower NS, Glaser T, Kosower EM. Membrane-motility agent-promoted fusion of erythrocytes: Fusibility is correlated with attack by calcium-activated cytoplasmic proteases on membrane proteins. Proc Natl Acad Sci 1983; 80:7542–7546.

1158. Kostic VS, Mojsilovi:c L, Stojanovi:c M. Degenerative neurological disorders associated with deficiency of glutamate dehydrogenase. J Neurol 1989; 236(2):111–114.

1159. Kostrzewa RM, Jacobowitz DM. Pharmacological actions of 6-hydroxydopamine. Pharmacol Rev 1974; 26:199–288.

1160. Krabbe K,H., Munch-Petersen CJ. Angioblastic meningioma with symptoms of Parkinsonism. Confin Neurol 1939; 2:312–319.

1161. Krauss JK, Mohadjer M, Wakhloo AK, Mundinger F. Dystonia and akinesia

due to pallidoputaminal lesions after disulfiram intoxication. Mov Disord 1991; 6:166–170.
1162. Kreiss P. Aus der inneren Abteilung des stadtischen St. Rochus-Krankenhauses Mainz (Oberarzt Dr. H. Curschmann). Z Nervenheilk 1912; 44:111–123.
1163. Krige D, Cooper JM, Schapira AHV. Platelet mitochondrial function in Parkinson's disease. Neurology 1992; 42 (Suppl 3):173.
1164. Kristensen M. Progressive supranuclear palsy—20 years later. Acta Neurol Scand 1985; 71:177–189.
1165. Krul JM, Wokke JH. Bilateral subdural hematoma presenting as subacute Parkinsonism. Clin Neurol Neurosurg 1987; 89:107–109.
1166. Kuhl DE, Metter EJ, Riege WH. Patterns of local cerebral glucose utilization determined in Parkinson's disease by the [18F] fluorodeoxyglucose method. Ann Neurol 1984; 15:419–424.
1167. Kume A, Takahashi A, Hashizume Y, Asai J. A histometrical and comparative study on Purkinje cell los and olivary nucleus cell loss in multiple system atrophy. J Neurol Sci 1991; 101(2):178–186.
1168. Kupsch A, Löschmann P-A, Sauer H, et al. Do NMDA receptor antagonists protect against MPTP-toxicty? Biochemical and immunocytochemical analyses in black mice. Brain Res 1992; 592:74–83.
1169. Kurihara T, Landau W, Torack R. Progressive supranuclear palsy with action myoclonus seizures. Neurology 1974; 24:219–223.
1170. Kurland AA. Genetic determinants of extrapyramidal motor effects from psychotropic drugs. In: Brill, ed. International Congress on Neuro-Psycho Pharm. 1990:616–618.
1171. Kurland LT, Hauser W, Okazaki H, Nobrega FT. Epidemiologic studies of parkinsonism with special reference to the cohort hypothesis. In: Gillingham FJ, Donaldson I, Fraser J, eds. Third Symposium on Parkinson's Disease. Edinburgh: F.S. Livingstone, 1969:12–17.
1172. Kurland LT. Epidemiology: Incidence, geographic distribution and genetic considerations. In: Field WS, ed. Pathogenesis and treatment of Parkinsonism. Springfield, Illinois: Charles C. Thomas, 1958:5–43.
1173. Kurland LT. An appraisal of epidemiologic and genetic developments in amyotrophic lateral sclerosis and Kuru. Proceedings of the 5th International Congress of Neuropathology 1966; 182–189.
1174. Kurland LT. An appraisal of the neurotoxicity of Cycad and the etiology of amyotrophic lateral sclerosis on Guam. Fed Proc 1972; 31:1540–1542.
1175. Kurland LT. Amyotrophic lateral sclerosis and Parkinson's disease complex on Guam linked to an environmental neurotoxin. TINS 1988; 11:51–54.
1176. Kurland LT, Brian DD. Contributions to neurology from records linkage in Olmsted County, Minnesota. In: Neurological epidemiology: Principles and clinical applications—Advances in Neurology, Vol 19. New York: Raven Press, 1978:93–105.
1177. Kurland LT, Hirano A, Malamud N, Lessell S. Parkinsonism-dementia complex, an endemic disease on the island of Guam. Clinical, pathological, genetic and epidemiological features. Trans Amer Neurol Asso 1961; 115–120.
1178. Kurland LT, Kurtzke JF, Goldberg ID, Choi NW, Williams G. Parkinsonism.

In: Epidemiology of Neurologic and Sense Organ Disorders. Cambridge: Harvard University Press, 1973:41–63.

1179. Kurland LT, Molgaard CA. Guamanian ALS: Hereditary or acquired? In: Roland LP, ed. Human Motor Neuron Disease. New York: Raven Press, 1982:165–177.

1180. Kurland LT, Mulder D. Epidemiologic investigations of amyotrophic lateral sclerosis. 2. Familial aggregations indicative of dominant inheritance. Neurology 1955; 5:182–196.

1181. Kurland LT, Mulder DW. Epidemiologic investigations of amyotrophic lateral sclerosis. I. Preliminary report on geographic distribution, with special reference to the Mariana Island, including clinical and pathologic observations. Neurology 1954; 4:355–378.

1182. Kurth JH, Kurth MC, Poduslo SE, Schwankhaus JD. Association of a monoamine oxidase B allele with Parkinson's disease. Ann Neurol 1993; 33(4):368–372.

1183. Kurth MC, Kurth JH. Variant cytochrome P450 CYP2D6 allelic frequencies in Parkinson's disease. Am J Med Genet 1993; 48:166–168.

1184. Kurtzke JF, Goldberg ID. Parkinsonism death rates by race, sex, and geography. Neurology 1988; 38:1558–1561.

1185. Kurtzke JF, Kurland LT. The epidemiology of neurologic disease. In: Baker AB, Baker LH, eds. Clinical Neurology. Philadelphia: Harper & Row, 1985:455–460.

1186. Kurtzke JF, Murphy FM. The changing patterns of death rates in parkinsonism. Neurology 1990; 40:42–49.

1187. Kwak S, Masaki T, Ishiura S, Sugita H. Multicatalytic proteinase is present in Lewy bodies and neurofibrillary tangles in diffuse Lewy body disease brain. Neurosci Lett 1991; 128:21–24.

1188. La Torre E, Forni C. [Parkinson's syndrome caused by meningioma of the sphenoid ala]. Riv Neurol 1968; 14:519–530.

1189. Laaksonen H, Riekkinen P, Rinne UK, Sonninen V. Brain glutamic acid decarboxylase and gamma-aminobutyric acid in Parkinson's disease. In: Birkmayer W, Hornykiewicz O, eds. Advances in Parkinsonism:Biochemistry, Physiology, Treatment. Stocholm: Roche, 1975:205–214.

1190. Ladero JM, Jimenez FJ, Benitze J, et al. Acetylator polymorphism in Parkinson's disease. Eur J Clin Pharmacol 1989; 37:391–393.

1191. Laing P, Knight J, Hill J, et al. Influenzaviruses induce autoantibodies to a brain-specific 37-kDa protein in rabbit. Proc Natl Acad Sci 1989; 86:1998–2002.

1192. Laitinen L. [Some views on the etiology of Parkinsonism]. Gerontology 1966; 18:24–29.

1193. Lampert PW, Hardman JM. Morphological changes in brains of boxers. JAMA 1984; 251:2676–2679.

1194. Lance J, Schwab R, Peterson E. Action tremor and the cogwheel phenomenon in PD. Brain 1963; 86:95–110.

1195. Lang A, Marsden C, Obeso J. Alcohol and Parkinson's disease. Ann Neurol 1982; 12:254–256.

1196. Lang A, Meadows J, Parkes J, Marsden C. Early onset of the "on-off" phenomenon in children with symptomatic parkinsonism. J Neurol Neurosurg Psychiatry 1982; 45:823–825.

1197. Lang AE. Genetics. In: Koller WC, ed. Handbook of Parkinson's Disease. New York: Marcel Dekker, Inc., 1987:81–97.
1198. Lang AE. Miscellaneous drug-induced movement disorders. In: Lang AE, Weiner WJ, eds. Drug-induced movement disorders. Mt Kisco: Futura, 1992:339–381.
1199. Lang AE, Blair RD. Parkinson's disease in 1984: An update. Can Med Assoc J 1984; 131:1031–1037.
1200. Lang AE, Garnett ES. Dopa-responsive parkinsonism with normal 6[18F]-fluorodopa positron emission tomography scans [letter]. Ann Neurol 1990; 28:592–593.
1201. Lang AE, Kierans C, Blair RD. Family history of tremor in Parkinson's disease compared with those of controls and patients. In: Parkinson's disease—Advances in neurology, Vol 45. New York: Raven Press, 1987:313–316.
1202. Langston JW. MPTP and Parkinson's disease. TINS 1985; 8:79–83.
1203. Langston JW. MPTP-Induced Parkinsonism: How good a model is it? In: Fahn S, Marsden CD, Teychenne PS, Jenner P, eds. Recent developments in Parkinson's disease. New York: Raven Press, 1986:119–126.
1204. Langston JW. Etiology. In: Koller WC, ed. Handbook of Parkinson's Disease. New York: Marcel Dekker, 1987:297–307.
1205. Langston JW. MPTP: Insights into the etiology of Parkinson's disease. Eur Neurol 1987; 26:2–10.
1206. Langston JW. Parkinson's disease: Current view. Am Fam Physician 1987; 35:201–206.
1207. Langston JW. Mechanisms underlying neuronal degeneration in Parkinson's disease: An experimental and theoretical treatise. Mov Disord 1989; 4:S15–S25.
1208. Langston JW. Current theories on the cause of Parkinson's disease. J Neurol Neurosurg Psychiatry 1989; 13–17.
1209. Langston JW. Predicting Parkinson's disease. Neurology 1990; 40(suppl):70–74.
1210. Langston JW. MPTP as it relates to the etiology of Parkinson's disease. In: Ellenberg JH, Koller WC, Langston JW, eds. Etiology of Parkinson's disease. New York: Marcel Dekker, 1994:367–399.
1211. Langston JW, Ballard PA. Parkinson's disease in a chemist working with 1-methl-4-phenyl- 1,2,5,6-tetrahydropyridine (MPTP). N Engl J Med 1983; 310.
1212. Langston JW, Ballard PA. Parkinsonism induced by 1-methyl-4-phenyl-1,2,5,6-tetrahydropyridine: Implications for treatment and the pathophysiology of Parkinson's disease. Can J Neurol Sci 1984; 11:160–165.
1213. Langston JW, Ballard PA, Tetrud JW, Irwin I. Chronic Parkinsonism in humans due to a product of meperidine-analog synthesis. Science 1983; 219:979–980.
1214. Langston JW, Forno LS, Rebert CS, Irwin I. Selective nigral toxicity after systemic administration of 1-methyl-4-phenyl-1,2,3,6-tetrahydropyridine (MPTP) in the squirrel monkey. Brain Res 1984; 292:390–394.
1215. Langston JW, Irwin I. MPTP: Current concepts and controversies. Clin Neuropharmacol 1986; 9:485–507.
1216. Langston JW, Irwin I, DeLanney LE. Factors that affect the expression of neurotoxicity: Lessons from MPTP. In: Rose FC, Norris FH, eds. ALS: New advances in toxicology and epidemiology. New York: Smith-Gordon, 1990:247–255.
1217. Langston JW, Irwin I, Forno LS, DeLanney LE. Parkinson's disease, aging,

and MPTP: Clinical and experimental observations. In: Fahn S, Marsden CD, Goldstein M, Calne DB, eds. Recent Developments in Parkinson's Disease. Florham Park, New Jersey: Macmillan Healthcare Information, 1987:59–74.

1218. Langston JW, Irwin I, Langston EB, DeLanney LE, Ricaurte GA. MPTP-induced parkinsonism in humans: A review of the syndrome and observations relating to the phenomenon of tardive toxicity. In: Markey SP, Castagnoli N, Jr., Trevor AJ, Kopin IJ, eds. MPTP: A neurotoxin producing a Parkinsonian syndrome. New York: Academic Press, 1986:9–21.

1219. Langston JW, Irwin I, Langston EB, Forno LS. 1-Methyl-4-phenyl-pyridinium ion (MPP+): Identification of a metabolite of MPTP, a toxin selective to the substantia nigra. Neurosci Lett 1984; 48:87–92.

1220. Langston JW, Irwin I, Langston EB, Forno LS. Pargyline prevents MPTP-induced parkinsonism in primates. Science 1984; 225:1480–1482.

1221. Langston JW, Irwin I, Ricaurte GA. Neurotoxins, parkinsonism, and Parkinson's disease. Pharmac Ther 1987; 32:19–46.

1222. Langston JW, Koller W. The next frontier in Parkinson's disease: Presymptomatic detection. Neurology 1991; 41(5) (Suppl 2):5–7.

1223. Langston JW, Tetrud JW. MPTP-induced parkinsonism in humans: New insights into Parkinson's disease. In: Kennard C, ed. Recent Advances in Clinical Neurology. London: Churchill Livingstone, 1988:153–173.

1224. Laplante M, Tran-Manh N. [Etiology and pathogenesis of idiopathic Parkinsonism: a model]. Agressologie 1973; 14:287–307.

1225. LaPresle J, Annabi A. Olivopontocerebellar atrophy with velopharyngolaryngeal paralysis: A contribution to the somatotopy of the nucleus ambiguous. J Neuropathol Exp Neurol 1979; 38:401–406.

1226. Laqueur G, Michelsen O, Whiting M, Kurland L. Carcinogenic properties of nuts from Cycas circinalis L. indigenous to Guam. J Natl Cancer Inst 1963; 31:919–933.

1227. Larsson T, Sjogren T. Essential tremor a clinical and genetic population study. Copenhagen: Ejnar Munksgaard, 1960.

1228. Lauterbach EC, Duvoisin RC. Anxiety disorders in familial parkinsonism [letter]. Am J Psychiatry 1991; 148:274.

1229. Lauterburg BH, Smith CV, Hughes H, Mitchell JR. Determinants of hepatic glutathione turnover: Toxicological significance. TIPS 1982; 3:245–248.

1230. Lavoie B, Parent A. Immunohistochemical study of the serotoninergic innervation of the basal ganglia in the squirrel monkey. J Comp Neurol 1990; 299:1–16.

1231. Lazzarini AM, Zimmerman TR, Mark MH, et al. Genetic studies in Parkinson disease multicase families. Neurology 1994; (in press)

1232. Lazzarini AM, Myers RH, Zimmerman TR, Jr., et al. A clinical genetic study of Parkinson's disease: Evidence for dominant transmission. Neurology 1994; 44:499–506.

1233. Lee CS, Snow BJ, Takahashi H, Calne DB. Progression of PET asymmetry in idiopathic Parkinsonism. Neurology 1992; 42, (Suppl 3):296.

1234. Leenders KL, Antonini A, Schwartz J, Oertel WH, Hess K, Weinddle A. Striatal dopamine D2-Receptors in 'De Novo' Parkinsonian patients measured using PET and [11C] Raclopride. Neurology 1992; 42, Suppl 3:295–296.

1235. Leenders KL, Salmon EP, Tyrrell P, et al. The nigrostriatal dopaminergic system assessed in vivo by positron emission tomography in healthy volunteer subjects and patients with Parkinson's disease. Arch Neurol 1990; 47:1290–1298.

1236. Lees AJ. Early diagnosis of Parkinson's disease. Br J Hosp Med 1981; 26:511–512, 517–518.

1237. Leheny WA, Davidson DL, deVane P, House AO, Lenman JA. HLA antigens in Parkinson's disease. Tissue Antigens 1983; 21:260–261.

1238. Lehninger AL. Biochemistry. 2nd ed. New York: Worth Publishers, 1975:

1239. Leibowitz U, Feldman S. Age shift in parkinsonism. Isr J Med Sci 1973; 9:599–602.

1240. Leigh AD. Infection of the nervous system occuring during an epidemic of influenza B. Br Med J 1946; ii:937–939.

1241. Lennox G, Lowe J, Landon M, Byrne EJ, Mayer RJ, Godwin-Austen RB. Diffuse Lewy body disease: Correlative neuropathology using anti-ubiquitin immunocytochemistry. J Neurol Neurosurg Psychiatry 1989; 52:1236–1247.

1242. Lennox G, Lowe J, Morrell K, Landon M, Mayer RJ. Anti-ubiquitin immunocytochemistry is more sensitive than conventional techniques in the detection of diffuse Lewy body disease. J Neurol Neurosurg Psychiatry 1989; 52:67–71.

1243. Leonhard D. Lange intervalle zwischen akuter encephalitis epidemica und dem parkinsonistischen folegezustand. Nervenarzt 1937; 10:568–572.

1244. Lepore FE, Steele JC, Cox TA, et al. Supranuclear disturbances of ocular motility in Lytico-Bodig. Neurology 1988; 38:1849–1853.

1245. Lerner MR, Goldman RS. Skin colour, MPTP, and Parkinson's disease. Lancet 1987; 1:212.

1246. Lesser RP, Fahn S, Snider SR, Cote LJ, Isgreen WP, Barrett RE. Analysis of the clinical problems in parkinsonism and the complications of long-term therapy. Neurology 1979; 29:1253–1260.

1247. Lestienne P, Nelson I, Riederer P, Reichmann H, Jellinger K. Mitochondrial DNA in postmortem brain from patients with Parkinson's disease. J Neurochem 1991; 56:1819.

1248. Lestienne P, Nelson J, Riederer P, Jellinger K, Reichmann H. Normal mitochondrial genome in brain from patients with Parkinson's disease and complex I defect. J Neurochem 1990; 55:1810–1812.

1249. Levaditi C. Etiology of epidemic enchephalitis its relation to herpes, epidemic poliomyelitis and post-vaccinal encephalopathy. Arch Neurol Psychiatry 1929; 22:767–803.

1250. Levaditi C, Harvier P. Recherches experimentales dur lencephalite epidemique. Comptes Rendus des Scances 1921; 84:388–390.

1251. Leverenz J, Sumi SM. Parkinson's disease in patients with Alzheimer's disease. Arch Neurol 1986; 43:662–664.

1252. Levin BE, Llabre MM, Ansley J, Weiner WJ, Sanchez-Ramos J. Do parkinsonians exhibit visuospatial deficits. In: Parkinson's disease: anatomy, pathology and therapy—Advances in neurology, Vol 53. New York: Raven Press, 1990:311–315.

1253. Levin BE, Llabre MM, Reisman S, et al. Visuospatial impairment in Parkinson's disease. Neurology 1991; 41:365–369.

1254. Levine RL, Jones JC, Bee N. Stroke and Parkinson's disease. Stroke 1992; 23(6):839–842.

1255. Levitt P, Pintar JE, Breakefield XO. Immunocytochemical demonstration of monoamine oxidase B in brain astrocytes and serotonergic neurons. Proc Natl Acad Sci 1982; 79:6385–6389.

1256. Lewin R. Trail of ironies to Parkinson's disease [news]. Science 1984; 224:1083–1085.

1257. Lewin R. Parkinson's disease: An environmental cause. Science 1985; 229:257–258.

1258. Lewin R. Metabolic profile of a neurotoxin. Science 1986; 5 December: 1201.

1259. Lewin R. Age factors loom in parkinsonian research [news]. Science 1986; 234:1200–1201.

1260. Lewin R. Environmental hypothesis for brain diseases strengthened by new data. Science 1987; 483–484.

1261. Lewin R. More clues to the cause of Parkinson's disease [news]. Science 1987; 237:978.

1262. Lewin R. Big first scored with nerve diseases. Science 1989; 245:467.

1263. LeWitt PA, Martin SD. Dystonia and hyperkinesis with putaminal necrosis after methanol intoxication. Clin Neuropharmacol 1988; 11:161–167.

1264. Lewy FH. Paralysis agitans. I Pathologische Anatomie. In: Lewandowsky M, ed. Handbuch der Neurologie. Berlin: Springer-Verlag, 1912:920–933.

1265. Lewy FH. Psychische Storungen. Monogr Neurol Psychiat 1922; 34:32–40.

1266. Lewy FH. Die Lehre vom Tonus und der Bewegung. Berlin: Springer-Verlag, 1923.

1267. Lewy FH. Diagnosis and differential diagnosis of CS2 intoxication. In: Bashore RM, Staley AL, eds. Survey of carbon disulphide and hydrogen sulphide hazards in the viscose rayon industry. Bulletin #46. Harrisburg: Commonwealth of Pennsylvania, Dept. of Labor and Industry, 1938:52–53.

1268. Lewy FH. Survey of carbon disulphide and hydrogen sulphide hazards in the viscose rayon industry. Bulletin #46. In: Bashore RM, Staley AL, eds. Neurological aspects of CS2 intoxication. Harrisburg: Commonwealth of Pennsylvania, Dept. of Labor and Industry, 1938:31–37.

1269. Li Sc, Schoenberg BS, Wang CC, et al. A prevalence survey of Parkinson's disease and other movement disorders in the People's Republic of China. Arch Neurol 1985; 42:655–657.

1270. Li TM, Swash M, Alberman E. Morbidity and mortality in motor neuron disease: Comparison with multiple and sclerosis and Parkinson's disease: Age and sex specific rates and cohort analyses. J Neurol Neurosurg Psychiatry 1985; 48:320–327.

1271. Liang YO, Plotsky PM, Adams RN. Isolation and identification of an in vivo reaction product of 6-hydroxydopamine. J Med Chem 1977; 20(4):581–583.

1272. Lichter D, Kurlan R, Miller C, Shoulson I. Does pergolide slow the progression of Parkinson's disease? A 7-year follow-up study. Neurology 1988; 38: 122. (abstract)

1273. Lidy C, Priollet P, Pepin B. Syndrome pyramidal et extra-pyramidal apparu au d'ecours d'une intoxication aiguee par le disulfiram. Nouv Presse Med 1979; 8:3561.

1274. Lieberman A, Dziatolowski M, Kupersmith M. Dementia in Parkinson's disease. Ann Neurol 1979; 6:355–359.
1275. Lieberman A, Goldstein M. Reversible parkinsonism related to meperidine. N Engl J Med 1985; 8:509.
1276. Lilienfeld DE, Chan E, Ehland J, et al. Two decades of increasing mortality from Parkinson's disease among the US elderly. Arch Neurol 1990; 47:731–734.
1277. Lilienfeld DE, Sprafka JM, Pham D-L, Baxter J. Parkinson's and motoneuron disease morbidity in the Twin Cities metropolitan area: 1979–1984. Neuroepidemiology 1991; 10:112–116.
1278. Lilienfeld DE, Sekkor D, Simpson S, et al. Parkinsonism death rates by race, sex and geography: A 1980s update. Neuroepidemiology 1990; 9:243–247.
1279. Lima B, Neves G, Nora M. Juvenile Parkinsonism: Clinical and methobolic characteristics. J Neurol Neurosurg Psychiatry 1987; 5-:345–348.
1280. Lindenberg R. Die Schadigungsmechanismen der Substantia nigra bei Hirntraumen und das Problem des posttraumatischen Parkinsonismus. Dtsch Z Nervenheilk 1964; 185:637–663.
1281. Lindquist NG, Larsson BS, Lyden-Sokolowski A. Neuromelanin and its possible protective and destructive properties. Pigment Cell Res 1987; 1:133–136.
1282. Lindquist NG, Larsson BS, Lyden-Sokolowski A. Autoradiography of [14C]paraquat or [14C]diquat in frogs and mice: accumulation in neuromelanin. Neurosci Lett 1988; 93:1–6.
1283. Lindquist NG, Lyden-Sokolowski A, Larsson BS. Accumulation of a parkinsonism-inducing neurotoxin in melanin-bearing neurons: Autoradiographic studies on 3H-MPTP. Acta Pharmacol Toxicol 1986; 59:161–164.
1284. Linnane AW, Marzuki S, Ozawa T, Tanaka M. Mitochondrial DNA mutations as an important contributor to ageing and degenerative diseases. Lancet 1989; 1:642–645.
1285. Lipczynska-Lojkowska W. [Etiology of parkinsonism. A verification of Poskanzer's and Schwab's hypothesis]. Neurol Neurochir Pol 1979; 13:593–599.
1286. Lippke KP, Schunack WG, Wenning W, Muller WE. Beta-carbolines as benzodiazepine receptor ligands. 1. Synthesis and benzodiazepine receptor interaction of esters of beta-carboline-3-carboxylic acid. J Med Chem 1983; 26:499–503.
1287. Lohr JB. Oxygen radicals and neuropsychiatric illness. Some speculations. Arch Gen Psychiatry 1991; 48:1097–1106.
1288. Lombard A, Gelfand M. Parkinson's disease in the African. Cent Afr J Med 1978; 24:5–8.
1289. Loranger AW, Goodell H, McDowell FH, Lee JE, Sweet RD. Intellectual impairment in Parkinson's syndrome. Brain 1972; 95:405–412.
1290. Lou J-S, Jankovic J. Essential tremor: Clinical correlates in 350 patients. Neurology 1991; 41:234–238.
1291. Lowe J, McDermott H, Landon M, Mayer J, Wilkinson KD. Ubiquitin carboxyl-terminal hydrolase (PGP 9.5) is selectively present in ubiquitinated inclusion bodies characteristic of human neurodegenerative diseases. J Pathol 1992; 161:153–160.
1292. Ludin SM, Ludin HP. Is Parkinson's disease of early onset a separate disease entity. J Neurol 1989; 236:203–207.
1293. Ludolph AC, He F, Spencer PS, Hammerstad J, Sabri MI. 3-Nitropropionic

acid - exogenous animal neurotoxin and possible human striatal toxin. Can J Neurol Sci 1991; 18:492–498.

1294. Ludolph AC, Seelig M, Ludolph A, et al. 3-Nitropropionic acid decreases cellular energy levels and causes neuronal degeneration in cortical explants. Neurodegeneration 1992; 1:155–161.

1295. Lutz E. Acute lithium-induced parkinsonism precipitated by liquid protein diet. J Med Soc MJ 1978; 75:165–166.

1296. Lux WE, Kurtzke JF. Is Parkinson's disease acquired? Evidence from a geographic comparison with multiple sclerosis. Neurology 1987; 37:467–471.

1297. Lycke E, Modigh K, Roos B. The monoamine metabolism in viral encephalitides of the mouse. I. Virological and biochemical results. Brain Res 1970; 23:235–246.

1298. Lycke E, Roos B. Some virological and biochemical aspects of the pathogenesis of Parkinson's disease. In: Gillingham: JFGillingham F, Donaldson I, eds. In Third Symposium of Parkinson's. Edinburgh/Livingston: 1969:16–19.

1299. Lycke E, Roos B. The monoamine metabolism in viral encephalitides of he mouse. II. Turn over of monoamines in mice infected with herpes simplex virus. Brain Res 1991; 44:603–613.

1300. Lyden A, Bondesson U, Larsson BS, Lindquist NG. Melanin affinity of 1-methyl-4-phenyl-1,2,3,6-tetrahydropyridine, and inducer of chronic parkinsonism in humans. Acta Pharmacol 1983; 53:429–432.

1301. Machetanz E. Postencephalitischer Parkinsonismus mit bickkrampfen im kindesalter. Zeitschrift fur Kinderheilkunde, 1958; 81:555–566.

1302. Mackay AVP, Iversen LL, Rossor M. Increased brain dopamine and dopamine receptors in schizophrenia. Arch Gen Psychiatry 1982; 39:991–997.

1303. Maher E, Lees A. The clinical features and natural history of the Steele-Richardson-Olszewski syndrome (progressive supranuclear palsy). Neurology 1986; 36:1005–1008.

1304. Mahgoub A, Dring LG, Idle JR, Lancaster R, Smith RL. Polymorphic hydroxylation of debrisoquine in man. Lancet 1977; 584–586.

1305. Maier HW. Uber traumatischen Parkinsonismus. Klin Wschr 1827; 5:1827–1830.

1306. Maki T, Sonoda Y, Sugita K. [Plasma atrial natriuretic peptide (ANP) levels in Parkinson's disease—with special reference to foot edema]. Rinsho Shinkeigaku 1990; 30:605–609.

1307. Makino Y, Ohta S, Tachikawa O, Hirobe M. Presence of tetrahydroisoquinoline and 1-methyl-tetrahydro-isoquinoline in foods: compounds related to Parkinson's disease. Life Sci 1988; 43:373–378.

1308. Makino Y, Tasaki Y, Kashiwasake M, Tachikawa O, Ohta S, Hirobe M. Formation of a novel and neurotoxic tetrahydrisoquinoline derivative, 1,3-dimethyltetrahydroisoquinoline (1,3DiMeTIQ). A condensation product of amphetamines and acetaldehyde in vivo. In: Nagatsu T, Fisher A, Yoshida M, eds. Basic, clinical, and therapeutic aspects of Alzheimer's and Parkinson's diseases. New York: Plenum Press, 1990:325–328.

1309. Makino Y, Tasaki Y, Ohta S, Hirobe M. Confirmation of the enantiomers of 1-methyl-1,2,3,4-tetrahydroisoquinoline in the mouse brain and foods applying gas chromatography/mass spectrometry with negative ion chemical ionization. Biomed Environ Mass Spectrom 1990; 19:415–419.

1310. Makishita H, Inoue K, Kagaya H, Yanagisawa N, Tsukagoshi H. [Familial juvenile parkinsonism with retinitis pigmentosa and vitiligo (author's transl)]. Rinsho Shinkeigaku 1978; 18:143–148.
1311. Makowiec RL, Abin RL, Cha JH, Young AB, Gilman S. Two types of quisqualate receptors are decreased in human olivopontocerebellar atrophy cerebellar cortex. Brain Res 1990; 523 (2):309–312.
1312. Mallie AH. Psychological problems among Parkinson's disease patients. These de Bordeaux 1908;
1313. Man'kovskii NB, Vainshtok AB, Litovchenko SV. [Experimental psychological research in parkinsonism]. Zh Nevropatol Psikhiatr 1974; 74:355–360.
1314. Mann DMA. Dopamine neurones of the vertebrate brain: Some aspects of anatomy and pathology. In: Winlow W, Markstein R, eds. The neurobiology of dopamine systems. Manchester: Manchester University Press, 1984:87–103.
1315. Mann DMA, Yates PO. Lipoprotein pigments—their relationship to ageing in the human nervous sytem—II. The melanin content of pigmented nerve cells. Brain 1974; 97:489–498.
1316. Mann DMA, Yates PO. Pathogenesis of Parkinson's disease. Arch Neurol 1982; 39:545–549.
1317. Mann DMA, Yates PO. Possible role of neuromelanin in the pathogenesis of Parkinson's disease. Mech Age Dev 1983; 21:193–203.
1318. Mann DMA, Yates PO. Pathological basis for neurotransmitter changes in Parkinson's disease. Neuroipathol Appl Neurobiol 1983; 8:3–19.
1319. Mann DMA, Yates PO, Barton CM. Neuromelanin and RNA in cells of substantia nigra. J Neuropathol Exp Neurol 1977; 36:379–383.
1320. Mann DMA, Yates PO, Davies JS, Hawkes J. Viruses, Parkinsonism and Alzheimer's disease [letter]. J Neurol Neurosurg Psychiatry 1981; 44:651.
1321. Mann VM, Cooper JM, Krige D, Daniel SE, Schapira AHV, Marsden CD. Brain, skeletal muscle and platelet homogenate mitochondrial function in Parkinson's disease. Brain 1992; 115:333–342.
1322. Mann VM, Cooper JM, Schapira AHV. Quantitation of a mitochondrial DNA deletion in Parkinson's disease. FEBS lett 1992; 299 (3):218–222.
1323. Manyam BV, Giacobini E, Colliver JA. Cerebrospinal fluid choline levels are decreased in Parkinson's disease. Ann Neurol 1990; 27:683–685.
1324. Maraganore D, Harding A, Marsden C. A clinical and genetic study of familial Parkinson's disease. Mov Disord 1991; 6:205–211.
1325. Marder K, Leary D, Tang M. Are demented patients with Parkinson's disease accurately reflected in prevalence surveys? A survival analysis. Neurology 1991; 41:1240–1243.
1326. Marder K, Flood P, Cote L, Mayeux R. A pilot study of risk factors for dementia in Parkinson's disease. Mov Disord 1990; 5:156–161.
1327. Marder K, Mayeux R. The epidemiology of dementia in patients with Parkinson's disease. Adv Exp Med Biol 1991; 295:439–445.
1328. Marek GJ, Vosmer G, Seiden LS. Pargyline increases 6-hydroxydopamine levels in the neostriatum of methamphetamine-treated rats. Pharmacol Biochem Behavior 1990; 36:187–190.
1329. Marek GJ, Vosmer G, Seiden LS. The effects of monoamine uptake inhibitors and methamphetamine on neostriatal 6-hydroxydopamine (6-OHDA) formation,

short-term monoamine depletions and locomotor activity in the rat. Brain Res 1990; 516:1–7.

1330. Maret G, Testa B, Jenner P, el Tayar N, Carrupt PA. The MPTP story: MAO activates tetrahydropyridine derivatives to toxins causing parkinsonism. Drug Metab Rev 1990; 22:291–332.

1331. Margulies ME. Parkinsonism and brain tumor. Arch Neurol Psychiatry 1953; 70:112–113.

1332. Marino A. [Parkinsonian and neurodysleptic syndromes during treatment with neuroleptic drugs]. Riv Sper Freniatr 1965; 89:892–926.

1333. Mark M. Personal communication, 1992.

1334. Mark MH, Burn DJ, Playford ED, et al. Parkinson's disease and twins: An F-Dopa PET study. Neurology 1991; 41(suppl 1):255.

1335. Mark MH, Dickson DW. The spectrum of Lewy body disease. Ann Clin Lab Sci 1992; 22:270.

1336. Mark MH, Dickson DW, Schwarz KO. Familial diffuse Lewy body disease. Tenth International Symposium on Parkinson's disease 1991; 56.

1337. Markey SP, Johannessen JN, Chiueh CC, Burns RS, Herkenham MA. Intraneuronal generation of a pyridinium metabolite may cause drug-induced parkinsonism. Nature 1984; 311:464–467.

1338. Markham CH, Diamond SG. Long-term follow-up of early dopa treatment in Parkinson's disease. Ann Neurol 1986; 19:365–372.

1339. Markham CH, Treciokas LJ, Diamond SG. Parkinson's disease and levodopa. A five-year follow-up and review. Western J Med 1974; 121:188–206.

1340. Marmot M. Mortality and Parkinson's disease. In: Rose FC, Capildeo R, eds. Research progress in Parkinson's disease. Kent: Tunbridge Wells, 1981:9–16.

1341. Marsden C, Tarsy D, Baldessarini RJ. Spontaneous and drug-induced movement disorders. In: Benson D, Blumer D, eds. Psychiatric aspects of neurologic disease. New York: Grune & Stratton, 1975:219–266.

1342. Marsden CD. Basal ganglia disease. Lancet 1982; 2:1141–1147.

1343. Marsden CD. Neuromelanin and Parkinson's disease. J Neural Transm Suppl 1983; 19:121-141.

1344. Marsden CD. Homen lecture. The cause of Parkinson's disease. UNKNOWN 1986; 9-17.

1345. Marsden CD. Parkinson's disease in twins [letter]. J Neurol Neurosurg Psychiatry 1987; 50:105–106.

1346. Marsden CD, Jenner PG. The Significance of 1-Methyl-4-Phenyl-1,2,3,6-Tetrahydropyridine. Ciba Found Symp 1987; 126:239–256.

1347. Marsden CD, Sandler M. The MPTP Story: An Introduction. J Neural Transm 1986; 1–3.

1348. Marshall J. Observations on essential tremor. J Neurol Neurosurg Psychiatry 1962; 25:122–125.

1349. Martin W. Parkinson's disease: Positron emission tomographic studies. Semin Neurol 1991; 9, (4):345–350.

1350. Martin WE, Loewenson RB, Resch JA, Baker AB. Parkinson's disease. Clinical analysis of 100 patients. Neurology 1973; 23:783–790.

1351. Martin WE, Resch JA, Baker AB. Juvenile parkinsonism. Arch Neurol 1971; 25:494–500.

1352. Martin WE, Young WI, Anderson VE. Parkinson's disease. A genetic study. Brain 1973; 96:495–506.
1353. Martin WRW. Parkinson's disease and aging: Presynaptic nigrostriatal function. In: Martin WRW, ed. Functional imaging in movement disorders. Boca Raton: CRC Press, 1990:103–113.
1354. Martin WRW, Palmer MR, Patlak CS, Calne DB. Nigrostriatal function in humans studied with positron emission tomography. Ann Neurol 1989; 26:535–542.
1355. Martin WRW, Stoessel AJ, Adam MJ, et al. Imaging of dopamine systems in human subjects exposed to MPTP. In: Markey SP, Castagnoli N, Jr., Trevor AJ, Kopin IJ, eds. MPTP: A neurotoxin producing a Parkinsonian syndrome. New York: Academic Press, 1986:315–325.
1356. Martinelli P, Gabellini AS, Gulli MR, Lugaresi E. Different clinical features of essential tremor: A 200 patient study. Acta Neurol Scand 1987; 75:106–111.
1357. Martinelli P, Gabellini AS, Martinelli A, Contin M. Gardening and Young Onset Parkinson Disease. Ital J Neurol Sci 1989; 10:465–466.
1358. Martinez A, Utterback R. Unilateral Parkinson's disease, clinical and neuropathologic findings. A case report. Neurology 1973; 23 (February):164–170.
1359. Martinovits G, Melamed E, Cohen O, Rosenthal J, Uzzan A. Systemic administration of antioxidants does not protect mice against the dopaminergic neurotoxicity of 1-methyl-4-phenyl-1,2,3, 6-tetrahydropyridine (MPTP). Neurosci Lett 1986; 69:192–197.
1360. Martland HS. Punch drunk. JAMA 1928; 91:1103–1107.
1361. Marttila RJ, Rinne UK, Halonen PE, Madden DL, Sever JL. Herpesviruses and parkinsonism. Arch Neurol 1981; 38:19–21.
1362. Marttila RJ. Poliomyelitis and arteriosclerosis in the etiology of Parkinson's disease [letter]. N Engl J Med 1978; 299:313.
1363. Marttila RJ. Epidemiology. In: Koller WC, ed. Handbook of Parkinson's disease. New York: Marcel Dekker, 1992:35–57.
1364. Marttila RJ, Arstila P, Nikoskelainen J, Halonen PE, Rinne UK. Viral antibodies in the sera from patients with Parkinson's disease. Eur Neurol 1977; 15:25–33.
1365. Marttila RJ, Halonen P, Rinne UK. Influenza virus antibodies in parkinsonism. Arch Neurol 1977; 34:99–100.
1366. Marttila RJ, Kalimo KOK, Ziola BR, Halonen PE, Rinne UK. Herpes simplex virus subunit antibodies in patients with Parkinson's disease. Arch Neurol 1978; 35:668–671.
1367. Marttila RJ, Kaprio J, Koskenvuo M, Rinne. Finnish Parkinson's disease twin study: Preliminary results. Upsala J Med Sci 1986; 43(suppl):93.
1368. Marttila RJ, Kaprio J, Koskenvuo M, Rinne UK. Parkinson's disease in a nationwide twin cohort. Neurology 1988; 38:1217–1219.
1369. Marttila RJ, Lorentz H, Rinne UK. Oxygen toxicity protecting enzymes in Parkinson's disease: Increase of superoxide dismutase-like activity in the substantia nigra and basal nucleus. J Neurol Sci 1988; 86:321–331.
1370. Marttila RJ, Rautakorpi I, Rinne UK. The relation of essential tremor to Parkinson's disease. J Neurol Neurosurg Psychiatry 1984; 47:734–735.
1371. Marttila RJ, Rinne U. Epidemiology of Parkinson's disease in Finland. Acta Neurol Scand 1976; 53:81–102.
1372. Marttila RJ, Rinne U, Tiilikainen A. Virus antibodies in Parkinson's disease.

Herpes simplex and measles virus antibodies in serum and CSF and their relation to HLA types. J Neuro Sci 1982; 54:227–238.

1373. Marttila RJ, Rinne UK. Arteriosclerosis, heredity, and some previous infections in the etiology of Parkinson's disease. A case-control study. Clin Neurol Neurosurg 1976; 79:46–56.

1374. Marttila RJ, Rinne UK. Dementia in Parkinson's disease. Acta Neurol Scand 1976; 54:431–441.

1375. Marttila RJ, Rinne UK. Level of blood pressure in patients with Parkinson's disease. Eur Neurol 1977; 16:73–78.

1376. Marttila RJ, Rinne UK. Disability and progression in Parkinson's disease. Acta Neurol Scand 1977; 56:159–169.

1377. Marttila RJ, Rinne UK. Herpes simplex virus antibodies in patients with Parkinson's disease. J Neurol Sci 1978; 35:375–379.

1378. Marttila RJ, Rinne UK. Smoking and Parkinson's disease. Acta Neurol Scand 1980; 62:322–325.

1379. Marttila RJ, Rinne UK. Epidemiology of Parkinson's disease—an overview. J Neural Transm 1981; 51:135–148.

1380. Marttila RJ, Rinne UK. Clues from epidemiology of Parkinson's disease. In: Parkinson's disease—Advances in Neurology, Vol 45. New York: Raven Press, 1987:285–288.

1381. Marttila RJ, Rinne UK. Parkinson's disease and essential tremor in families of patients with early-onset Parkinson's disease. J Neurol Neurosurg Psychiatry 1988; 51:429–431.

1382. Marttila RJ, Rinne UK. Epidemiological approaches to the etiology of Parkinson's disease. Acta Neurol Scand 1989; 126:13–18.

1383. Marttila RJ, Rinne UK. Progression and survival in Parkinson's disease. Acta Neurol Scand 1991; 84 (suppl 136):24–28.

1384. Marttila RJ, Rinne UK, Siirtola T, Sonninen V. Mortality of patients with Parkinson's disease treated with Levodopa. J Neurol 1977; 216:147–153.

1385. Marttila RJ, Viljanen M, Toivonen E, Lorentz H, Rinne UK. Superoxide dismutase-like activity in the Parkinson's disease brain. In: Parkinson's disease: Anatomy, pathology and therapy—Advances in Neurology, Vol 53. New York: Raven Press, 1990:141–144.

1386. Mash DC, Pablo J, Buck BE, Sanchez-Ramos J, Weiner WJ. Distribution and number of transferrin receptors in Parkinson's disease and in MPTP-treated mice. Exp Neurol 1991; 114:73–81.

1387. Mastaglia F, Grainger K, Kee F, Sadka M, Lefroy R. Progressive supranuclear palsy: The Steele-Richardson-Olszewski syndrome: Clinical and electrophysiological observations in eleven cases. Proc Aust Assoc Neurol 1973; 10:35–44.

1388. Mathai KV. Amyotrophic lateral sclerosis and parkinsonism dementia in the Marianas. Am J Trop Med Hyg 1970; 19:151–154.

1389. Matsumoto H. Cycasin. In: Rechcigl M, ed. CRC Handbook of naturally occurring food toxicants. Boca Raton: CRC Press, 1985:45–61.

1390. Mattock CH, Marmot M, Stern G. Could Parkinson's disease follow intra-uterine influenza? A speculative hypothesis. J Neurol Neurosurg Psychiatry 1988; 51:753–756.

1391. Mattock GL. Reactions of adrenochrome with some thiols. Arch Biochem Biophys 1967; 120:170–174.
1392. Mattock GL, Heacock RA. The chemistry of aminochromes. VI. The reaction of adrenochrome with glutathione. Can J Chem 1965; 43:119–125.
1393. Matuso F, Cummins JW, Anderson RE. Neurological sequelae of massive hydrogen sulfide inhalation. Arch Neurol 1979; 36:451.
1394. Mauri JA, Asensio M, Jimenez A, Huerta JR, Redondo MJ, del Villar V. [Familial Parkinson disease]. Neurologia 1990; 5:45–47.
1395. Maurizi CP. Why was the 1918 influenza pandemic so lethal? The possible role of a neurovirulent neuraminidase. Med Hypotheses 1985; 16:1–5.
1396. Maurizi CP. Was a neurovirulent influenza virus the cause of amyotrophic lateral sclerosis and parkinsonism-dementia on Guam. Med Hypotheses 1987; 23:325–326.
1397. Mavridis M, Degryse A-D, Lategan AJ, Marien MR, Colpaert FC. Effects of locus coeruleus lesions on parkinsonian signs, striatal dopamine and substantia nigra cell loss after 1-methyl-4-phenyl-1,2,3,6-tetrahydropyridine in monkeys: A possible role for the locus coeruleus in the progression of Parkinson's disease. Neuroscience 1991; 41:507–523.
1398. Mawdsley C, Manc MB, Ferguson FR. Neurological disease in boxers. Lancet 1963; 2:795–801.
1399. May T, Rommelspacher H, Pawlik M. [3H]Harman binding experiments. I: A reversible and selective radioligand for monoamine oxidase subtype A in the CNS of the rat. J Neurochem 1991; 56:490–499.
1400. Mayer JM, Mikol J, Haguenau M, Dellanave J, Pepin B. Familial juvenile parkinsonism with multiple systems degenerations: A clinicopathological study. J Neurol Sci 1986; 72:91–101.
1401. Mayer RA, Jarvis MF, Wagner GC. Cocaine blocks the dopamine depletion induced by MPTP. Res Commun Chem Pathol Pharmacol 1985; 49:145–148.
1402. Mayer RA, Kindt MV, Heikkila RE. Prevention of the nigrostriatal toxicity of 1-methyl-4-phenyl-1,2,3,6-tetrahydropyridine by inhibitors of 3,4-dihydroxyphenylethylamine transport. J Neurochem 1986; 47:1073–1079.
1403. Mayer RJ, Lowe J, Lennox G, Landon M, MacLennan K, Doherty FJ. Intermediate filament-Ubiquitin diseases: Implications for cell sanitization. Biochem Soc Symp 1989; 193–201.
1404. Mayeux R, Denaro J, Hemenegildo N, Marder K. A population-based investigation of Parkinson's disease with and without dementia. Relationship to age and gender. Arch Neurol 1992; 49(5):492–497.
1405. Mayeux R, Sano M, Chen J, Tatemichi T, Stern Y. Risk of dementia in first-degree relatives of patients with Alzheimer's disease and related disorders. Arch Neurol 1991; 48:269–273.
1406. Mayeux R, Stern Y, Rosen J, Leventhal J. Depression, intellectual impairment, and Parkinson disease. Neurology 1981; 31:645–650.
1407. Mayeux R, Stern Y, Rosenstein R, et al. An estimate of the prevalence of dementia in idiopathic Parkinson's disease. Arch Neurol 1988; 45:260–262.
1408. Mayeux R, Stern Y, Spanton S. Heterogeneity in dementia of the Alzheimer type: Evidence of subgroups. Neurology 1985; 35:453–461.

1409. Mayeux R, Tang MX, Marder K, Côtè LJ, Stern Y. Smoking and Parkinson's disease. Mov Disord 1994; 9(2):207–212.
1410. Mazza S, Laudisio A, Bergonzi P. Occult normal pressure hydrocephalus with parkinsonian symptomatology. Eur Neurol 1976; 14:39–42.
1411. McBrien DCH, Slater TF. Free radicals, lipid peroxidation and cancer. London: Academic Press, 1982:
1412. McClelland H. Discussion on assessment of drug-induced extrapyramidal reactions. Br J Clin Pharmacol 1976; 3:401–403.
1413. McConkey DJ, Hartzell P, Duddy SK, Hakansson H, Orrenius S. 2,3,7,8-tetrachlorodibenzo-p-dioxin kills immature thymocytes by Ca2+-mediated endonuclease activation. Science 1988; 242:256–259.
1414. McConkey DJ, Hartzell P, Nicotera P, Orrenius S. Calcium-activated DNA fragmentation kills immature thymocytes. FASEB J 1989; 3:1843–1849.
1415. McConkey DJ, Nicotera P, Hartzell P, Bellomo G, Wyllie AH, Orrenius S. Glucocorticoids activate a suicide process in thymocytes through an elevation of cytosolic CA^{2+} concentration. Arch Biochem Biophys 1989; 269:365–370.
1416. McCrank E, Rabheru K. Four cases of progressive supranuclear palsy in patients exposed to organic solvents. Canadian Journal of Psychiatry 1989; 34(9):934–936.
1417. McCrodden JM, Tipton KF, Sullivan JP. The neurotoxicity of MPTP and the relevance to Parkinson's disease. Pharmacol Toxicol 1990; 67:8–13.
1418. McDowell FH. Changes in behaviour and mentation in L-dopa and parkinsonism. In: Barbeau A, McDowell FH, eds. L-Dopa and parkinsonism. Philadelphia: FA Davis, 1970:321–325.
1419. McGeer PL. Tyrosine hydroxylase and parkinsonism. Lancet 1971; 2:165.
1420. McGeer PL, Itagaki S, Akiyama H, NcGeer G. Rate of cell death in parkinsonism indicates active neuropathological process. Ann Neurol 1988; 24:574–576.
1421. McGeer PL, McGeer EG, Suzuki JS. Aging and extrapyramidal function. Neurology 1977; 34:33–35.
1422. McIsaac WM. Formation of 1-methyl-6-methoxy-1,2,3,4-tetrahydro-2-carboline under physiological conditions. Biochem Biophys Acta 1961; 52:607–609.
1423. McLean D, Jacobs H, Mielke B. Methanol poisoning: A clinical and pathological study. Ann Neurol 1980; 8:161–167.
1424. McNeill TH, Koek LL. Differential effects of advancing age on neurotransmitter cell loss in the substantia nigra and striatum of C57BL/6N mice. Brain Res 1990; 521:107–117.
1425. Meador KJ, Meador MP, Loring DW, Feldman DS, Sethi KD. Neuroepidemiology of Parkinson's disease. Neurology 1987; 37:120.
1426. Megro F. Les syndromes Parkinsoniens par intoxication sulfocarbonee. Revue Neurologique 1930; 49:518.
1427. Meillard MN, Bentué-Ferrer D, Brunet-Bourgin F, Morel G, Allain H. Étude de l'hydroxylation de la débrisoquine dans la maladie de Parkinson. La Presse Médicale 1990; 19:947–949.
1428. Meister A. Selective modification of glutathione metabolism. Science 1983; 220:472–477.
1429. Melamed E, Bitton V, Kidron D. Parkinson's disease in Israelis:Relationship to

ethnic origin supports etiologic importance of genetic factors. Neurology 1987; 37:121.

1430. Melamed E, Pikarski E, Goldberg A, Rosenthal J, Uzzan A, Conforti N. Effect of serotonergic, corticostriatal and kainic acid lesions on the dopaminergic neurotoxicity of 1-methyl-4-phenyl-1,2,3,6-tetrahydropyridine (MPTP) in mice. Brain Res 1986; 399:178–180.

1431. Melamed E, Rosenthal J, Cohen O, Globus M, Uzzan A. Dopamine but not norepinephrine or serotonin uptake inhibitors protect mice against neurotoxicity of MPTP. Eur J Pharmacol 1985; 116:179–181.

1432. Melamed E, Rosenthal J, Globus M, Cohen O, Uzzan A. Suppression of MPTP-induced dopaminergic neurotoxicity in mice by nomifensine and L-dopa. Brain Res 1985; 342:401–404.

1433. Melamed E, Soffer D, Rosenthal J, Reches A, Pikarski E. Effect of intrastriatal and intranigral administration of synthetic neuromelanin on the dopaminergic neurotoxicity of MPTP in rodents. Neurosci Lett 1987; 83:41–46.

1434. Melchior C, Collins MA. The route and significance of endogenous synthesis of alkaloids in animals. Critical Reviews in Toxicology 1982; 9:313–354.

1435. Melchior CL. Interaction of salsolinol and tetrahydropapaveroline with catecholamines. Alcohol Clin Exp Res 1979; 3(4):364–367.

1436. Melo-Souza S, Ragazzo P. Neurologic side-effects of flunarizine. Neurology 1989; 39 supp 1:390.

1437. Mena I, Marin O, Fuenzalida S, Cotzias G. Chronic manganese poisoning. Clinical picture and manganese turnover. Neurology 1967; 17:128–136.

1438. Mena I. Manganese poisoning. In: Vinken PJ, Bruyn GW, Cohen MM, Klawans HL, eds. Handbook of clinical neurology, Vol 36: Intoxications of the nervous system, Part 1. Amsterdam: North Holland Publishing Company, 1979:217–237.

1439. Mendell JR, Chase TN, Engel WK. Amyotrophic lateral sclerosis. A study of central monoamine metabolism and therapeutic trial of levodopa. Arch Neurol 1971; 25:320–325.

1440. Menza M, Forman NE, Goldstein HE, Golbe LI. Parkinson's disease, personality and dopamine. J Neuropsychiatry Clin Neurosci 1990; 2:282–287.

1441. Merz PA, Rohwer RG, Kascak R, et al. Infection-specific particle from the uncoventional slow virus diseases. Science 1984; 225:437–440.

1442. Messert B, Wanamaker B. Reappraisal of the adult occult hydrocephalus syndrome. Neurology 1974; 24:224–231.

1443. Messert B, Van Nuis C. A syndrome of paralysis of downward gaze, dysarthria, pseudobulbar palsy, axial rigidity of neck and trunk and dementia. J Nerv Ment Dis 1966; 143:47–54.

1444. Mestre D, Blin O, Serratrice G, Pailhous J. Spatiotemporal contrast sensitivity differs in normal aging and Parkinson's disease. Neurology 1990; 40:1710–1714.

1445. Metzer WS, Newton JEO, Steele RW, et al. HLA antigens in drug-induced parkinsonism. Mov Disord 1989; 4:121–128.

1446. Meyboom R, Ferrari M, Dieleman P. Parkinsonism, tardive dyskinesia, akathisia, and depression induced by flunarizine. Lancet 1986; ii:292.

1447. Meyer A. Experimentelle erfahrungen uber die kohlinoxydvergiftung des zentralnervensystems. Ztschr f d ges. Neurol u Psychiat 1928; 112–187.
1448. Meyer B. Encephalitis after measles with severe parkinsonism rigidity: Recovery. Br Med J 1943; 1:508.
1449. Meyer J, Baron D. Ataxia of gait: A clinico-physiological study. Brain 1960; 83:261–284.
1450. Meyer JS, Magee KR. Current views concerning the etiology, pathophysiology, and treatment of Parkinson's disease. J Neuropsychiatry 1964; 5:284–290.
1451. Michaowicz R, Chmielik J, Ignatowicz R, Karkowska B. [Etiology and pathogenesis of Parkinson disease in children in the light of clinical observations]. Pediatr Pol 1982; 57:811–815.
1452. Michel D, Tommasi M, Laurent B, Trillet M, Schott B. Striato-nigral degeneration. A propos of 2 anatomo-clinical cases. Revue Neurologique 1976; 132(1):3–22.
1453. Michel PP, Agid Y. The glutamate antagonist, MK-801, does not prevent dopaminergic cell death induced by the 1-methyl-4-phenylpyridinium ion (MPP+) in rat dissociated mesencephalic cultures. Brain Res 1992; 597:233–240.
1454. Micheli F, Fernandez-Pardal M, Giannaula R. Movement disorders and depression due to flunarizine and cinnarizine. Mov Disord 1989; 4:139–146.
1455. Miller A, Perrild H, Pedersen H, Hier-Madsen M. Parkinson's disease and autoimmunity. Acta Neurol Scand 1989; 79:173–175.
1456. Miller DM, Buettner GR, Aust SD. Transition metals as catalysts of auto-oxidation reactions. Free Rad Biol Med 1990; 8:95–108.
1457. Miller L, Jankovic J. Neurologic approach to drug-induced movement disorders: A study of 125 patients. South Med J 1990; 83(5):525–532.
1458. Miller LG, Jankovic J. Metoclopramide-induced movement disorders. Clinical findings with a review of the literature. Arch Intern Med 1989; 149:2486–2492.
1459. Mims CA. Viral aetiology of diseases of obscure origin. Br Med Bull 1985; 41:63–69.
1460. Mindham RH, Ahmed SW, Clough CG. A controlled study of dementia in Parkinson's disease. J Neurol Neurosurg Psychiatry 1982; 45:969–974.
1461. Mindham RH, Marsden CD, Parkes JD. Psychiatric symptoms during L-dopa therapy for Parkinson's disease and their relationship to physical disability. Psychol Med 1976; 6:23–33.
1462. Mindham RHS. Psychiatric symptoms in parkinsonism. J Neurol Neurosurg Psychiatry 1970; 33:188–191.
1463. Minor L. About hereditary tremor. Zbl Neruol Psychiatr 1922; 28:514–516.
1464. Mintz U, Lieberman U, Vries A. Parkinsonian syndrome due to cephaloridine. JAMA 1971; 216:1200.
1465. Mirabelli F, Salis A, Marinoni V. Menadione-induced bleb formation in hepatocytes is associated with the oxidation of thiol groups in actin. Arch Biochem Biophys 1988; 264:261–269.
1466. Mirabelli F, Salis A, Viaretti M, Bellomo G, Thor H, Orrenius S. Cytoskeletal alterations in human platelets exposed to oxidative stress are mediated by oxidative and Ca2+-dependent mechanisms. Arch Biochem Biophys 1989; 270(2):478–488.

1467. Mircheva Y, Vidailhet M, Marconi R, Bonnet AM, Beaune P, Agid Y. Selective decrease in S-Methylation in Parkinson's disease. Neurology 1993; 43(4):Suppl:A154–A155.
1468. Mitchell IJ, Cross AJ, Sambrook MA, Crossman AR. Sites of the neurotoxic action of 1-methyl-4-phenyl-1,2,3,6-tetrahydropyridine in the macaque monkey include the ventral tegmental area and the locus ceruleus. Neurosci Lett 1985; 61:195–200.
1469. Mitchell IJ, Cross AJ, Sambrook MA, Crossman AR. N-methyl-4-phenyl-1,2,3,6-tetrahydropyridine-induced parkinsonism in the monkey: Neurochemical pathology and regional brain metabolism. J Neural Transm 1986; 41–46.
1470. Mitchell IJ, Sambrook MA, Crossman AR. Subcortical changes in the regional uptake of [3H]-2-deoxyglucose in the brain of the monkey during experimental choreiform dyskinesia elicited by injection of a gamma-aminobutyric acid antagonist into the subthalamic nucleus. Brain 1985; 108:405–422.
1471. Mitchell JR, Jollow DJ. Metabolic activation of drugs to toxic substances. Gastroenterology 1975; 68:392–410.
1472. Mitra N, Mohanakumar KP, Ganguly DK. Dissociation of serotoninergic and dopaminergic components in acute effects of 1-methy-4-phenyl-1,2,3,6-tetrahydropyridine in mice. Brain Res Bull 1992; 28:355–364.
1473. Miyake H, Chiueh CC. Effects of MPP+ on the release of serotonin and 5-hydroxyindoleacetic acid from rat striatum in vivo. Eur J Pharmacol 1989; 166:49–55.
1474. Miyasaki K, Takayoshi F. Parkinsonism following encephalitis of unknown etiology. J Neuropathol Exp Neurol 1977; 36:1–8.
1475. Mizuno Y. [Contribution of MPTP to studies on the pathogenesis of Parkinson's disease]. Rinsho Shinkeigaku 1989; 29:1494–1496.
1476. Mizuno Y, Ikebe S, Hattori N, Nakagawa-Hattori Y, Tanaka M, Ozawa T. Mitochondrial abnormalities in Parkinson's disease. Mov Disord 1992; 7(Supplement 1):11.
1477. Mizuno Y, Ohta S, Tanaka M, et al. Mitochondrial complex I deficiency in Parkinson's disease and MPTP-induced parkinsonism (Abstract). Mov Disord 1990; 5:30.
1478. Mizuno Y, Ohta S, Tanaka M, et al. Deficiencies in complex I subunits of the respiratory chain in Parkinson's disease. Biochem Biophys Res Commun 1989; 163:1450–1455.
1479. Mizuno Y, Suzuki K, Ohta S. Postmortem changes in mitochondrial respiratory enzymes in brain and a preliminary observation in Parkinson's disease. J Neurol Sci 1990; 96:49–57.
1480. Mizuno Y, Suzuki K, Sone N, Saitoh T. Inhibition of ATP synthesis by 1-methyl-4-phenylpridinium ion (MPP+) in isolated mitochondria from mouse brains. Neurosci Lett 1987; 81:204–208.
1481. Mizutani T, Inose T, Nakajima S, Gambetti P. Familial parkinsonism and dementia with "ballooned neurons". In: Narabayashi H, Nagatsu T, Yanagisawa N, Mizuno. Y., eds. Parkinson's disease: From basic research to treatment—Advances in Neurology, Vol.60. New York: Raven Press, 1993:613–617.
1482. Mizutani Y, Yokochi M, Oyanagi S. Juvenile parkinsonism: A case with first

clinical manifestation at the age of six years and with neuropathological findings suggesting a new pathogenesis. Clin neuropathol 1991; 10 (2):91–97.

1483. Mjönes H. Paralysis agitans: A clinical and genetic study. Acta Psychiatr Neurol 1949; 25 (supp 54):1–195.

1484. Moersch FP. Tumor of the frontal lobe presenting a parkinsonism syndrome. Minn Med 1928; 11:734–736.

1485. Moore G. Influenza and Parkinson's disease. Public Health Rep 1977; 92:79–80.

1486. Moraes CT, DiMauro S, Zeviani M, et al. Mitochondrial DNA deletions in progressive external ophthalmoplegia and Kearns-Sayre syndrome. N Engl J Med 1989; 320(20):1293–1299.

1487. Moratalla R, Quinn B, DeLanney LE, Langston JW, Graybiel AM. Differential vulnerability of primate caudate-putamen and striosome-matrix dopamine systems to the neurotoxic effect of MPTP. Proc Natl Acad Sci 1992; 89: 3859–3863.

1488. Morgan RO, Naglie G, Horrobin DF, Barbeau A. Erythrocyte protoporphyrin levels in patients with Friedreich's and other ataxias. Can J Neurol Sci 1979; 6(2):227–232.

1489. Mortimer JA, Hansch EC, Pirozzolo FJ, Webster DC. Continuum of intellectual deficit in Parkinson disease. Ann Neurol 1982; 12:402–404.

1490. Mortimer JA, June SP, Kuskowski MA, Webster R. Sybtypes of Parkinson's disease defined by intellectual impairment. J Neural Transm 1987; 24:101–104.

1491. Mortimer JA, Pirozzolo FJ, Hansch EC, Webster DD. Relationship of motor symptoms to intellectual deficits in Parkinson disease. Neurology 1982; 32(2):133–137.

1492. Morton NE, Lalouel JM, Jackson JF, Currier RD, Yee S. Linkage studies in spinocerebellar ataxia (SCA). Am J Med Genet 1980; 6(3):251–257.

1493. Moses H, Klawans HL. Bromide intoxication. In: Vinken PJ, Bruyn GW, eds. Handbook of clinical neurology, vol. 36, Intoxications of the nervous system, pt.1. Amsterdam: 1979:291–318.

1494. Moskowitz M, Winickoff R, Heinz E. Familial calcification of the basal ganglion. A metabolic and genetic study. N Engl J Med 1971; 280:72–77.

1495. Mölsä PK, Marttila RJ, Rinne UK. Extrapyramidal signs in Alzheimer's disease. Neurology 1984; 34:1114–1116.

1496. Muenter M, Howard JF, Okazaki H, Forno L, Kish S, Hornykiewicz O. A familial parkinson-dementia syndrome. Neurology 1986; 36:115.

1497. Muenter M, Whisnant J. Basal ganglia calcifications, hypoparathyroidism, and extrapyramidal motor manifestations. Neurology 1968; 18:1075–1083.

1498. Mulder D, Parrott M, Thaler M. Sequelae of western equine encephalitis. Neurology 1951; 1:318–327.

1499. Muller R, Benker G, Windeck R, Reinwein D, Jorg J. [Hemiparkinson syndrome in hyperparathyroidism (letter)]. Dtsch Med Wochenschr 1985; 110:1231–1232.

1500. Murphy SD. Pesticides. In: Doull J, Klaassen CD, Amdur MO, eds. Cassarett and Doull's toxicology. 2nd ed. New York: Macmillan, 1980:357–408.

1501. Murrow R, Schweiger G, Kepes J, Koller W. Parkinsonism due to a basal ganglia lacunar state: Clinicopathologic correlation. Neurology 1990; 40:897–900.

1502. Mutch WJ, Dingwall-Fordyce I, Downie AW, Paterson JG, Roy SK. Parkinson's disease in a Scottish city. Br Med J 1986; 292:534–536.

1503. Mutch WJ, Strudwick A, Roy SK, Downie AW. Parkinson's disease: disability, review, and management. Br Med J 1986; 293:675–677.
1504. Myers RD. Tetrahydroisoquinolines in the brain: the basis of an animal model of alcoholism. Alcohol Clin Exp Res 1978; 2(2):145–154.
1505. Myers RD, Melchior CL. Differential actions on voluntary alcohol intake of tetrahydroisoquinolines or a beta-carboline infused chronically in the ventricle of the rat. Pharmacol Biochem Behavior 1977; 7:381–392.
1506. Myllyla VV, Sotaniemi KA, Vuorinen JA, Heinonen EH. Selegiline as a primary treatment of Parkinson's disease. Acta Neurol Scand 1991; 84 (Supplement 136):70–72.
1507. Myllyla VV, Sotaniemi KA, Vuorinen JA, Heinonen EH. Selegiline as initial treatment in de novo parkinsonian patients. Neurology 1992; 42:339–343.
1508. Myrianthopoulos N, Kurland A, Kurland L. Hereditary predisposition in drug-induced parkinsonism. Arch Neurol 1962; 6:5.
1509. Myrianthopoulos NC, Waldrop IN, Vincent BL. A repeat study of hereditary predisposition in drug-induced parkinsonism. In: Barbeau A, Brunette JB, eds. Progress in neurogenetics. Amsterdam: Excerpta Medica, 1969:486–491.
1510. Nagatsu T. [Pathogenic substances in Parkinson disease and new therapeutics considering the etiologic nechanism]. Nippon Rinsho 1988; 46:2086–2097.
1511. Nagatsu T. Change of tyrosine hydroxylase in the parkinsonian brain and in the brain of MPTP-treated mice as revealed by homospecific activity. Neurochem Res 1990; 15:425–429.
1512. Nagatsu T. Changes of tyrosine hydroxylase in parkinsonian brains and in the brains of MPTP-treated mice. In: Parkinson's disease: anatomy, pathology and therapy—Advances in neurology, Vol 53. New York: Raven Press, 1990:207–214.
1513. Nagatsu T, Hirata Y. Inhibition of the tyrosine hydroxylase system by MPTP, 1-methyl-4-phenylpyridinium ion (MPP+) and the structurally related compounds in vitro and in vivo. Eur Neurol 1987; 26(Supplement 1):11–15.
1514. Nagatsu T, Yoshida M. An endogenous substance of the brain, tetrahydroisoquinoline, produces parkinsonism in primates with decreased dopamine, tyrosine hydroxylase and biopterin in the nigrostriatal regions. Neurosci Lett 1988; 87:178–182.
1515. Nakagawa-Hattori Y, Yoshino H, Kondo T, Mizuno Y, Horai S. Is Parkinson's disease a mitochondrial disorder. J Neurol Sci 1992; 107:29–33.
1516. Nakazato Y, Yamazaki H, Hirato J, Ishida Y, Yamaguchi H. Oligodendroglial microtubular tangles in olivopontocerebellar atrophy. J Neuropathol Exp Neurol 1990; 49(5):521–530.
1517. Naoi M, Hirata Y, Nagatsu T. Inhibition of monoamine oxidase by N-methylisoquinolinium. J Neurochem 1987; 48:709–712.
1518. Naoi M, Matsuura S, Parvez H, et al. Oxidation of N-methyl-1,2,3,4-tetrahydoisoquinoline into the N-methyl-isoquinolinium ion by monoamine oxidase. J Neurochem 1989; 52:653–655.
1519. Naoi M, Matsuura S, Takahashi T, Nagatsu T. A N-methyltransferase in human brain catalyses N-methylation of 1,2,3,4-tetrahydroisoquinoline into N-methyl-1,2,3,4-tetrahydroisoquinoline, a precursor of a dopaminergic neurotoxin, N-methylisoquinolinium ion. Biochem Biophys Res Commun 1989; 161:1213–1219.

1520. Naoi M, Matsuura S, Takahashi T, Nagatsu T. Biosynethesis of N-methylisoquinolinium ion, a potent inhibitor of catecholamine metabolism, from 1,2,3,4-tetrahydroisoquinoline through N-methyl-1,2,3,4-tetrahydroisoquinoline in human brain. In: Nagatsu T, Fisher A, Yoshida M, eds. Basic, clinical, and therapeutic aspects of Alzheimer's and Parkinson's diseases, Volume 1. New York: Plenum Press, 1990:317–320.

1521. Naoi M, Nagatsu T. Inhibition of type A monoamine oxidase by methylquinones and structurally related compounds. J Neurochem 1988; 50:1105–1110.

1522. Naoi M, Takahashi T, Parvez H. N-methylisoquinolinium ion as an inhibitor of tyrosine hydroxylase, aromatic L-amino acid decarboxylase and monoamine oxidase. Neurochem Int 1989; 15:315–320.

1523. Narabayashi H, Yokochi M, Iizuka R, Nagatsu T. Juvenile parkinsonism. In: Vinken PJ, Bruyn GW, Klawans HL, eds. Handbook of clinical neurology, Vol. 5: Extrapyramidal disorders. 49th ed. Amsterdam: Elsevier Science Publishers, 1986:153–165.

1524. Nath A, Jankovic J, Pettigrew L. Movement disorders and AIDS. Neurology 1987; 37:37–41.

1525. National Academy of Sciences. Medical and biologic effects of environmental pollutants. Washington, D.C.: National Academy of Sciences, 1973.

1526. Navarro A. Parkinsonism due to corpus callosum astrocytoma: case report. J Neurol Neurosurg Psychiatry 1986; 49:1457–1458.

1527. Nayernouri T. Posttraumatic parkinsonism. Surg Neurol 1985; 24:263–264.

1528. Neafsey EJ, Drucker G, Raikoff K, Collins MA. Striatal dopaminergic toxicity following intranigral injection in rats of 2-methyl-norharman, a B-carbolinium analog of N-methyl-4-phenylpyridinium ion (MPP+). Neurosci Lett 1989; 105:344–349.

1529. Nee L, Brown R, Polinsky R. HLA in autonomic failure. Arch Neurol 1989; 46:758–759.

1530. Neff NH, Barrett RE, Costa E. Selective depletion of caudate nucleus dopamine and serotonin during chronic manganese dioxide administration to squirrel monkeys. Experientia 1969; 25:1140–1114.

1531. Nefzger MD, Quadfasel FA, Karl VC. A retrospective study of smoking in Parkinson's disease. Am J Epidemiol 1968; 88:149–158.

1532. Neill K. An unusual case of syphilitic Parkinsonism. Br Med J 1953; August 8:320–322.

1533. Neiman J, Borg S, Wahlund LO. Parkinsonism and dyskinesias during ethanol withdrawal. Br J Addict 1988; 83:437–439.

1534. Neiman J, Lang AE, Fornazzari L, Carlen PL. Movement disorders in alcoholism: A review. Neurology 1990; 40:741–746.

1535. Nerl C, Mayeux R, O'Neill GJ. HLA-linked complement markers in Alzheimer's and Parkinson's disease: C4 variant (C4B2) a possible marker for senile dementia of the Alzheimer type. Neurology 1984; 34:310–314.

1536. Netter P. Relationships between lethargic encephalitis and Parkinson's disease. Revue Neurologique 1921; 37(6):573–575.

1537. Neumayer E. [Parkinson's disease concurring with other diseases of the central nervous system]. Z Neurol 1971; 199:306–318.

1538. Newman G. Treatment of progressive supranuclear palsy with tricyclic antidepressants. Neurology 1985; 35:1189–1193.
1539. Ngim CH, Devathasan G. Epidemiologic study on the association between body burden mercury level and idiopathic Parkinson's disease. Neuroepidemiology 1989; 8:128–141.
1540. Nicholls P. Formate as an inhibitor of cytochrome c oxidase. Biochem Biophys Res Commun 1975; 67:610–616.
1541. Nicholson AN, Turner EA. Parkinsonism produced by parasaggital meningiomas. J Neurosurg 1964; 21:104–113.
1542. Nicklas W, Vyas I, Heikkila E. Inhibition of NADH-linked oxidation in brain mitochondria by 1-methyl-4-phenyl-pyridine, a metabolite of the neurotoxin, 1-methyl-4-phenyl-1,2,5,6-tetrahydropyridine. Life Sci 1985; 36: 2503–2508.
1543. Nicotera P, Hartzell P, Baldi C, Svensson SA, Bellomo G, Orrenius S. Cystamine induces toxicity in hepatocytes through the elevation of cytosolic Ca2+ and the stimulation of a nonlysosomal proteolytic system. J Biol Chem 1986; 261(31):14628–14635.
1544. Nicotera P, Hartzell P, Davis G, Orrenius S. The formation of plasma membrane blebs in hepatocytes exposed to agents that increase cytosolic Ca2+ is mediated by the activation of a non-lysomal proteolytic system. FEBS lett 1986; 209(1):139–144.
1545. Nielsen J. Complications of encephalitis of the von Economo type. Bull L A Neurol Soc 1953; 18:84–90.
1546. Nielsen SL. Striatonigral degeneration disputed in familial disorder [letter]. Neurology 1977; 27(3):306.
1547. Nies A, Robinson DS, Davis JM, Ravaris CL. Changes in monoamine oxidase with aging. In: Eisdorfer C, Fann WE, eds. Advances in Behavioral Biology, Volume 6. Psychopharmacology and aging. New York: Plenum Press, 1973:41–54.
1548. Nieto MA, Lopez-Rivas A. IL-2 protects T lymphocytes from glucocorticoid-induced DNA fragmentation and cell death. J Immunol 1989; 143:4166–4170.
1549. Nigro N. [The viral etiology of some chronic neurologic diseases in childhood (letter)]. Minerva Pediatr 1981; 33:45–46.
1550. Nino HE, Noreen HJ, Dubey DP, et al. A family with hereditary ataxia: HLA typing. Neurology 1980; 30(1):12–20.
1551. Nishino N, Noguchi-Kuno S, Sugiyama T, Tanaka C. [3H] Nitrendipine binding sites are decreased in the substantia nigra and striatum of the brain from patients with Parkinson's disease. Brain Res 1986; 377:186–189.
1552. Niwa T, Takeda N, Kaneda N, Hashizume Y, Nagatsu T. Presence of tetrahydroisoquinoline and 2-methyl-tetrahydroquinoline in parkinsonian and normal human brains. Biochem Biophys Res Commun 1987; 144:1084–1089.
1553. Niwa T, Takeda N, Sasaoka T. Detection of tetrahydroisoquinoline in parkinsonian brain as an endogenous amine by use of gas chromatography-mass spectrometry. J Chromatogr 1989; 491:397–403.
1554. Niwa T, Takeda N, Tatematsu A, Matsuura S, Yoshida M, Nagatsu T. Migration of tetrahydroisoquinoline, a possible Parkinsonian neurotoxin, into monkey brain

from blood as proved by gas chromatography-mass spectrometry. J Chromatogr 1988; 452:85–91.

1555. Niwa T, Takeda N, Yoshizumi H, et al. Presence of 2-methyl-6,7-dihydroxy - 1,2,3,4-tetrahydroisoquinoline and 1,2-dimethyl-6,7-dihydroxy-1,2,3,4-tetrahydroisoquinoline, novel endogenous amines, in parkinsonian and normal human brains. Biochem Biophys Res Commun 1991; 177:603–609.

1556. Niwa T, Yoshizumi H, Takeda N, Tatematsu A, Matsuura S, Nagatsu T. Detection of tetrahydroisoquinoline, a parkinsonism-related compound, in parkinsonian brains and foods by gas chromatography-mass spectrometry. In: Nagatsu T, Fisher A, Yoshida M, eds. Basic, clinical, and therapeutic aspects of Alzheimer's and Parkinson's diseases, Volume 1. New York: Plenum Press, 1990:313–316.

1557. Niwa T, Yoshizumi H, Tatematsu A. Endogenous synthesis of N-methyl-1,2,3,4-tetrahydroisoquinoline, a precursor of N-methylisoquinolinium ion, in the brains of primates with parkinsonism after systemic administration of 1,2,3,4-tetrahydroisoquinoline. J Chromatogr Biomed Appl 1990; 533:145–151.

1558. Niwa T, Yoshizumi H, Tatematsu A, Matsuura S, Nagatsu T. Presence of tetrahydroisoquinoline, a parkinsonism-related compound, in foods. J Chromatogr 1989; 493:347–352.

1559. Niznik HB, Fogel EF, Fassos FF, Seeman P. The dopamine transporter is absent in parkinsonian putamen and reduced in the caudate nucleus. J Neurochem 1991; 56:192–198.

1560. Niznik HB, Tyndale RF, Sallee FR, et al. The dopamine transporter and cytochrome P450IID1 (Debrisoquine 4-hydroxylase) in brain: Resolution and identification of two distinct [3H]GBR-12935 binding proteins. Arch Biochem Biophys 1990; 276(2):424–432.

1561. Nobrega FT, Glattre E, Kurland LT, Okazaki H. Comments on the epidemiology of parkinsonism including prevalence and incidence statistics for Rochester, Minnesota, 1935–1966. In: Barbeau A, Brunette JR, eds. Progress in neuro-genetics: Proceedings of the International Congress of Neuro-genetics and Neuro-opthalmology. Amsterdam: Exerpta Medica, 1969:474–485.

1562. Noel S, Guillaume M-P, Telerman-Toppet N, Cogan E. Movement disorders due to cerebral toxoplasma gondii infection in patients with the acquired immunodeficiency syndrome (AIDS). Acta Neurol Belg 1992; 92:148–156.

1563. Nomoto M, Igata A. Do parkinsonian patients have a greater resistance to the common cold? J Neurol Neurosurg Psychiatry 1983; 46:1153–1154.

1564. Novelli A, Reilly JA, Lysko PG. Glutamate becomes neurotoxic via the N-methyl-D-aspartate receptor when intracellular energy levels are reduced. Brain Res 1988; 451:205–212.

1565. Nukada H, Kowa H, Saitoh T, Tazaki Y, Miura S. [A big family of paralysis agitans (author's transl)]. Rinsho Shinkeigaku 1978; 18:627–634.

1566. Nunn PB, Seelig M, Zagoren JC, Spencer PS. Stereospecific acute neuronotoxicity of ''uncommon'' plant amino acids linked to human motor-system diseases. Brain 1987; 410:375–379.

1567. Nutt JG, Mrox EA, Leeman SE, Williams AC, Engel WK, Chase TN. Substance P in human cerebrospinal fluid: reductions in peripheral neuropathy and autonomic dysfunction. Neurology 1980; 30(12):1280–1285.

1568. Nygaard TG, Duvoisin RC. Hereditary dystonia-parkinsonism syndrome of juvenile onset. Neurology 1986; 36:1424–1428.
1569. O'Brien C, Sung J, McGeachie R, Lee M. Striatonigral degeneration: Clinical, MRI, and pathologic correlation. Neurology 1990; 40:710–711.
1570. Oertel WH, Gasser T, Ippisch R, Trenkwalker C, Poewe W. Apomorphine test for dopaminergic responsiveness. Lancet 1989; 1:1262–1263.
1571. Ogawa M, Araki M, Nagatsu I, Nagatsu T, Yoshida M. The effect of 1,2,3,4-tetrahydroisoquinoline (TIQ) on mesencephalic dopaminergic neurons in C57BL/6J mice: Immunohistochemical studies—Tyrosine hydroxylase. Biogenic Amines 1989; 6:427–436.
1572. Ohkubo S, Hiraro T, Oka K. Methyltetrahydro-beta-carbolines and Parkinson's disease. Lancet 1985; 1:1272–1273.
1573. Ohlson C.G., Hogstedt C. Parkinson's disease and occupational exposure to organic solvents, agricultural chemicals and mercury-a case referrant study. Scand J Work Environ Health 1981; 7:252–256.
1574. Ohta S, Kohno M, Makino Y, Tachikawa O, Hirobe M. Tetrahydroisoquinoline and 1-methyl-tetrahydroisoquinoline are present in the human brain: Relation to Parkinson's disease. Biomed Res 1987; 8(6):453–456.
1575. Ohta S, Tachikawa O, Makino Y, Tasaki Y, Hirobe M. Metabolism and brain accumulation of tetrahydroisoquinoline (TIQ): A possible Parkinsonism inducing substance, in an animal model of a poor debrisoquine metabolizer. Life Sci 1990; 46:599–605.
1576. Ohta S, Tasaki Y, Makino Y, Tachikawa O, Hirobe M. Importance of 1-methyltetrahydroisoquinoline (1MeTIQ) in Parkinson's disease. In: Nagatsu T, Fisher A, Yoshida M, eds. Basic, clinical, and therapeutic aspects of Alzheimer's and Parkinson's diseases, Volume 1. New York: Plenum Press, 1990:321–324.
1577. Oishi M, Takasu T, Tateno M, Uchida H. Hair trace elements in cerebellar degeneration: low copper levels in late cortical cerebellar atrophy. J Neurol 1990; 237(3):163–165.
1578. Okada K, Kobayashi S, Tsunematsu T. Prevalence of Parkinson's disease in Izumo City, Japan. Gerontology 1990; 36:340–344.
1579. Okaya N. A case of paralysis agitans in the Chamorro people (Micronesian) of the U.S. Territory of Guam. Tokyo Med J 1936; 2997:2517–1518.
1580. Okeda R, Funata N, Takano T, et al. The pathogenesis of carbon monoxide encephalopathy in the acute phase—physical and morphological correlation. Acta Neuropathol(Berlin) 1981; 54:1–10.
1581. Olanow CW. Oxidation reactions in Parkinson's disease. Neurology 1990; 40(supplement):32–37.
1582. Olanow CW, Calne D. Does selegiline monotherapy in Parkinson's disease act by symptomatic or protective mechanisms? Neurology 1991; 42(supp 4):13–26.
1583. Olanow CW, Cohen G, Perl DP, Marsden CD. Role of iron and oxidant stress in the normal and Parkinsonian brain: Proceedings of a symposium sponsored by the University of Florida, November 14–17, 1991. Ann Neurol, 32(Supplement), 1992:
1584. Oleinik LI, Palamarchuk LA. [Features of catecholamine metabolism in the

families of patients with idiopathic parkinsonism]. Zh Nevropatol Psikhiatr 1980; 80:353–358.
1585. Oliver L. Parkinsonism due to midbrain compression. Lancet 1959; 2:817–819.
1586. Olney JW. Excitotoxic mechanisms of neurotoxicity. In: Spencer PS, Schaumburg HH, eds. Experimental and clinical neurotoxicology. Baltimore: Williams and Wilkins, 1980:272–294.
1587. Olsson JE, Brunk U, Lindvall B, Eeg-Olofsson O. Dopa-responsive dystonia with depigmentation of the substantia nigra and formation of Lewy bodies. J Neurol Sci 1992; 112:90–95.
1588. Omata S, Sugano H. Methyl mercury: Effects on protein synthesis in nervous tissue. In: Blum K, Manzo L, eds. Neurotoxicology. New York: Marcel Dekker, 1985:369–384.
1589. Onofrj M, Ghilardi MF. MPTP induced parkinsonian syndrome: Long term follow-up and neurophysiological study. Ital J Neurol Sci 1990; 11:445–458.
1590. Oppenheimer D. Diseases of the basal ganglia, cerebellum and motor neurons. In: Adam J, Corsellis J, eds. Greenfield's Neuropathology. London: Edward Arnold, 1984:700–747.
1591. Origitano T, Hannigan J, Collins MA. Rat brain salsolinol and blood-brain barrier. Brain Res 1981; 224:446–451.
1592. Orrenius S, McConkey DJ, Jones DP, Nicotera P. CA2 + -activated mechanisms in toxicity and programmed cell death. ISI Atlas Sci Pharmacol 1988; 2:319–324.
1593. Orzechowski C, Mitkus W. De la forme parkinsonienne des tumeurs de la region infundulo-hypophysaire. Rev Neurol (Paris) 1925; 2:1–17.
1594. Osswald W, Azevedo I. Chemical sympathectomy due to tetrahydroisoquinolines derived from adrenaline. In: Begleiter H, ed. Biological effects of alcohol. New York: Plenum Press, 1980:131–146.
1595. Osswald W, Polonia J, Polonia MA. Preparation and pharmacological activity of the condensation product of adrenaline with acetaldehyde. Arch Pharmacol 1975; 275:290.
1596. Osuntokum BO, Adeuja AOG, Schoenberg BS, et al. Prevalence of neurological disorders in a community in Nigeria. J Neurol 1985; 232(suppl):196.
1597. Osuntokun BO. The pattern of neurological illness in tropical Africa. Experience at Ibadan, Nigeria. J Neurol Sci 1971; 12:417–442.
1598. Osuntokun BO. Psychiatric symptoms in typhoid fever. Br Med J 1973; 26:436–437.
1599. Osuntokun BO, Bademosi O. Parkinsonism in the Nigerian African: A prospective study of 217 patients. East Afr Med J 1979; 56:597–607.
1600. Osuntokun BO, Bademosi O, Ogunremi K, Wright SG. Neuropsychiatric manifestations of typhoid fever in 959 patients. Arch Neurol 1972; 27:7–13.
1601. Ota Y, Miyoshi S, Ueda O, Mukai T, Maeka A. Familial paralysis agitans juvenils. A clinical anatomical and genetic study. Neurology 1958; 12:112–121.
1602. Otsuka M, Ichiya Y, Kuwabara Y, et al. Cerebral blood flow, oxyegen and glucose metabolism with PET in progressive supranuclear palsy. Ann Nucl Med 1989; 3(3):111-118.
1603. Otto FG. [Familial aggregation in the occurrence of cases of parkinsonism]. Nervenarzt 1983; 54:423–425.

1604. Ozawa T, Tanaka M, Ikebe S, Ohno K, Kondo T, Mizuno Y. Quantitative determination of deleted mitochondrial DNA relative to normal DNA in parkinsonian striatum by a kinetic PCR analysis. Biochem Biophys Res Commun 1990; 172:483–489.
1605. Ozawa T, Tanaka M, Ino H, et al. Distinct clustering of point mutations in mitochondrial DNA among patients with mitochondrial encephalomyopathies and with Parkinson's disease. Biochem Biophys Res Commun 1991; 176(2):938–946.
1606. Ozawa T, Tanaka M, Sugiyama S, et al. Patients with idiopathic cardiomyopathy belong to the same mitochondrial DNA gene family of Parkinson's disease and mitochondrial encephalomyopathy. Biochem Biophys Res Commun 1991; 177 (1):518–525.
1607. Paddison RM, Griffith RP. Occurrence of Parkinson's disease in black patients at Charity Hospital in New Orleans. Neurology 1974; 24:688–690.
1608. Pahwa R, Koller WC. Defining Parkinsonism and Parkinson's disease. In: Ellenberg JH, Koller WC, Langston JW, eds. Etiology of Parkinson's disease. New York: Marcel Dekker, 1994:1–54.
1609. Pahwa R, Busenbark K, Gray C, Koller WC. Identical twins with similar onset of Parkinson's disease: A case report. Neurology 1993; 43:1159–1161.
1610. Pakkenberg H, Brody H. The number of nerve cells in the substantia nigra in paralysis agitans. Acta Neuropathol 1965; 5:320–324.
1611. Palakurthy P, Iyer V, Meckler R. Unusual neurotoxicity associated with amiodarone therapy. Arch Intern Med 1987; 147:881–884.
1612. Pall HS, Brailsford S, Williams AC, Lunec J, Blake DR. Ferritin in the cerebrospinal fluid of patients with Parkinson's disease [letter]. J Neurol Neurosurg Psychiatry 1990; 53:803.
1613. Pall HS, Williams A. 74 year old lady who developed bilateral parkinsonism secondary to an intrinsic cerebral tumour [letter]. J Neurol Neurosurg Psychiatry 1987; 50:1386–1387.
1614. Palmer R, Finley K. Sequelae of encephalitis: Report of a study after the California epidemic. California Medicine 1956; 84:98–100.
1615. Palombo E, Porrino LJ, Bankiewicz KS, Crane AM, Sokoloff L, Kopin IJ. Local cerebral glucose utilization in monkeys with hemiparkinsonism induced by intracarotid infusion of the neurotoxin MPTP. J Neurol Sci 1990; 10:860–869.
1616. Papavasiliou PS, Miller ST, Thal LJ. Age-related motor and catecholamine alterations in mice on levodopa supplemented diet. Life Sci 1981; 28:2945–2952.
1617. Papeschi R. Dopamine, extrapyramidal system, and psychomotor function. Psychiatr Neurol Neurochir 1972; 75:13–48.
1618. Papp MI, Kahn JE, Kantos PL. Glial cytoplasmic inclusions in the CNS of patients with multiple system atrophy (striatonigral degeneration, olivopontocerebellar atrophy and Shy-Drager syndrome). J Neurol Sci 1989; 94(1–3):79–100.
1619. Parant V. La paralysie agitante examinee comme cause de folie. Ann Med Psychol 1883; 10:45–62.
1620. Parent A, Hazrati LN. Anatomical aspects of information processing in primate basal ganglia. TINS 1993; 16:111–116.
1621. Parisi JE, Burns RS. The neuropathology of MPTP-induced parkinsonism in man and experimental animals. In: Markey SP, Casragnoli NJr, Trevor AJ, Kopin IJ,

eds. MPTP: A neurotoxin producing a Parkinsonian syndrome. Orlando: Academic Press, 1986:141–148.

1622. Park BE, Netsky MG, Betsill WL. Pathogenesis of pigment and spheriod formation in Hallervorden-Spatz syndrome and related disorders. Neurology 1975; 25:1172–1178.
1623. Parker WD. Preclinical detection of Parkinson's disease: Biochemical approaches. Neurology 1991; 41(suppl 2):34–37.
1624. Parker WD, Boyson SJ, Parks JK. Deficient NADH: Ubiquinone oxidoreductase activity in idiopathic Parkinson's disease. Meeting of the American Neurological Association 1989.
1625. Parker WDJr, Boyson SJ, Parks JK. Abnormalities of the electron transport chain in idiopathic Parkinson's disease. Ann Neurol 1989; 26:719–723.
1626. Parkes J, Marsden C, Rees J, Carjon M. Parkinson's disease, cerebral arteriosclerosis, and senile dementia. Q J Med 1974; 43:49–61.
1627. Parkinson J. An essay on the shaking palsy. London: Whittingham and Rowland for Sherwood, Neely, Jones, 1817.
1628. Pastakia B, Polinsky R, DiChiro G, Simmons JT, Brown R, Wener L. Multiple system atrophy (Shy-Drager syndrome): MR imaging. Radiology 1986; 159(2):499–502.
1629. Patrick HT, Levy DM. Parkinson's disease: A clinical study of one hundred and forty-six cases. Arch Gen Psychiatry 1922; 7:711–720.
1630. Patrick RL, Barchas JD. Regulation of catecholamine synthesis in rat brain synaptosomes. J Neurochem 1974; 23:7–15.
1631. Pauleikhoff B, Muller-Fahlbusch H, Mester H, Meissner U. [Late sequelae, especially weakness of memory, following carbon monoxide poisoning]. Fortschr Neurol Psychiatr Grenzgeb 1971; 39:349–377.
1632. Paulson G, Dadmehr N. Is there a premorbid personality typical for Parkinson's disease? Neurology 1991; 41 (suppl 2):73–76.
1633. Paulson G, Lowery H, Taylor G. Progressive supranuclear palsy: Pneumoencephalography, electronystagmography and treatment with methysergide. Eur Neurol 1981; 20:13–16.
1634. Paulus W, Jellinger K. The neuropathologic basis of different clinical subgroups of Parkinson's disease. J Neuropathol Exp Neurol 1991; 50(6):743–755.
1635. Pearce FS. Trauma as an exciting cause of paralysis agitans. Philadelphia Med J 1901; 1017–1019.
1636. Pearce J, Pearce I. Current concepts of Parkinsonism. Postgrad Med J 1971; 47:794–799.
1637. Pearce JM. Aetiology and natural history of Parkinson's disease. Br Med J 1978; 2:1664–1666.
1638. Pembrey ME. Discordant identical twins. II. Parkinsonism. Practitioner 1972; 209:240–243.
1639. Penalver R. Manganese poisoning. Ind J Med Surg 1955; 14:1–7.
1640. Peppard RF, Byrne E, Nye D. Chronic subdural haematomas presenting with parkinsonian signs. Clin Exp Neurol 1986; 22:19–23.
1641. Peppard RF, Martin WR, Clark CM, Carr GD, McGeer PL, Calne DB. Cortical

glucose metabolism in Parkinson's and Alzheimer's disease. J Neurosci Res 1990; 27(4):561–568.

1642. Perez-Otano I, Herrero MT, Oset C. Extensive loss of brain dopamine and serotonin induced by chronic administration of MPTP in the marmosest. Brain Res 1991; 567:127–132.

1643. Perkin G, Lees A, Stern G, Kocen R. Problems in the diagnosis of progressive supranuclear palsy. Can J Neurol Sci 1978; 5:167–173.

1644. Perl D. An appraisal of recent cases of ALS/PDC in Guam. Int ALS-MND Update 1989; 14.

1645. Perl DP, Gajdusek DC, Garruto RM, Yanagihara RT, Gibbs CT, Jr.. Intraneuronal aluminum accumulation in amyotrophic lateral sclerosis and parkinsonism-dementia of Guam. Science 1982; 217:1053–1055.

1646. Perl DP, Good PF. Comparative techniques for determining cellular iron distribution in brain tissues. Ann Neurol 1992; 32:s76–s81.

1647. Perlmutter JS. New insights into the pathophysiology of Parkinson's disease: the challenge of positron emission tomography. TINS 1988; 11:203–208.

1648. Perry EK, Curtis M, Dick DJ, et al. Cholinergic correlates of cognitive impairment in Parkinson's disease: Comparisons with Alzheimer's disease. J Neurol Neurosurg Psychiatry 1985; 48:413–421.

1649. Perry RH, Irving D, Blessed G, Fairbairn A, Perry EK. Senile dementia of Lewy body type: A clinically and neuropathologically distinct form of Lewy body dementia in the elderly. J Neurol Sci 1990; 95:119–139.

1650. Perry TL. Hereditary mental depression with taurine deficiency: Further studies, including a therapeutic trial of taurine administration. In: Huxtable R, Barbeau A, eds. Taurine. New York: Raven Press, 1976:365–374.

1651. Perry TL. Four biochemically different types of dominantly inherited olivopontocerebellar atrophy. In: Duvoisin R, Plaitakis A, eds. The olivocerebellar atrophies—Advances in neurology, Vol 41. New York: Raven Press, 1984:205–216.

1652. Perry TL, Agid FJ, Agid Y, Fibiger HC. Striatal GABAergic neuronal activity is not reduced in Parkinson's disease. J Neurochem 1983; 40:1120–1123.

1653. Perry TL, Bergeron C, Biro A, Hansen S. B-N-methylamino-L-alanine—chronic oral administration is not neurotoxic to mice. J Neurol Sci 1989; 94:173–180.

1654. Perry TL, Bergeron C, Steele JC, McLachlan DR, Hansen S. Brain amino acid contents are dissimilar in sporadic and Guamanian amyotrophic lateral sclerosis. J Neurol Sci 1990; 99:3–8.

1655. Perry TL, Bratty P, Hansen S, Kennedy J, Urquhart N, Dolman C. Hereditary mental depression and parkinsonism with taurine deficiency. Arch Neurol 1975; 32:108–113.

1656. Perry TL, Currier R, Hansen S, MacLean J. Aspartate-taurine imbalance in dominantly inherited olivopontocerebellar atrophy. Neurology 1977; 27:257–261.

1657. Perry TL, Godin DW, Hans. Parkinson's disease: A disorder due to nigral glutathione deficiency. Neurosci Lett 1982; 33:305–310.

1658. Perry TL, Jones K, Hansen S. Tetrahydroisoquinoline lacks dopaminergic nigrostriatal neurotoxicity in mice. Neurosci Lett 1988; 85:101–104.

1659. Perry TL, Jones K, Hansen S, Wall RA. 4-phenylpyridine and three other ana-

logues of 1-methyl-4-phenyl-1,2,3,6-tetrahydropyridine neurotoxicity in mice and marmosets. Neurosci Lett 1987; 75:65–70.
1660. Perry TL, Jones K, Hansen S, Wall RA. 2-Phenylpyridine and 3-Phenylpyridine, constituents of tea, are unlikely to cause idiopathic Parkinson's disease. J Neurol Sci 1988; 85:309–317.
1661. Perry TL, Kish S, Hansen C, Currier R. Neurotransmitter amino acids in dominantly inherited cerebellar disorders. Neurology 1981; 31:237–242.
1662. Perry TL, Krieger C, Hansen S, Tabatabaei A. Amyotrophic lateral sclerosis: Fasting plasma levels of cysteine and inorganic sulfate are normal, as are brain contents of cysteine. Neurology 1991; 41:487–490.
1663. Perry TL, Norman MG, Yong VW, et al. Hallervorden-Spatz disease: Cysteine accumulation and cysteine dioxygenase deficiency in the globus pallidus. Ann Neurol 1985; 18:482–489.
1664. Perry TL, Wright J, Berry K, Hansen S, Perry TLJr. Dominantly inherited apathy, central hypoventilation, and Parkinson's syndrome: Clinical, biochemical, and neuropathologic studies of 2 new cases. Neurology 1990; 40:1882–1887.
1665. Perry TL, Yong VW. Idiopathic Parkinson's disease, progressive supranuclear palsy and glutathione metabolism in the substantia nigra. Neurosci Lett 1986; 67:269–274.
1666. Perry TL, Yong VW, Clavier RM, et al. Partial protection from the dopaminergic neurotoxin N-methyl-4-phenyl-1,2,3,6-tetrahydropyridine by four different antioxidants in the mouse. Neurosci Lett 1985; 60:109–114.
1667. Perry TL, Yong VW, Ito M. Nigrostriatal dopaminergic neurons remain undamaged in rats given high doses of L-dopa and carbidopa chronically. J Neurochem 1984; 43:990–993.
1668. Perry TL, Yong VW, Jones K, Wright JM. Manipulation of glutathione contents fails to alter dopaminergic nigrostriatal neurotoxicity of N-methyl-4-phenyl-1,2,3,6-tetrahydropyridine (MPTP) in the mouse. Neurosci Lett 1986; 70:261–265.
1669. Perry TL, Yong VW, Wall RA, Jones K. Paraquat and two endogenous analogues of the neurotoxic substance N-methyl-4-phenyl-1,2,3,6-tetrahydropyridine do not damage dopaminergic nigrostriatal neurons in the mouse. Neurosci Lett 1986; 69:285–289.
1670. Perticoni GF, Pezzella F, Ferroni A. The problem of Parkinsonism associated with motor neuron disease. Clinical report on 11 sporadic cases. Rivista Di Patologia Nervosa E Mentale 1977; 98:159–170.
1671. Petelin LS. [Current problems of Parkinsonism]. Klin Med (Mosk) 1973; 51:9–16.
1672. Peters HA, Goemen A, Cripps DJ, Bryan GT, Dogramaci I. Epidemiology of hexachlorobenzene-induced porphyria in Turkey. Arch Neurol 1982; 39:744–749.
1673. Peters HA, Johnson SAM, Cam S. Hexachlorobenzene-induced porphyria: Effect of chelation on the disease, porphyrin and mental methabolism. Am J Med Sci New Series 1966; 251:314–322.
1674. Peters HA, Levine RL, Matthews CG, Chapman LJ. Extrapyramidal and other neurologic manifestations associated with carbon disulfide fumigant exposure. Arch Neurol 1988; 45:537–540.

1675. Peters HA, Levine RL, Matthews CG, Sauter SL, Chapman L. Synergistic neurotoxicity of carbon tetrachloride/carbon disulfide (80/20 fumigants) and other pesticides in grain storage workers. Acta Pharmacol Toxicol 1986; 59:535–546.
1676. Peters HA, Levine RL, Matthews CG, Sauter SL, Rankin JH. Carbon disulfide-induced neuropsychiatric changes in grain storage workers. Am J Ind Med 1982; 3:373–391.
1677. Petersen EN. DMCM: a potent convulsive benzodiazepine receptor ligand. Eur J Pharmacol 1983; 94:117–124.
1678. Petersen EN, Jensen LH. Proconflict effect of benzodiazepine receptor inverse agonists and other inhibitors of GABA function. Eur J Pharmacol 1984; 103:91–94.
1679. Peterson LA, Caldera PS, Trevor AJ, Chiba K, Castagnoli N,Jr.. Studies on the 1-methyl-4-phenyl-2,3-dihydropyridinium species 2, 3-MPDP+, the monoamine oxidase catalyzed oxidation product of the nigrostriatal toxin 1-methyl-4-phenyl-1,2,3,6-tetrahydropyridine (MPTP). J Med Chem 1986; 28:1432–1436.
1680. Peura P, Johnson JV, Yost RA, Faull KF. Concentrations of tryptoline and methtryptoline in rat brain. J Neurochem 1989; 52:847–852.
1681. Pezzoli G, Barbieri S, Ferrante C, Zecchinelli A. Parkinsonism Due to N-hexane exposure. Lancet 1989; 2:874–870.
1682. Pezzoli G, Ricciardi S, Masotto C, Mariani CB, Carenzi A. N-hexane induces parkinsonism in rodents. Brain Res 1990; 531:355–357.
1683. Piechocki DW. [Parkinsonism following lethargic encephalitis]. Neurol Neurochir Pol 1977; 11:603–605.
1684. Pifl C, Bertel O, Schingnitz G, Hornykiewicz O. Extrastriatal dopamine in symptomatic and asymptomatic rhesus monkeys treated with 1-methyl-4-phenyl-1,2,3,6-tetrahydropyridine (MPTP). Neurochem Int 1990; 17:263–270.
1685. Pifl C, Schingnitz G, Hornykiewicz O. Effect of 1-methyl-4-phenyl-1,2,3,6-tetrahydropyridine on the regional distribution of brain monoamines in the rhesus monkey. Neuroscience 1991; 44:591–605.
1686. Pifl CH, Schingnitz G, Hornykiewicz O. The neurotoxin MPTP does not reproduce in the rhesus monkey the interregional pattern of striatal dopamine loss typical of human idiopathic Parkinson's disease. Neurosci Lett 1988; 92:228–233.
1687. Pilas B, Sarna T, Kalyanaraman B, Swartz HM. The effect of melanin on iron associated decomposition of hydrogen peroxide. Free Rad Biol Med 1988; 4:285–293.
1688. Pileblad E, Cardenas A. The Ca++-antagonist nimodipine decreases and the Ca++-agonist Bay K 8644 increases catecholamine synthesis in mouse brain. Neuropharmacology 1987; 26:101-105.
1689. Pileblad E, Carlsson A. Catecholamine-uptake inhibitors prevent the neurotoxicity of 1-methyl-4-phenyl-1,2,3,6-tetrahydropyridine (MPTP) in mouse brain. Neuropharmacology 1985; 24(7):689-692.
1690. Pileblad E, Slivka A, Bratvold D, Cohen G. Studies on the autoxidation of dopamine: Interaction with ascorbate. Arch Biochem Biophys 1988; 263(2):447–452.
1691. Pillon B, Dubois B, Ploska A, Agid Y. Severity and specificity of cognitive

impairment in Alzheimer's, Huntington's and Parkinson's diseases and progressive supranuclear palsy. Neurology 1991; 41:634–643.
1692. Pinsky C, Bose R. Pyridine and other coal tar constituents as free radical-generating environmental neurotoxicants. Mol Cell Biochem 1988; 84:217–222.
1693. Pirozzolo FJ, Hansch EC, Mortimer JA, Webster DD, Kuskowski MA. Dementia in Parkinson disease: A neuropsychological analysis. Brain & Cognition 1982; 1:71–83.
1694. Pirozzolo FJ, Swihart A, Rey G, Jankovic J, Mortimer JA. Cognitive impairments associated with Parkinson's disease and other movement disorders. In: Jankovic J, Tolosa E, eds.. Baltimore: Urban & Schwarzenberg, 1988:425–440.
1695. Pitcairn TK, Clemie S, Gray JM, Pentland B. Impressions of parkinsonian patients from their recorded voices. Br J Disord Commun 1990; 25:85–92.
1696. Plaitakis A. The olivopontocerebellar atrophies. New York: Thieme-Stratton, 1982:
1697. Plaitakis A. Abnormal metabolism of neuroexcitatory amino acids in olivopontocerebellar atrophy. In: Duvoisin RC, Plaitakis A, eds. The olivopontocerebellar atrophies—Advances in Neurology, Vol 41. New York: Raven Press, 1984:225–243.
1698. Plaitakis A, Berl L, Yahr M. Neurological disorders associated with deficiency of glutamate dehydrogenase. Ann Neurol 1984; 15:144–153.
1699. Plaitakis A, Nicklas W, Desnick R. Glutamate dehydrogenase deficiency in three patients with spinocerebellar syndrome. Ann Neurol 1980; 7:297–303.
1700. Plaitakis A, Berl S. Oral glutamate loading in disorders with spinocerebellar and extrapyramidal involvement: Effect on plasma glutamate, aspartate and taurine. J Neural Transm 1983; 19(suppl):65–74.
1701. Plaitakis A, Berl S, Yahr M. Abnormal glutamate metabolism in an adult onset degenerative neurological disorder. Science 1982; 216:193–196.
1702. Plato CC, Cruz MT, Kurland LT. Amyotrophic lateral sclerosis-Parkinsonism dementia complex of Guam: Further genetic investigations. Am J Hum Genet 1969; 21:133–141.
1703. Plato CC, Garruto R, Fox K. Familial and epidemiological studies of amyotrophic lateral sclerosis and parkinsonism-dementia of Guam: A twenty-five year prospective patient control study. Am J Epidemiol 1984; 120:478.
1704. Plato CC, Garruto R, Yanagihara R, Chen K, Wood J. Cortical bone loss and measurements of the second metacarpal bone. I. Comparisons between adult Guamanian Chamorros and American Caucasians. Am J Phys Anthropol 1982; 59:461–465.
1705. Plato CC, Garruto RM, Fox KM, Gajdusek DC. Amyotrophic lateral sclerosis and parkinsonism-dementia on Guam: A 25-year prospective case-control study. Am J Epidemiol 1986; 124:643–656.
1706. Plato CC, Grelich W, Garruto R, Yanagihara R. Cortical bone loss and measurements of the second metacarpal bone. II. Hypodense bone in post-war Guamanian children. Am J Phys Anthropol 1984; 63:57–63.
1707. Plato CC, Reed DM, Elizan TS, Kurland LT. Amyotrophic lateral sclerosis-Parkinsonism-dementia complex of Guam. IV. Familial and genetic investigations. Am J Hum Genet 1967; 19:617–632.

1708. Poeck K. [Letter: Paralysis agitans]. Dtsch Med Wochenschr 1976; 101:1077.
1709. Poewe W, Gerstenbrand F, Ransmayr G, Plörer S. Premorbid personality of Parkinson patients. J Neural Transm 1983; 19(suppl):215–224.
1710. Poewe W, Karamat E, Kemmler GW, Gerstenbrand F. The premorbid personality of patients with Parkinson's disease: A comparative study with healthy controls and patients with essential tremor. In: Parkinson's disease: anatomy, pathology and therapy. New York: Raven Press, 1990:339–342.
1711. Poirier J, Roy M, Campanella G, Cloutier T, Paris S. Debrisoquine metabolism in parkinsonian patients treated with antihistamine drugs. Lancet 1987; ii:386.
1712. Poirier J, Barbeau A. 1-Methyl-4-phenyl-pyridinium-induced inhibition of nicotinamide adenosine dinucleotide cytochrome c reductase. Neurosci Lett 1985; 62:7–11.
1713. Poirier J, Kogan S, Gauthier S. Environment, genetics and idiopathic Parkinson's disease. Can J Neurol Sci 1991; 18:70–76.
1714. Polinsky RJ. Multiple system atrophy. Clinical aspects pathophysiology, and treatment. Neurol Clin 1984; 2(3):487–498.
1715. Pollanen MS, Bergeron C, Weyer L. Detergent-insoluble cortical Lewy body fibrils share epitopes with neurofilament and tau. J Neurochem 1992; 58:1953–1956.
1716. Pollanen MS, Dickson DW, Bergeron C. Pathology and biology of the Lewy body. J Neuropathol Exp Neurol 1993; 52:183–191.
1717. Pollock M, Hornabrook RW. The prevalence, natural history and dementia of Parkinson's disease. Brain 1966; 89:429–448.
1718. Polyzoidis KS, McQueen JD, Rajput AH, MacFadyen DJ. Parkinsonism as a manifestation of brain tumor. Surg Neurol 1985; 23:59–63.
1719. Popovitch ER, Wisniewski HM, Kaufman MA, Grundke-Iqbal I, Wen GY. Young adult-form of dementia with neurofibrillary changes and Lewy bodies. Acta Neuropathol(Berlin) 1987; 74:97–104.
1720. Porrino LJ, Viola JJ, Crane AM, Pontieri FE. Alterations in opiate receptor binding in MPTP-induced hemiparkinsonian. Neurosci Lett 1991; 127:155–159.
1721. Porta EA. Advances in pigment research. Arch Gerontol Geriatr 1991; 12:303–320.
1722. Poser C. Epidemiology: Incidence, geographic distribution and genetic considerations by Kurland, L.T. Discussion: Varicella encephalitis as causing Parkinsonism (Posen 47-49). In: Field W, ed. Pathogenesis and treatment of parkinsonism. Springfield: Charles C. Thomas, 1958:5–49.
1723. Poser CM, Huntley CI, Poland ID. Para-encephalitic parkinsonism. Report of an acute case due to coxsackie virus type B2 and re-examination of the etiologic concepts of post-encephalitic parkinsonism. Acta Neurol Scand 1969; 45:199–215.
1724. Posey W. Paralysis of the upward movements of the eyes. Ann Opthalmol 1904; 13:523–529.
1725. Poskanzer D, Schwab R. Cohort analysis of parkinson's syndrome; evidence for a single etiology related to subclinical infection about 1920. J Chron Dis 1963; 16:961–973.
1726. Poskanzer DC, Schwab RS. Studies in the epidemiology of Parkinson's disease

predicting its disappearance as a major clinical entity by 1980. Trans Am Neurol Assoc 1961; 86:234–235.

1727. Poskanzer DC, Schwab RS, Fraser DW. The cohort phenomenon in Parkinson's syndrome. In: Gillingham FJ, Donaldson I, Fraser J, eds. Third Symposium on Parkinson's Disease. Edinburgh: F. S. Livingstone, 1969:8–12.

1728. Poskanzer DC, Schwab RS, Fraser DW. Further observations on the cohort phenomenon in Parkinson's syndrome. In: Barbeau A, Brunette JR, eds. Progress in neuro-genetics: Proceedings of the International Congress of Neuro-genetics and Neuro-opthalmology. Amsterdam: Exerpta Medica, 1969:497–505.

1729. Powell H, London G, Lampert P. Neurofibrillary tangles in progressive supranuclear palsy: Electron microscopic observations. J Neuropathol Exp Neurol 1974; 33:98–106.

1730. Powell W, Heacock RA. Chemistry of the aminochromes. XVII. Formation of addition products with bisulphite and thiols. J Chem Soc 1973; 509–515.

1731. Powell W, Heacock RA, Mattock GL, Wilson DL. Chemistry of the aminochromes. X. Some further observations on the reactions of aminochromes with thiols. Can J Chem 1969; 47:467–476.

1732. Prasher D, Bannister R. Brain stem auditory evoked potentials in patients with multiple system atrophy with progressive autonomic failure (Shy-Drager syndrome). J Neurol Neurosurg Psychiatry 1986; 49(3):278–289.

1733. Prell GD, Khandelwal JK, Burns RS, Blandina P, Morrishow AM, Green JP. Levels of pros-methylimidazoleacetic acid: Correlation with severity of Parkinson's disease in CSF of patients and with the depletion of striatal dopamine and its metabolites in MPTP-treated mice. J Neural Transm 1991; 3:109–125.

1734. Preziosi TJ, Lindenberg R, Levy D, Christenson M. An experimental investigation in animals of the functional and morphological effects of single and repeated exposures of high and low concentrations of carbon monoxide. Ann N Y Acad Sci 1970; 174:369–384.

1735. Prick JJG. Thallium poisoning. In: Vinken PI, Bruyn GW, eds. Handbook of clinical neurology, vol. 36, Intoxication of the nervous system, pt.1. Amsterdam: 1979:239–278.

1736. Pritchard PB, 3d., Netsky MG. Prevalence of neoplasms and causes of death in paralysis agitans. A necropsy study. Neurology 1973; 23:215–222.

1737. Prusiner SB. Prions and neurodegenerative diseases. N Engl J Med 1987; 317:1571–1581.

1738. Pruskauer-Apostol B, Popescu-Pretor R, Plaiasu D, Tataru E, Ciobanu I, Voiculescu V. The present status of encephalitis lethargica. Neurol Psychiatr (Bucur) 1977; 15:125–128.

1739. PSG Study Group on Environmental Influences. Smoking and age at onset of Parkinson's disease: Analysis of the DATATOP cohort. Ann Neurol 1990; 28:295.

1740. Purdy A, Hahn A, Barnett HJM, et al. Familial fatal parkinsonism with alveolar hypoventilation and mental depression. Ann Neurol 1979; 6:523–531.

1741. Qualman SJ, Haupt KM, Yang P, Hamilton SR. Esophageal Lewy bodies associated with ganglion cell loss in achalasia: Similarity to Parkinson's disease. Gastroenterology 1984; 87:848–856.

1742. Quarelli G. L'intossicazione professionaledu CS2. Bericht d.5. Internat Kongr f Berufskrankh. Budapest, 1928.
1743. Quarelli G. Solfocarbonismos professionale. Ressegna d Previd Sociale 1930; 21:10.
1744. Quattrini A, Paggi A, Del Pesce M, et al. [Anatomo-clinical investigations on 100 parkinsonian patients examined by CAT (author's transl)]. Riv Patol Nerv Ment 1978; 99:207–234.
1745. Quinn N. Disproportionate antecollis in multiple system atrophy [Letter to Editor]. Lancet 1989; 1:844.
1746. Quinn N. Multiple system atrophy—the nature of the beast. J Neurol Neurosurg Psychiatry 1989; Supp: 78–89.
1747. Quinn N, Critchley P, Marsden C. Young onset Parkinson's disease. Mov Disord 1987; 2:73–91.
1748. Quinn NP, Luthert P, Honavar M, Marsden CD. Pure akinesia due to Lewy body Parkinson's disease: A case with pathology. Mov Disord 1989; 4:85–89.
1749. Quinn NP, Parkes D, Janota I, Marsden CD. Preservation of the substantia nigra and locus ceruleus in a patient receiving levodopa (2kg) plus decarboxylase inhibitor over a four-year period. Mov Disord 1986; 1:65–68.
1750. Rabey JM, Grynberg E, Graff E. Cholinergic muscarinic binding of blood lymphocytes in patients with Parkinson's disease. In: Parkinson's disease: Anatomy, pathology and therapy—Advances in Neurology, Vol 53. New York: Raven Press, 1990:129–134.
1751. Rafal R, Grimm R. Progressive supranuclear palsy: Functional analysis of the response to methysergide and antiparkinsonian agents. Neurology 1981; 31:1507–1518.
1752. Ragozzino MW, Kurland LT, Rajput AH. Investigation of the association between herpes zoster and Parkinson's disease. Neuroepidemiology 1983; 2:89–92.
1753. Rail D, Scholtz C, Swash M. Post-encephalitic parkinsonism: Current experience. J Neurol Neurosurg Psychiatry 1981; 44:670–676.
1754. Rajasekhran Nair K, Bhaskaran R. Familial parkinsonism. Acta Neurol (Napoli) 1986; 8:633–638.
1755. Rajput AH. Epidemiology of Parkinson's disease. Can J Neurol Sci 1984; 11:156–159.
1756. Rajput AH. Frequency and cause of Parkinson's disease. Can J Neurol Sci 1992; 19:103–107.
1757. Rajput AH, Bennett VL, Uitti RJ. Early rural exposure as a risk to Parkinson's disease onset in later age (Abstract). 9th International Symposium on Parkinson's Disease 1988; 11.
1758. Rajput AH, Offord K, Beard CM, Kurland L. Essential tremor in Rochester, Minnesota: A 45 year study. J Neurol Neurosurg Psychiatry 1984; 47: 466–470.
1759. Rajput AH, Offord K, Beard CM, Kurland LT. Epidemiological survey of dementia in parkinsonism and control population. In: Parkinson-specific motor and mental disorders, role of the pallidum: pathophysiological, biochemical, and therapeutic aspects—Advances in neurology, Vol 40. New York: Raven Press, 1984:229–234.

1760. Rajput AH, Offord KP, Beard CM, Kurland LT. Epidemiology of parkinsonism: Incidence, classification, and mortality. Ann Neurol 1984; 16:278–282.

1761. Rajput AH, Offord KP, Beard CM, Kurland LT. A case-control study of smoking habits, dementia, and other illnesses in idiopathic Parkinson's disease. Neurology 1987; 37:226–232.

1762. Rajput AH, Rozdilsky B. Parkinsonism and dementia: Effects of levodopa. Lancet 1975; i:1084.

1763. Rajput AH, Rozdilsky B, Ang L, Rajput A. Clinicopathologic observations in essential tremor: Report of six cases. Neurology 1991; 41:1422–1424.

1764. Rajput AH, Rozdilsky B, Hornykiewicz O. Reversible drug-induced parkinsonism. Arch Neurol 1982; 39:644–646.

1765. Rajput AH, Rozdilsky B, Rajput A. Alzheimer's disease with idiopathic Parkinson's disease: Clinical, pharmacological, and pathological observations. Neurology 1990; 40(suppl. 1):339.

1766. Rajput AH, Rozdilsky B, Rajput A. Accuracy of clinical diagnosis in parkinsonism—a prospective study. Can J Neurol Sci 1991; 18:275–278.

1767. Rajput AH, Rozdulsky A. Occurrence of resting tremor in Parkinson's disease. Neurology 1991; 41:1298–1299.

1768. Rajput AH, Thiessen B. Parkinson's disease onset age in sibships. Ann Neurol 1989; 26:143.

1769. Rajput AH, Thiessen B, Munoz D, Laverty D, Desai H. Consideration of age and environments and number of substantia nigra cells. 9th International Symposium on Parkinson's Disease 1988; 11.

1770. Rajput AH, Uitti RJ. Paraquat and Parkinson's disease [letter]. Neurology 1987; 37:1820–1821.

1771. Rajput AH, Uitti RJ. Neurological disorders and services in Saskatchewan—A report based on provincial health care records. Neuroepidemiology 1988; 7:145–151.

1772. Rajput AH, Uitti RJ, Stern W, Laverty W. Early onset Parkinson's disease in Saskatchewan—environmental considerations for etiology. Can J Neurol Sci 1986; 13:312–316.

1773. Rajput AH, Uitti RJ, Stern W, Laverty W. Early onset Parkinson's disease and childhood environment. In: Parkinson's disease—Advances in Neurology, Vol 45. New York: Raven Press, 1986:295–297.

1774. Rajput AH, Uitti RJ, Stern W, et al. Geography, drinking water chemistry, pesticides and herbicides and the etiology of Parkinson's disease. Can J Neurol Sci 1987; 14:414–418.

1775. Ramsay RR, Kowal AT, Johnson K, Salach JI, Singer TP. The inhibition site of MPP+ the neuotoxic bioactivation product of 1-methyl-4-phenyl-1,2,3,6-tetrahydropyridine is near the Q-binding site of NADH dehydrogenase. Arch Biochem Biophys 1987; 259:645–649.

1776. Ramsay RR, Krueger MJ, Youngster SK, Gluck MR, Casida JE, Singer TP. Interaction of 1-methyl-4-phenylpyridinium ion (MPP+) and its analogs with the rotenone/piericidin binding site of NADH dehydrogenase. J Neurochem 1991; 56:1184–1190.

1777. Ramsay RR, Salach JI, Dadgar J, Singer TP. Inhibition of mitochondrial NADH dehydrogenase by pyridine derivatives and its possible relation to experimental and idiopathic parkinsonism. Biochem Biophys Res Commun 1986; 135(1):269–275.

1778. Ramsay RR, Youngster SK, Nicklas WJ. Structural dependence of the inhibition of mitochondrial respiration and of NADH oxidase by 1-methyl-4-phenylpyridinium (MPP+) analogs and their energized accumulation by mitochondria. Proc Natl Acad Sci 1989; 86:9168–9172.
1779. Ramsden DB, Williams AC. Production in nature of compound resembling methylphenyltetrahydropyridine, a possible cause of Parkinson's disease. Lancet 1985; 1:215–216.
1780. Ranelletti A. Die berufliche Schwefelkohlenstoff Vergiftung in Italien. Arch f Gewerbepath u Gewerbehyg 1931; 2:664.
1781. Ransom BR, Kunis DM, Irwin I, Langston JW. Astrocytes convert the parkinsonism-inducing neurotoxin, MPTP, to its active metabolite, MPP+. Neurosci Lett 1987; 75:323–328.
1782. Raps SP, Lai JCK, Hertz L, Cooper AJL. Glutathione is present in high concentrations in cultured astrocytes but not in cultured neurons. Brain Res 1989; 493:398–401.
1783. Rascol O, Clanet M, Montastruc JL, et al. Abnormal ocular movements in Parkinson's disease. Evidence for involvement of dopaminergic systems. Brain 1989; 112:1193–1214.
1784. Raskin SA, Borod JC, Wasserstein J, Bodis-Wollner I, Coscia L, Yahr MD. Visuospatial orientation in Parkinson's disease. Int J Neurosci 1990; 51:9–18.
1785. Rathus EM, Landy PJ. Methyl bromide poisoning. Br J Indust Med 1961; 18:53–57.
1786. Rausch WD, Hirata Y, Nagatsu T, Riederer P, Jellinger K. Tyrosine hydroxylase activity in caudate nucleus from Parkinson's disease: Effects of iron and phosphorylating agents. J Neurochem 1988; 50:202–208.
1787. Rautakorpi I, Takala J, Marttila RJ, Sievers K, Rinne UK. Essential tremor in a Finnish population. Acta Neurol Scand 1982; 66:58–67.
1788. Ravenholt R, Foege W. 1918 Influenza, encephalitis lethargica, parkinsonism. Lancet 1982; ii:860–864.
1789. Rawat AK. Ethanol and psychotropic drug interaction during pregnancy and lactation. Biochem Pharmacol 1981; 30(17):2457–2460.
1790. Rebeiz J, Kolodny E, Richardson E. Corticodentatonigral degeneration with neuronal achromasia. Arch Neurol 1968; 18:20–33.
1791. Reches A, Burk R, Kuhn C, Fahn S. Tetrabenazine, an amine-depleting drug, also blocks dopamine receptors in rat brain. J Pharmacol Exp Ther 1983; 225:515–521.
1792. Reden J, Ripka WC, Rice KC, Brossi A. 4-Hydroxy-1,2,3,4-tetrahydroisoquinolines: Potential reaction products of norepinephrine. In: Begleiter H, ed. Biological effects of ethanol. New York: Plenum Press, 1980:69–84.
1793. Reed D, Labarthe D, Chen KM, Stallones R. A cohort study of amyotrophic lateral sclerosis and parkinsonism-dementia on Guam and Rota. Am J Epidemiol 1987; 125:92–100.
1794. Reed D, Plato C, Elizan T, Kurland LT. The amyotrophic lateral sclerosis/

parkinsonism-dementia complex: A ten year follow-up on Guam. I. Epidemiology studies. Am J Epidemiol 1966; 83:54–73.

1795. Reed DM, Brody JA. Amyotrophic lateral sclerosis and parkinsonism-dementia on Guam, 1945–1972. I. Descriptive epidemiology. Am J Epidemiol 1975; 101:287–301.

1796. Reed DM, Torres JM, Brody JA. Amyotrophic lateral sclerosis and parkinsonism-dementia on Guam, 1945–1972. II. Familial and genetic studies. Am J Epidemiol 1975; 101:320–310.

1797. Reed E, Lewison A, Mayeux R, Suciu-Foca N. HLA antigens in Parkinson's disease. Tissue Antigens 1983; 21:161–163.

1798. Reef HE. 11th World Congress of Neurology, International Congress Series 427. In: Jager HWA, Bruyn GW, Heihstee APJ, eds. Prevalence of Parkinson's disease in a multiracial community. Amsterdam: Excerpta Medica, 1977:125.

1799. Reiderer P, Lange KW. Pathogenesis of Parkinson's disease. Curr Opin Neurol Neurosurg 1992; 5:295–300.

1800. Reisner H. [Enzymopathies with psychiatric and neurologic symptoms]. Wein Klin Wochenschr 1971; 83:303–306.

1801. Reshef JM, Rabey P, Bar A, Schlosberg A, Korczyn AD. Smoking and drug-induced parkinsonism. Neurology 1987; 37:121.

1802. Riachi NJ, Behmand RA, Harik SI. Correlation of MPTP neurotoxicity in vivo with oxidation of MPTP by the brain and blood-brain barrier in vitro in five rat strains. Brain Res 1991; 555:19–24.

1803. Riachi NJ, Harik SI. Strain differences in systemic 1-methyl-4-phenyl-1,2,3,6-tetrahydropyridine neurotoxicity in mice correlate best with monoamine oxidase activity at the blood-brain barrier. Life Sci 1988; 42:2359–2363.

1804. Riachi NJ, Harik SI, Kalaria RN, Sayre LM. On the mechanisms underlying 1-methyl-4-phenyl-1,2,3,6-tetrahydropyridine neurotoxicity. II. Susceptibility among mammalian species correlates with the toxin's metabolic patterns in brain microvessels and liver. J Pharmacol Exp Ther 1988; 244(2):443–448.

1805. Riachi NJ, LaManna JC, Harik SI. Entry of 1-methyl-4-phenyl-1,2,3,6-tetrahydropyridine into the rat brain. J Pharmacol Exp Ther 1989; 249:744–748.

1806. Ricaurte GA, DeLanney LE, Irwin I, Langston JW. Older dopaminergic neurons do not recover from the effects of MPTP. Neuropharmacology 1987; 26(1):97–99.

1807. Ricaurte GA, Irwin I, Forno LS, DeLanney LE, Langston EB, Langston JW. Aging and MPTP-induced degeneration of dopaminergic neurons in the substantia nigra. Brain Res 1987; 403:43–51.

1808. Ricaurte GA, Langston JW, DeLanney LE, Irwin I, Brooks JD. Dopamine uptake blockers protect against the dopamine depleting effects of 1-methyl-4-phenyl-1,2,3,6-tetrahydropyridine (MPTP) in the mouse striatum. Neurosci Lett 1985; 59:259–264.

1809. Ricaurte GA, Langston JW, DeLanney LE, Irwin I, Peroutka SJ, Forno LS. Fate of nigrostriatal neurons in young mature mice given 1-methyl-4-phenyl-1,2,3,6-tetrahydropyridine: A neurochemical and morphological reassessment. Brain Res 1986; 376:117–124.

1810. Richardson EP Jr. Parkinson's disease [editorial]. Ann Neurol 1986; 20:447–448.

1811. Richardson J, Steele J, Olszewski J. Supranuclear ophthalmoplegia, pseudobulbar palsy, nuchal dystonia and dementia. Trans Am Neurol Assoc 1963; 88:25–29.
1812. Richter R. Degeneration of the basal ganglia in monkeys from chronic carbon disulfide poisoning. J Neuropathol Exp Neurol 1945; 4:324–353.
1813. Richter R, Shimojyo S. Neurologic sequelae of Japanese B encephalitis. Neurology 1961; 11:553–559.
1814. Riederer P, Dirr A, Goetz M, Sofic E, Jellinger K, Youdim MBH. Distribution of iron in different brain regions and subcellular compartments in Parkinson's disease. Ann Neurol 1992; 32 Suppl.:S101–S104.
1815. Riederer P, Rausch WD, Schmidt B. Biochemical fundamentals of Parkinson's disease. Mt Sinai J Med 1988; 55(1):21–28.
1816. Riederer P, Sofic E, Rausch WD, et al. Transition metals, ferritin, glutathione, and ascorbic acid in parkinsonian brains. J Neurochem 1989; 52:515–520.
1817. Riederer P, Wuketich St. Time course of nigrostriatal degeneration in Parkinson's disease: A detailed study of influential factors in human brain amine analysis. J Neural Transm 1976; 38:277–301.
1818. Riggs JE. Longitudinal Gompertzian analysis of Parkinson's disease mortality in the U.S., 1955–1986: The dramatic increase in overall mortality since 1980 is the natural consequence of deterministic mortality dynamics. Mech Age Dev 1990; 55:221–233.
1819. Riggs N, Finley K. Sequelae of Western Encephalitis and St. Louis Encephalitis. California Vector Views 1960; 7:35–41.
1820. Riley D, Lang A, Lewis A, et al. Cortical-basal ganglionic degeneration. Neurology 1990; 40:1203–1212.
1821. Ringel S, Klawans H. Carbon monoxide induced parkinsonism. J Neurol Sci 1972; 16:245–251.
1822. Ringwald E. What causes Parkinson's disease? (Letter). Lancet 1984; February 11:336.
1823. Rinne JO, Halonen T, Riekkinen PJ, Rinne UK. Free amino acids in the brain of patients with Parkinson's disease. Neurosci Lett 1988; 94:182–186.
1824. Rinne JO, Laihinen A, N angren K, et al. PET demonstrates different behaviour of striatal dopamine D-1 and D-2 receptors in early Parkinson's disease. J Neurosci Res 1990; 27:494–499.
1825. Rinne JO, Rummukainen J, Paljarvi L, Sako E, Molsa P, Rinne UK. Neuronal loss in the substantia nigra in patients with Alzheimer's disease and Parkinson's disease in relation to extrapyramidal symptoms and dementia. Prog Clin Biol Res 1989; 317:325–332.
1826. Rinne UK. Recent advances in research on parkinsonism. In: Marttila RJ, ed. Proceedings of the 22nd Scandinavian Congress of Neurology. Acta Neurologica Scandinavica, 1978:77–113.
1827. Rinne UK, Laihinen A, Rinne JO, Ñagren K, Bergman J, Ruotsalainen U. Positron emission tomography demonstrates dopamine D2 receptor supersensitivity in the striatum of patients with early Parkinson's disease. Mov Disord 1990; 5:55–59.
1828. Robbins JH. Alkaloid formation by condensation of biogenic amines with acetaldehyde. Clinical Research 1968; 16:350.

1829. Robbins JH. Possible alkaloid formation in alcoholism and other diseases. Clinical Research 1968; 15:554.

1830. Robbins JH. Parkinson's disease, twins, and the DNA-damage hypothesis [letter]. Ann Neurol 1987; 21:412.

1831. Robbins JH, Otsuka F, Tarone RE, Polinsky RJ, Brumback RA, Nee LE. Parkinson's disease and Alzheimer's disease: Hypersensitivity to X rays in cultured cell lines. J Neurol Neurosurg Psychiatry 1985; 48:916–923.

1832. Roberts AH. Brain damage in boxers. London: Pitman Medical and Scientific Pubishing Co., Ltd, 1969.

1833. Robertson RG, Clarke CA, Boyce S, Sambrook MA, Crossman AR. The role of striatopallidal neurones utilizing gamma-aminobutyric acid in the pathophysiology of MPTP-induced parkinsonism in the primate: Evidence from [3H]flunitrazepam autoradiography. Brain Res 1990; 531:95–104.

1834. Robins AH. Tyrosine hydroxylation in Parkinsonism. Lancet 1971; 1:1350.

1835. Robinson DS, Davis JM, Nies A, Ravaris CL, Sylwester D. Relation of sex and aging to monoamine oxidase activity of human brain, plasma, and platelets. Arch Gen Psychiatry 1971; 24:536–539.

1836. Robinson DS, Sourkes TL, Nies A. Monoamine metabolism in human brain. Arch Gen Psychiatry 1977; 34:89–92.

1837. Rocca WA, Morgante L, Grigoletto F, et al. Prevalence of Parkinson's disease (PD) and other parkinsonisms: A door-to-door survey in two Sicilian communities. Neurology 1990; 40(suppl 1):422.

1838. Rodgers AD, Curzon G. Melanin formation by human brain in vitro. J Neurochem 1975; 24:1123–1129.

1839. Rodgers-Johnson P, Garruto R, Yanagihara R. Amyotrophic lateral sclerosis and parkinsonism-dementia on Guam: A 30 year evaluation of clinical and neuropathological trends. Neurology 1986; 36:7–13.

1840. Rogers JD, Brogan D, Mirra SS. The nucleus basalis of Meynert in neurological disease: a quantitative morphological study. Ann Neurol 1985; 17:163–170.

1841. Rogers R, Powell-Griner E. Life expectancies of cigarette smokers and nonsmokers in the United States. Soc Sci Med 1991; 32:1151–1159.

1842. Rollema H, Alexander GM, Grothusen JR, Matos FF, Castagnoli N,Jr.. Comparison of the effects of intracerebrally administered MPP+ (1-methyl-4-phenylpyridinium) in three species: Microdialysis of dopamine and metabolites in mouse, rat and monkey striatum. Neurosci Lett 1989; 106:275–281.

1843. Rollema H, De Vries JB, Damsma G, et al. The use of in vivo brain dialysis of dopamine, acetylcholine, aminoacids and lactic acid in studies on the neurotoxin 1-methyl-4-phenyl-1,2,3,6-tetrahydropyridine (MPTP). Toxicology 1988; 49:503–511.

1844. Rollema H, De Vries JB, Westerink BHC, Van Putten FMS, Horn AS. Failure to detect 6-hydroxydopamine in rat striatum after the dopamine releasing drugs dexamphetamine, methylamphetamine and MPTP. Eur J Pharmacol 1986; 132:65–69.

1845. Rollema H, Johnson EA, Booth RG, et al. In vivo dopaminergic neurotoxicity of the 2-beta-mehylcarbolinium ion, a potential endogenous MPP+ analog. Eur J Pharmacol 1988; 153:131–134.

1846. Rollema H, Johnson EA, Booth RG, et al. In vivo intracerebral microdialysis studies in rats of MPP+ analogues and related charged species. J Med Chem 1990; 33:2221–2230.
1847. Rollema H, Kuhr WG, Kranenborg GL, De Vries JB, Van Den Berg C. MPP+-induced efflux of dopamine and lactate from rat striatum have similar time courses as shown by in vivo brain dialysis. J Pharmacol Exp Ther 1988; 245(3):858–866.
1848. Romàn GC, Zhang Z-X, Ellenberg JH. The neuroepidemiology of Parkinson's disease. In: Ellenberg JH, Koller WC, Langston JW, eds. Etiology of Parkinson's disease. New York: Marcel Dekker, 1994:203–243.
1849. Romberg MH. Lehrbuch der Nervenkrankheiten des Menschen. Berlin: Dunker, 1851.
1850. Rommelspacher H, Coper H, Strauss S. On the mode of formation of tetrahydro-beta-carbolines. Life Sci 1976; 18:81–88.
1851. Rommelspacher H, Nanz C, Borbe HO, Fehske KJ, Muller WE, Wollert U. 1-Methyl-beta- carboline (harmane), a potent endogenous inhibitor of benzodiazepine receptor binding. Arch Pharmacol 1980; 314:97–100.
1852. Rommelspacher H, Nanz C, Borbe HO, Fehske KJ, Muller WE, Wollert U. Benzodiazepine antagonism by harmane and other beta-carbolines in vitro and in vivo. Eur J Pharmacol 1981; 70:409–416.
1853. Rommelspacher H, Susilo R. Tetrahydroisoquinolines and beta-carbolines: Putative natural substances in plants and animals. In: Jucker E, ed. Progress in drug research, Volume 29. Basel: Burkhauser-Verlag, 1985:415–459.
1854. Roos B, Lycke E. Viral infections in the central nervous system and 5-hydroxytryptamine metabolism. Adv Biochem Psychopharmacol 1974; 2:115–117.
1855. Roos RAC, Steenvoorden JMC, Mulder GJ, Van Kempen GMJ. Acetaminophen sulfation in patients with Parkinson's disease or Huntington's disease is not impaired. Neurology 1993; 43:1373–1376.
1856. Rosati G, Granieri E, Pinna L, et al. Parkinson's disease. Prevalence and incidence in the province of Sassari, North Sardinia. Acta Neurol (Napoli) 1978; 33:201–207.
1857. Rosati G, Granieri E, Pinna L, et al. The risk of Parkinson's disease in Mediterranean people. Neurology 1980; 30:250–255.
1858. Rosati G, Granieri E, Pinna L, Devoto MC. The frequency of Parkinson's disease in the province of Nuoro (Sardinia). Acta Neurol Scand 1979; 1:303–308.
1859. Rosenberg NL, Myers JA, Martin WR. Cyanide-induced parkinsonism: Clinical, MRI, and 6-fluorodopa PET studies. Neurology 1989; 39:142–144.
1860. Rosenberg R, Banner C. Normal cerebellar glutamate dehydrogenase protein in spinocerebellar degeneration. J Neurol Sci 1989; 52:666–668.
1861. Rosenberg RN, Nyhan WL, Bay C, Shore P. Autosomal dominant striatonigral degeneration. A clinical, pathologic, and biochemical study of a new genetic disorder. Neurology 1976; 26:703–714.
1862. Rosenblum A, Montgomery E. Exacerbation of parkinsonism by methyldopa. JAMA 1980; 224:2727–2728.
1863. Rosengren E, Linder-Eliasson E, Carlsson A. Detection of 5-s-cysteinyl-DA in human brain. J Neural Transm 1985; 63:247–253.
1864. Rosenthal G, Gilman S, Koeppa RA, et al. Motor dysfunction in olivopontocere-

bellar atrophy is related to cerebralmetabolic rate studied with positron emission tomography. Ann Neurol 1988; 24(3):414–419.

1865. Rosetti ZL, Sotgiu A, Sharp D, Hadjiconstantinou M, Neff MH. 1-Methyl-4-phenyl-1,2,3,6-tetrahydropyridine (MPTP) and free radicals in vitro. Biochem Pharmacol 1988; 37:4573–4574.

1866. Rosing HS, Hopkins LC, Wallace DC, Epstein CM, Weidenheim K. Maternally inherited mitochondrial myopathy and myoclonic epilepsy. Ann Neurol 1985; 17:228–237.

1867. Ross CA, McInnis MG, Margolis RL, Li SH. Genes with triple repeats: Candidate mediators of meuropsychiatric disorders. TINS 1993; 16, No.7:254–260.

1868. Ross GW, Mahler ME, Cummings JL. The dementia syndromes of Parkinson's disease: Cortical and subcortical features. In: Huber SJ, Cummings JL, eds. Parkinson's disease: neurobehavioral aspects. New York: Oxford University Press, 1992:132–148.

1869. Ross RT. Young age Parkinsonism and common drugs: To the Editor (Letter). Can J Neurol Sci 1989; 16:366–367.

1870. Ross RT. Drug-induced parkinsonism and other movement disorders. Can J Neurol Sci 1990; 17:155–162.

1871. Ross S, Spencer P. Specific antagonism of behavioral action of ''uncommon'' amino acids linked to motor-system disease. Synapse 1987; 1:248–253.

1872. Ross SM, Seelig M, Spencer PS. Specific antagonism of excitotoxic action of 'uncommon' amino acids assayed by organotypic mouse cortical cultures. Brain Res 1987; 425:120–127.

1873. Rouillard C, Bédard PJ, Di Paolo T. Effects of chronic treatment of MPTP monkeys with bromocriptine alone or in combination with SKF 38393. Eur J Pharmacol 1990; 185:209–215.

1874. Roy M, Boyer L, Barbeau A. A prospective study of 50 cases of familial Parkinson's disease. Can J Neurol Sci 1983; 10:37–42.

1875. Roy S, Datta C, Hirano A, Ghatak N, Zimmerman H. Electron microscopic study of neurofibrillary tangles in Steele-Richardson-Olszewski syndrome. Acta Neuropathol(Berlin) 1974; 29:175–179.

1876. Rub H, Henning K, Ekhardt H, Przuntek H. The influence of N-methyl-4-phenyl-1,2,3,6-tetrahydropyridine on the levels of dopamine, serotonin and their metabolites in the caudate nucleus of the rat. Arzneim-Forsch/Drug Research 1985; 35(1):481.

1877. Rubenstein A, Brust JC. Parkinsonian syndrome as complication of post-thyroidectomy hypoparathyroidism. N Y State J Med 1974; 74:2029–2030.

1878. Ruberg M, Javoy-Agid F, Agid Y. What causes Parkinson's disease? (Letter). Lancet 1984; February 11:336–337.

1879. Ruberg M, Javoy-Agid F, Hirsch E. Dopaminergic and cholinergic lesions in progressive supranuclear palsy. Ann Neurol 1985; 18:523–529.

1880. Rutledge JN. Magnetic resonance of movement disorders. In: Jankovic J, Tolosa E, eds. Parkinson's disease and movement disorders. Baltimore: Urban & Schwartzenberg, 1988:441–460.

1881. Ruttenber AJ, Garbe PL, Kalter HD, et al. Meperidine analog exposure in California narcotics abusers: Initial epidemiologic findings. In: Markey SP, Castagnoli

N Jr, Trevor AJ, Kopin IJ, eds. MPTP: A neurotoxin producing a parkinsonian syndrome. New York: Academic Press, 1986:339–353.

1882. Rybicki BA, Johnson CC, Uman J, Gorell JM. Parkinson's disease mortality and the industrial use of heavy metals in Michigan. Mov Disord 1993; 8,(1):87–92.

1883. Sachdev KK, Singh N, Krishnamoorthy MS. Juvenile parkinsonism treated with levodopa. Arch Neurol 1977; 34:244–245.

1884. Sacks OW, Kohl MS, Messelloff CR, Schwartz WF. Effects of levodopa in parkinsonism patients with dementia. Neurology 1972; 22:516–519.

1885. Sadibelouiz A, Sadibelouiz M. Parkinson's disease in Algiers: Report of 183 cases (Abstract). Mov Disord 1990; 5:11.

1886. Sagar HJ. Clinical similarities and differences between Alzheimer's disease and Parkinson's disease. J Neural Transm 1987; (Suppl)24:87–99.

1887. Sage JI. Tomatoes and Parkinson's disease. Med Hypotheses 1989; 28:75–79.

1888. Sage JI, Mark MA. Diffuse Lewy body disease. In: Stern MB, Koller WC, eds. Parkinsonian syndromes. New York: Marcel Dekker, 1993:393–411.

1889. Sage JI, Miller DC, Golbe LI, Walters A, Duvoisin RC. Clinically atypical expression of pathologically typical Lewy-body parkinsonism. Clin Neuropharmacol 1990; 13:36–47.

1890. Saggu H, Cooksey J, Dexter DT. A selective increase in particulate superoxide dismutase activity in parkinsonian substantia nigra. J Neurochem 1989; 53:692–697.

1891. Saheb SE, Dajani RM. 1-Methyl-6-hydroxytetrahydrocarboline: a possible product of ethanol and tryptophan metabolism. Comp Gen Pharmac 1973; 4:225–227.

1892. Sahgal A, Andrews JS, Biggins JA, et al. N-methyl-4-phenyl-1,2,3,6-tetrahydropyridine (MPTP) affects locomotor activity without producing a nigrostriatal lesion in the rat. Neurosci Lett 1984; 48:179–184.

1893. Saito T, Mizuno Y, Yoshida M. [Differential diagnosis of parkinsonism based on a semiquantitative scoring system—chiefly to discriminate two major causes, paralysis agitans and vascular parkinsonism]. Rinsho Shinkeigaku 1985; 25:591–596.

1894. Saitoh T, Mizuno Y, Nagatsu T, Yoshida M. Effect of long-term administration of 1,2,3,4-tetrahydroisoquinoline (TIQ) on striatal dopamine and 3,4-dihydroxyphenylacetic acid (DOPAC) content in mice. Neurosci Lett 1988; 92:321–324.

1895. Saitoh T, Niijima K, Mizuno Y. Long-term effect of 1-methyl-4-phenyl-1,2,3,6-tetrahydropyridine (MPTP) on striatal dopamine content in young and mature mice. J Neurol Sci 1987; 77:229–235.

1896. Salazar M, Sokoloski TD, Patil PN. Binding of dopaminergic drugs by the neuromelanin of the substantia nigra, synthetic melanins and melanin granules. Fed Proc 1978; 37:2403–2407.

1897. Salganik I, Korczyn. Risk factors for dementia in Parkinson's disease. In: Parkinson's disease: Anatomy, pathology and therapy—Advances in Neurology, Vol 53. New York: Raven Press, 1990:343–347.

1898. Salisachs P, Findley LJ. Problems in the differential diagnosis of essential tremor. In: Findley LJ, Capildeo R, eds. Movement disorders: Tremor. London: Macmillan, 1984:219–224.

1899. Samiy E. Chronic subdural hematoma presenting a Parkinsonian syndrome. J Neurosurg 1963; 20:903.
1900. Samorajski T, Rolsten C. Age and regional differences in the chemical composition of brain of mice, monkeys and humans. Proc Brain Res 1973; 40:253–265.
1901. Sampaio C, Castro Caldas A. [Etiopathogeny of Parkinson disease. The MPTP revolution]. Acta Med Port 1988; 1:304–307.
1902. Sanchez-Ramos JR, Barrett JN, Goldstein M, Weiner WJ, Hefti F. 1-Methyl-4-phenylpyridinium (MPP+) but not 1-methyl-4-phenyl-1,2, 3,6-tetrahydropyridine (MPTP) selectively destroys dopaminergic neurons in cultures of dissociated rat mesencephalic neurons. Neurosci Lett 1986; 72:215–220.
1903. Sanchez-Ramos JR, Factor SA, Weiner WJ. Paraquat and Parkinson's Disease: Reply from the Authors (Letter). Neurology 1987; 37:1820–1821.
1904. Sanchez-Ramos JR, Hefti F, Weiner WJ. Paraquat and Parkinson's disease [letter]. Neurology 1987; 37:728.
1905. Sandler M, Carter SB, Hunter KR, Stern GM. Tetrahydroisoquinoline alkaloids: In vivo metabolites of L-dopa in man. Nature 1973; 241:439–443.
1906. Sandow BA, West NB, Norman RJ, Brenner RM. Hormonal control of apoptosis in hamster uterine luminal epithelium. Am J Anat 1979; 156:15–35.
1907. Sandy MS, Langston JW, Smith MT, Di Monte DA. PCR analysis of platelet mtDNA: Lack of specific changes in Parkinson's disease. Mov Disord 1993; 8(1):74–82.
1908. Sandy MS, Smith J, Langston W, Di Monte D. Comparison of mitochondrial DNA from platelets of Parkinsonian patients and controls. (Neurotoxins and their potential role in neurodegeneration). The New York Academy of Sciences, May 6–8 1991; PI–29.(abstract)
1909. Sandyk R. Parkinsonism after hysterectomy: To the Editor (Letter). S Afr Med J 1982; 61:574.
1910. Sandyk R. Parkinsonism caused by chronic subdural hematoma. S Afr Med J 1982; 17:595–596.
1911. Sandyk R. Parkinsonism secondary to neurosyphilis. A case report. S Afr Med J 1983; 63:665–666.
1912. Sandyk R. Parkinson's disease and thalassalmia in a South African family of Greek origin [letter]. S Afr Med J 1983; 63:141.
1913. Sandyk R. Autoimmune mechanisms in Parkinson's disease. Int J Neurosci 1989; 48:369–375.
1914. Sandyk R. Pineal melatonin functions: Possible relevance to Parkinson's disease. Int J Neurosci 1990; 50:37–53.
1915. Sandyk R. Pineal melatonin functions and the depression of Parkinson's disease: A hypothesis. Int J Neurosci 1990; 51:73–77.
1916. Sandyk R, Iacono RP. Hypothalamic-mediated immune mechanisms and their relevance to the pathoetiology of Parkinson's disease [letter]. Int J Neurosci 1987; 32:979–981.
1917. Sandyk R, Iacono RP. The relationship of the reticular system to the primary pathoetiology of Parkinson's disease. Int J Neurosci 1988; 42:297–300.
1918. Sandyk R, Iacono RP. The neurotoxicity of MPTP and its relationship to the pathophysiology of Parkinson's disease. Int J Neurosci 1989; 44:165–167.

1919. Sandyk R, Iacono RP. Early versus late-onset Parkinson's disease: The role of the locus coeruleus [letter]. Int J Neurosci 1990; 52:243–247.
1920. Sandyk R, Kahn I. Parkinsonism due to subdural hematoma. Case report. J Neurosurg 1983; 58:298–299.
1921. Sandyk R, Kay SR. Relationship of neuroleptic-induced akathisia to drug-induced parkinsonism. Ital J Neurol Sci 1990; 11:439–442.
1922. Sandyk R, Pardeshi R. Pyridoxine improves drug-induced parkinsonism and psychosis in a schizophrenic patient. Int J Neurosci 1990; 52:225–232.
1923. Santamaria J, Tolosa E, Valles A. Parkinson's disease with depression: A possible subgroup of idiopathic parkinsonism. Neurology 1986; 36:1130–1133.
1924. Santiago M, Rollema H, De Vries JB, Westerink BHC. Acute effects of intranigral application of MPP+ on nigral and bilateral striatal release of dopamine simultaneously recorded by microdialysis. Brain Res 1991; 538:226–230.
1925. Santiago M, Westerink BHC, Rollema H. Responsiveness of striatal dopamine release in awake animals after chronic 1-methyl-4-phenylpyridinium ion-induced lesions of the substantia nigra. J Neurochem 1991; 56:1336–1342.
1926. Saper CB, Sorrentino DM, German DC, deLacalle S. Medullary catecholaminergic neurons in the normal human brain and in Parkinson's disease. Ann Neurol 1991; 29:577–584.
1927. Sarna T, Duleba A, Korytowksi W, Swartz HM. Interaction of melanin with oxygen. Arch Biochem Biophys 1980; 200:140–148.
1928. Sasaki H, Hamada T, Wakisaka A, Tashiro K. A clinical study of a family affected with HLA-linked hereditary spinocerebellar ataxia. No To Shinkei. Brain Nerve 1990; 42(11):1103–1111.
1929. Sasaki H, Sudoh K, Hamada K, Manada T, Tashiro K. Skeletal myoclonus in olivopontocerebellar atrophy: Treatment with trihexphenidyl. Neurology 1987; 37(7):1258–1262.
1930. Sasco A, Paffenbarger R. Smoking and Parkinson's disease. Epidemiology 1990; 6:460–465.
1931. Sasco AJ, Paffenbarger RS,Jr.. Measles infection and Parkinson's disease. Am J Epidemiol 1985; 122:1017–1031.
1932. Sato T, Ikuta F. Neuropathology of methylmercury intoxication in Niigata and chronic effects in monkeys. In: Roizin L, Shiraki H, Grcevic N, eds. Neurotoxicology. New York: Raven Press, 1977:261–274.
1933. Satoyashi E, Narabayashi H, Tsubaki T, Mozai T, Sobue I. [Round table discussion: topics on neuromuscular disease]. Naika 1971; 28:538–552.
1934. Savill JS, Wyllie AH, Hensen JE, Walport MJ, Hensen PM, Haslett C. Macrophage phagocytosis of ageing neutrophils in inflammation: Programmed cell death in the neutrophil leads to its recognition by macrophages. J Clin Invest 1989; 83:865–875.
1935. Savoiardo M, Steada L, Girotti F, et al. MR imaging in progressive supranuclear palsy and Shy-Drager syndrome. J Comput Assist Tomogr 1989; 13:555–560.
1936. Savoiardo M, Strada L, Girotti F, et al. Olivopontocerebellar atrophy: MR diagnosis and relationship to multisystem atrophy. Radiology 1990; 174:693–696.
1937. Sawle GV, Colebatch JG, Brooks DJ, Marsden CD, Frackowiak RSJ. PET studies of the aging nigrostriatal system (Abstract). Mov Disord 1990; 5:18.

1938. Sawle GV, Colebatch JG, Shah A, Brooks DJ, Marsden CD, Frackowiak RS. Striatal function in normal aging: Implications for Parkinson's disease. Ann Neurol 1990; 28:799–804.

1939. Sawle GV, Wroe SJ, Lees AJ, Brooks DJ, Frackowiak RSJ. The identification of presymptomatic Parkinsonism: Clinical and [18F] dopa positron emission tomography studies in an Irish kindred. Ann Neurol 1992; 32,No5:609–617.

1940. Sayre LM. Biochemical mechanism of action of the dopaminergic neurotoxin 1-methyl-4-phenyl-1,2,3,6-tetrahydropyridine (MPTP). Toxicol Lett 1989; 48:121–149.

1941. Sayre LM, Arora PK, Iacofano LA, Harik SI. Comparative toxicity of MPTP, MPP+ and 3,3-dimethyl-MPDP+ to dopaminergic neurons of the rat substantia nigra. Eur J Pharmacol 1986; 124:171–174.

1942. Sayre LM, Singh MP, Arora PK, Wang F, McPeak RJ, Hoppel CL. Inhibition of mitochondrial respiration by analogues of the dopaminergic neurotoxin 1-methyl-4-phenylpyridinium: Structural requirements for accumulation-dependent enhanced inhibitory potency on intact mitochondria. Arch Biochem Biophys 1990; 280:274–283.

1943. Scarr S. Progress in Human Behavior genetics -Recent reports on genetic syndromes, twin studies, and statistical advances. In: Vandenberg SG, ed. Environmental bias in twin studies. Baltimore: Johns Hopkins Press, 1968:205–219.

1944. Schapira AH, Holt IJ, Sweeney M, Harding AE, Jenner P, Marsden CD. Mitochondrial DNA analysis in Parkinson's disease. Mov Disord 1990; 5:294–297.

1945. Schapira AHV. MPTP and other Parkinson-inducing agents. Current Science 1992; 5:396–400.

1946. Schapira AHV, Cooper JM, Dexter CD, Clark JB, Jenner P, Marsden CD. Mitochondrial complex I deficiency in Parkinson's disease (Abstract). Ann Neurol 1989; 26:122–123.

1947. Schapira AHV, Cooper JM, Dexter D, Clark JB, Jenner P, Marsden CD. Mitochondrial complex I deficiency in Parkinson's disease. J Neurochem 1990; 54(3):823–827.

1948. Schapira AHV, Cooper JM, Dexter D, Jenner P, Clark JB, Marsden CD. Mitochondrial complex I deficiency in Parkinson's disease (Letter). Lancet 1989; i:1269.

1949. Schapira AHV, Mann VM, Cooper JM, et al. Anatomic and disease specificity of NADHCoQ1 reductase (complex I) deficiency in Parkinson's disease. J Neurochem 1990; 55:2142–2145.

1950. Schapira AHV, Mann VM, Cooper JM, Krige D, Jenner PJ, Marsden CD. Mitochondrial function in Parkinson's disease. Ann Neurol 1992; 32 Suppl.:S116–S124.

1951. Schaumburg HH, Berger AR, Thomas PK. Disorders of peripheral nerves. 2nd ed. Philadelphia: Davis, 1982.

1952. Schaumburg HH, Spencer PS. Environmental hydrocarbons produce degeneration in cat hypothalamus and optic tract. Science 1978; 199:199–200.

1953. Scheithauer BW. Symptomatic subependymoma. J Neurosurg 1978; 49:689–696.

1954. Scherman D, Desnos C, Darchen F, Pollak P, Javoy-Agid F, Agid Y. Striatal dopamine deficiency in Parkinson's disease: Role of aging. Ann Neurol 1989; 26:551–557.

1955. Schinelli S, Zuddas A, Kopin IJ, Barker JL, Di Porzio U. 1-Methyl-4-phenyl-1,2,3,6-tetrahydropyridine metabolism and 1-methyl-4-phenylpyridinium uptake in dissociated cell cultures from the embryonic mesencephalon. J Neurochem 1988; 50:1900–1907.
1956. Schirger A, Sheps S, Thomas J, Fealey R. Midodrine, a new agent in the management of idiopathic orthostatic hypotension and Shy-Drager syndrome. Mayo Clin Proc 1981; 56:429–433.
1957. Schmidt CJ, Bruckwick E, Lovenberg W. Lack of evidence supporting a role for dopamine in 1-methyl-4-phenyl-1,2,3,6-tetrahydropyridine neurotoxicity. Eur J Pharmacol 1985; 113:149–150.
1958. Schmidt WR, Jarcho LW. Persistent dyskinesias following phenothiazine therapy Report of five cases and a review. Arch Neurol 1966; 14:369–377.
1959. Schmitt HP, Emser W, Heimes C. Familial occurrence of amyotrophic lateral sclerosis, parkinsonism, and dementia. Ann Neurol 1984; 16:642–648.
1960. Schneider E, Fischer PA, Jacobi P, Becker H, Hacker H. The significance of cerebral atrophy for the symptomatology of Parkinson's disease. J Neurol Sci 1979; 42:187–197.
1961. Schneider JS. Levodopa-induced dyskinesias in Parkinsonian monkeys: Relationship to extent of nigrostriatal damage. Pharmacol Biochem Behavior 1989; 34:193–196.
1962. Schneider JS. Chronic exposure to low doses of MPTP. II. Neurochemical and pathological consequences in cognitively-impaired, motor asymptomatic monkeys. Brain Res 1990; 534:25–36.
1963. Schoenberg BS. Descriptive epidemiology of Parkinson's disease: Disease distribution and hypothesis formulation. In: Parkinson's disease—Advances in Neurology, Vol 45. New York: Raven Press, 1986:277–283.
1964. Schoenberg BS. Environmental risk factors for Parkinson's disease: The epidemiologic evidence. Can J Neurol Sci 1987; 14:407–413.
1965. Schoenberg BS, Anderson DW, Haerer AF. Prevalence of Parkinson's disease in the biracial population of Copiah County, Mississippi. Neurology 1985; 35:841–845.
1966. Schoenberg BS, Osuntokun BO, Adeuja AO, et al. Comparison of the prevalence of Parkinson's disease in black populations in the rural United States and rural Nigeria: Door-to-door community studies. Neurology 1988; 38:645–646.
1967. Schott GP. Induction of involuntary movements by peripheral trauma. An analogy with causalgia. Lancet 1986; 2:712–715.
1968. Schouten MJ, Bruinvels J. Endogenously formed nonharman (beta-carboline) in platelet rich plasma obtained from porphyric rats. Pharmacol Biochem Behavior 1986; 24:1219–1223.
1969. Schultz DR, Barthal JS, Garrett G. Western equine encephalitis with rapid onset of parkinsonism. Neurology 1977; 27:1095–1096.
1970. Schultz W, Scarnati E, Sundstrom E, Romo R. Protection against 1-methyl-4-phenyl-1,2,3,6-tetrahydropyridine-induced Parkinsonism by the catecholamine

uptake inhibitor nomifensine: Behavioral analysis in monkeys with partial striatal dopamine depletions. Neuroscience 1989; 31:219–230.

1971. Schultz W, Scarnati E, Sundstrom E, Tsutsumi T, Jonsson G. The catecholamine uptake blocker nomifensine protects against MPTP-induced parkinsonism in monkeys. Exp Brain Res 1986; 63:216–220.

1972. Schut J, Haymaker W. Hereditary Ataxia. A pathological study of five cases of common ancestry. J Neuropathol Clin Neurol 1951; 1:183–213.

1973. Schwab R. Personal communication, 1991.

1974. Schwab R, England A, Peterson A. Akinesia in Parkinson's disease. Neurology 1959; 9:65–72.

1975. Schwab RS, Doshay LJ, Garland H, Bradshaw P, Garvey E, Crawford B. Shift to older age distribution in parkinsonism: A report on 1,000 patients covering the past decade from three centers. Neurology 1956; 6:783–790.

1976. Schwab RS, England A.C.. Parkinson syndromes due to various specific causes. In: Vinken PJ, Bruyn GW, eds. Handbook of clinical neurology. Amsterdam: North-Holland, 1968:227–247.

1977. Schwartz J, Elizan TS. Search for viral particles and virus-specific products in idiopathic Parkinson disease brain material. Ann Neurol 1979; 6:261–263.

1978. Sciarra D, Sprofkin B. Symptoms and signs referable to the basal ganglia in brain tumor. Arch Neurol Psychiatry 1953; 69:450–461.

1979. Scott M. Parkinsonism-like tremor and cogwheel rigidity in child secondary to massive ependymoma of the frontal lobe and caudate necleus: Prefrontal lobectomy with cessation of tremor and rigidity. Arch Neurol Psychiatry 1974; 57:649–654.

1980. Scott R, Brody JA. Benign early onset of Parkinson's disease: A syndrome distinct from classic postencephalitic parkinsonism. Neurology 1971; 21:366–368.

1981. Scott RM, Brody JA. Benign early-onset Parkinson's disease: A syndrome distinct from classic postencephalitic parkinsonism. Neurology 1970; 20:400.

1982. Sealy RC, Felix CC, Hyde JS, Swartz HM. Structure and reactivity of melanins: Influence of free radicals and metal ions. In: Pryor W, ed. Free radicals in biology, Volume IV. New York: Academic Press, 1980:209–259.

1983. Seawright A, Brown A, Nolan C. Selective degeneration of cerebellar cortical neurons caused by cycad neurotoxin, L-B-methylaminoalanine (1-BMAA), in rats. Neuropathol Appl Neurobiol 1990; 16:153–169.

1984. Sechi GP, Agnetti V, Piredda M, et al. Acute and persistent parkinsonism after use of diquat. Neurology 1992; 42:261–263.

1985. Seegal RF. Polychlorinated Biphenyls (PCBS) yield persistent decreases in dopamine in the non-human primate nigroneostriatal system (Neuro-toxins and their potential role in neurodegeneration. The New York Academy of Sciences,May 6-8 1991; PII-15. (abstract)

1986. Segawa M, Hosaka A, Miyagawi T. Hereditary progressive dystonia with marked diurnal fluctuation. In: Dystonia—Advances in Neurology, Vol 14. New York: Raven Press, 1976:215–233.

1987. Seiden LS, Fischman MW, Schuster CR. Long-term methamphetamine-induced changes in brain catecholamines in tolerant rhesus monkeys. Drug Alc Depend 1975; 1:215–219.

1988. Seiden LS, Vosmer G. Formation of 6-hydroxydopamine in caudate nucleus of the rat brain after a single large dose of methylamphetamine. Pharmacol Biochem Behavior 1984; 21:29–31.

1989. Seitelberger F, Jellinger K. Neuropathologie der zeckenencephalitis. Neuropathologia 1966; 4:367–400.

1990. Semchuk KM, Love EJ, Lee RG. Parkinson's disease and exposure to rural environmental factors: A population based case-control study. Can J Neurol Sci 1991; 18:279–286.

1991. Semchuk KM, Love EJ, Lee RG. Parkinson's disease: A test of the multifactorial etiologic hypothesis. Neurology 1993; 43:1173–1180.

1992. Semchuk KM, Love ET, Lee RG. Parkinson's disease and exposure to agricultural work and pesticide chemicals. Neurology 1992; 42:1328–1335.

1993. Sengstock GJ, Olanow CW, Dunn AJ, Menzies R, Arendash GW. Iron induces degeneration of substantia nigra neurons. Mov Disord 1991; 6(3):272.

1994. Senoh S, Creveling CR, Udenfriend S, Witkop B. Chemical, enzymatic and metabolic studies on the mechanism of oxidation of dopamine. J Am Chem Soc 1959; 81:6236–6240.

1995. Senoh S, Daly J, Axelrod J, Witkop B. Enzymatic p-0-methylation by catechol-0-methyl transferase. J Am Chem Soc 1959; 81:6240–6245.

1996. Senoh S, Witkop B. Non-enzymatic conversions of dopamine to norepinephrine and trihydroxyphenethylamines. J Am Chem Soc 1959; 81:6222–6230.

1997. Senoh S, Witkop B. Formation and rearrangements of aminochromes from a new metabolite of dopamine and some of its derivatives. J Am Chem Soc 1959; 81:6231–6235.

1998. Seppalainen AM. Experimental and clinical neurotoxicology. In: Spencer PS, Schaumburg HH, eds. Carbon disulfide. Baltimore: Williams and Wilkins, 1980:356–373.

1999. Serratrice GT, Toga M, Pellissier JF. Chronic spinal muscular atrophy and pallidonigral degeneration: Report of a case. Neurology 1983; 33:301–310.

2000. Sershen H, Hashim A, Lajtha A. Behavioral and biochemical effects of nicotine in an MPTP-induced mouse model of Parkinson's disease. Pharmacol Biochem Behavior 1987; 28:299–303.

2001. Sershen H, Reith MEA, Hashim A, Lajtha A. Protection against 1-methyl-4-phenyl-1,2,3,6-tetrahydropyridine neurotoxicity by the antioxidant ascorbic acid. Neuropharmacology 1985; 24(12):1257–1259.

2002. Sethi KD, Meador KJ, Loring D, Meador MP. Neuroepidemiology of Parkinson's disease: Analysis of mortality data for the U.S.A. and Georgia. Int J Neurosci 1989; 46:87–92.

2003. Sethi KD, Patel B, Meador KJ. Metoclopramide-induced parkinsonism. South Med J 1989; 82:1581–1582.

2004. Severson JA, Marcusson J, Winblad B, Finch CE. Age-correlated loss of dopaminergic binding sites in human basal ganglia. J Neurochem 1982; 39:1623–1631.

2005. Shahi GS, Das NP, Moochhala SM. Parkinson's disease and cytochrome P450: A possible link. Med Hypotheses 1990; 32:277–282.

2006. Shahi GS, Moochhala SM. Smoking and Parkinson's disease - A new perspective. Rev Environ Hlt 1991; 9(3):123–136.

2007. Shahi GS, Moochhala SM, Lee EJ, Das NP. Studies on the interactions of MPTP(1-methyl-4-phenyl-1,2,3,6-tetrahydropyridine) with the cytochrome P-450 enzyme system—clues to a possible aetiological factor in Parkinson's disease. Ann Acad Med Singapore 1989; 18:93–97.

2008. Shandling M, Carlen PL, Lang AE. Parkinsonism in alcohol withdrawal: A follow-up study. Mov Disord 1990; 5:(1):36-(1):39.

2009. Shaw K, Lees A, Stern G. The impact of treatment with levodopa on Parkinson's disease. Q J Med 1980; 49:283–293.

2010. Shier WT, Koda LY, Bloom FE. A metabolic approach to the detection of tetrahydroisoquinoline formation from 3H-dopamine in rat brain following treatment with ethanol or chloral hydrate. Prog Clin Biol Res 1982; 90:191–200.

2011. Shimizu T, Yasuda N, Kono I. Hepatic and spinal lesions in goats chronically intoxicated with cycasin. Jpn J Vet Sci 1986; 8:1291–1295.

2012. Shimoyama M, Kito S, Itoga E, Kishida T, Nanba K. Binding experiments of muscarinic acetylcholine and dopamine receptors in human brains with emphasis on a case of striatonigral degeneration. J Pharmacology (Japanese) 1982; 32(6):1157–1166.

2013. Shipley MT. Transport of molecules from nose to brain: Transneuronal anterograde and retrograde labeling in the rat olfactory system by wheat germ agglutinin-horseradish peroxidase applied to the nasal epithelium. Brain Res Bull 1985; 15(2):129–142.

2014. Shiraki H, Goto A, Narabayashi H. Etat passe et present de l'encephalite japonaise au Japon. Revue Neurologique 1963; 108:633–696.

2015. Shiraki H, Yase Y. Amyotrophic lateral sclerosis. In: Vinken P, Bruyn G, eds. Handbook of clinical neurology, Vol. 22. System disorders and atrophies. Part II. Amsterdam: Elsevier, 1975:353–419.

2016. Shiraki H. Neuropathological aspects of organic mercury intoxication, including Minamata disease. In: Vinken PJ, Bruyn GW, eds. Handbook of clinical neurology, vol. 36, Intoxications of the nervous system, pt.1. Amsterdam: 1979:83–145.

2017. Shiraki H, Suzuki K, Mizyuno Y, Yoshida M. Selective inhibition of complex I of the brain electron transport system by tetrahydroisoquinoline. Biochem Biophys Res Commun 1989; 144:1541–1545.

2018. Shoemaker DW, Cummins JT, Bidder TG, Boettger HG, Evans M. Identification of harman in the rat arcuate nucleus. Arch Pharmacol 1980; 310:227–230.

2019. Shoffner JM, Watts RL, Juncos JL, Torroni A, Wallace DC. Mitochondrial oxidative phosphorylation defects in Parkinson's disease. Ann Neurol 1991; 30:332–339.

2020. Shoffner JM, Watts RL, Juncos JL, Torroni A, Wallace DC. Mitochondrial function in Parkinson's disease. Ann Neurol 1992; 32:227.

2021. Shoulson I, Chase T. Huntington's disease. Ann Rev Med 1975; 26:419–426.

2022. Shoulson I, Fahn S, Langston JW. Symposium on the etiology, pathogenesis, and Prevention of Parkinson's disease. Arch Neurol 1988; 45:807–811.

2023. Shuster S, Thody AJ, Goolamali SK, Burton JL, Plummer N, Bates D. Melanocyte-stimulating hormone and parkinsonism. Lancet 1973; March 3:463–464.

2024. Shy G, Drager G. A neurological syndrome associated with orthostatic hypotension. Arch Neurol 1960; 2:511–527.

2025. Siddique T, Figlewicz DA, Pericak-Vance MA, et al. Linkage of a gene causing familial amyotrophic lateral sclerosis to chromosome 21 and evidence of genetic-locus heterogeneity. N Engl J Med 1991; 324(20):1381–1384.

2026. Sieber SM, Correa P, Dalgard DW, McIntire RK, Adamson RH. Carcinogenicity and hepatotoxicity of cycasin and its aglycone methylazoxymethanolacetate in non-human primates. J Natl Cancer Inst 1986; 65:177–189.

2027. Siemers E, Robbins B, Hui S. Environmental agents associated with Parkinson's disease. Meeting of the American Neurological Association 1989; 13.

2028. Sigwald J, Jamet F. [Injury and Parkinson's syndrome. Nosological and medicolegal problems]. Ann Med Leg Criminol Police Sci Toxicol 1966; 46:239–249.

2029. Sima AA, Hoag G, Rozdilsky B. Shy-Ddrager syndrome: The transitional variant. Clin Neuropathol 1987; 6(2):49–54.

2030. Singer C, Weiner W. Could parkinson's disease follow intra-uterine influenza? A speculative hypothesis. J Neurol Neurosurg Psychiatry 1989; 52:931.

2031. Singer TP, Ramsay RR. Mechanism of the neurotoxicity of MPTP. An update. FEBS lett 1990; 274:1–8.

2032. Singer TP, Salach JI, Castagnoli N,Jr., Trevor AJ. Interactions of the neurotoxic amine 1-methyl-4-phenyl-1,2,3,6-tetrahydropyridine with monoamine oxidases. Biochem J 1986; 235:785–789.

2033. Sirvio J, Rinne JO, Valjakka A, Rinne UK, Riekkinen PJ, Paljarvi L. Different forms of brain acetylcholinesterase and muscarinic binding in Parkinson's disease. J Neurol Sci 1989; 90:23–32.

2034. Sjoquist B, Magnusson E. Analysis of salsolinol and salsoline in biological samples using deuterium-labelled standards and gas chromatography/mass spectrometry. J Chromatogr 1980; 183:17–22.

2035. Skre H. Current research in neuro-epidemiology. Some main trends. Acta Neurol Scand Suppl 1978; 67:11–36.

2036. Slater E. Expectation of abnormality on paternal and maternal sides: A computational model. J Med Genet 1966; 3:159–161.

2037. Slivka A, Cohen G. Hydroxyl attack on dopamine. J Biol Chem 1985; 260:15466–15472.

2038. Slivka A, Mytilineou C, Cohen G. Histochemical evaluation of glutathione in brain. Brain Res 1987; 409:275–284.

2039. Smith AD, Bolam JP. The neural network of the basal ganglia as revealed by the study of synaptic connections of identified neurones. TINS 1990; 13:259–265.

2040. Smith CAD, Gough AC, Leigh PN, et al. Debrisoquine hydroxylase gene polymorphism and susceptibility to Parkinson's disease. Lancet 1992; 339:1375–1377.

2041. Smith JS, Mellick RS. Neuropsychiatric relapse following acute carbon monoxide poisoning—the contribution of electroconvulsive therapy. Med J Aust 1975; 1:465–468.

2042. Smith MT, Ekström G, Sandy MS, Di Monte D. Studies on the mechanism of 1-methyl-4-phenyl-1,2,3,6-tetrahydropyridine cytotoxicity in isolated hepatocytes. Life Sci 1987; 40:741–748.

2043. Smythies JR. The previous personality in Parkinsonism. J Psychosom Res 1967; 11:169–171.

2044. Snider S, Sandyk N. Sensory dysfunction. In: Koller W, ed. Handbook of Parkinson's disease. New York: Marcel Dekker, 1987:171–180.

2045. Snider SR, Fahn S, Isgreen WP, Cote LJ. Primary sensory symptoms in parkinsonism. Neurology 1976; 26:423–429.

2046. Snow B, Wiens M, Hertzman C, Calne DB. A community survey of Parkinson's disease. Can Med Assoc J 1989; 141:418–422.

2047. Snow BJ, Peppard RF, Guttman M. Positron emission tomographic scanning demonstrates a presynaptic dopaminergic lesion in Lytico-Bodig. The amyotrophic lateral sclerosis parkinsonism dementia complex of Guam. Arch Neurol 1990; 47:870–874.

2048. Snyder AM, Stricker EM, Zigmond MJ. Stress-induced neurological impairments in an amimal model of parkinsonism. Ann Neurol 1985; 18:544–551.

2049. Snyder HR, Hansch CH, Katz L, Parmerter SM, Spaeth EC. The synthesis of derivatives of beta-carboline. II. Syntheses from di-tryptophan and aldehydes. J Am Chem Soc 1948; 70:219–221.

2050. Snyder HR, Parmerter SM, Katz L. The synthesis of derivatives of beta-carboline. III. The nitration of harmane. J Am Chem Soc 1948; 70:222–225.

2051. Snyder SH. Parkinson's Disease. Clues to aetiology from a toxin. Nature 1984; 311:514–517.

2052. Snyder SH, D'Amato RJ. Predicting Parkinson's Disease. Nature 1985; 317:198–199.

2053. Snyder SH, D'Amato RJ. MPTP: A neurotoxin relevant to the pathophysiology of Parkinson's disease. Neurology 1986; 36:250–258.

2054. Sobue G, Hashizume Y, Mitsuma T, Takahashi A. Size-dependent myelinated fiber loss in the corticospinal tract in Shy-Drager syndrome and amyotrophic lateral sclerosis. Neurology 1987; 37(3):529–532.

2055. Sobue G, Hashizume Y, Ohya M, Takahashi A. Shy-Drager syndrome: Neuronal loss depends on size, function, and topography in ventral spinal outflow. Neurology 1986; 36(3):404–407.

2056. Sofic E, Paulus W, Jellinger K, Riederer P, Youdim MB. Selective increase of iron in substantia nigra zona compacta of parkinsonian brains. J Neurochem 1991; 56:978–982.

2057. Sofic E, Riederer P, Heinsen H, et al. Increased iron (III) and total iron content in post mortem substantia nigra of parkinsonian brain. J Neural Transm 1988; 74:199–205.

2058. Sonsalla PK, Heikkila RE. Neurotoxic effects of 1-methyl-4-phenyl-1,2,3,6-tetrahydropyridine (MPTP) and methamphetamine in several strains of mice. Prog Neuropsychopharmacol Biol Psychiat 1988; 12:345–354.

2059. Sonsalla PK, Nicklas WJ, Heikkila RE. Role for excitatory amino acids in

methamphetamine-induced nigrostriatal dopaminergic toxicity (Abstract). Science 1989; 243:398–400. (abstract)
2060. Sonsalla PK, Riordan DE, Heikkila RE. Competitive and noncompetitive antagonists at N-methyl-D-aspartate receptors protect against methamphetamine-induced dopaminergic damage in mice. J Pharmacol Exp Ther 1991; 256:506–512.
2061. Sonsalla PK, Zeevalk GD, Manzino L, Giovanni A, Nichlas WJ. MK-801 fails to protect against the dopaminergic neuropathology produced by systemic 1-methyl-4-phenyl-1,2,3,6-tetrahydropyridine in mice or intranigral 1-methyl-4-phenylphyridinium in rats. J Neurochem 1992; 58:1979–1982.
2062. Sorbi S, Tonini S, Giannini E, Piacentini S, Marini P, Amaducci L. Abnormal platelet glutamate dehydrogenase activity and activation in dominant and nondominant olivopontocerebellar atrophy. Ann Neurol 1986; 19:239–245.
2063. Sorensen P, Jansen E, Gjerris F. Motor disturbances in normal-pressure hydrocephalus. Arch Neurol 1986; 43:34–38.
2064. Souques A. Rapport sur les syndromes Parkinsoniens. Revue Neurologique 1991; 28:534–573.
2065. Sourkes TL. Possible new metabolites mediating actions of L-dopa. Nature 1971; 229:413–414.
2066. Spagna VA, Maeder MC, Johson JC, Mazaferri EL. Normal pressure hydrocephalus, parkinsonism, and primary empty sella-coincidence or cause-effect? Neurology 1978; 28:1191–1193.
2067. Spatz H. Parkinson's Disease(Paralysis agitans) and postencephalitic parkinsonism: Attempt at a clinical-anatomical differential diagnosis. Archiv fur Psychiatrie und Nervenkrankheiten 1940; 111(2):251–321.
2068. Spatz H, Laqueur G. Transplacental induction of tumors in Sprague-Dawley rats with crude cycad material. J Natl Cancer Inst 1967; 38:233.
2069. Spehlmann R, Stahl SM. Dopamine acetylcholine imbalance in Parkinson's disease. Possible regenerative overgrowth of cholinergic axon terminals. Lancet 1976; 1:724–726.
2070. Spellman G. Report of familial cases of parkinsonism; Evidence of a dominant trait in a patient's family. JAMA 1962; 179:372–374.
2071. Spencer PS. Guam ALS/Parkinsonism-dementia: A long-latency neurotoxic disorder caused by "Slow Toxin(s)" in food. Can J Neurol Sci 1987; 14:347–357.
2072. Spencer PS. The grass pea—Threat and promise. New York/London: Third World Medical Research Foundation, 1989.
2073. Spencer PS, Allen C, Kisby G. Lathyrism and western Pacific ALS: Etiology of short- and long-latency motor-system disorders. In: Rowland L, ed. Proceedings of ALS conference. New York: Raven Press, 1991:287–299.
2074. Spencer PS, Butterfield P. Environmental agents and Parkinson's disease. In: Ellenberg JH, Koller WC, Langston JW, eds. Etiology of Parkinson's disease. New York: Marcel Dekker, 1994:319–365.
2075. Spencer PS, Kisby G, Ludolph A. Slow toxins, biologic markers, and long-latency neurodegenerative disease in the western Pacific region. Neurology 1991; 41 (suppl 2):62–66.
2076. Spencer PS, Nunn PB, Hugon J, Ludolph A, Dwijendra NR. Motor neurone disease on Guam: Possible role of a food neurotoxin. Lancet 1986; 1:965.

2077. Spencer PS, Nunn PB, Hugon J, et al. Guam Amyotrophic Lateral Sclerosis-parkinsonism-dementia linked to a plant excitant neurotoxin. Science 1987; 237:517–522.

2078. Spencer PS, Ohta M, Palmer VS. Cycad use and motor neurone disease in Kii peninsula of Japan. Lancet 1987; ii:1462–1463.

2079. Spencer PS, Palmer V, Ohta M, Herman A. Cycad, a suspect etiological factor for Guam ALS/P-D is associated with motor neuron disease in Irian Jaya,Indonesia, and Kii Peninsula,Japan. In: Tsubaki T, Yase Y, eds. Amyotrophic lateral sclerosis. New York, N.Y.: Elsevier Science Publishers B.V. (Biomedical Division), 1988:35–40.

2080. Spencer PS, Palmer VS, Herman A, Asmedi A. Cycad use and motor neurone disease in Irian Jaya. Lancet 1987; 2:1273–1274.

2081. Spencer PS, Peterson ER, Madrid RA, Raine CS. Effects of thallium salts on neuronal mitochondria in organotypic cordganglia-muscel combination cultures. J Cell Biol 1973; 58:79–95.

2082. Spencer PS, Ross S, Kisby G. Western Pacific amyotrophic lateral sclerosis: Putative role of cycad toxins. In: Hudson A, ed. Amyotrophic lateral sclerosis: Concepts in pathogenesis and etiology. Toronto: University of Toronto Press, 1990:263–295.

2083. Spencer PS, Ross SM, Kisby G, Roy DN, Nunn PB. Western Pacific Parkinsonism-dementia complex: Role of plant neurotoxic factors. 9th Iternational Symposium on Parkinson's Disease 1988; 10.

2084. Spencer PS, Schaumburg HH. Experimental and clinical neurotoxicology. Baltimore: Williams and Wilkins, 1980.

2085. Spencer PS, Schaumburg HH, Sabri MI, Veronesi B. The enlarging view of hexacarbon neurotoxicity. CRC Crit Rev Toxicol 1980; 7:279–356.

2086. Spiller W. The importance in clinical diagnosis of paralysis of associated movements of the eyeballs (Blick-laehmung), especially of upward and downward associated movements. Nerv Ment Dis 1905; 32:417–448,49.

2087. Spina MB, Cohen G. Dopamine turnover and glutathione oxidation: Implications for Parkinson disease. Proc Natl Acad Sci 1989; 86:1398–1400.

2088. Spokes E, Bannister R, Oppenheimer D. Multiple system atrophy with autonomic failure: Clinical, histological and neurochemical observations on four cases. J Neurol Sci 1979; 43:59–82.

2089. Srivastava R, Brouillet E, Beal MF, Storey E, Hyman BT. Blockade of 1-methyl-4-phenylpyridinium ion (MPP+) nigral toxicity in the rat by prior decortication or MK-801 treatment: A sterological estimate of neuronal loss. Neurobiol Aging 1993; 14:295–301.

2090. Sroka H, Elizan TS, Yahr MD, Burger A, Mendoza MR. Organic mental syndrome and confusional states in Parkinson's disease. Relationship to computerized tomographic signs of cerebral atrophy. Arch Neurol 1981; 38:339–342.

2091. Staal A, Meerwaldt JD, van Dongen KJ, Mulder PG, Busch HF. Non-familial degenerative disease and atrophy of brainstem and cerebellum. Clinical and CT data in 47 patients. J Neurol Sci 1990; 95(3):259–269.

2092. Stanhope JM, Brody JA, Morris CE. Epidemiologic features of amyotropic lateral sclerosis and parkinsonism-dementia in Guam, Mariana Islands. Int J Epidemiol 1972; 1:199–210.

2093. Stanzione P, Fattapposta F, Tagliati M, et al. Dopaminergic pharmacological manipulations in normal humans confirm the specificity of the visual (PERG-VEP) and cognitive (P300) electrophysiological alterations in Parkinson's disease. Electroencephalogr Clin Neurophysiol Suppl 1990; 41:216–220.

2094. Starke PE, Farber JL. Ferric iron and superoxide ions are required for the killing of cultured hepatocytes by hydrogen peroxide. Evidence for the participation of hydroxyl radicals formed by an iron-catalyzed Haber-Weiss reaction. J Biol Chem 1985; 260:10099–10104.

2095. Steck H. Le syndrome extra-pyramidal et diencephalique au cours des traitements au forgactil au Serpasil. Ann Med Psychol 1954; 1/2:737–743.

2096. Steece-Collier K, Collier TJ, Sladek CD, Sladek JRJ. Chronic levodopa impairs morphological development of grafted embryonic dopamine neurons. Exp Neurol 1990; 110:201–208.

2097. Steele JC. Progressive supranuclear palsy. Brain 1972; 95:693–704.

2098. Steele JC. Progressive supranuclear palsy. In: Vinken P, Bruyn G, eds. Handbook of clinical neurology: System disorders and atrophies. Amsterdam: 1975: 217–229.

2099. Steele JC, Guzman T. Observations about amyotrophic lateral sclerosis and the Parkinsonism-dementia complex of Guam with regard to epidemiology and etiology. Can J Neurol Sci 1987; 14:358–362.

2100. Steele JC, Guzman TQ, Driver MG. Nutritional factors in amyotrophic lateral sclerosis on Guam: Observations from Umatac. In: Hudson AJ, ed. Concepts in pathogenesis and etiology. Toronto: University of Toronto Press, 1990:193–223.

2101. Steele JC, Richardson J, Olszewski J. Progressive supranuclear palsy; a heterogenous degeneration involving the brainstem, basal ganglia and cerebellum with vertical gaze and pseudobulbar palsy, nuchal dystonia, and dementia. Arch Neurol 1964; 10:333–359.

2102. Stefanache F, Pendefunda L, Prodan R, Pendefunda G. [The physiopathology of the basal ganglia and the etiopathogenesis of Parkinson's diseases]. Rev Med Chir Soc Med Nat Iasi 1989; 93:145–154.

2103. Stefano E, Casali C, Caporali M, Sancesario G, Morocutti C. Parkinson disease in farm workers [letter]. Ital J Neurol Sci 1989; 10:379.

2104. Steiger MJ, Lledo P, Quinn NP, Marsden CD, Turner P, Jenner PG. Debrisoquine hydroxylation in Parkinson's disease. Acta Neurol Scand 1992; 86:159–164.

2105. Steinbusch HWM. Serotonin-immunoreactive neurons and their projections in the CNS. In: Bjorklund A, Hokfelt T, Kuhar MJ, eds. Handbook of clinical neuroanatomy: Volume 3: Classical transmitters and transmitter receptors in the CNS, Part II. Amsterdam: Elsevier Science Publishers, 1984:68–125.

2106. Stepanova VG. [Relation between the structure of akinetic-rigid syndromes and the level of the central nervous system lesion]. Zh Nevropatol Psikhiatr 1971; 71:481–484.

2107. Stern G. The effects of lesions in the substantia nigra. Brain 1966; 89:449–478.

2108. Stern G. MPTP: Clinical implications. J Neural Transm Suppl 1986; 20:77–81.

2109. Stern M, Dulaney E, Gruber S. Risk factors for Parkinson's disease: A case-control study in young and old onset PD patients. Ann Neurology (Abstract) 1990; 28:294.

2110. Stern M, Dulaney E, Gruber S, et al. The epidemiology of Parkinson's disease:

A case-control study of young-onset and old-onset patients. Arch Neurol 1991; 48:903–907.
2111. Stern M, Koller WC. Parkinsonian syndromes. New York: Marcel Dekker, 1993.
2112. Stern MB. Head trauma as a risk factor for Parkinson's disease. Mov Disord 1991; 6(2):95–97.
2113. Stern MB, Braffman BH, Skolnick BE, Hurtig HI, Grossman RI. Magnetic resonance imaging in Parkinson's disease and parkinsonian syndromes. Neurology 1989; 39(11):1524–1526.
2114. Stern MB, Koller WC. Parkinson's disease. In: Stern MB, Koller WC, eds. Parkinsonian syndromes. New York: Marcel Dekker, 1993:3–29.
2115. Stern SL, Hurtig HI, Mendels J, Balaban D. Psychiatric illness in relatives of patients with Parkinson's disease: A preliminary report. Am J Psychiatry 1977; 134:443–444.
2116. Stern Y. MPTP-induced parkinsonism. Prog Neurobiol 1990; 34:107–114.
2117. Stern Y, Langston JW. Intellectual changes in patients with MPTP-induced parkinsonism. Neurology 1985; 35:1506–1509.
2118. Stern Y, Marder K, Tang MX, Mayeux R. Antecedent clinical features associated with dementia in Parkinson's disease. Neurology 1993; 43:1690–1692.
2119. Stern Y, Tetrud JW, Martin WRW, Kutner SJ, Langston JW. Cognitive change following MPTP exposure. Neurology 1990; 40:261–264.
2120. Sternson AW, McCreery R, Feinberg B, Adams RN. Electrochemical studies of adrenergic neurotransmitters and related compounds. Electroanalytical Chemistry and Interfacial Electrochemistry 1973; 46:313–321.
2121. Steventon GB, Heafield MTE, Sturman SG, Waring RH, Williams AC, Ellingham J. Degenerative neurological disease and debrisoquine-4-hydroxylation capacity. Med Sci Res 1989; 17:163–164.
2122. Steventon GB, Heafield MTE, Waring RH, Williams AC. Xenobiotic metabolism in Parkinson's disease. Neurology 1989; 39:883–887.
2123. Steventon GB, Heafield MTE, Waring RH, Williams AC, Sturman SG, Green M. Metabolism of low-dose paracetamol in patients with chronic neurological disease. Xenobiotica 1990; 20:117–122.
2124. Steventon GB, Humfrey C, Sturman SG, Williams AC, Waring RH. Monoamine oxidase-B and Parkinson's disease. Lancet 1990; 335:180.
2125. Steventon GB, Sturman SG, Heafield MTE, Waring RH, Napier J, Williams AC. Platelet monoamine oxidase-B activity in Parkinson's disease. J Neural Transm 1989; 1:255–261.
2126. Stewart SS, Appel SH. Trophic factors in neurologic disease. Ann Rev Med 1988; 39:193–201.
2127. Still CN. Postmenopausal parkinsonism: Brain iron overload. Adv Exp Med Biol 1977; 90:291–296.
2128. Stoddard SL, Tyce GM, Ahlskog JE, Zinsmeister AR, Carmichael SW. Decreased catecholamine content in parkinsonian adrenal medullae. Exp Neurol 1989; 104:22–27.
2129. Storey E, Hyman BT, Jenkins B, et al. 1-Methyl-4- Phenylpyridinium produces excitotoxic lesions in rat striatum as a result of impairment of oxidative metabolism. J Neurochem 1992; 58:1975–1978.

2130. Strang RR. ABO blood-groups in Parkinson's disease. Acta Pathol Microbiol Scand 1965; 65:653.

2131. Strang RR. The ABO blood-group distribution of 450 Swedish patients with Parkinson's disease. Neurology 1966; 16:1051–1052.

2132. Strang RR. Conjugal parkinsonism. Dis Nerv Syst 1967; 28:814–815.

2133. Strang RR. The etiology of Parkinson's disease. Dis Nerv Syst 1970; 31:381–390.

2134. Strong G. Parkinson's syndrome following severe herpes ophthalmicus. Br Med J 1952; 1:533.

2135. Struck LK, Rodnitzky RL, Dobson JK. Stroke and its modification in Parkinson's disease. Stroke 1990; 21:1395–1399.

2136. Sturman SG, Steventon GB, Waring RH, Williams AC. MAO-B and Parkinson's disease [letter]. Mov Disord 1990; 5:338–339.

2137. Sturman SG, Williams AC, Steventon GB, Waring RH. Metabolism of MPTP and benzylamine in Parkinson's disease. 1994. (in press)

2138. Sudarsky L, Morris J, Romero J, Walshe TM. Dementia in Parkinson's disease: The problem of clinicopathological correlation. J Neuropsychiatry Clin Neurosci 1989; 1:159–166.

2139. Sundstrom E, Fredriksson A, Archer T. Chronic neurochemical and behavioral changes in MPTP-lesioned C57BL/6 mice: A model for Parkinson's disease. Brain Res 1990; 528:181–188.

2140. Sundstrom E, Jonsson G. Pharmacological interference with the neurotoxic action of 1-methyl-4-phenyl-1,2,3,6-tetrahydropyridine (MPTP) on central catecholamine neurons in the mouse. Eur J Pharmacol 1985; 110:293–299.

2141. Sung JH, Mastri AR, Segal E. Pathology of Shy-Drager syndrome. J Neuropathol Exp Neurol 1979; 38(4):353–368.

2142. Sunohara N, Mano Y, Ando K, Satoyoshi B. Idiopathic dystonia—parkinsonism with marked diurnal fluctuations of symptoms. Ann Neurol 1985; 17:39–45.

2143. Susilo R, Damm H, Rommelspacher H, Hofle G. Biotransformation of 1-methyl-1,2,3,4-tetrahydro-beta carboline-1-carboxylic acid to harmalan, tetrahydroharman and harman in rats. Neurosci Lett 1987; 81:325–330.

2144. Sutcliffe RL, Prior R, Mawby B, McQuillan WJ. Parkinson's disease in the district of the Northampton Health Authority, United Kingdom. A study of prevalence and disability. Acta Neurol Scand 1985; 72(4):363–379.

2145. Sutherland JM. Parkinson's syndrome: Aetiological factors and certain clinical features. Aust N Z J Med 1971; 1:Suppl 1:29-Suppl 1:34.

2146. Suzuki K, Mizuno Y, Yoshida M. Inhibition of mitochondrial NADH-ubiquinone oxidoreductase and ATP synthesis by tetrahydroisoquinoline. Neurosci Lett 1988; 86:105–108.

2147. Suzuki K, Mizuno Y, Yoshida M. The effect of tetrahydroisoquinoline on the mitochondrial respiration. In: Nagatsu T, Fisher A, Yoshida M, eds. Basic, clinical, and therapeutic aspects of Alzheimer's and Parkinson's diseases, Volume 1. New York: Plenum Press, 1990:309–312.

2148. Svenson LW. Geographic distribution of deaths due to Parkinson's disease in Canada: 1979–1986. Mov Disord 1990; 5:322–324.

2149. Svenson LW. Regional disparities in the annual prevalence rates of Parkinson's disease in Canada. Neuroepidemiology 1991; 10:205–210.

2150. Swartz HM, Sarna T, Zecca L. Modulation by neuromelanin of the availability and reactivity of metal ions. Ann Neurol 1992; 32 Suppl.:S69–S75.

2151. Sweet RD. Parkinson's disease: Current diagnosis and treatment pp. 51–73. A Non-Journal Reference 1990.

2152. Sweet RD, McDowell F. Five years' treatment of Parkinson's disease with levodopa. Ann Intern Med 1975; 83:456–463.

2153. Sweet RD, McDowell FH, Feigenson JS, Loranger AW, Goodell H. Mental symptoms in Parkinson's disease during chronic treatment with levodopa. Neurology 1976; 26:305–310.

2154. Sypert GW, Leffman H, Ojemann GA. Occult normal pressure hydrocephalus manifested by parkinsonism-dementia complex. Neurology 1973; 23:234–238.

2155. Szulc-Kuberska J, Stepien H, Klimek A, Cieslak D. Effect of bromocriptine and metoclopramide on serum prolactin levels in patients with amyotrophic lateral sclerosis. J Neurol Neurosurg Psychiatry 1988; 51:643–645.

2156. Tabatabaei A, Perry TL, Hansen S, Krieger C. Partial protective effect of MK-801 on MPTP-induced reduction of striatal dopamine in mice. Neurosci Lett 1992; 141:192–194.

2157. Taddei IM, Ludin HP. Essential tremor: A follow-up study. Schweizer Archiv Fur Neurologie Und Psychiatrie 1988; 139:33–46.

2158. Takada K, Nakamura H, Igo M. An autopsy case of diffuse Lewy body disease diagnosed as having familial PD [in Japanese]. 30th Annual Congress of Neuropathologists in Japan, Tokyo 1993; 196.

2159. Takagi S, Shinohara Y, Tsuji K. Histocompatibility antigens in Parkinson's disease. Acta Neurol Scand 1982; 66:590–593.

2160. Taketomi T, Hara A, Kitazawa N, Takada K, Nakamura H. An adult case of adrenoleukodystrophy with features of olivo-ponto-cerebellar atrophy: II. Lipid biochemical studies. J Exp Med (Japanese) 1987; 57(1):59–70.

2161. Takeuchi T. Neuropathology of Minamata disease in Kumanoto: Especially at the chronic stage. In: Roizin L, Shiraki H, Grcevic N, eds. Neurotoxicology. New York: Raven Press, 1977:235–260.

2162. Tanaka J, Nakamura H, Honda S,Takada K, Kato S. Neuropathological study on 1-methyl-4-phenyl-1,2,3,6-tetrahydropyridine of the crab-eating monkey. Acta Neuropathol (Berlin) 1988; 75:370–376.

2163. Tanaka M, Sotomatsu A, Kanai H, Hirai S. Dopa and dopamine cause cultured neuronal death in the presence of iron. J Neurol Sci 1991; 101:198–203.

2164. Tanner C, Goetz C, Klawans H. Autonomic nervous system disorders. In: Koller W, ed. Handbook of Parkinson's disease. New York: Marcel Dekker, 1987:145–170.

2165. Tanner CM, Langston JW. Do environmental toxins cause Parkinson's disease? A critical review. Ann Neurol 1990; 40(suppl 3):17–30.

2166. Tanner CM. Influence of environmental factors on the onset of Parkinson's disease (PD). Neurology 1986; 36:215.

2167. Tanner CM. The role of environmental toxins in the etiology of Parkinson's disease. TINS 1989; 12:49–54.

2168. Tanner CM. Environmental toxins and Parkinsons disease (Reply to letter). TINS 1989; 12:182–183.

2169. Tanner CM. Abnormal liver enxyme-mediated metabolism in Parkinson's disease: A second look. Neurology 1991; 41 (suppl 2):89–92.
2170. Tanner CM. Epidemiology of Parkinson's disease. Neurol Clin 1992; 10:317–329.
2171. Tanner CM. Occupational and environmental causes of Parkinsonism. Occup Med 1992; 7:503–513.
2172. Tanner CM, Chen B, Cohen JA, et al. Dietary anti-oxidant vitamins and the risk of developing Parkinson's disease. Neurology 1989; 39:181.
2173. Tanner CM, Chen B, Wang WZ, et al. Environmental factors and Parkinson's disease: A case-control study in China. Neurology 1989; 39:660–664.
2174. Tanner CM, Chen B, Wang WZ, et al. Environmental factors in the etiology of Parkinson's disease. Can J Neurol Sci 1987; 14:419–423.
2175. Tanner CM, Chen B, Wang WZ, et al. Environmental factors in the etiology of Parkinson's disease (Letter). Neurology 1988; 38:349–340.
2176. Tanner CM, Cohen JC, Summerville BC, Goetz CG. Vitamin use and Parkinson's disease. Ann Neurology (Abstract) 1988; 23:182.
2177. Tanner CM, Grabler P, Goetz CG. Occupation and the risk of Parkinson's disease (PD): A case control study in young onset patients. Neurology 1990; 40:422.
2178. Tanner CM, Koller WC, Gilley DC, et al. Cigarette smoking, alcohol drinking and Parkinson's disease: Cross-cultural risk assessment (Abstract). Mov Disord 1990; 5:11.
2179. Tanner CM, Thelen JA, Offord KP, Rademacher D, Goetz CG, Kurland LT. Parkinson's disease (PD) incidence in Olmsted County, MN:1935–1988. Neurology 1992; (Supplement 3):194.
2180. Tanner CM, Zack MM. Comorbidity as it relates to the cause of Parkinson's disease. In: Ellenberg JH, Koller WC, Langston JW, eds. Etiology of Parkinson's disease. New York: Marcel Dekker, 1994:245–275.
2181. Tasaki Y, Makino Y, Ohta S, Hirobe M. 1-Methyl-1,2,3,4-tetrahydroisoquinoline, decreasing in 1-methyl-4-phenyl-1,2,3,6-tetrahydropyridine-treated mouse, prevents parkinsonsim-like behavior abnormalities. J Neurochem 1991; 57:1940–1943.
2182. Teelken AW, Lakke JPW. Amino acid abnormalities in CSF: A possible biochemical support for the hypothesized existence of a continuun of neurological heredodegenerative diseases. In: Lakke JPWF, Korf J, Wesseling H, eds. Parkinson's disease: Concepts and prospects. Amsterdam: Exerpta Medica, 1977:85–97.
2183. Teillet R. Traumatismes des membres et syndromes Parkinsoniens. These de Toulouse, Faculte de medecine. Universite de Toulouse, 1952.
2184. Teitelbaum JS, Zatorre RJ, Carpenter S, Gendron D. Neurologic sequelae of domoic acid intoxication due to the ingestion of contaminated mussels. N Engl J Med 1990; 322:1781–1787.
2185. Tellez-Nagel I, Wisniewski H. Ultrastructure of neurofibrillary tangles in Steele-Richardson-Olszewski syndrome. Arch Neurol 1973; 29:324–327.
2186. Tenovuo O, Kolhinen O, Laihinen A, Rinne UK. Brain substance P receptors in Parkinson's disease. In: Parkinson's disease: Anatomy, pathology and therapy—Advances in Neurology, Vol 53. New York: Raven Press, 1990:145–148.
2187. Teravainen H, Forgach L, Hietanen M, Schulzer M, Schoenberg BS, Calne DB.

The age of onset of Parkinson's disease: Etiological implications. Can J Neurol Sci 1986; 13:317–319.
2188. Teravainen H, Hietanen M, Stoessl J, Calne DB. Dementia in movement disorders. Can J Neurol Sci 1986; 13 (4 suppl):546–558.
2189. Teravainen H, Schoenberg BS, Calne DB. Age of onset of Parkinson's disease: Authors' reply. Can J Neurol Sci 1987; 14:180.
2190. Terry R, Katzman R. Alzheimer disease and cognitive loss. In: Katzman R, Rowe JW, eds. Principles of Geriatric Neurology. Philadelphia: Davis, 1992:207–265.
2191. Testa B, Naylor R, Costall B, Jenner P, Marsden CD. Does an endogenous methylpyridinium analogue cause Parkinson's disease. J Pharm Pharmacol 1985; 37:679–680.
2192. Tetrud JW. Preclinical Parkinson's disease: Detection of motor and nonmotor manifestations. Neurology 1991; 41(suppl.2):69–72.
2193. Tetrud JW, Langston JW. Early parkinsonism in humans due to MPTP exposure (Abstract). Neurology 1986; 36(Suppl 1):308.
2194. Tetrud JW, Langston JW. MPTP-induced parkinsonism as a model for Parkinson's disease. Acta Neurol Scand Suppl 1989; 126:35–40.
2195. Tetrud JW, Langston JW. The effect of deprenyl (selegiline) on the natural history of Parkinson's disease. Science 1989; 245:519–522.
2196. Tetrud JW, Langston JW. Tremor in MPTP-induced parkinsonism. Neurology 1992; 42:407–410.
2197. Tetrud JW, Langston JW, Garbe PL, Ruttenber AJ. Mild parkinsonism in persons exposed to 1-methyl-4-phenyl-1,2,3,6-tetrahydropyridine (MPTP). Neurology 1989; 39:1483–1487.
2198. Teusink JP, Alexopoulos GS, Shamoian CA. Parkinsonian side effects induced by a monamine oxidase inhibitor. Am J Psychiatry 1984; 141:118–119.
2199. The Parkinson Study Group. Effect of deprenyl on the progression of disability in early Parkinson's disease. N Engl J Med 1989; 321:1364–1371.
2200. Thiessen B, Rajput AH, Laverty W, Desai H. Age, environments, and the number of substantia nigra neurons. In: Parkinson's disease: Anatomy, pathology and therapy—Advances in Neurology, Vol 53. New York: Raven Press, 1990:201–206.
2201. Thomison JB. Addled brains and coffin nails [editorial]. South Med J 1989; 82:541–542.
2202. Tiller-Borcich JK, Forno LS. Parkinson's disease and dementia with neuronal inclusions in the cerebral cortex: Lewy bodies or Pick bodies. J Neuropathol Exp Neurol 1988; 47:526–535.
2203. Todes CJ. Idiopathic Parkinson's disease and depression: A psychosomatic view. J Neurol Neurosurg Psychiatry 1984; 47:298–301.
2204. Todes CJ, Lees AJ. The pre-morbid personality of patients with Parkinson's disease. J Neurol Neurosurg Psychiatry 1985; 48:97–100.
2205. Tohgi H, Abe T, Hashiguchi K, Takahashi S, Nozaki Y, Kikuchi T. A significant reduction of putative transmitter amino acids in cerebrospinal fluid of patients with Parkinson's disease and spinocerebellar degeneration. Neurosci Lett 1991; 126(2):155–158.
2206. Tohgi H, Abe T, Takahashi S, Ueno M, Nozaki Y. Cerebrospinal fluid dopamine,

norepinephrine, and epinephrine concentrations in Parkinson's disease correlated with clinical symptoms. In: Parkinson's disease: Anatomy, pathology and therapy - Advances in Neurology, Vol 53. New York: Raven Press, 1990:277–282.

2207. Tohgi H, Tabuchi M, Tomonaga M, Izumiyama N. Selective loss of small myelinated and unmyelinated fibers in Sky-Drager syndrome. Acta Neuropathol 1982; 57(4):282–286.

2208. Tolosa E, Santamaria J. Parkinsonism and basal ganglia infarcts. Neurology 1984; 34:1516–1518.

2209. Tomlinson AH, Esiri MM. Herpes simplex encephalitis. Immunohistological demonstration of spread of virus via olfactory pathways in mice. J Neurol Sci 1983; 60(3):473–484.

2210. Tommasi M, Berger G, Kopp N, Carrier H. [Slow viruses and the nervous system]. Arch Anat Pathol (Paris) 1972; 20:229–242.

2211. Tomokane N, Kitamoto T, Tateishi J, Sato Y. Immunohistochemical quantification of substance P in spinal dorsal horns of patients with multiple system atrophy. J Neurol Neurosurg Psychiatry 1991; 54(6):535–541.

2212. Tomonaga M. Neuropathology of the locus ceruleus: A semi-quantitative study. J Neurol 1983; 230 (4):231–240.

2213. Traub RD, Rains TC, Garruto RM, Gajdusek DC, Gibbs CJJr. Brain destruction alone does not elevate brain aluminum. Neurology 1981; 31(8):986–990.

2214. Trelles JO, Cuba JM, Palomino L. [Demential forms of chronic subdural hematomas]. Rev Neuropsiquiatr 1968; 31:1–16.

2215. Treves TA, Chandra V, Korczyn AD. Parkinson's and Alzheimer's disease: Epidemiological comparison. 2. Persons at risk. Neuroepidemiology 1994; 12:345–349.

2216. Treves TA, Cuesta J. Time-Space Patterns in Parkinsonism (PD) Mortality in the US, 1971–78 (Abstract). 9th International Symposium on Parkinson's Disease 1988; 57–50.

2217. Treves TA, de Pedro Cuesta J. Parkinsonism mortality in the US, 1. Time and space distribution. Acta Neurol Scand 1991; 84:389–397.

2218. Treves TA, Rabey JM, Korczyn AD. Case-control study, with use of temporal approach, for evaluation of risk factors for Parkinson's disease (PD) (Abstract). Mov Disord 1990; 5:11.

2219. Trevor AJ, Castagnoli N,Jr., Caldera PS, Ramsay RR, Singer TP. III. Bioactivation of MPTP: Reactive metabolites and possible biochemical sequelae. Life Sci 1987; 40:713–719.

2220. Trevor AJ, Castagnoli N, Jr., Singer TP. The formation of reactive intermediates in the MAO-catalyzed oxidation of the nigrostriatal toxin 1-methyl-4-phenyl-1,2,3,6-tetrahydropyridine (MPTP). Toxicology 1988; 49:513–519.

2221. Trétiakoff C. Contribution a l'etude de l'anatomie pathologique du locus niger de Soemmering avec quelques deductions relatives a la pathogenie des troubles du tonus musculaire et de la maladie de Parkinson. 1919: These de Paris.

2222. Tse DCS, McCreery R, Adams RN. Potential oxidative pathways of brain catecholamines. J Med Chem 1976; 19(1):37–40.

2223. Tsubaki T, Irukayama K. Minamata disease. Tokyo: Kodansha, 1977.

2224. Tsuneoka Y, Matsuo Y, Iwahashi K, Takeuchi H, Ichikawa Y. A novel cytochrome P-450IID6 mutant gene associated with Parkinson's disease. J Biochem 1993; 114:263–266.

2225. Turski L, Bressler K, Rettig K-J, Löschmann P-A, Wachtel H. Protection of substantia nigra from MPP+ neurotoxicity by N-methyl-D-aspartate antagonists. Nature 1991; 349:414–418.

2226. Tyndel M. Zur Frage des intervalles zwischen encephalitis und beginn des postencephalitischen parkinsonismus. Nervenarzt 1938; 11:305–306.

2227. Tyrer P, Alexander M, Regan A, Lee I. An extrapyramidal syndrome after lithium therapy. Br J Psychiatry 1980; 136:191–194.

2228. Tzeng WF, Chen YH. Suppression of snake-venom cardiotoxin-induced cardiomyocyte degeneration by blockage of CA2+ influx or inhibition on non-lysosomal proteinases. Biochem J 1988; 256:89–95.

2229. Ueki A, Willoughby J, Glover V, Sandler M, Stibbe K, Stern GM. Endogenous urinary monoamine oxidase inhibitor excretion in Parkinson's disease and other neurological disorders. J Neural Transm Park Dis Dement Sect 1989; 1:263–268.

2230. Uematsu D, Hamada J, Gotoh F. Brainstem auditory evoked responses and CT findings in multiple system atrophy. J Neurol Sci 1987; 77(2–3):161–171.

2231. Uhl GR, Kitayama S, Cerruti C, et al. Dopamine transporter: Correlates with Parkinsonian pathogenesis. Mov Disord 1993; 8, No.3:403–404.

2232. Uitti RJ, Rajput A, Ashenhurst E, Rozdilsky B. Cyanide-induced parkinsonism. A clinicopathologic report. Neurology 1985; 35:921–925.

2233. Uitti RJ, Rajput AH, Rozdilsky B, Bickis M, Wollin T, Yuen WK. Regional metal concentration in Parkinson's diseases other chronic neurological diseases, and control brains. Can J Neurol Sci 1989; 16:310–314.

2234. Umeda Y, Sakata E. A case of progressive supranuclear palsy—neurotoxicological findings and etiology. J Otolaryngol 1978; 7(5):409–414.

2235. Umehara F, Nomoto M, Usuki F, Matsumoto W, Osame M. Juvenile parkinsonism in monozygotic twins. Clin Neurol 1991; 31:306–309.

2236. Uncini A, Tartaro A, Di Stefano E, Gambi D. Parkinsonism, basal ganglia calcification and epilepsy as late complications of postoperative hypoparathyroidism. J Neurol 1985; 232:109–111.

2237. Ung-Chhun N, Cheng BY, Pronger DA. Alkaloid adducts in human brain: Coexistence of 1-carboxylated and noncarboxylated isoquinoline and beta carbolines in alcoholics and nonalcoholics. In: Collins MA, ed. Adducts in alcoholism. New York: Alan R. Liss, 1985:125–136.

2238. Ungerstedt U. 6-hydroxy-dopamine induced degeneration of central monoamine neurons. Eur J Pharmacol 1968; 5:107–110.

2239. Uono M, Segawa M, Aoyama M. [Symposium: Metabolism in neurological disorders. 1. Parkinsonism. Four pedigrees of familial Parkinsonism-mainly on DOPA metabolism]. In:. Nippon Naika. Gakkai. Zasshi, 1972:1136–1138.

2240. Urakami K, Masaki N, Shimoda K, Nishikawa S, Takahashi K. Increase of striatal dopamine turnover by stress in MPTP-treated mice. Clin Neuropharmacol 1988; 11:360–368.

2241. Vaidya AB, Rajagopalan TG, Mankodi NA, et al. Treatment of Parkinson's disease with the cowhage plant—Mucuna pruriens Bak. Neurology (India) 1978; 26:171–176.

2242. Valanis B. Epidemiology in nursing and health care. Norwalk, CT: Appleton-Century-Crofts, 1986.
2243. Van Bogaert L. The thalamic and parkinsonian types of infundibular tumors. Arch Neurol Psychiatry 1928; 19:377–393.
2244. Van Bogaert L, Radermecker MA. Typical amyotrophic lateral sclerosis and paralysis agitans inherited in the same family with a type of possible transmission of both diseases. Monatsschr Psychiatr Neurol 1954; 127:185–203.
2245. Van der Wende C, Spoerlein MT. Oxidation of dopamine to melanin by an enzyme of rat brain. Life Sci 1963; 6:386–392.
2246. van Leeuwen RB, Perquin WV. Striatonigral degeneration. A case report and a review of the literature. Clin Neurol Neurosurg 1988; 90(2):121–124.
2247. Van Rossum J, Veenama H, Went LN. Linkage investiations in two families with hereditary ataxia. J Neurol Neurosurg Psychiatry 1981; 44(6):516–522.
2248. Van Woert MH. DPNH oxidation by melanin: Inhibition by phenothiazines. Proc Soc Exp Biol Med 1968; 129:165–171.
2249. Van Woert MH, Prasad KN, Borg DC. Spectroscopic studies of substantia nigra pigment in human subjects. J Neurochem 1967; 14:707–716.
2250. Van Wolferen WJ, Bruyn GW, Teepen JL. Letter: Pathogenesis of Huntington's chorea, Pick's disease, and paralysis agitans. Lancet 1974; 1:1112.
2251. Vandenberg SG. Human behavior genetics. In: Kaplan AR, ed. Twin studies. Springfield: Thomas, C.C., 1976:90–150.
2252. Vandervort WJ. Are Alzheimer's disease, Parkinson's disease, and amyotrophic lateral sclerosis caused by neurotoxins. Del Med J 1987; 59:533–4, 537.
2253. vanDuijn CM, Hofman A. Relation between nicotine intake and Alzheimer's disease. Br Med J 1991; 302:1491–1494.
2254. Vassilopoulos D, Spengos M, Ilias A, Stamboulis E, Karabellas G. Morbidity risks for the relatives of patients with Parkinson's disease (Abstract). 9th International Symposium on Parkinson's Disease 1988; 118.
2255. Vatassery GT, Schut LJ. Changes in vitamin E concentration in red blood cells and plasma of patients with olivopontocerebellar atoxia within the Schut-Swier kindred. J Am Coll Nutr 1987; 6(2):151–156.
2256. Velasco Suarez MM. [Dyskinesia, neurosurgery and its future]. Cir 1969; 37:582–604.
2257. Vernon GM. Parkinson's Disease. J Neurol Sci 1989; 21:273–284.
2258. Verslegers W, DePotter W, Lowenthal A. Toxic Parkinsonism: Three Cases (Abstract). 9th International Symposium on Parkinson's Disease 1988; 11.
2259. Vescovi A, Gebbia M, Cappelletti G, Parati EA, Santagostino A. Interactions of managanese with human brain glutathione-s-transferase. Toxicology 1989; 57:183–191.
2260. Viader F, Poncelet AM, Chapon F, et al. Les formes neurologiques de la maladie de lyme: 12 cas. Rev Neurol (Paris) 1989; 145(5):362–368.
2261. Victor M, Adams RD, Cole M. The acquired (non-Wilsonian) type of chronic hepatocerebral degeneration. Medicine 1965; 44:345–396.
2262. Vieregge P, Schiffke A, Kompf D. Parkinson's disease in twins. Neurology 1991; 41(suppl 1):255.
2263. Vieregge P, Glaese A, Ulm G, Kompf D. Familial Parkinson's disease. Mov Disord 1992; 7(supp. 1):23.

2264. Vieregge P, Kleinhenz J, Fassl H, Jorg J, Kompy D. Epidemiology and outpatient care in Parkinson's disease: Results from a pilot-study in Northern Germany (Schleswig-Holstein). J Neurol Transm 1991; 33(suppl):115–118.
2265. Vigliani EC. Carbon disulphide poisoning in viscose rayon workers. Br J Indust Med 1954; 11:325–344.
2266. Vincent F, Myers W. Poliomyelitis and parkinsonism. N Engl J Med 1978; March 23:688–689.
2267. Viola M, Frazier M, White L, Brody JA, Spiegelman S. RNA-instructed DNA polymerase activity in a cytoplasmic particulate fraction in brain from Guamanian patients. J Exp Med 1975; 142:483–494.
2268. Viola M, Myers J, Gibbs C, Jr., Roos R. Failure to detect poliovirus genetic information in amyotrophic lateral sclerosis. Ann Neurol 1979; 5:402–403.
2269. Voller GW. [Clinical aspects and treatment of diseases of the extrapyramidal system]. Z Allgemeinmed 1969; 45:859–869.
2270. von Economo C. The sequelae of encephalitis lethargica. In: Newman K, ed. Encephalitis Lethargica its sequelae and treatment. London: Oxford Univ Press, 1931:105–156.
2271. Vuia O. Striato-nigral degeneration and Shy-Drager syndrome (idiopathic orthostatic hypotension). Clin Neurol Neurosurg 1975; 78(3):196–203.
2272. Vyas I, Heikkila RE, Nicklas WJ. Studies on the neurotoxicity of 1-methyl-4-phenyl-1,2,3,6-tetrahydropyridine: Inhibition of NAD-linked substrate oxidation by its metabolite, 1-methyl-4-phenylpyridinium. J Neurochem 1986; 46:1501–1507.
2273. Waggener J, Beggs J, Sidell A. Virus-like filaments in juvenile parkinsonism. J Neuropathol Exp Neurol 1972; 31:187.
2274. Wagner GC, Jarvis MF, Carelli RM. Ascorbic acid reduces the dopamine depletion induced by MPTP. Neuropharmacology 1985; 24(12):1261–1262.
2275. Wagner GC, Ricaurte GA, Seiden LS, Schuster CR, Miller RJ, Westley J. Long-lasting depletion of striatal dopamine and loss of dopamine uptake sites following repeated administration of methamphetamine. Brain Res 1980; 181:151–160.
2276. Wakabayashi K, Takahashi H, Takeda S, Ohama E, Ikuta F. Parkinson's disease: The presence of Lewy bodies in Auberbach's and Meissner's plexuses. Acta Neuropathol 1988; 76:217–221.
2277. Wakabayashi K, Takahashi H, Takeda S, Ohama E, Ikuta F. Lewy bodies in the enteric nervous system in Parkinson's disease. Arch Histol Cytol 1989; 52:191–194.
2278. Wallace DC. Mitochondrial genetics: A paradigm for aging and neurodegenerative diseases. Science 1992; 256:628–632.
2279. Wallace DC, Shoffner JM, Watts RL, Juncos JL, Torroni A. Mitochondrial oxidative phosphorylation defects in Parkinson's disease. Ann Neurol 1992; 32:113–114.
2280. Wallace DC, Singh G, Lott MT, et al. Mitochondrial DNA mutation associated with Leber's hereditary optic neuropathy. Science 1988; 242:1427–1430.
2281. Wallace RA, Boldry R, Schmittgen T, Miller D, Uretsky N. Effect of 1-methyl-4-phenyl-1,2,3,6-tetrahydropyridine (MPTP) on monoamine neurotransmitters in mouse brain and heart. Life Sci 1984; 35:285–291.
2282. Walshe J. Wilson's disease. In: Vinken P, Bruyn G, eds. Handbook of clinical neurology. Amsterdam: North-Holland Publishing Co., 1976:379–414.

2283. Walters J. Postencephalitic Parkinson Syndrome after Meningoencephalitis due to Coxsackie Virus Group B, Type 2. N Engl J Med 1960; 263:744–747.
2284. Wang JD, Huang CC, Hwang YH, Chiang JR, Lin JM, Chen JS. Manganese induced parkinsonism: an outbreak due to an unrepaired ventilation control system in a ferromanganese smelter. Br J Ind Med 1989; 46:856–859.
2285. Wang SL, Huang JD, Lai MD, Liu BH, Lai ML. Molecular basis of genetic variation in debrisoquin hydroxylation in Chinese subjects: Polymorphism in RFLP and DNA sequence of CYP2D6. Clin Pharmacol Ther 1993; 53:410–418.
2286. Wang Y, Hamburger M, Cheng CHK, et al. Neurotoxic sesquiterpenoids from the yellow star thistle. Helv Chimica Acta 1991; 74:117–123.
2287. Wang Y, Shi Y, Wu S HeY, Zhang B. Parkinson's Disease in China. Chin Med J 1991; 960–964.
2288. Wang YS, Shi YM, Wu ZY, He Y, Zhang BZ. Epidemiologic survey—Parkinson's disease in China. Chin Med J 1991; 104(11):960–964.
2289. Ward CD, Duvoisin RC, Ince SE, Nutt JD, Eldridge R, Calne DB. Parkinson's disease in 65 pairs of twins and in a set of quadruplets. Neurology 1983; 33:815–824.
2290. Ward CD, Duvoisin RC, Ince SE, et al. Parkinson's disease in twins. In: Parkinson-specific motor and mental disorders, role of the pallidum: pathophysiological, biochemical, and therapeutic aspects—Advances in Neurology, Vol 40. New York: Raven Press, 1984:341–344.
2291. Ward CD, Gibb WR. Research diagnostic criteria for Parkinson's disease. Advances in Neurology. Vol. 53. In: Streifler MB, Korczyn AD, Melamed E, Youdim MBH, eds. Parkinson's disease: Anatomy. Pathology and Therapy. Advances in Neurology. Vol. 53. New York: Raven Press, 1990:245–247.
2292. Ward CD, Hess WA, Calne DB. Olfactory impairment in Parkinson's disease. Neurology 1983; 33:943–946.
2293. Warembourg H, Niquet G, Pauchant M, Ducloux G. Syndrome parkinsonien. Sequelle d'une poliomyèlite aiguë a forme d'encephalite lethargique chez un enfant de 20 mois. Semaine des hopitaux de Paris 1962; 38:2299–2307.
2294. Waring RH, Sturman SG, Smith MCG, Steventon GB, Heafield MTE, Williams AC. S-Methylation in motor neurone disease and Parkinson's disease. Lancet 1989; ii:356–357.
2295. Warren J. Encephalitis lethargica. In: Rivers T, Horsfall Jr F, eds. Virus and rickettsial infections of man. 3rd ed. Philadelphia: Lippincott, JB, 1959:1174–1176.
2296. Wasik A, Roslawski A. [Mental disturbances in ankylosing spondylitis]. Wiad Lek 1966; 19:1057–1062.
2297. Wastiaux JP, Lamoureux G, Bouchard JP, Durivage A, Barbeau C, Barbeau A. HLA and complement typing in olivo-ponto-cerebellar atrophy. Can J Neurol Sci 1978; 5(1):75–81.
2298. Waters CH, Miller CA. Autosomal dominant transmission of Parkinson's disease in a four generation family. Ann Neurol 1994; 35:59–64.
2299. Waterson A, Almeida J. Virological aspects of neurological disease. Postgrad Med J 1969; 45:351–360.
2300. Watson A, Yunnanfu B. The origin of encephalitis lethargica. China Med J 1928; 42:427–432.

2301. Watson D, Carpenter C, Marks S, Greenberg D. Striatal calcium channel antagonist receptors in Huntington's disease. Ann Neurol 1988; 23:303–305.
2302. Watson JS. Parkinsonism diagnosed as postencephalitic in 1930 and 1931 in a brother and sister. Proc R Soc Med 1970; 63:457–458.
2303. Watts RL, Mandir AS, Ahn KJ, Juncos JL, Zakers GO, Freeman A. Electrophysiologic analysis of early Parkinson's disease. Neurology 1991; 41 (suppl 2):44–49.
2304. Weber WW, Hein DW. N-acetylation pharmacogenetics. Pharmacol Rev 1985; 37(1):25–79.
2305. Weihmuller FB, Hadjiconstantinou M, Bruno JP. Acute stress or neuroleptics elicit sensorimotor deficits in MPTP-treated mice. Neurosci Lett 1988; 85:137–142.
2306. Weiner W, Bergen D. Prevention and management of the side effects of levodopa. In: Klawans HL, ed. Clinical Neuropharmacology. New York: Raven Press, 1977:1–20.
2307. Weiner W, Lang A. Other akinetic-rigid syndromes. In: Weiner W, Lang A, eds. Movement disorders, A comprehensive reivew. NY: Futura, 1989:117–219.
2308. Weiner WJ, Lang AE. Movement disorders: a comprehensive survey. Mount Kisco, New York: Futura Publishing Company, 1989.
2309. Weiner WJ, Sanchez-Ramos J, Singer C, et al. The aircraft industry and Parkinson's disease—Any relationship? Meeting of the American Neurological Association 1989; 1989:14.
2310. Weinmann R. Heterogenous system degeneration of the central nervous system associated with peripheral neuropathy. Neurology 1967; 17:597–603.
2311. Weiss J, Koh J, Choi D. Neurotoxicity of B-N-methyl-amino-L-alanine (BMAA) and B-N-oxalylamino-L-alanine (BOAA) on cultured cortical neurons. Brain Res 1989; 497:64–71.
2312. Weiss JH, Choi DW. Beta-N-methylamino-L-alanine neurotoxicity: Requirement for bicarbonate as a cofactor. Science 1988; 241:973–975.
2313. Weller RO, Swash M, McLellan DL, Scholtz CL. Clinical neuropathology. 72nd ed. Berlin: Springer-Verlag, 1983.
2314. Wender M, Kabschowa B, Owsianowski M. [Nervous system diseases in workers of a large metallurgic plant]. Neurol Neurochir Pol 1976; 10:613–620.
2315. Wender M, Pruchnik D, Kowal P, Florczak J, Zalejski M. [Epidemiology of Parkinson disease in the Pozna'n province]. Przegl Epidemiol 1989; 43:150–155.
2316. Werner E, Olanow C. Parkinsonism and amiodarone therapy. Ann Neurol 1989; 25:630–632.
2317. Werner P, Cohen G. Intramitochondrial formation of oxidized glutathione during the oxidation of benzylamine by monoamine oxidase. FEBS lett 1991; 280(1):44–46.
2318. Westerink BHC, Damsma G, Rollema H, De Vries JB, Horn AS. Scope and limitations of in vivo brain dialysis: A comparison of its application to various neurotransmitter systems. Life Sci 1987; 41:1763–1776.
2319. Westlund K. Distribution and mortality time trend of multiple sclerosis and some other diseases in Norway. Acta Neurol Scand 1970; 46:455–483.
2320. Westlund KN, Denney RM, Kochersperger LM, Rose RM, Abell CW. Distinct monoamine oxidase A and B populations in primate brain. Science 1985; 230:181–183.

2321. Wetmur JG, Schwartz J, Elizan TS. Nucleic acid homology studies of viral nucleic acids in idiopathic Parkinson's disease. Arch Neurol 1979; 36:462–464.
2322. Whitehouse PJ. The concept of subcortical and cortical dementia: Another look. Ann Neurol 1986; 19:1–6.
2323. Whitehouse PJ. Parkinson's disease and Alzheimer's disease: new neurochemical parallels. Mov Disord 1989; 4:S57–S62.
2324. Whitehouse PJ, Hedreen JC, White CLIII, Price DL. Basal forebrain neurons in the dementia of Parkinson disease. Ann Neurol 1983; 12:243–248.
2325. Whiting MG. Food practices in ALS foci in Japan, the Marianas and New Guinea. Fed Proc 1964; 23:1343–1345.
2326. Williams A. CSF biochemical studies on some extrapyramidal diseases. In: Rose F, Capildeo R, eds. Research progress in Parkinson's disease. London: Pitman, 1981:170–180.
2327. Williams A. MPTP Toxicity: Clinical Features. J Neural Transm 1986; 5–9.
2328. Williams A. Xenobiotics and inherited risk factors. In: Ellenberg JH, Koller WC, Langston JW, eds. Etiology of Parkinson's disease. New York: Marcel Dekker, 1994:141–152.
2329. Williams A, Houff S, Lees A, Calne DB. Oligoclonal banding in the cerebrospinal fluid of patients with postencephalitic Parkinsonism. J Neurol Neurosurg Psychiatry 1979; 42:790–792.
2330. Williams A, Steventon G, Sturman S, Waring R. Xenobiotic enzyme profiles and Parkinson's disease. Neurology 1991; 41(suppl 2):29–33.
2331. Williams A, Sturman S, Steventon G. Metabolic biomarkers of Parkinson's disease. Acta Neurol Scand 1991; 136(suppl):19–23.
2332. Williams A. Hypersusceptibility to chemicals: risk factors for neurological disease? J Neurol Neurosurg Psychiatry 1993; 56:943–946.
2333. Williams A, Waring R. The MPTP tale: Pathway to prevention of Parkinson's disease? Br J Hosp Med 1993; 49(10):716–719.
2334. Williams AC. Ecogenetics, xenobiotic biochemistry and neurological disease. J Neurology 1991; 238:187–190.
2335. Williams AC. Ecogenetics. J R Coll Physicians Lond 1994; 28:2–3.
2336. Williams AC. Toxins, polymorphisms and Parkinson's disease. Focus on Parkinson's disease 1991; 3:12–15.
2337. Williams AC, Pall HS, Steventon GB, et al. N-Methylation of pyridines and Parkinson's disease. In: Narabayashi H, Nagatsu T, Yanagisawa N, Mizuno Y, eds. Parkinson's disease: From basic research to treatment. Advances in Neurology, Vol 60. New York: Raven Press, 1993:194–196.
2338. Williams AC, Steventon GB, Sturman SG, Waring RH. Hereditary variation of liver enzyme involved with detoxification and neurodegenerative disease. J Inher Metab Dis 1991; 14:431–435.
2339. Williams AC, Sturman SG, Steventon GB, Waring RH. Metabolic markers of Parkinson's disease. In: Int Workshop Berlin Parkinson's disease. How to proceed today in treatment; from basic research and early diagnosis to long-term treatment. Netherlands: Medicom, 1991:117–125.
2340. Williams DB, Annegers JP, Kokeman E, O'Brien PC, Kurland LT. Brain injury and neurologic sequelae: A cohort study of dementia, parkinsonism, and amyotrophic lateral sclerosis. Neurology 1991; 41:1554–1557.

2341. Wilson JA, MacLennan WJ. Review: Drug-induced parkinsonism in elderly patients. Age Ageing 1989; 18:208–210.
2342. Wilson JA, Wilson JS, Weight FF. MPDP+ causes a non-reversible decrease in neostriatal synaptic transmission in mouse brain slice. Brain Res 1987; 425:376–379.
2343. Wilson S. Progressive lenticular degeneration. A familial necrosis disease associated with cirrhosis of the liver. Brain 1971; 34:295–509.
2344. Wilson S, Cobb S. Mesencephalitis syphilitica. J Neurol Psychopath 1924; 5:44–60.
2345. Winokur A, Dugan J, Mendels J, Hurtig HI. Psychiatric illness in relatives of patients with Parkinson's disease: An expanded survey. Am J Psychiatry 1978; 135:854–855.
2346. Wisniewski T, Haltia M, Ghiso J, Frangione B. Lewy bodies are immunoreactive with antibodies raised to Gelsolin related Amyloid—Finnish type. Am J Pathol 1991; 138:1077–1083.
2347. Wolters EC, Huang CC, Clark C, et al. Positron emission tomography in manganese intoxication. Ann Neurol 1989; 26:647–651.
2348. Wong GF, Gray CS, Hassanein RS, Koller WC. Environmental risk factors in siblings with Parkinson's disease. Arch Neurol 1991; 48:287–289.
2349. Woodruff AW, Ansdell VE, Bowen ETW. Le Dantec virus infection in a patient who had not been to West Africa. Br Med J 1977; 2:1632–1633.
2350. Woods B, Schaumberg H. Nigro-spino-dentatal degeneration with nuclear ophthalmoplegia: A unique and partially treatable clinicopathological entity. J Neurol Sci 1972; 17:149–166.
2351. Wöhrle D, Hennig I, Vogel W, Steinbach P. Mitotic stability of fragile X mutations in differentiated cells indicates early post-conceptional trinucleotide repeat expansion. Nature Genetics 1993; 4:140–142.
2352. Wright AD. Parkinsonism secondary to cerebral tumors. J Neurol Neurosurg Psychiatry 1957; 20:71–72.
2353. Wszolek Z, Monsour H, Smith P, Pfeiffer R. Cryptococcal meningoencephalitis with parkinsonian features. Mov Disord 1988; 3:271–273.
2354. Wszolek ZK, Pfeiffer RF, Bhatt MH, et al. Rapidly progressive autosomal dominant parkinsonism and dementia with pallido-ponto-nigral degeneration. Ann Neurol 1992; 32:312–320.
2355. Wu E, Shinka T, Caldera-Munoz P, Yoshizumi H, Trevor A, Castagnoli N, Jr. Metabolic studies on the nigrostriatal toxin MPTP and its MAO B generated dihydropyridinium metabolite MPDP+. Chem Res Toxicol 1988; 1:186–194.
2356. Wu EY, Chiba K, Trevor AJ, Castagnoli N, Jr.. Interactions of the 1-methyl-4-phenyl-2,3-dihydropyridinium species with synthetic dopamine-melanin. Life Sci 1986; 39:1695–1700.
2357. Wyllie AH. Glucocorticoid-induced thymocyte apoptosis is associated with endogenous endonuclease activation. Nature 1980; 284:555–556.
2358. Xuereb JH, Tomlinson BE, Irving D, Perry RH, Blessed G, Perry EK. Cortical and subcortical pathology in Parkinson's disease: Relationship to parkinsonian dementia. In: Streifler MB, Korczyn AD, Melamed E, Youdim MBH, eds. Parkinson's disease: Anatomy, pathology and therapy. Advances in Neurology, Vol. 53. New York: Raven Press, 1990:35–40.

2359. Yahr M. Encephalitis lethargica (VonEconomo's disease, epidemic encephalitis. In: Vinken P, Bruyn G, eds. Handbook of clinical neurology. Amsterdam: Excerpta Medica, 1978:451–457.
2360. Yahr M. Evaluation of long-term therapy in Parkinson's disease. Mortality and therapeutic efficacy. In: Birkmayer W, Hornykiewicz O, eds. Advances in Parkinsonism. Basle: Editiones Roche, 1991:435–443.
2361. Yahr MD. Parkinson's disease—overview of its current status. Mt Sinai J Med 1977; 44:183–191.
2362. Yakura H, Wakisaka A, Fujimoto S, Itakura K. Hereditary ataxia and HL-A genotypes. N Engl J Med 1974; 291:154–155.
2363. Yamada M, Ohno S, Okayasu I, et al. Chronic managanese poisoning: A neuropathological study with determination of manganese distribution in the brain. Acta Neuropathol(Berlin) 1986; 70:273–278.
2364. Yamada T, McGeer PL, Baimbridge KG, McGeer EG. Relative sparing in Parkinson's disease of substantia nigra dopamine neurons containing calbindin-D28K. Brain Res 1990; 526:303–307.
2365. Yamaguchi T, Hayaski K, Murakami H. Glutamate dehydrogenase deficiency in spinocerebellar degeneration. Neurochem Res 1982; 7, No 5:627–636.
2366. Yamamura Y, Sobue I, Ando K, Iida M, Yanagi T. Paralysis agitans of early onset with marked diurnal fluctuation of symptoms. Neurology 1973; 23:239–244.
2367. Yanagihara R. Heavy metals and essential minerals in motor neuron disease. In: Rowland L, ed. Human motor neuron diseases—Advances in Neurology, Vol 36. New York: Raven Press, 1982:233–247.
2368. Yanagihara R, Garruto R, Gajdusek D, Tomita A, Uchikawa T. Calcium and Vitamin D metabolism in Guamanian Chammorros with amyotrophic lateral sclerosis and parkinsonism-dementia. Ann Neurol 1984; 15:42–48.
2369. Yanagihara RT, Garruto RM, Gajdusek DC. Epidemiological surveillance of amyotrophic lateral sclerosis and parkinsonism-dementia in the commonwealth of the Northern Mariana Islands. Ann Neurol 1983; 13:79–86.
2370. Yang M, Michelsen O, Campbell M. Cycad flour used by Guamanians: Effect produced in rats by long term feeding. J Nutr 1966; 90:153–156.
2371. Yaryura-Tobias J, Diamond B, Merlis S. Psychiatric manifestations of levodopa. Can Psychiatr Assoc J 1972; 17SS:123–128.
2372. Yase Y. The pathogenesis of amyotrophic lateral sclerosis. Lancet 1972; 2:292–296.
2373. Yase Y. The role of aluminum in CNS degeneration with interaction of calcium. Neurotoxicology 1980; 1:101–109.
2374. Yesalis CE, Lemke JH, Wallace RB, Kohout FJ, Morris MC. Health status of the rural elderly according to farm work history: The Iowa 65 + Rural Health Study. Environ Health 1985; 40:245–253.
2375. Yokochi M. Juvenile Parkinson's disease—Part I. Clinical aspects. Adv Neurol Sci 1979; 23:1048–1059.
2376. Yokochi M, Narabayashi H, Iizuka R, Nagatsu T. Juvenile parkinsonism: Some clinical, pharmacological, and neuropathological aspects. In: Hassler RG, Christ JF, eds. Parkinson-specific motor and mental disorders, role of Pallidum: Pathological, Biochemical, and therapeutic aspects. Advances in Neurology, Vol. 40. New York: Raven Press, 1984:407–413.

2377. Yokota T, Tanabe H. Serum antibodies to HTLV-I in autonomic failure with multisystem atrophy. Ann Neurol 1990; 27:110–111.
2378. Yong VW, Perry TL. Monoamine oxidase B, smoking, and Parkinson's disease. J Neurol Sci 1986; 72:265–272.
2379. Yoshida M, Niwa T, Nagatsu T. Parkinsonism in monkeys produced by chronic administration of an endogenous substance of the brain, tetrahydroisoquinoline: The behavioral and biochemical changes. Neurosci Lett 1990; 119:109–113.
2380. Yoshimura N, Ikuta F. [Chronic cerebral diseases secondary to head injury; neuropathological review and investigation, part II (author's transl)]. No To Shinkei 1976; 28:129–140.
2381. Yoshimura N, Yoshimura I, Asada M, et al. Juvenile Parkinson's disease with widespread Lewy bodies in the brain. J Neuropathol 1988; 77:213–218.
2382. Yoshino H, Nakagawa-Hattori Y, Kondo T, Mizuno Y. Mitochondrial complex I and II activities of lymphocytes and platelets in Parkinson's disease. J Neural Transm 1992; 4:27–34.
2383. Youdim MB. Iron in the brain: Implications for Parkinson's and Alzheimer's diseases [published erratum appears in Mt Sinai J Med (NY) 1988 Mar; 55(2):inside back cover]. Mt Sinai J Med 1988; 55:97–101.
2384. Youdim MB, Ben-Shachar D, Eshel G, Finberg JP, Riederer P. The neurotoxicity of iron and nitric oxide. Relevance to the etiology of Parkinson's disease. In: Narabayashi H, Nagatsu T, Yanakisawa N, Mizuno Y, eds. Parkinson's disease: From basic research to treatment. Advances in Neurology, Vol. 60. New York: Raven Press, 1993:259–266.
2385. Youdim MB, Ben-Shachar D, Riederer P. The possible role of iron in the etiopathology of Parkinson's disease. Mov Disord 1993; 8:1–12.
2386. Youdim MB, Ben-Shachar D, Riederer R. Iron-melanin interaction can explain the selectivity and vulnerability of substantia nigra dopamine neurons to degeneration in Parkinson's disease. Meeting of the American Neurological Association 1989; 5.
2387. Youdim MBH, Ben-Shachar D, Eshel G, Riederer P, Jellinger K. Iron, glia, oxidative stress, and Parkinson's disease. Mov Disord 1992; 7(3):289.
2388. Youdim MBH, Ben-Shachar D, Riederer P. Is Parkinson's disease a progressive siderosis of substantia nigra resulting in iron and melanin induced neurodegeneration? Acta Neurol Scand Suppl 1989; 126:47–54.
2389. Youdim MBH, Ben-Shachar D, Riederer P. Iron in brain function and dysfunction with emphasis on Parkinson's disease. Eur Neurol 1991; 31 Suppl. 1:34–40.
2390. Young WI, Martin WE, Anderson VE. The distribution of ancestral secondary cases in Parkinson's disease. Clin Genet 1977; 11:189–192.
2391. Yurek DM, Sladek JR, Jr.. Dopamine cell replacement: Parkinson's disease. Annu Rev Neurosci 1990; 13:415–440.
2392. Zack MM, Langston WJ. Multiple system involvement and multifactorial cause as they relate to the etiology of Parkinson's disease. In: Ellenberg JH, Koller WC, Langston JW, eds. Etiology of Parkinson's disease. New York: Marcel Dekker, 1994:55–63.
2393. Zack MM, Tanner CM. Infectious diseases as they relate to the etiology of Parkinson's disease. In: Ellenberg JH, Koller WC, Langston JW, eds. Etiology of Parkinson's disease. New York: Marcel Dekker, 1994:401–423.

2394. Zayed J, Ducic S, Campanella G, et al. [Environmental factors in the etiology of Parkinson's disease]. Can J Neurol Sci 1990; 17:286–291.
2395. Zetusky W, Jankovic J, Pirozzolo F. The heterogenicity of Parkinson's disease. Clinical and prognostic implications. Neurology 1985; 35:522–526.
2396. Zhang ZX, Anderson DW, Lavine L, Mantel N. Patterns of acquiring Parkinsonism-dementia complex on Guam:1944 through 1985. Arch Neurol 1990; 47:1019–1024.
2397. Zhang ZX, Anderson DW, Mantel N. Geographic patterns of Parkinsonism-dementia complex on Guam: 1956 through 1985. Arch Neurol 1990; 47:1069–1074.
2398. Zhang ZX, Romàn GC. Worldwide occurrence of Parkinson's disease: An updated review. Neuroepidemiology 1993; 12:195–208.
2399. Ziegler DK, Schimke RN, Kepes JJ, Rose DL, Klinkenfuss G. Late onset ataxia, rigidity and peripheral neuropathy. A familial syndrome with variable therapeutic response to levodopa. Arch Neurol 1972; 27:52–66.
2400. Ziegler L. Follow-up studies on persons who have had epidemic encephalitis. JAMA 1928; July 21:138–141.
2401. Zigmond MJ, Hastings TG. Neurochemical responses to 6-hydroxydopamine and L-dopa therapy: implications for Parkinson's disease. Ann N Y Acad Sci 1992; 648:71–86.
2402. Zigmond MJ, Stricker EM. Parkinson's disease: Studies with an animal model. Life Sci 1984; 35:5–18.
2403. Zimmerman HM. Monthly report to medical officer in command. U S Naval Medical Research 1945; 2.
2404. Zimmerman T, Sage JI. Long-term pergolide treatment and progression of Parkinson's disease. Neurology 1989; 39:200.
2405. Zimmerman T, Sage JI. Comparison of combination pergolide and levodopa to levodopa alone after 63 months of treatment. Clin Neuropharmacol 1991; 14:165–169.
2406. Zimmerman TR. Personal communication, 1992.
2407. Zimmerman TR, Bhatt MH, Calne DB, Duvoisin RC. Parkinson's disease in monozygotic twins: A follow-up. Neurology 1991; 41(Suppl 1):255.
2408. Zinsser H. The present state of knowledge regarding epidemic encephalitis. Archives of Pathology 1928; 6:271–301.
2409. Zuber M, Verdier-Taillefer M-H, Alperovitch M, de Recondo J. Smoking and Parkinson's disease: Differences according to age at disease onset (Meetings of Research Group on Neuroepidemiology, April 22, 1991). World Federation of Neurology 1991; Abstract #22:103–104.(abstract)
2410. Zuddas A, Oberto G, Vaglini F, Fascetti F, Fornai F, Corsini GU. MK-801 prevents 1-methyl-4-phenyl-1,2,3,6-tetrahydropyridine-induced Parkinsonism in primates. J Neurochem 1992; 59:733–739.
2411. Zuddas A, Vaglini F, Fornai F, Fascetti F, Corsini GU. MK-801 prevents MPTP-induced nigrostriatal neuronal death in monkeys and mice. Soc Neurosci 1991; 17(1):716.(abstract)
2412. Zweig R, Whitehouse P, Casanova M, Walker L, Jankel W, Price D. Loss of pendunculopontine neurons in progressive supranuclear palsy. Ann Neurol 1987; 22:18–25.

2413. Zweig RM, Singh A, Cardillo JE, Langston JW. The familial occurrence of Parkinson's disease—Lack of evidence for maternal inheritance. Arch Neurol 1992; 49:1205–1207.

Index

About the Editors

JONAS H. ELLENBERG is Chief of the Biometry and Field Studies Branch, National Institute of Neurological Disorders and Stroke, National Institutes of Health, Bethesda, Maryland. The author or coauthor of over 85 professional publications and the coeditor of two books, Dr. Ellenberg is a Fellow of both the American Statistical Association and the American Association for the Advancement of Science, as well as Past President of the International Biometric Society and an elected member of the International Statistical Institute. He received the B.Sc. degree (1963) in economics from the University of Pennsylvania, Philadelphia, and the A.M. (1964) and Ph.D. (1970) degrees in statistics from Harvard University, Cambridge, Massachusetts.

WILLIAM C. KOLLER is a Professor in and Chairman of the Department of Neurology and a Professor of Pharmacology at the University of Kansas Medical Center, Kansas City. A Fellow of the American Academy of Neurology and a member of the American Neurological Association and the Movement Disorder Society, Dr. Koller is the coauthor, editor, or coeditor of several books, including the *Handbook of Parkinson's Disease, Second Edition*; *Therapy of Parkinson's Disease, Second Edition* (with George Paulson); and (with Leslie J. Findley) the *Handbook of Tremor Disorders* (all titles, Marcel Dekker, Inc.). He is also the editor of the Neurological Disease and Therapy series (Marcel Dekker, Inc.) and the author or coauthor of over 200 journal articles. Dr. Koller received the M.S. (1971) and Ph.D. (1974) degrees in pharmacology and the M.D. degree (1976) from Northwestern University Medical School, Chicago, Illinois.

J. WILLIAM LANGSTON is President of the Parkinson's Institute, Sunnyvale, California. The author or coauthor of more than 210 professional publications, Dr. Langston is the North American Editor of the journal *Neurodegeneration*. He is a member of the American Academy of Neurology, the Movement Disorders Society, the Society for Neuroscience, and the American Neurological Association, among others. Dr. Langston received the B.S. degree from the University of Missouri—Columbia and the M.D. degree (1967) from the University of Missouri—Columbia School of Medicine.